ENDOCRINOLOGY
ADULT AND PEDIATRIC

ENDOCRINOLOGY

ADULT AND PEDIATRIC 6TH EDITION

THE ADRENAL GLAND

Volume Editor

Ashley Grossman, BA, BSc, MD, FRCP, FMedSci

Professor of Neuroendocrinology
Endocrinology
St. Bartholomew's Hospital
London, United Kingdom

ELSEVIER
SAUNDERS

1600 John F. Kennedy Blvd.
Ste 1800
Philadelphia, PA 19103-2899

Endocrinology, Adult and Pediatric: The Adrenal Gland

ISBN: 978-0-323-22157-3
POD ISBN: 978-0-323-24059-8

Content for this eBook is derived from a book that may have contained additional digital media. Media content is not included in this eBook purchase.

Library of Congress Cataloging-in-Publication Data
Endocrinology / senior editors, Leslie J. De Groot, J. Larry Jameson ; section editors Ashley Grossman ... [et al.].—6th ed.
  p. ; cm.
  Includes bibliographical references and index.
  ISBN-13: 978-1-4160-5593-9 (v.1 & v.2 : hardback : alk. paper)
  ISBN-13: 978-9996074479 (v.1 : hardback : alk. paper)
  ISBN-10: 9996074471 (v.1 : hardback : alk. paper)
  ISBN-13: 978-9996074417 (v.2 : hardback: alk. paper)
  [etc.]
  1. Endocrine glands–Diseases.   2. Endocrinology.   I. De Groot, Leslie J.   II. Jameson, J. Larry.
  [DNLM: 1. Endocrine System Disease.   2. Endocrine Glands.   3. Hormones.   WK 140 E5595 2010]
  RC648.E458 2010
  616.4—dc22

Acquisitions Editor: Helene Caprari
Developmental Editor: Mary Beth Murphy
Publishing Services Manager: Anne Altepeter
Project Manager: Jennifer Nemec
Design Direction: Ellen Zanolle

Transferred to Digital Printing in 2013

Senior Editors

J. Larry Jameson, MD, PhD
Professor of Medicine, Dean
Northwestern University Feinberg School of Medicine
Northwestern University
Chicago, Illinois

David de Kretser, AO, FAA, FTSE, MD, FRACP
Emeritus Professor
Monash Institute of Medical Research
Monash University
Clayton, Melbourne, Victoria, Australia

Ashley Grossman, BA, BSc, MD, FRCP, FMedSci
Professor of Neuroendocrinology
Endocrinology
St. Bartholomew's Hospital
London, United Kingdom

John C. Marshall, MD, PhD
Andrew D. Hart Professor of Internal Medicine
Director, Center for Research in Reproduction
Department of Medicine
University of Virginia School of Medicine
Charlottesville, Virginia

Shlomo Melmed, MD
Senior Vice President, Academic Affairs and Dean of
   the Faculty
Cedars Sinai Medical Center
Los Angeles, California

Leslie J. De Groot, MD
Research Professor
Cellular and Life Sciences
University of Rhode Island, Providence Campus
Providence, Rhode Island

John T. Potts, Jr, MD
Jackson Distinguished Professor of Clinical Medicine
Harvard Medical School;
Director of Research and Physician-in-Chief Emeritus
Department of Medicine
Massachusetts General Hospital
Boston, Massachusetts

Gordon C. Weir, MD
Head, Section on Islet Transplantation and Cell Biology
Diabetes Research and Wellness Foundation Chair
Joslin Diabetes Center;
Professor of Medicine
Harvard Medical School
Boston, Massachusetts

Harald Jüppner, MD
Professor of Pediatrics
Endocrine Unit and Pediatric Nephrology Unit
   Massachusetts General Hospital and Harvard Medical
   School
Boston, Massachusetts

Contributors

Bruno Allolio, MD
Professor of Medicine
Department of Endocrinology and Diabetes
University Hospital
University of Würzburg
Würzburg, Germany

Richard J. Auchus, MD, PhD
The Charles A. and Elizabeth Ann Sanders Chair
 in Translational Research
Professor, Internal Medicine
Division of Endocrinology and Metabolism
The University of Texas Southwestern Medical
 Center at Dallas
Dallas, Texas

Lloyd Axelrod, MD
Associate Professor of Medicine
Department of Medicine
Harvard Medical School;
Physician and Chief of the James Howard Means
 Firm Medical Services
Massachusetts General Hospital
Boston, Massachusetts

Chuong Bui, MBBS, FRACP, DDU
Staff Specialist
Nuclear Medicine Department
Nepean Hospital
Kingswood, New South Wales, Australia

Robert M. Carey, MD, MACP
David A. Harrison III Distinguished Professor of
 Medicine;
Dean, Emeritus and University Professor
Division of Endocrinology and Metabolism
University of Virginia Health System
Charlottesville, Virginia

Francesco Cavagnini, MD
Professor of Endocrinology
Chair of Endocrinology
University of Milan;
Chief, Divisione di Medicina Generale ad Indirizzo
 Endocrino-Metabolico, Ospedale
San Luca, Istituto Auxologico Italiano
Milan, Italy

V. Krishna Chatterjee, MD, FRCP
Professor of Endocrinology
Department of Medicine
Institute of Metabolic Science
University of Cambridge
Cambridge, United Kingdom

Kyung J. Cho, MD
Professor
Department of Radiology
University of Michigan Medical School
Ann Arbor, Michigan

Teng-Teng Chung, MBBS, MRCP
MRC Clinical Research Fellow
Centre for Endocrinology
Barts & the London School of Medicine &
 Dentistry
London, United Kingdom

John A. Cidlowski, PhD
Chief, Laboratory of Signal Transduction
National Institute of Environmental Health
 Sciences, National Institutes of Health
Research Triangle Park, North Carolina

Adrian J.L. Clark, DSc, FRCP
Professor of Medicine
Endocrinology
Barts & the London School of Medicine &
 Dentistry
London, United Kingdom

Leslie J. De Groot, MD
Research Professor
Cellular and Life Sciences
University of Rhode Island, Providence Campus
Providence, Rhode Island

Graeme Eisenhofer, PhD
Professor and Chief
Division of Clinical Neurochemistry
Institute of Clinical Chemistry and Laboratory
 Medicine and Department of Medicine
Universitätsklinikum Carl Gustav Carus Dresden
Dresden, Germany

Martin Fassnacht, MD
Max Eder Senior Research Fellow
Consultant Endocrinologist
Professor for Medicine
Department of Internal Medicine I, Endocrine and
 Diabetes Unit
University Hospital of Würzburg
Würzburg, Germany

Peter Fuller, BMedSci, MBBS, PhD, FRACP
NHRMC Senior Principal Research Fellow,
 Associate Director
NHMRC Senior Principal Research Fellow
Associate Director, Prince Henry's Institute of
 Medical Research
Director, Endocrinology Unit, Southern Health
Adjunct Professor in Medicine and Biochemistry
 and Molecular Biology
Monash University
Clayton, Victoria, Australia

Milton D. Gross, MD
Professor, Division of Nuclear Medicine
Department of Radiology
University of Michigan
Ann Arbor, Michigan

**Ashley Grossman, BA, BSc, MD, FRCP,
 FMedSci**
Professor of Neuroendocrinology
Endocrinology
St. Bartholomew's Hospital
London, United Kingdom

John B. Hanks, MD
C Bruce Morton Professor
Chief, Division of General Surgery
Department of Surgery
University of Virginia Health System
Charlottesville, Virginia

**Ieuan A. Hughes, MA, MD, FRCP, FRCP(C),
 FRCPCH, F Med Sci**
Professor of Paediatrics, University of Cambridge;
 Honorary Consultant Paediatrician, Cambridge
 University Hospitals NHS Foundation Trust
Cambridge, United Kingdom

Hero K. Hussain, MBChB, FRCR
Associate Professor
MRI/Abdominal Division
Department of Radiology
University of Michigan
Ann Arbor, Michigan

J. Larry Jameson, MD, PhD
Professor of Medicine, Dean
Northwestern University Feinberg School of
 Medicine
Northwestern University
Chicago, Illinois

Melvyn Korobkin, MD
Professor of Radiology
University of Michigan
Ann Arbor, Michigan

Laura J. Lewis-Tuffin, PhD
Intramural Research Associate
Laboratory of Signal Transduction
National Institute of Environmental Health
 Sciences, NIH, HHS
Research Triangle Park, North Carolina;
Senior Research Fellow
Department of Cancer Biology
Mayo Clinic
Jacksonville, Florida

Carl D. Malchoff, MD, PhD
Professor of Medicine
Division of Endocrinology and Metabolism and
 Neag Comprehensive Cancer Center
University of Connecticut Health Center
Farmington, Connecticut

Diana Mark Malchoff, PhD
Chair
Department of Science
Avon Old Farms School
Avon, Connecticut

Walter L. Miller, MD
Distinguished Professor of Pediatrics
Chief of Endocrinology
University of California San Francisco
San Francisco, California

Damian G. Morris, MBBS, PhD, FRCP
Department of Diabetes and Endocrinology
The Ipswich Hospital
Ipswich, Suffolk, United Kingdom

Allan U. Munck, PhD
Emeritus Professor of Physiology
Department of Physiology
Dartmouth Medical School
Lebanon, New Hampshire

Anikó Náray-Fejes-Tóth, MD
Professor of Physiology
Department of Physiology
Dartmouth Medical School
Lebanon, New Hampshire

Maria I. New, MD
Professor of Pediatrics
Professor of Genetics and Genomic Sciences
Director, Adrenal Steroid Disorders Program
Department of Pediatrics
Mount Sinai School of Medicine
New York, New York

Lynnette K. Nieman, MD
Senior Investigator
Intramural Research Program on Reproductive and
    Adult Endocrinology
The Eunice Kennedy Shriver National Institute of
    Child Health and Human Development,
    National Institutes of Health
Bethesda, Maryland

Robert H. Oakley, PhD
Laboratory of Signal Transduction
National Institute of Environmental Health
    Sciences
National Institutes of Health, Department of
    Health and Human Services
Research Triangle Park, North Carolina

Karel Pacak, MD, PhD, DSc
Professor of Medicine
Senior Investigator
Chief, Section on Medical Neuroendocrinology
    National Institute of Child Health and Human
    Development
National Institutes of Health
Bethesda, Maryland

Shetal H. Padia, MD
Division of Endocrinology and Metabolism
Department of Medicine
University of Virginia School of Medicine
Charlottesville, Virginia

Francesca Pecori Giraldi, MD
University Researcher
University of Milan Divisione di Medicina
    Generale ad Indirizzo Endocrino-Metabolico,
    Ospedale San Luca,
Istituto Auxologico Italiano
Milan, Italy

Marcus Quinkler, MD
Doctor
Department of Clinical Endocrinology
Charité Campus Mitte
Charité University Medicine Berlin
Berlin, Germany

Philip W. Smith, MD
Chief Resident
Department of Surgery
University of Virginia
Charlottesville, Virginia

**Paul M. Stewart, MB, ChB, MD, FRCP,
    FMedSci**
Professor
University of Birmingham
Queen Elizabeth Hospital
Edgbaston, Birmingham, United Kingdom

Henri J.L.M. Timmers, MD, PhD
Clinical Endocrinologist
Assistant Professor, Endocrinology
Radboud University Nijmegen Medical Centre
Nijmegen, The Netherlands

Michael P. Wajnrajch, MD
Senior Medical Director
Specialty Care
Pfizer, Inc;
Associate Professor
Department of Pediatrics
New York University
New York, New York

Preface

Publishing has never stood still, ever since printing was invented by Gutenberg and introduced into the English language by William Caxton. However, the greatest challenge has only arisen in the opening years of the twenty-first century, with the explosion of Internet-related resources and the exponential access to new information channels. We need to respond to these changes in a positive way: there remains the need for accurate, informed, and expert information, even as—and maybe especially as—so much other information becomes generally available. We have decided to produce the highly respected Jameson and De Groot's *Endocrinology, Adult and Pediatric* as an ebook to increase the availability and visibility of expert information. It has been my pleasure to collate and edit the adrenal section of this book, and I do hope that the exposure to a yet wider audience will increase the sum total of accurate and relevant information to all those managing adrenal disease. In the end, we have the responsibility to our patients to make available to scientists and clinicians all that is best, and if publication of the ebook helps better achieve this aim, then I, my contributors, and the other editors will have been successful in our task.

Ashley Grossman, BA, BSc, MD, FRCP, FMedSci

Contents

Chapter 1

THE PRINCIPLES, ENZYMES, AND PATHWAYS OF HUMAN STEROIDOGENESIS

RICHARD J. AUCHUS and WALTER L. MILLER

Overview of the Human Steroidogenic Enzymes and Steroidogenesis
Cytochrome P450 Enzymes
Hydroxysteroid Dehydrogenases and Reductases
Acute Regulation of Steroidogenesis
Chronic Maintenance of the Steroidogenic Machinery

Human Steroidogenic P450s
P450scc
P450c17
P450c21
P450c11β and P450c11AS
P450aro (Aromatase)

Redox Partner Proteins
Adrenodoxin (Ferredoxin)
Adrenodoxin (Ferredoxin) Reductase
P450 Oxidoreductase
Cytochrome b_5

Steroidogenic Dehydrogenases and Reductases
3β-Hydroxysteroid Dehydrogenase/Δ^5-Δ^4-Isomerases
17β-Hydroxysteroid Dehydrogenases
Steroid 5α-Reductases
3α-Hydroxysteroid Dehydrogenases
11β-Hydroxysteroid Dehydrogenases

Pathways
Adrenal Steroidogenic Pathways
Gonadal Steroidogenic Pathways

Overview of the Human Steroidogenic Enzymes and Steroidogenesis

All steroid hormones derive from cholesterol in a process that can be conceptualized as having six distinct components:

1. *The conversion of cholesterol to pregnenolone.* Although viewed superficially as a single chemical transformation, the mobilization of cholesterol into the steroidogenic pathways is a complex event that serves as a key locus of regulation and also conventionally defines a tissue as "steroidogenic." In humans, only the adrenal cortex, testicular Leydig cells, ovarian theca cells, trophoblast cells of the placenta, and specific glial and neuronal cells of the brain possess the capacity to cleave cholesterol into pregnenolone (the C_{21} precursor of all active steroid hormones) and isocaproaldehyde. The differences in how this process is regulated and in how pregnenolone is subsequently metabolized define the roles of the various steroidogenic cells and tissues in human physiology. Unlike peptide-secreting glands, steroidogenic cells do not store steroid hormones and intermediates, and it is the activation of this first step that enables the rapid production of steroids in response to hormonal and environmental stimuli.

2. *The transformation of pregnenolone to active hormones, intermediates, and exported steroid derivatives.* The repertoire of enzymes and cofactor proteins present in a given steroidogenic cell is responsible for the characteristic steroid profile of that cell type, and the coordinate regulation of their expression promotes the completion of all steps of a given pathway. Thus, these enzymes determine qualitatively what steroids are made, but since these steps are not kinetically limiting, it is step 1 that quantitatively regulates how much steroid is made at a given moment. Steroids diffuse into the bloodstream, although the sulfation of Δ^5 steroids helps promote their binding to proteins and prolong their half-lives in the circulation.

3. *Peripheral metabolism of hormones and precursors.* Although not "steroidogenic" as defined earlier, some organs, such as the liver and skin, possess tremendous capacity to transform various steroids. For example, 70% to 80% of circulating testosterone in normally cycling women derives from the conversion of adrenal dehydroepiandrosterone (DHEA). Steroids can be activated in target tissues, such as the conversion of testosterone to dihydrotestosterone (DHT) in the prostate. In contrast, active androgens and estrogens are inactivated in the uterus and in other peripheral tissues.

4. *Multiple layers of regulation.* The regulation of steroidogenesis by trophic hormones, such as adrenocorticotropin (ACTH), angiotensin II, and luteinizing hormone (LH) is well known; less well appreciated are the multiple levels

at which such regulation may occur. These include the transcriptional regulation of the genes encoding steroidogenic enzymes and co-factors; regulation of mitochondrial protein import; transfer of electrons from NADPH; post-translational modification of steroidogenic enzymes; and subcellular localization and/or targeting.

5. *Catabolism and unproductive metabolism.* A panoply of steroids can be isolated from human plasma and tissues, many of which have negligible biological activity. Most inactive byproducts derive from hepatic transformations (e.g., $6\alpha/6\beta$-hydroxylation of C_{19} steroids, 5β-reduction of C_{21} and C_{19} steroids, and 4-hydroxylation of estrogens), which promote renal excretion of these steroids.

6. *More than one pathway to specific steroids.* Particularly for the terminal steps of long pathways, such as the synthesis of DHT or estradiol, two or more routes may yield the same final product. Often the different routes utilize different enzymes, and these enzymes may be found in different tissues under different regulatory mechanisms. The relative importance of these pathways differ with age, sex, and physiologic state.

Steroids are molecules derived from the cyclopentanoperhydrophenanthrene four-ring hydrocarbon nucleus (Fig. 1-1). Most enzymes involved in steroid biosynthesis are either cytochrome P450s or hydroxysteroid dehydrogenases (Fig. 1-2). All of these reactions are functionally if not absolutely unidirectional, so the accumulation of products does not drive flux back to the precursor. All P450-mediated hydroxylations and carbon-carbon bond cleavage reactions are mechanistically and physiologically irreversible.[1] Hydroxysteroid dehydrogenase reactions are mechanistically reversible and can run in either direction under certain conditions in vitro, but each hydroxysteroid dehydrogenase drives steroid flux predominantly in either the oxidative or reductive mode in vivo.[2] However, two or more hydroxysteroid dehydrogenases drive the flux of a steroid pair in opposite directions, some favoring ketosteroid reduction and others favoring hydroxysteroid oxidation.

CYTOCHROME P450 ENZYMES

Mammalian cytochrome P450 enzymes fall into two broad classes, type 1 and type 2.[3] Type 1 enzymes and their electron-transfer proteins reside in the mitochondria (Table 1-1) of eukaryotes; almost all bacterial P450s are also type 1 enzymes. Human type 1 P450 enzymes include the cholesterol side-chain cleavage enzyme P450scc; the two isozymes of 11-hydroxylase

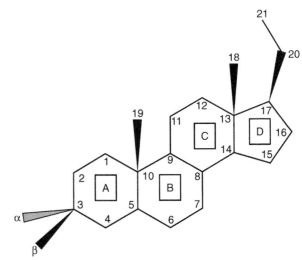

FIGURE I-I. Cyclopentanoperhydrophenanthrene steroid nucleus. Steroid rings are identified with *boxed capital letters*, and carbon atoms are *numbered*. Substituents and hydrogens are labeled as α or β if they are positioned behind or in front of the plane of the page, respectively.

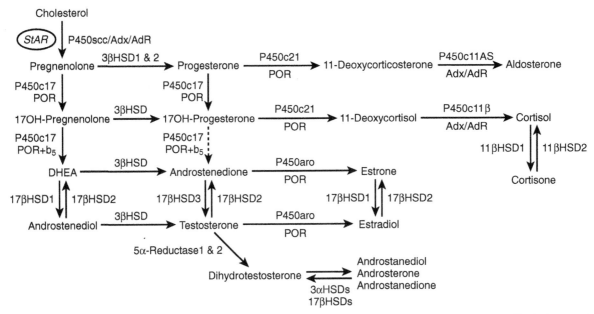

FIGURE I-2. Major human steroidogenic pathways. Key enzymes and cofactor proteins are shown near arrows indicating chemical reactions. The StAR protein *(oval)* mobilizes cholesterol from the outer mitochondrial membrane to the inner mitochondrial membrane, where P450scc cleaves cholesterol to pregnenolone, the first committed intermediate in steroid biosynthesis. The steroids in the first column are Δ^5-steroids, which constitute the preferred pathway to C_{19} steroids in human beings, and the *dashed arrow* indicates poor flux from 17α-hydroxyprogesterone to androstenedione. Steroids in the second column and farther right are Δ^4-steroids, except the C_{18} estrogens (estrone and estradiol) and 5α-reduced steroids, including the potent androgen DHT and other androstanes *(bottom row)*. Not all intermediate steroids, pathways, and enzymes are shown.

Table 1-1. Intracellular Location of Steroidogenic Proteins

Mitochondria	Cytoplasm	Endoplasmic Reticulum
P450scc		P450c17
P450c11β		P450c21
P450c11AS		P450aro
Adrenodoxin reductase		P450-oxidoreductase
Adrenodoxin		
StAR	StAR	Cytochrome b_5
3β-HSD1 and 2	3β-HSD1 and 2	3β-HSD1 and 2
	17β-HSD1	17β-HSD1–3*
	Reductive 3α-HSDs	Oxidative 3α-HSD
	includes 17β-HSD5	5α-Reductase 1 and 2
		11β-HSD1 and 2

HSD, Hydroxysteroid dehydrogenase.
*17β-HSD4 is located in peroxisomes.

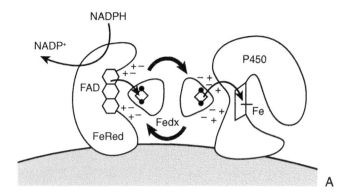

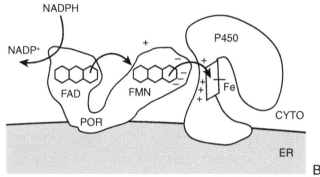

FIGURE 1-3. Electron transfer pathways for steroidogenic cytochrome P450 enzymes. **A,** In type 1 (mitochondrial) enzymes, the two electrons from the reduced form of nicotinamide adenine dinucleotide phosphate (NADPH) pass from the flavin (FAD) of ferredoxin (adrenodoxin) reductase (FeRed) to the iron-sulfur (Fe_2S_2, *diamond with dots*) cluster of ferredoxin (adrenodoxin, Fedx) and then to the heme of the P450 (*square with iron atom* [Fe]). Negatively-charged residues in Fedx (–) guide docking and electron transfer with positively-charged residues (+) in both Fedx and the P450. **B,** In type 2 (microsomal) enzymes, the flavoprotein P450-oxidoreductase (POR) receives electrons from NADPH to its FAD moiety, transfers electrons to its FMN moiety, and after a conformational rearrangement, directly transfers electrons from the FMN to the P450. Negative charges on POR (–) and positive charges (+) on the P450 guide the interaction as with the type 1 P450; phosphorylation and cytochrome b_5 also regulate electron transfer and catalysis. Heme of P450 is indicated by *square with iron atom* (Fe).

(i.e., P450c11β and P450c11AS); and two of the three principal enzymes in vitamin D metabolism (i.e., 1α-hydroxylase and 24-hydroxylase). Type 1 enzymes receive electrons from the reduced form of nicotinamide adenine dinucleotide phosphate (NADPH) via adrenodoxin, a small, soluble, iron-sulfur protein. Adrenodoxin does not oxidize NADPH directly, however, but receives the two electrons from NADPH via the flavoprotein adrenodoxin reductase (Fig. 1-3). Type 2 enzymes, in contrast, receive electrons from NADPH via the flavin adenine dinucleotide (FAD)-flavin mononucleotide (FMN) two-flavin protein, P450 oxidoreductase (POR). Type 2 enzymes are exclusively located in the smooth endoplasmic reticulum and constitute the majority of the human P450 enzymes.

P450 enzymes activate molecular oxygen using their heme center and electrons from NADPH. Substrate binding is required prior to heme reduction with one electron, which enables oxygen binding, the second one-electron transfer, and formation of the iron-oxygen complex which oxygenates the substrate. Thus, P450 reactions on steroids are limited to oxygen insertion (hydroxylation) reactions and, in a few notable cases, oxidative carbon-carbon bond cleavage reactions (Table 1-2).

HYDROXYSTEROID DEHYDROGENASES AND REDUCTASES

All hydroxysteroid dehydrogenases (HSDs) and related enzymes use nicotinamide cofactors either to reduce or to oxidize the steroid by two electrons through a hydride transfer mechanism.[2] Most examples involve the conversion of a secondary alcohol to a ketone or vice versa, and in the case of the 3β-hydroxysteroid dehydrogenase/$\Delta^{5/4}$-isomerases, the dehydrogenation is accompanied by the isomerization of the adjacent carbon-carbon double bond from the Δ^5 (between carbons 5 and 6) to the Δ^4 positions (see Figs. 1-1 and 1-2). The human steroid 5α-reductases types 1 and 2, which are included with the HSDs for convenience, reduce olefinic carbon-carbon double bonds to the saturated state rather than acting on carbon centers bonded to oxygen.

The HSDs can be categorized according to either structural or functional classification schemes. *Structurally*, HSDs are members of either the short-chain dehydrogenase reductase (SDR) or aldo-keto reductase (AKR) families.[4] The SDR enzymes are β-α-β proteins where up to seven parallel β-strands fan across the center of the molecule, forming the "Rossman fold" characteristic of oxidation/reduction enzymes that use nicotinamide cofactors. The AKR enzymes are soluble proteins that contain a beta-barrel or triosephosphate isomerase (TIM-barrel)

motif in which eight parallel β-strands lie in a slanted circular distribution like the staves of a barrel. In both cases, the active site contains a critical tyrosine and lysine pair of residues involved in proton transfer from or to the steroid alcohol during catalysis. *Functionally*, HSDs act either as true dehydrogenases, using NAD^+ as a cofactor to convert hydroxysteroids to ketosteroids, or as ketosteroid reductases, utilizing predominantly NADPH to reduce ketosteroids. Many HSDs catalyze either oxidation or reduction in vitro based on the pH and cofactor concentrations, but these enzymes, when expressed in intact mammalian cells, drive steroid flux primarily in one direction.[4] These directional preferences derive primarily from the relative abundance of the oxidized and reduced form of cofactors and the relative affinity of each enzyme for NAD(H) versus NADP(H), because cofactor concentrations exceed steroid concentrations by many orders of magnitude.[2,5] Consequently, the directional preference of some "reductive" enzymes can be reduced or reversed by depleting cells of NADPH or by mutations that impair NADPH binding.[6]

ACUTE REGULATION OF STEROIDOGENESIS

Every time that a pulse of corticotrophin (adrenocorticotropic hormone [ACTH]) reaches the adrenal cortex, or a pulse of luteinizing hormone (LH) reaches the gonad, a subsequent pulse

Table 1-2. Key Human Steroidogenic Enzymes and Cofactor Proteins

Protein	Gene	Gene Size (kb)	Chromosomal Locus	Location	Principal Substrates	Major Activities	Deficiency Syndromes
P450scc	CYP11A1	>20	15q23-q24	ZG/ZF/ZR Gonads (L,T), placenta, brain	Cholesterol Hydroxysterols	22R-Hydroxylase 20R-Hydroxylase 20,22-Lyase	Atypical lipoid CAH
P450c17	CYP17A1	6.6	10q24.3	ZF/ZR Gonads (L,T), brain	Preg, 17OH-Preg, Prog [17OH-Prog] 5α-reduced C_{21} steroids	17α-Hydroxylase 17,20-Lyase [16α-Hydroxylase] [Δ^{16}-Synthase]	17-Hydroxylase deficiency Isolated 17,20-lyase deficiency
P450c21	CYP21A2	3.4	6p21.1	ZG/ZF/ZR	Prog, 17OH-Prog	21-Hydroxylase	21-Hydroxylase deficiency
P450c11β	CYP11B1	9.5	8q21-q22	ZF/ZR, brain	11-Deoxycortisol 11-DOC	11β-Hydroxylase [18-Hydroxylase]	11-Hydroxylase deficiency
P450c11AS	CYP11B2	9.5	8q21-q22	ZG, brain, heart	Corticosterone 11-DOC 18OH-Corticosterone	11β-Hydroxylase 18-Hydroxylase 18-Oxidase	CMO I deficiency CMO II deficiency
P450aro	CYP19A1	>52	15q21.1	Gonads (L,G), placenta, brain, bone, fat	Androstenedione Testosterone	19-Hydroxylase 19-Oxidase, aromatization	Aromatase deficiency
3β-HSD1	HSD3B1	7.8	1p13.1	Placenta, liver, brain	Preg, 17OH-Preg DHEA, Δ^5-A	3β-Dehydrogenase $\Delta^{5/4}$-Isomerase	Not described (presumed lethal)
3β-HSD2	HSD3B2	7.8	1p13.1	ZG/ZF>ZR Gonad (L,T)	Preg, 17OH-Preg DHEA, Δ^5-A	3β-Dehydrogenase $\Delta^{5/4}$-Isomerase	3β-HSD deficiency
17β-HSD1	HSD17B1	3.3	17q11-q21	Gonad (G), placenta, breast	Estrone, [DHEA]	17β-Ketosteroid reductase	Not described
17β-HSD2	HSD17B2	>40	16q24.1-q24.2	Endometrium, broadly	Testosterone, estradiol, DHT	17β-Hydroxysteroid dehydrogenase	Not described
17β-HSD3	HSD17B3	>60	9q22	Gonad (L)	Androstenedione, 5α-A, 5α/3α-A [DHEA]	17β-Ketosteroid reductase	17-Ketosteroid reductase deficiency
Reductive 3α-HSDs	AKR1C1-4	13-25 each	10p14-p15	Liver, broadly	DHT, 5α-A 5α-reduced C_{21} steroids [17β-HSD: DHEA, Androstenedione, 5α/3α-A]	3α-Ketosteroid reductase, 17β-ketosteroid reductase	Not described
Oxidative 3α-HSD	HSD17B6	>23	12q13	Liver, prostate, broadly	Adiol, 5α/3α-A, 5α/3α-reduced C_{21} steroids, (products)	3α-Hydroxysteroid dehydrogenase (3α-, 20α-, and 17β-ketosteroid reductase)	Not described
5α-Reductase 1	SRD5A1	>35	5p15	Liver, brain, skin	Testosterone, Δ^4/C_{21}-steroids	5α-Reductase	Not described
5α-Reductase 2	SRD5A2	>35	2p23	Prostate, genital skin	Testosterone, Δ^4/C_{21}-steroids	5α-Reductase	5α-Reductase deficiency
11β-HSD1	HSD11B1	9	1q32-q41	Liver, brain, placenta, fat, broadly	Cortisone, 11-dehydro-corticosterone [products]	11β-Ketosteroid reductase	?Cortisone reductase deficiency
11β-HSD2	HSD11B2	6.2	16q22	Kidney, gut, placenta	Cortisol, corticosterone	11β-Hydroxysteroid dehydrogenase	Syndrome of apparent mineralocorticoid excess
Adrenodoxin	ADX	>30	11q22	Ubiquitous	Mitochondrial P450s	Electron transfer	Not described (presumed lethal)
Adrenodoxin reductase	ADR	11	17q24-q25	Ubiquitous	Adrenodoxin	Electron transfer	Not described (presumed lethal)
StAR	STAR	8	8p11.2	ZF/ZG/ZR, gonad (L,T)	Cholesterol flux within mitochondria	Cholesterol delivery to P450scc	Lipoid CAH
P450 oxido-reductase	POR	73	7q11.2	Ubiquitous	Microsomal P450s	Electron transfer	Multiple steroidogenic defects ± ABS
Cytochrome b_5	CYB5	32	18q23	ZR>ZG/ZF gonad (L, T)	P450c17	Augments 17,20-lyase activity	?17,20-Lyase deficiency with methemoglobinemia
H6PD6	H6PD6	9.6	1p36	Liver, muscle, broadly	11-βHSD1	Generate NADPK	Cortisone reductase deficiency

Δ^5-A, Androsta-5-ene-3β,17β-diol; 5α-A, 5α-androstane-3,20-dione; 5α/3α-A, androsterone; 17OH-Preg, 17α-hydroxypregnenolone; 17OH-Prog, 17α-hydroxyprogesterone; ABS, Antley-Bixler syndrome; Adiol, 5α-androstane-3α,17β-diol; CAH, congenital adrenal hyperplasia; CMO, corticosterone methyl oxidase; DHEA, dehydroepiandrosterone; DHT, dihydrotestosterone; DOC, deoxycorticosterone; G, granulosa cells; L, Leydig cells; T, theca cells; ZG/ZF/ZR, adrenal zona glomerulosa/fasciculata/reticularis, respectively. Steroids in brackets are poor substrates.

of steroid hormone production is observed within minutes. Although it has long been known that the loss of trophic hormones from the pituitary gland leads to adrenal and gonadal atrophy, the action of ACTH and LH to promote organ survival and to maintain steroidogenic capacity occurs at three distinct levels. First, as seen in long-term exposure to ACTH (e.g., in Cushing's disease), ACTH promotes adrenal growth. This growth occurs primarily by ACTH stimulating the production of cyclic adenosine monophosphate (cAMP), which in turn promotes the synthesis of insulin-like growth factor 2 (IGF-2),[7,8] basic fibroblast growth factor,[9] and epidermal growth factor.[10] Together, these growth factors stimulate adrenal cellular hypertrophy and hyperplasia. Second, ACTH acts long term through cAMP, and angiotensin II acts through the calcium/calmodulin pathway to promote the transcription of genes encoding various steroidogenic enzymes and electron-donating cofactor proteins. Third, ACTH fosters the increased flow of cholesterol into mitochondria, where it becomes substrate for the first and rate-limiting enzyme, P450scc. This acute response occurs within minutes and is inhibited by inhibitors of protein synthesis (e.g., puromycin or cycloheximide), indicating that a short-lived protein species mediates this process. Although other proteins are involved in the chronic replenishment of mitochondrial cholesterol, abundant biochemical, clinical, and genetic evidence implicates the steroidogenic acute regulatory protein (StAR) as this labile protein mediator.[11]

StAR is a 37-kilodalton (kD) phosphoprotein that is cleaved to a 30-kD form when it enters the mitochondrion. Overexpression of mouse StAR in mouse Leydig MA-10 cells increased their basal steroidogenic rate,[12] and cotransfection of expression vectors for both StAR and the P450scc system in nonsteroidogenic COS-1 cells augmented pregnenolone synthesis above that obtained with the P450scc system alone.[13] Mutations in StAR cause the most common form of congenital lipoid adrenal hyperplasia,[13,14] in which very little steroid is made, and targeted disruption of the *Star* gene in the mouse causes a similar phenotype.[15]

The mechanism of StAR's action is not known in detail.[16] StAR acts exclusively on the outer mitochondrial membrane (OMM),[17,18] and its activity in promoting steroidogenesis is proportional to its residency time on the OMM.[18] When expressed in cytoplasm or added to mitochondria in vitro, both the 37-kD "precursor" and the 30-kD "mature form" of StAR are equally active, but StAR is inactive in the mitochondrial intramembranous space or matrix.[18] Thus, it is StAR's cellular localization, not its cleavage, that determines whether or not it is active. StAR has a sterol-binding pocket that accommodates a single molecule of cholesterol.[19] The interaction of StAR with the OMM involves conformational changes[20,21] that are necessary for StAR to accept and discharge cholesterol molecules. Although StAR can transfer cholesterol between synthetic membranes in vitro,[22] suggesting that other protein molecules are not needed for its action, this activity can also be seen with the inactive mutant R182L, which causes lipoid CAH.[23] Thus, StAR's action to promote steroidogenesis is distinct from its cholesterol-transfer activity. StAR appears to interact with the peripheral benzodiazepine receptor (PBR)[24] voltage-dependent anion channel 1 (VDAC1) and phosphate carrier protein,[25] all proteins found on the outer mitochondrial membrane. Each molecule of StAR appears to be recycled, moving hundreds of molecules of cholesterol before the cleavage/inactivation event.[26] Although StAR is required for the acute steroidogenic response, steroidogenesis will persist in the absence of StAR at about 14% of the StAR-induced rate,[27] accounting for the steroidogenic capacity of tissues that lack StAR (e.g., the placenta and the brain).

CHRONIC MAINTENANCE OF THE STEROIDOGENIC MACHINERY

While the acute regulation of steroidogenesis is determined by access of cholesterol to the P450scc enzyme, which is mediated by StAR, P450scc is the enzymatic rate-limiting step in steroidogenesis. Thus the chronic regulation of steroidogenesis is quantitatively (how much) determined by P450scc gene expression[28] and qualitatively (which steroids) determined by the expression of downstream enzymes. The episodic bursts of cAMP resulting from the binding of ACTH and LH to their respective receptors are necessary but not sufficient for the continued expression of the steroidogenic enzymes and the production of steroids. Patients with inactivating mutations in the ACTH receptor[29] or LH receptor[30] make negligible steroids from the affected glands. Conversely, activating mutations of the $G_s\alpha$ protein, which couples receptor binding to cAMP generation, and activating mutations of the LH receptor cause hypersecretion of steroids.[31] Indeed, cAMP-responsive elements have been identified in the genes for most of the human steroidogenic P450 enzymes, but this mechanism alone does not allow for the diversity of steroid production observed in the various zones of the adrenal cortex, the gonads of both sexes, the placenta, and the brain.

Other transcription factors (e.g., AP-2, SP-1, SP-3, NF1C, NR4A1, NR4A2, GATA4, and GATA6) aid in defining the basal- and cAMP-stimulated transcription of each gene, which is also regulated in a tissue-specific manner by the regulatory elements unique to each gene. Among these factors, steroidogenic factor-1 (SF-1, NR5A1), an orphan nuclear receptor, coordinates the expression of steroidogenic enzymes in adrenal and gonadal cells.[32] By contrast, steroidogenesis in the brain[33] and placenta[34,35] is independent of SF-1. Targeted disruption of SF-1 in the mouse not only disrupts steroid biosynthesis but also blocks the development of the adrenal glands, gonads, and the ventromedial hypothalamus in homozygous animals.[36] Furthermore, SF-1 does not act in isolation, but its action is modified by other transcription factors (e.g., WT-1 and DAX-1[37]) or by sumoylation and phosphorylation.[38] The development of steroidogenic organs is intimately related to the capacity to produce steroids, and multiple factors acting on the genes for steroidogenic enzymes yield both common features and diversity among the steroidogenic tissues.

Most steroidogenic enzymes derive from a single mRNA species. The most prominent exception to this paradigm is aromatase, whose gene has four different promoters that enable vastly different regulation of expression of the same aromatase protein in many different tissues.[39] Although different transcripts of several genes (including 17β-HSDs types 1, 2, and 3) have been described, the encoded proteins derived from "exon skipping" are inactive if translated.[40]

Human Steroidogenic P450s

P450SCC

Encoded by the *CYP11A1* gene, P450scc consumes three equivalents of NADPH and molecular oxygen during the conversion of cholesterol to pregnenolone. Although the enzyme is named for the cleavage of the cholesterol side chain, this process consists of three discrete steps: (1) the 22-hydroxylation of cholesterol; (2) the 20-hydroxylation of 22(R)-hydroxycholesterol; and

(3) the oxidative scission of the C20-C22 bond of 20(R), 22(R)-dihydroxycholesterol—the side-chain cleavage event. The enzyme will utilize free hydroxysterol intermediates as substrates for the side-chain cleavage reaction, a tool that is used experimentally because the hydroxysterols are much more soluble than cholesterol and because their access to P450scc is independent of StAR.[13] In vivo, however, little of these free intermediates probably accumulate because their k_{cat}/K_m ratios are much higher than for cholesterol,[41] and the high K_d for pregnenolone (about 3000 nM) drives product dissociation. This complex process is the rate-limiting step in steroidogenesis, with turnover numbers of only about 20 molecules of cholesterol per molecule P450scc per minute.[41] P450scc will also cleave the side chain of other hydroxysterols (e.g., 7-dehydrocholesterol), and 20- and 22-hydroxylates vitamin D.[42]

The single human gene for P450scc[43] encodes an mRNA of 2 kb.[44] A 39-amino-acid mitochondrial leader peptide that targets P450scc to the mitochondria is then proteolytically removed to yield a 482-amino-acid protein. Forms of P450scc targeted to the endoplasmic reticulum are inactive,[45] demonstrating that the mitochondrial environment is required for activity. Expression of P450scc is induced in the adrenal zona fasciculata/reticularis,[46] testis,[47] and ovary by cAMP; and in the zona glomerulosa by intracellular calcium/protein kinase C.[48,49] In contrast, placental P450scc expression is constitutive[50] and is caused at least in part by the LBP family of transcription factors.[35,51] Side-chain cleavage activity and pregnenolone biosynthesis have been demonstrated in the rat and human brain[52]; and abundant P450scc expression is found in the rodent brain, especially in fetal life. Deletion of the gene for P450scc has been described in rabbits[53] and mice,[54] abrogating all steroidogenesis and thus proving that P450scc is the only enzyme that can convert cholesterol to pregnenolone. While homozygous mutations in P450scc are expected to be embryonic lethal by eliminating placental progesterone synthesis, a small number of patients has been described having P450scc mutations that typically retain partial enzymatic activity.[55,56]

P450C17

For investigators studying the enzymology and genetics of the steroidogenic pathways, P450c17 is especially interesting. Clinical observations showed that adrenal 17α-hydroxylase activity (reflected by serum cortisol concentrations) was fairly constant throughout life, whereas adrenal 17,20-lyase activity (reflected by serum DHEA and DHEAS concentrations) was low in early childhood but rose abruptly during adrenarche at ages 8 to 10 years.[57,58] This dissociation between adrenal secretion of 17α-hydroxylase products (cortisol) and 17,20-lyase products (DHEA) suggested that distinct enzymes performed the two transformations, a hypothesis that was reinforced by the description of patients with putative isolated 17,20-lyase deficiency. Consequently, reports[59] that the 17α-hydroxylase and 17,20-lyase activities of neonatal pig testes copurified were initially received with great skepticism. This controversy of "one enzyme or two" persisted until the cDNA for bovine P450c17 was cloned and shown to confer both 17-hydroxylase and 17,20-lyase activities when expressed in nonsteroidogenic COS-1 cells.[60] The human genome has one gene for P450c17,[61] which is expressed in the adrenals and gonads,[62] and not two tissue-specific isozymes as had been thought. A single 2.1-kb mRNA species yields a 57-kD protein in these tissues, and mutations in this gene produce a spectrum of deficiencies in 17-hydroxysteroids and C_{19} steroids.

Human P450c17 17-hydroxylates both pregnenolone and progesterone with approximately equal efficiency,[63,64] but all other reactions show prominent differences between Δ^4 and Δ^5 substrates. The 17,20-lyase activity is about 50 times more efficient for the 17α-hydroxypregnenolone-to-DHEA reaction than for the 17α-hydroxyprogesterone-to-androstenedione reaction.[63,64] Although the rate of the lyase reaction can be increased more than 10-fold by the addition of a molar excess of cytochrome b_5,[63-65] the Δ^5 preference persists, and the lyase rate never quite reaches the rate of the hydroxylase reactions. In addition, human P450c17 16α-hydroxylates progesterone but not pregnenolone[64]; in the presence of cytochrome b_5, it diverts about 10% of pregnenolone metabolism to a Δ^{16} andiene product[63] that is also formed by this pathway in pigs and that acts as a pheromone in that species. Although experiments to study the chemistry of human P450c17 often require manipulations that could be considered nonphysiologic, the remarkable consistency for substrate preferences and kinetic constants observed for the modified, solubilized P450c17 expressed in *Escherichia coli*[63,65] and native P450c17 expressed in yeast microsomes,[64] or intact COS-1 cells,[66] or that obtained from human tissues and cells,[64,67] serve to verify these conclusions.

Given the diverse repertoire of reactions catalyzed by P450c17 in the classical pathways, it is not surprising that synthetic steroids such as dexamethasone[68] and the enantiomer of progesterone,[69] as well as planar drugs such as troglitazone,[70] also bind to and inhibit P450c17. In addition, the 5α-reduced C_{21} steroids dihydroprogesterone (5α-pregnane-3,20-dione) and allopregnanolone (5α-pregnan-3α-ol-20-one) are excellent substrates for the 17α-hydroxylase activity of P450c17[71] (Fig. 1-4A). Furthermore, 17α-hydroxylated allopregnanolone (5α-pregnane-3α,17α-diol-20-one; 17OH-Allo) is the most efficient substrate yet identified for the 17,20-lyase activity of human P450c17, and its cleavage to androsterone is minimally dependent on cytochrome b_5,[71] unlike 17α-hydroxypregnenolone metabolism to DHEA.[63-65] The conversion of 17OH-Allo to androsterone by the 17,20-lyase activity of P450c17, first described in the testes of tammar wallaby pouch young,[72] provides an alternative or "backdoor" pathway to DHT, by which DHT is produced without utilizing DHEA, androstenedione, and testosterone as intermediates[73] (see Fig. 1-4B). Consequently, the presence of 5α-reductases in steroidogenic cells does not preclude the production of C_{19} steroids but rather paradoxically enhances the production of DHT by directing flux to 5α-reduced precursors of DHT.

The backdoor pathway enables production of C_{19} steroids in the presence of abundant 3β-HSD activity, despite the poor 17,20-lyase activity of human P450c17 for 17α-hydroxyprogesterone, by using 17OH-Allo as the substrate for the 17,20-lyase reaction. The presence of 5α-reductase activity is a key requirement for the backdoor pathway. The best-studied example of 5α-reduction in a human steroidogenic tissue is the production of 5α-dihydroprogesterone in human corpus luteum by the type 1 enzyme.[74] Human enzymes catalyze all of the other reactions required to complete this alternate route to DHT, and good evidence documents production of 5α-reduced androgens by the fetal adrenal, at least in some pathologic states. Consequently, it is possible that the backdoor pathway is the principal route to DHT in pathologic states in which 17α-hydroxyprogesterone accumulates, including 21-hydroxylase deficiency and P450 oxidoreductase deficiency (see the following). Androgen production by the backdoor pathway may explain why newborn girls with 21- and 11-hydroxlase deficiencies can

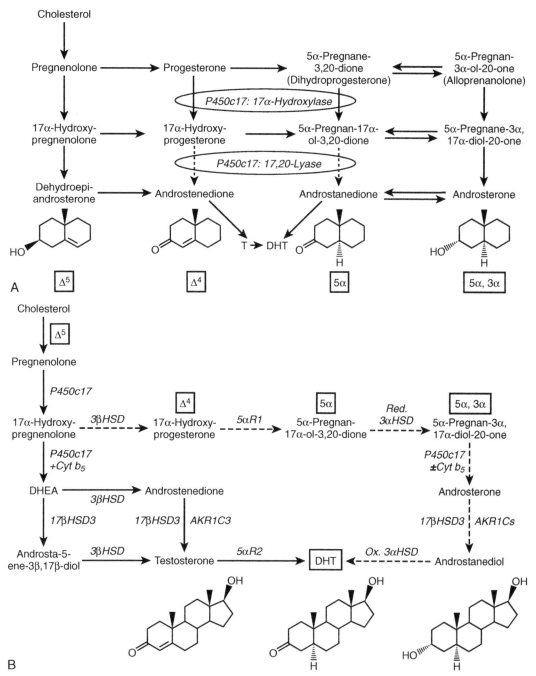

FIGURE 1-4. Reactions catalyzed by human P450c17 and pathways to C_{19} steroids. **A,** The four principal A/B-ring configurations of active endogenous steroids and their precursors: Δ^5, Δ^4, 5α, and $5\alpha,3\alpha$ *(boxes and structures at bottom)*. Progesterone and 17α-hydroxyprogesterone can be 5α-reduced, and once the A-ring is saturated, these 5α-reduced steroids are substrates for reductive 3α-HSDs of the AKR1C family. Human P450c17 17α-hydroxylates all four classes of C_{21} steroids, but the 17,20-lyase activity is robust only with 17α-hydroxypregnenolone and 5α-pregnane-3α,17α-diol-20-one (Δ^5- and 5α,3α-pathways, respectively). **B,** Two pathways to DHT using the different 17,20-lyase activities of human P450c17. In the conventional or Δ^5-pathway *(solid arrows)*, the 17,20-lyase activity of P450c17 requires cytochrome b_5 to efficiently convert 17α-hydroxyprogesterone to DHEA, and testosterone is reduced in target tissues by 5α-reductase 2 (5αR2) to DHT. In the "backdoor" or 5α,3α-pathway *(broken arrows)*, 5α-reduction by 5αR1 and 3α-reduction of C_{21} steroids occurs in the steroidogenic tissue prior to the 17,20-lyase reaction. In the best characterized pathway, 5α-pregnane-3α,17α-diol-20-one is cleaved to androsterone without requiring cytochrome b_5 and reduced to androstanediol. Androstanediol is exported from the testis and metabolized to DHT by oxidative 3α-HSDs (Ox. 3α-HSD). Note that testosterone is *not* an intermediate in the backdoor pathway to DHT, that different isoforms of 5α-reductase appear to be involved in the two pathways, and that both reductive and oxidative 3αHSDs are required for the "backdoor" pathway. Structures of testosterone, DHT, and androstanediol are shown at bottom.

be severely virilized, while those with 3β-HSD2 deficiency, whose adrenals cannot make 17α-hydroxyprogesterone, are minimally virilized.[75] The fractional contributions of the conventional and backdoor pathways to DHT production during human sexual differentiation (at 8 to 12 weeks of gestation) and the

expression of 5α-reductase in fetal adrenal and gonad tissues,[76] however, are only beginning to be determined.

The chemistry of P450c17-mediated hydroxylations is believed to proceed via the common iron oxene species and "oxygen rebound" mechanism proposed for prototypical P450 hydroxylations.[77] The mechanism of the 17,20-lyase reaction involving a carbon-carbon bond cleavage, however, is not known despite considerable study. The failure of hydrogen peroxide alone to support catalysis (as has been shown for some other P450-mediated deacylation reactions) and computer modeling studies suggest that the same heme-oxygen complex might participate in both hydroxylations and the 17,20-lyase reaction,[78] but no conclusive evidence to exclude proposed mechanisms exist.

One consequence of the Δ^5 preference of the human enzyme for the 17,20-lyase reaction is that most human C_{19} and C_{18} steroids derive from DHEA as an intermediate.[67] This Δ^5 preference allows for the phenomenon of adrenarche to occur in humans, an event that only takes place in large primates.[79,80] However, Δ^5-lyase activity is not sufficient for adrenarche to occur, because some monkeys (e.g., rhesus macaques) produce high amounts of DHEA throughout life, but most mammals (e.g., cattle, dogs, cats, etc.) never produce much DHEA.[79] The biochemistry of P450c17, with its differential regulation of the 17α-hydroxylase and 17,20-lyase activities, provides clues to the genesis of this enigmatic process of adrenarche. P450c17 is a phosphoprotein, and phosphorylation selectively enhances the 17,20-lyase activity.[81,82] It appears likely that the regulation of P450c17 phosphorylation, which is a dynamic balance between phosphorylation and dephosphorylation, plays an important role in adrenarche and pathologic hyperandrogenic states such as polycystic ovary syndrome.[83] Whereas the kinase(s) responsible for P450c17 phosphorylation remain unknown, it is now apparent that the kinase activity is counterbalanced by protein phosphatase 2A, which in turn is regulated by cAMP via phosphoprotein SET.[84] Cytochrome b_5 also augments 17,20-lyase activity,[64,82] and high expression of b_5 in the zona reticularis of monkeys[85] and humans[86] suggests that the developmentally regulated expression of b_5 might be a key event. The transcriptional regulation of cytochrome b_5 in the adrenal is similar to that of P450c17,[87] but mechanisms enabling zone-specific expression have not been elucidated. Finally, limiting steroid flux to the Δ^5 pathway by lowering 3β-HSD activity in the zona reticularis (where most DHEA derives) potentiates the effect of increased 17,20-lyase activity.[86,88]

The initial description of 17α-hydroxylase deficiency was a case in which both 17α-hydroxylase and 17,20-lyase products were absent.[89] When the gene for human P450c17 was cloned,[61] patients with 17α-hydroxylase deficiency were found to harbor mutations in the *CYP17A1* gene, and more than 40 mutations scattered throughout the *CYP17A1* gene have been characterized,[90] with mutations W406R and R362C being the most common and accounting for the high prevalence of 17α-hydroxylase deficiency in Brazil.[91] The identification of *CYP17A1* mutations causing apparent isolated 17,20-lyase deficiency is fraught with difficulty,[92] but in the past decade, five cases of isolated 17,20-lyase deficiency caused by mutations in arginines 347 and 358 have been confirmed.[93,94] Computer modeling studies demonstrate that R347H and R358Q neutralize positive charges in the redox-partner binding site.[78,93] Biochemical studies confirm that mutations R347H and R358Q impair interactions of P450c17 with its electron donor POR and with cytochrome b_5.[95] Therefore, these cases of isolated 17,20-lyase deficiency are not caused by an inability of the mutant enzymes to bind the intermediate 17α-hydroxypregnenolone but rather are caused by subtle disturbances in interactions with redox partners.[93,95] In contrast, mutation E305G has been shown to cause 17,20-lyase deficiency by selectively disrupting binding of 17α-hydroxypregnenolone and DHEA synthesis despite

enhanced conversion of 17α-hydroxyprogesterone to androstenedione.[96] This unusual variant of isolated 17,20-lyase deficiency provides further genetic evidence that the flux of androgens derived from conversion of 17α-hydroxyprogesterone to androstenedione in the minor Δ^4 pathway is not sufficient to form normal male external genitalia. One of the first patients reported to have isolated 17,20 lyase deficiency was recently found to have a homozygous mutation in P450 oxidoreductase (G539R), further emphasizing the crucial role of efficient electron transfer in the 17,20 lyase reaction.[97]

P450C21

Microsomal P450c21 performs the 21-hydroxylation of the Δ^4 steroids 17α-hydroxyprogesterone and progesterone, an essential step in the biosynthesis of both mineralocorticoids and glucocorticoids (see Fig. 1-2). The human P450c21 protein is found only in the adrenal glands; the extra-adrenal 21-hydroxylase activity found in other organs such as the liver and the aorta[98] is not catalyzed by P450c21[99] but appears to be catalyzed by CYP2C9, CYP3A4, and possibly CYP2C19 and other enzymes as well.[100,101]

The locus containing the *CYP21* genes is among the most complex in the human genome and explains why 21-hydroxylase deficiency (affecting 1 of 14,000 live births) is one of the most common autosomal-recessive diseases. The *CYP21A2* gene and the *CYP21A1* pseudogene lie on chromosomal locus 6p21.1 in the midst of the human leukocyte antigen (HLA) locus. Because the HLA locus is highly recombinogenic, exchange between the *CYP21A1* and *CYP21A2* loci is common. Thus 85% of cases of 21-hydroxylase deficiency derive from micro- or macrogene conversion events where some or all of the *CYP21A1* pseudogene replaces the corresponding area of the *CYP21A2* gene, thus reducing the expression of the encoded P450c21 protein and/or impairing its activity.[102] In addition, at least eight additional genes lie in this locus (Fig. 1-5), including the liver-specific *C4A* and *C4B* genes; the adrenal-specific "ZA" and "ZB" genes; and the ubiquitously expressed tenascin X or *TNXB* gene,[103] the disruption of which is one cause of Ehlers-Danlos syndrome.[104] Occasionally, a patient with 21-hydroxylase deficiency and Ehlers-Danlos syndrome will have a contiguous gene syndrome with tenascin X deficiency as well.[105]

Much less is known about the enzymology of P450c21 than of P450c17, but the available evidence suggests that unlike P450c17, P450c21 is not very sensitive to the abundance of POR or cytochrome b_5. It is clear that genotype consistently predicts phenotype in very severe and very mild cases of 21-hydroxylase deficiency. In contrast, patients with P450c21 variants (e.g., the common Pro30Leu and Val281Leu mutations and less common mutations Arg339His and Pro453Ser), which have 20% to 50% of wild-type activity,[102,106] can have various phenotypes, implying additional factors that can modify the clinical manifestations of 21-hydroxylase deficiency.

P450C11β AND P450C11AS

The classical descriptions of distinct deficiencies in 11β-hydroxylase, 18-hydroxylase (also called *corticosterone methyl oxidase I*, or CMOI), and 18-oxidase (CMOII) suggested that three enzymes executed these three respective transformations.[107,108] Analogous to the scenario for P450c17, a single enzyme[109] and corresponding gene[110] were found in bovine adrenals that possessed all three activities. In contrast, humans have two genes named *CYP11B1* and *CYP11B2*[111] that encode the mitochondrial enzymes 11β-hydroxylase (P450c11β) and aldo-

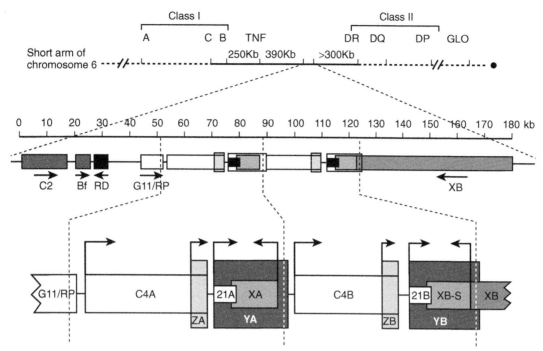

FIGURE I-5. Genetic map of the human leukocyte antigen (HLA) locus containing the genes for P450c21. The *top line* shows the p21.1 region of chromosome 6, with the telomere to the left and the centromere to the right. Most HLA genes are found in the class I and class II regions; the class III region containing the *CYP21* genes lies between these two. The *second line* shows the scale (in kb) for the diagram immediately below, showing (from left to right) the genes for complement factor C2, properdin factor Bf, and the *RD* and *G11/RP* genes of unknown function; *arrows* indicate transcriptional orientation. The *bottom line* shows the 21-hydroxylase locus on an expanded scale, including the *C4A* and *C4B* genes for the fourth component of complement, the "*CYP21A*" pseudogene (*CYP21A1*, 21A), and the active "*CYP21B*" gene (*CYP21A2*, 21B) that encodes P450c21. XA, YA, and YB are adrenal-specific transcripts that lack open reading frames. The *XB* gene encodes the extracellular matrix protein tenascin-X; *XB-S* encodes a truncated adrenal-specific form of the tenascin-X protein whose function is unknown. ZA and ZB are adrenal-specific transcripts that arise within the *C4* genes and have open reading frames, but it is not known if they are translated into protein; however, the promoter elements of these transcripts are essential components of the *CYP21A1* and *CYP21A2* promoters. The *arrows* indicate transcriptional orientation. The *vertical dotted lines* designate the boundaries of the genetic duplication event that led to the presence of A and B regions.

sterone synthase (P450c11AS), respectively, and rats but not mice have three functional *CYP11B* genes.[112] Although P450c11β and P450c11AS both possess 11β-hydroxylase activities, P450c11AS also performs the two oxygenations at C_{18} required for aldosterone biosynthesis.[113,114] Mutations in *CYP11B1* cause 11β-hydroxylase deficiency,[115] whereas defects in *CYP11B2* cause either CMOI or CMOII deficiencies.[116] Severe defects can impair all P450c11AS activities, leading to the clinical phenotype of CMOI deficiency,[113] whereas P450c11β provides 11β-hydroxylase activity in the zona fasciculata. Fortuitous site-directed mutagenesis experiments of nature have found amino acid substitutions such as Arg181Trp plus Val386Ala, which mainly impair 18-oxidase activity and lead to CMOII deficiency.[117]

The coding regions of the *CYP11B1* and *CYP11B2* genes share 93% amino acid identity and the same exonic gene structure found in all mitochondrial P450 genes.[118] Despite the sequence similarities of these tandem genes, located within 40 kb on chromosome 8q24.3, the expression of P450c11AS is restricted to the adrenal zona glomerulosa, whereas P450c11β is found in the zona fasciculata and zona reticularis. The regulation of P450c11β is driven mainly by cAMP in response to ACTH, whereas P450c11AS expression derives from potassium and angiotensin II activation of the protein kinase C pathway.[119] Thus, under normal circumstances, 18-hydroxylase and 18-oxidase activities are restricted to the zona glomerulosa, where 17-hydroxylase activity is low, limiting the repertoire of steroids that can undergo 18-oxygenation.

Although the organization of two highly homologous, adjacent *CYP11B1* and *CYP11B2* genes on chromosome 8 is reminiscent of the genetics of the *CYP21A1* and *CYP21A2*, gene conversion in the *CYP11B* locus occurs rarely.[120] Instead, a clinical entity called *glucocorticoid remediable aldosteronism* (GRA) arises when an unequal crossing over of the *CYP11B1* and *CYP11B2* genes creates a third, hybrid gene in which the ACTH-regulated promoter of *CYP11B1* drives expression of a chimeric protein with aldosterone synthase activity.[121,122] As a result, 18-hydroxylase and 18-oxidase activities are ectopically expressed in the zona fasciculata, leading to elevated renin-independent production of aldosterone, as well as 18-oxygenated metabolites of cortisol. The expression of this gene is suppressed by blunting ACTH production with glucocorticoids such as dexamethasone, which is used for diagnosis and treatment.[123] The prevalence of GRA varies from nil to as high 2% of referred patients with hypertension.[124]

The genetics of GRA has assisted in the precise identification of residues in P450c11AS that enable 18-oxygenase activities. Residues 288, 296, 301, 302, 325, and perhaps most importantly, 320 are critical for 18-oxygenase activities.[125,126] Therefore, crossovers 3′ to codon 320 do not enable aldosterone synthase activity. These key residues lie in or near the I-helix, which contains the catalytically important threonine residue implicated in oxygen activation for almost all P450s; thus, these mutations would be expected to alter active site geometry.

P450ARO (AROMATASE)

The oxidative demethylation of C_{19} steroids, mainly androstenedione and testosterone, consumes three equivalents of molecular oxygen and NADPH, yielding formic acid and C_{18} steroids with an aromatic A-ring, hence the common name for this enzyme, *aromatase*. As is the case for P450scc, each subsequent oxygenation proceeds with greater efficiency, aiding in the completion of this transformation that is essential for estrogen biosynthesis in all animals.[127] The mechanism of this aromatization must account for the incorporation of the final oxygen atom from molecular oxygen into the formic acid byproduct. The weight of evidence favors a hydroxylation at C2 of 19-oxo-androstenedione, followed by an enzyme-assisted rearrangement and tautomerization of the intermediate dienone to the phenolic A-ring.[128]

P450aro is expressed in steroidogenic tissues (ovarian granuloma cells, placenta), in brain, and in nonsteroidogenic tissues, especially fat and bone.[127] The *CYP19A1* gene for P450aro spans over 75 kb[129] and contains five different transcriptional start sites[130] with individual promoters that permit the tissue-specific regulation of expression in diverse tissues. P450aro is a glycoprotein, but glycosylation per se does not appear to affect activity.

Studies of patients with aromatase deficiency confirm that biologically significant estrogen synthesis derives entirely from this enzyme,[131,132] although dietary phytoestrogens can provide some estrogen action in mice with targeted deletion of the aromatase gene.[133] Although very few cases of aromatase deficiency have been described, they are highly informative "knockouts of nature" that illustrate principles of fetoplacental steroidogenesis. In fetuses homozygous for aromatase deficiency, the principal manifestation results from its deficiency in the placenta,[131] because ovarian steroidogenesis is quiescent during fetal life.[134] The fetal adrenal makes large amounts of C_{19} steroids, principally DHEA-S, much of which is 16α-hydroxylated in the fetal liver before undergoing metabolism via steroid sulfatases, 3β-HSD1, aromatase, and 17β-HSD1 in the placenta to produce estriol, the characteristic estrogen of pregnancy. Although huge amounts of estriol and estradiol are produced by the fetoplacental unit, estrogens are not needed for fetal development, the maintenance of pregnancy, or the onset of parturition; all of these processes proceed normally in fetuses lacking StAR, P450c17, or aromatase, or even in fetuses wholly lacking adrenal glands because of mutations in SF-1 or DAX-1.[135] However, in the absence of placental aromatase activity, androgenic C_{19} steroids derived from the fetal adrenal are passed into the maternal circulation, causing marked virilization of the mother.[131]

Furthermore, in pregnancies in which the mother has poorly treated 21-hydroxylase deficiency, maternal testosterone values can exceed 300 ng/dL (a midpubertal value for males), yet the fetus is not virilized[136] because the maternal testosterone is efficiently metabolized to estradiol by placental aromatase. Thus, placental aromatase is a key enzyme in protecting the fetus and mother from unwanted androgen exposure. After birth, individuals with aromatase deficiency grow normally and continue linear growth after completion of puberty, with males producing normal amounts of testosterone. However, when treated with estrogens, aromatase-deficient subjects fuse their epiphyses and cease linear growth.[137] These observations provide powerful evidence that bony maturation and epiphyseal fusion in children is mediated by estrogens, not androgens, even in males. These observations have led to the experimental use of aromatase inhibitors in various disorders of accelerated bone maturation.

Redox Partner Proteins

The proteins collectively referred to as *redox partners* channel reducing equivalents from NADPH to the heme centers of P450

enzymes.[3] Recent studies, however, suggest that these proteins act to promote catalysis by more than just their electron-transfer properties. Because of this, the precise nature of the interactions of the P450s with their redox partners is of considerable importance. Our understanding of these interactions has been greatly advanced by the x-ray crystal structures of these four proteins.

ADRENODOXIN (FERREDOXIN)

Adrenodoxin (Adx), also known as *ferredoxin*, is encoded by a gene on chromosome 11q22 that spans over 30 kb. Adx is a small (14 kD), soluble, Fe_2S_2 electron shuttle protein that resides either free in the mitochondrial matrix or is loosely bound to the inner mitochondrial membrane.[138] Adx is expressed in many tissues, and its expression in steroidogenic tissues is induced by cAMP in parallel with P450scc.[139]

Bovine Adx consists of two domains,[140] a core region and an interaction domain. The core region contains residues 1-55 and 91-end (bovine numbering), including the four cysteines whose sulfur atoms tether the Fe_2S_2 cluster to the protein. Residues 56 to 90 form the interaction domain, which is a hairpin containing a helix at its periphery that includes acidic residues critical for the interaction of Adx with P450scc[141] (specifically, aspartates 72, 76, and 79, plus glutamate 73). The Fe_2S_2 cluster lies in a protuberance in the molecule at the junction of its two domains. The charged residues of Adx cluster in the interaction domain, giving the molecule a highly negatively charged surface above the Fe_2S_2 cluster (see Fig. 1-3A). This description of the Adx molecule concurs with earlier studies that showed that overlapping sets of negative charges on Adx drive Adx interactions with positive charges on both P450scc and adrenodoxin reductase (AdR).[142] Because a preponderance of the evidence favors a model in which the same surface of Adx shuttles between AdR and the P450 to transport electrons,[142,143] a model of how Adx interacts with AdR would approximate how mitochondrial P450s interact with Adx.

ADRENODOXIN (FERREDOXIN) REDUCTASE

Like Adx, adrenodoxin reductase (AdR) is widely expressed in human tissues, but its expression is two orders of magnitude higher in steroidogenic tissues.[144] The primary RNA transcript from the 11-kb *AdR* gene[145] on chromosome 17q24-q25[146] is alternatively spliced, generating two mRNA species that differ by only 18 bp,[147] but only the protein encoded by the shorter mRNA is active in steroidogenesis.[148] Unlike most steroidogenic genes, the promoter for AdR contains six copies of GGGCGGG sequences,[145] which is the canonical binding site for the transcription factor SP-1 typically found in "housekeeping genes." Accordingly, cAMP does not regulate transcription of the AdR gene, as is the case for Adx and P450scc,[144] implying that AdR plays additional roles in human physiology beyond steroidogenesis. Given their essential roles in the conversion of cholesterol to pregnenolone, no null mutations in AdR or Adx have been described in humans, and impairment of the *Drosophila* AdR homologue *dare* causes developmental arrest and degeneration of the adult nervous system owing to the loss of ecdysteroid production.[149]

Bovine AdR also consists of two domains, each comprising a β-sheet core surrounded by α-helices.[150] The NADP(H)-binding domain is a compact region composed of residues 106 to 331 (bovine numbering), whereas the more open FAD domain, formed by the remaining amino- and carboxy-terminal residues, binds the dinucleotide portion of FAD across a Rossman fold, with the redox-active flavin isoalloxazine ring abutting the

NADP(H) domain. By analogy to related structures, including glutathione and thioredoxin reductases, the nicotinamide ring of NADPH is modeled to lie adjacent to the flavin ring in a position to transfer its two electrons to the FAD. Intramolecular electron transfer occurs in the cleft formed by the angled apposition of these two domains. Within this cleft, basic residues abound, including arginines 240 and 244, which are important for interactions with Adx.[142,151] Hypothetical docking of the two structures suggests that the negative surface of Adx fits elegantly into the positive surface of AdR, even with NADP(H) bound.[150] Basic residues are also critical for the interaction of P450scc with the negative surface charges on Adx,[143] so that AdR-Adx docking is expected to share some key features with the mitochondrial P450-Adx interaction.

P450 OXIDOREDUCTASE

The flavoprotein P450 oxidoreductase (POR) is expressed widely in human tissues and serves as the sole electron-transfer protein for all microsomal P450s, including xenobiotic-metabolizing hepatic P450s, steroidogenic P450s, and P450s found in other tissues such as the kidney and brain. POR contains two lobes, one binding FAD and the other binding FMN, and a flexible amino terminus that tethers it to the endoplasmic reticulum. NADPH is bound to the cofactor-binding domain above the FAD in a β-sheet-rich FAD domain, and an α-helical connecting domain joins the FAD and the FMN domains.[152] A disordered "hinge" of about 25 residues lies between the FMN domain and the connecting domain, suggesting that the FMN and FAD domains can move substantially relative to each other. In the x-ray structure of rat liver POR,[152] the FMN and FAD lie at the base of a cleft formed by the butterfly-shaped apposition of the FAD and FMN domains, reminiscent of the electron transfer surface of AdR.[150] It is not clear how the surface containing the FMN docks into the redox partner-binding surface of the P450, but the flexible hinge region on which the FMN domain resides suggests that the FMN domain can reorient itself significantly to accommodate docking to the P450 (see Fig. 1-3).[3,64] The surface of the electron-donating FMN domain is dominated by acidic residues, whereas the redox-partner binding site of P450 enzymes contain numerous basic residues.

The crystal structure of the complex between the P450 and flavoprotein domains of the bacterial protein P450BM3 serves as a model of this flavoprotein-P450 interaction.[153] Negative charges of the FMN domain guide interactions with positive charges on the P450. The FMN approaches no closer than 18 Å from the heme, similar to the 16 Å distance of FAD from the Fe_2S_2 cluster in the modeled AdR-Adx complex, and presumably similar to the distance of the heme from the Fe_2S_2 cluster in the P450-Adx complex.[150] These distances are too far for electrons to "jump" directly to the heme; rather, electron transfer apparently uses the polypeptide chain as a conduit.[153] Basic residues in the redox-partner binding surface are crucial for interactions with POR and for electron transfer,[3,154] and these positive charges in human P450c17 are critical for maximal 17,20-lyase activity.[78,95] Thus, these structures demonstrate several key principles of the electron transfer proteins involved in human steroidogenesis: NADPH and prosthetic groups lie at the interfaces of protein domains in which electron transfer occurs; the electron transfer surfaces are negatively charged to pair with positive charges on the P450s; the terminal electron transfer moiety (FMN domain or Adx) must be mobile or soluble to pass electrons on to the P450; and electrons flow from the FMN or Fe_2S_2 cluster along the adjacent polypeptide chain to the heme.

Cytochrome P450 Oxidoreductase Deficiency: A Disorder Affecting Multiple P450 Enzymes

Beginning with a clinical report in 1985,[155] several patients have been described with clinical and hormonal findings suggesting partial deficiencies of both 17α-hydroxylase and 21-hydroxylase.[156] Some of these individuals were born to mothers who had become virilized during pregnancy, suggesting fetoplacental aromatase deficiency, and many also had the Antley-Bixler congenital malformation syndrome characterized by craniosynostosis and radioulnar synostosis. About half of patients with Antley-Bixler syndrome have normal steroidogenesis and normal genitalia; these subjects have dominant gain-of-function mutations in the gene for fibroblast growth factor receptor type 2 (FGFR2); however, patients with Antley-Bixler syndrome who also have genital anomalies and disordered steroidogenesis do not have FGFR2 mutations.[157] The initial report described three patients with Antley-Bixler syndrome, genital ambiguity, and hormonal findings suggestive of partial deficiencies of 17α-hydroxylase and 21-hydroxylase, as well as a fourth patient who was phenotypically normal but had a similar hormonal profile. All had recessive loss-of-function amino acid replacement mutations in POR.[158] One of these patients was born to a woman who had become virilized during the pregnancy, suggesting partial fetoplacental aromatase deficiency.

In vitro biochemical assays of the recombinant mutant proteins showed that the mutations in the Antley-Bixler subjects had severely impaired but not totally absent activity, whereas the mutations found in the phenotypically normal subject with amenorrhea were less severe.[158] Examination of the POR and FGFR2 genes in a series of 32 patients established that the recessive POR mutations and the dominant FGFR2 mutations segregate completely.[159] To date, approximately 50 POR-deficient patients have been described.[160] It appears unlikely that subjects will be found who are homozygous for null POR alleles, because knockouts of POR in mice cause embryonic lethality.[161,162] On the other hand, liver-specific ablation of the Por gene in mice results in phenotypically and reproductively normal animals with profoundly impaired drug metabolism,[163,164] because POR is required for the activities of all hepatic drug-metabolizing P450 enzymes. Consequently, it seems likely that patients with POR deficiency will also metabolize drugs poorly. Reports of Antley-Bixler syndrome in some infants of mothers who ingested fluconazole (an azole drug that inhibits the fungal P450 lanosterol-14-demethylase and also inhibits some human P450s) suggest that haploinsufficiency of POR may be a risk factor for teratogenic effects of some drugs, particularly those that inhibit P450s involved with embryogenesis.[158]

The human POR gene, located on chromosome 7, consists of 16 exons.[160,165] The sequence of this gene in 842 normal persons from four ethnic groups revealed a high degree of polymorphism; most notably, the coding sequence variant A503V was found on ~28% of all alleles.[166] This sequence variant reduces the 17α-hydroxylase and 17,20 lyase activities of P450c17 to ~60% of normal[159,166] but has no measurable effect on the activities of P450c21[167] or hepatic CYP1A2 or CYP2C19.[168]

CYTOCHROME b_5

The small (12 to 17 kD) hemoprotein cytochrome b_5 (b_5) is found in many tissues (e.g., as a membrane-bound cytochrome in liver and as a soluble protein lacking the C-terminal membrane anchor in erythrocytes). Importantly, b_5 is expressed in both the adrenals and gonads, where it can interact with P450c17; the adrenal expression is zone specific and may contribute to the genesis of adrenarche.[85,86] Much evidence has shown that b_5 can augment some activities of certain P450 enzymes, and the mechanism of this effect has been presumed to involve electron transfer from b_5 to the P450 for the second electron during the P450 cycle.[169] Although b_5 can certainly receive electrons from flavoproteins like POR, the redox potentials of b_5 and one-electron-reduced P450 are unfavorable for b_5-to-P450 electron transfer. Indeed, some of the actions of b_5 in experimental systems can be observed with apo-b_5[170] or Mn^{2+}-b_5 (which do not transfer electrons), including the stimulation of 17,20-lyase activity of human P450c17.[63,64] These experiments suggest that b_5 does not act alone as an electron donor but rather functions in concert with POR to somehow aid catalysis.

The soluble form of bovine b_5 was one of the first proteins studied by x-ray crystallography, and a wealth of structural data for b_5 have been acquired using molecular dynamics and nuclear magnetic resonance (NMR) spectroscopy for both the holo- and apo-b_5.[171,172] Analogous to Adx, b_5 consists of two domains: (1) a heme-liganding core 1 domain (residues 40 to 65, bovine numbering) and (2) a structural core 2 domain, from which the C-terminal membrane-anchoring helix extends. The heme extends more to the periphery of b_5 than does the Fe_2S_2 cluster of Adx, and the entire surface is dominated by negatively charged residues rather than just one cluster of negative charges near the heme. In addition, the core 1 domain acquires considerable conformational flexibility in apo-b_5, whereas the core 2 domain remains folded as in holo-b_5.[172] Finally, the C-terminal membrane-spanning helix (exiting the core 2 domain) is required to stimulate the 17,20-lyase activity of human P450c17, but the signal peptide is not.[173] Genetic and biochemical studies have implicated basic residues in P450c17, including R347, R358, and perhaps R449 and K89, as important for its interaction with b_5,[78,95,173] while E48 and E49 of b_5 are required for high 17,20-lyase activity.[174] The molecular details of how addition of b_5 to the P450c17 POR complex augments 17,20-lyase activity, however, is not yet known.

Steroidogenic Dehydrogenases and Reductases

3β-HYDROXYSTEROID DEHYDROGENASE/Δ^5-Δ^4-ISOMERASES

Conversion of Δ^5 steroids into their Δ^4 congeners, a step required for the production of progestins, mineralocorticoids, glucocorticoids, and sex steroids, consists of two chemical transformations, both performed by the 3β-hydroxysteroid dehydrogenase/$\Delta 5/4$-isomerase (3β-HSD) enzymes. The first reaction is the oxidation of the 3β-hydroxyl group to the ketone, and during this process NAD^+ is converted to NADH. The intermediate Δ^5, 3-ketosteroid remains tightly bound to the enzyme with nascent NADH, and the presence of NADH in the cofactor binding site activates the enzyme's second activity, the $\Delta^5 \rightarrow \Delta^4$-isomerase activity.[175] Competition experiments have shown that the dehydrogenase and isomerase activities reside in a single active site,[176] yet these enzymes are often referred to by their dehydrogenase activity alone.

Although rodents contain multiple 3β-HSD isoforms, only two active genes have been identified in humans. The type 1 enzyme (3β-HSD1) is expressed in the placenta, liver, brain, and some other tissues.[177] This isoform is required for placental pro-

gesterone production during pregnancy, which may explain why a deficiency of 3β-HSD1 has never been described. In contrast, the type 2 enzyme (3β-HSD2) is by far the principal isoform in the adrenals and gonads.[178] Deficiency of 3β-HSD2 causes the rare form of congenital adrenal hyperplasia known as *3β-HSD deficiency*.[75] The presence of the type 1 isozyme in these patients helps to explain the paradox of why 46,XX individuals born with severe 3β-HSD2 deficiency can virilize slightly in utero: The 3β-HSD block in the adrenal diverts Δ^5-steroids away from cortisol and toward DHEA; extra-adrenal 3β-HSD1 enables testosterone synthesis despite 3β-HSD2 deficiency in the adrenal.

The types 1 and 2 enzymes share 93.5% amino acid identity, and all biochemical studies comparing the two enzymes yield very similar results. The enzymes are strongly inhibited by Δ^4 products[179] and by synthetic Δ^4 steroids such as medroxyprogesterone acetate.[68] Both enzymes have very similar affinities for the Δ^5,17-ketosteroid pregnenolone, 17α-hydroxypregnenolone, and DHEA of about 5 μM[68,176] and also convert the 17β-hydroxysteroid androsta-5-ene-3β,17β-diol to testosterone. The enzymes are primarily membrane bound and are found both in the microsomal and mitochondrial fractions during subcellular fractionation.[176] Ultrastructural studies using immunogold labeling confirm that at least in bovine adrenal zona glomerulosa cells, 3β-HSD immunoreactivity is indeed found not only in mitochondria and the endoplasmic reticulum but also in the cytoplasm.[180]

Considerable evidence suggests that 3β-HSD activity is an important factor in regulating adrenal dehydroepiandrosterone sulfate (DHEA-S) production. The human fetal adrenal, which produces vast amounts of DHEA-S, contains little 3β-HSD immunoreactivity.[181] Furthermore, the expression of 3β-HSD in the innermost regions of the adrenal cortex declines as the zona reticularis develops in childhood,[86,182] and 3β-HSD immunoreactivity is low in the zona reticularis of the adult rhesus macaque[85] and of humans.[86] Thus the development of an adrenal cell type (reticularis) that is relatively deficient in 3β-HSD activity appears to be a necessary component of adrenarche, in which adrenal production of the Δ^5 steroids DHEA and DHEA-S rises exponentially.[183]

17β-HYDROXYSTEROID DEHYDROGENASES

There are at least 14 human 17β-hydroxysteroid dehydrogenase (17β-HSD) isoforms; these isoforms vary widely in size, structure, substrate specificity, cofactor utilization, and physiologic functions.[184] This section focuses on the human isoforms that possess significant, rather than gratuitous, 17β-HSD activity.

17β-HSD Type I

The interconversion of estrone and estradiol by 17β-HSD1 has been studied more extensively than any other human steroidogenic enzyme, and in the late 1980s, three independent groups reported the cloning of its cDNA, the first of any human HSD.[185] Located on chromosome 17q25[186] adjacent to a pseudogene, the *HSD17B1* gene[187] encodes a 34-kD protein subunit that is expressed primarily in the placenta and in ovarian granulosa cells of developing follicles.[186] The enzyme, which is active only as a dimer, accepts mainly estrogens such as estrone, although it also has low catalytic activity for the conversion of androstenedione to testosterone and DHEA to androsta-5-ene-3β,17β-diol.[188] Although the enzyme can oxidize 17β-hydroxysteroids in the presence of NAD^+ in vitro at a high pH, the enzyme functions in vivo to reduce estrone to estradiol and 16α-hydroxyestrone to estriol.[188]

Detailed kinetic analyses of 17β-HSD1 began in the late 1960s, and attempts to identify active-site residues using affinity labels and mechanism-based inactivators followed.[189] Sequence alignments with other members of the SDR family identified a Tyr-X-X-X-Lys active-site motif in residues 155 to 159. These predictions were verified when the x-ray structure of 17β-HSD1 was solved.[190] The structure demonstrates that cofactor lies across the β-sheet core of the protein in a Rossman fold characteristic of all SDR enzymes. Steroid appears to dangle from the top of the enzyme almost perpendicular to the cofactor, with a hydrophobic pocket holding the body of the steroid in place while the 3-hydroxyl forms hydrogen bonds with His 221 and Glu 282. At the place where the steroid and cofactor meet, Ser 142, Tyr 155, and Lys 159 help to form a proton-relay system that drives catalysis.

Because steroid flux to estrogens preferentially occurs via the aromatization of androstenedione to estrone, 17β-HSD1 appears to be required for the conversion of estrone to biologically active estradiol in the ovary and placenta.[186] This role has not been proven unequivocally, because no cases of human 17β-HSD1 deficiency have been reported. Such a disease is theoretically compatible with life, because fetuses with aromatase deficiency and estrogen insensitivity (ER-α mutations) are viable.[132] Nevertheless, this enzyme is probably critical for ovulation and may be important in the pathogenesis and progression of estrogen-dependent breast cancers.[191]

17β-HSD Type 2

In contrast to the "activating" role of 17β-HSD1 in the placenta and ovary, human endometrium was known to inactivate estradiol by the conversion to estrone. This activity, which was induced by progestins, was not 17β-HSD1, because 17β-HSD1 mRNA was not detected in the human uterus.[186] Instead, a cDNA encoding microsomal *HSD17B2* was cloned[192] and found to be expressed in endometrium, placenta, and other tissues.[193] In fact, 17β-HSD2 not only converts estradiol to estrone but also oxidizes testosterone and DHT to their inactive 17-ketosteroid homologues, androstenedione and 5α-androstanedione, respectively. The widespread tissue distribution and broad substrate specificity of 17β-HSD2 suggests that its role in human physiology is to protect tissues from excessive exposure to active steroid hormones by oxidation to inactive 17-ketosteroids.[184] This role is again somewhat speculative, given that a human deficiency of this enzyme has not been described; but 17β-HSD2 is certainly the most active human inactivating (oxidizing) 17β-HSD that has been described to date. The type 2 enzyme also oxidizes 20α-dihydroprogesterone to progesterone, but this activity is low relative to its 17β-HSD activity.[192]

17β-HSD Type 3

Because 17β-HSD1 shows poor activity with C_{19} steroids, at least one other 17β-HSD enzyme capable of reducing androstenedione to testosterone was postulated to complete testosterone biosynthesis. Furthermore, reports of male pseudohermaphrodites lacking this putative androgenic "17-ketosteroid reductase" activity surfaced in the 1970s.[194] When the large, complex gene for 17β-HSD3 was cloned, patients with "17-ketosteroid reductase deficiency" were found to harbor mutations in this *HSD17B3* gene,[195,196] proving the central role of this enzyme in male sexual differentiation and marking 17β-HSD3 as the only 17β-HSD enzyme whose role in human physiology is genetically established by a deficiency syndrome. Nonetheless, patients with 17β-HSD3 deficiency make small amounts of testosterone, suggesting

that one or more additional human 17β-HSD enzymes convert androstenedione to testosterone. Similarly, the human ovary exports some testosterone despite an absence of 17β-HSD3 expression, and women with 17β-HSD3 deficiency produce normal amounts of androgens and estrogens.[197]

Unlike 17β-HSD1, which has been the subject of intense biochemical study, relatively little is known about 17β-HSD3 enzymology. This knowledge gap is at least in part caused by the very hydrophobic nature of the encoded 310-amino-acid protein, hampering the expression of this enzyme in bacteria. From experiments in transiently transfected HEK-293 cells, we know that 17β-HSD3 reduces all of the C_{19} 17-ketosteroids that serve as precursors of testosterone and DHT in human beings, including DHEA, 5α-androstanedione, and androsterone.[196] The conversion of DHEA to androsta-5-ene-3β,17β-diol by 17β-HSD3 may contribute significantly to testicular testosterone synthesis. Estrogens such as estrone are poor substrates for human 17β-HSD3.[188]

17β-HSD Types 4 and 5

Many additional 17β-HSD isoforms have been described in rodents and in humans, but the activities of these isoforms for steroids are generally poor. For example, the type 4 enzyme is a trifunctional protein located in peroxisomes,[198] but its (oxidative) HSD activity toward estradiol is 10^6 times slower than its 3-hydroxyacyl-coenzyme A dehydrogenase activity.[199] Deficiency of the type 4 enzyme causes Zellweger syndrome, in which bile acid synthesis is disturbed, but steroidogenesis is not affected.[200] Thus, this enzyme has 17β-HSD activity as one of its repertoire of transformations, but steroidogenesis is not its principal physiologic function.

Unlike 17β-HSDs types 1 to 4, which are SDR enzymes, the type 5 enzyme is an AKR enzyme, which is expressed both in steroidogenic and non-steroidogenic tissues.[201] There has been some confusion about the nature of the type 5 enzyme because of its multiple activities and inconsistent results from different laboratories. Originally described as hepatic 3α-HSD type 2 for its ability to reduce DHT to 3α-androstanediol,[202] this protein was later found to also have 17β-HSD activity,[201] including reducing androstenedione to testosterone.[203] This enzyme, now known as *AKR1C3* (see 3α-HSDs), may account for much of the extratesticular androstenedione-to-testosterone conversion, although its catalytic efficiency as a 17β-HSD is poor[204] compared to its 20α-HSD activity with progesterone and 11-deoxycorticosterone[205] or its prostaglandin dehydrogenase activity, reducing PGH_2 to $PGF_{2\alpha}$.[206] Nevertheless, AKR1C3 is more highly expressed in the human fetal adrenal during the time of sexual differentiation than 17β-HSD3[207] and may participate in testosterone production, particularly in virilizing congenital adrenal hyperplasias.

STEROID 5α-REDUCTASES

The conversion of testosterone to 5α-dihydrotestosterone (DHT) in target tissues was described in the 1960s,[208] and studies using fibroblasts suggested that at least two human enzymes with different pH optima and genetics performed these transformations.[209] These initial results were confirmed when the genes encoding the type 1[210] and type 2[211] enzymes were cloned, and patients with clinical 5α-reductase deficiency were found to have mutations in the *SRD5A2* gene. The two isoforms are very hydrophobic 30-kD microsomal proteins that share 50% identity. The type 1 enzyme is limited to the nongenital skin and liver, and it is not expressed significantly in peripheral tissues of the fetus, which explains why a deficiency of the type 2 enzyme is not compensated for by the type 1 enzyme.[212] The type 2 enzyme remains the predominant enzyme in genital skin, male accessory sex glands, and prostate, whereas the type 1 enzyme accounts for most of the hepatic 5α-reduction.

Although 5α-reductase activity is generally discussed in the context of male genital differentiation and androgen action, both isoenzymes reduce a variety of steroids in what are believed to be degradative pathways in human beings. In fact, progesterone, 17α-hydroxyprogesterone and related C_{21} steroids are the best substrates for both 5α-reductases, particularly the type 1; cortisol, cortisone, corticosterone, and related compounds are also good substrates.[213] The 5α- (and 5β-) reduced steroids may be metabolized further and conjugated for excretion in the urine. Given the importance of 5α-reductase type 2 in prostate growth, inhibitors of the type 2 enzyme have been developed for the treatment of prostatic hyperplasia and the prevention of its recurrence after surgery.[214] Finasteride selectively inhibits human 5α-reductase type 2, whereas dutasteride inhibits both the type 1 and type 2 isoenzymes. Both drugs are approved for treatment of prostatic hyperplasia in the United States.

Although the function of 5α-reductase type 2 is firmly established from the studies of male pseudohermaphrodites with this deficiency, the role of the type 1 isoform in human beings is less clear. Given the abundant expression of the type 1 isoform in liver and its high activity with C_{21} steroids, this enzyme has been ascribed a role of degrading circulating C_{21} steroids in preparation for excretion in the urine. However, disruption of *Srd5a1* in mice results in delayed parturition, a defect that can be rescued with 5α-androstane-3α,17β-diol.[215] In immature mice, 5α-reductase type 1 is expressed both in the ovary and in the Leydig cells, and this enzyme participates in the testicular synthesis of 5α-androstanediol via two pathways.[216] Whether 5α-reductases are expressed in human adrenal or gonads in normal physiology or in pathologic states is not known.

3α-HYDROXYSTEROID DEHYDROGENASES

The four major human 3α-hydroxysteroid dehydrogenases (3α-HSDs) are AKR enzymes with reductive preferences that belong to the AKR1C family. The 3α-HSDs types 1, 2, 3, and 4 are trivial names for AKR1C4, 1C3, 1C2, and 1C1, respectively, which are located in tandem on chromosome 10p14-p15. Each enzyme has its characteristic tissue distribution[217,218] and repertoire of catalytic activities.[204] AKR1C3 also performs the 17β-HSD reaction with androstenedione and is known also as 17β-HSD5. All of the AKR1C isoforms catalyze additional reactions, such as the 20α-reduction of pregnanes. In the brain, 3α-HSDs reduce 5α-dihydroprogesterone to tetrahydroprogesterone (allopregnanolone), which is an allosteric activator of the GABA_A receptor-chloride channel complex, with a nanomolar affinity.[219] AKR1C4 is abundant in liver but has been found in adrenal and gonads; AKR1C3 was cloned from liver, prostate, and brain; AKR1C2 is found in the prostate and brain; and AKR1C1 is abundant in the uterus. Furthermore, the amino acid compositions of isozymes of the type 2 and 3 enzymes differ by a few residues. These minor differences in composition, however, cannot be neglected, because these differences might alter substrate utilization.

Recent studies have indicated an important role for 3α-HSDs in the nervous system. Antidepressant drugs in the selective serotonin reuptake inhibitor class (e.g., fluoxetine and paroxetine) directly lower the K_m of rat brain type 2 3α-HSD for 5α-dihydroprogesterone by almost 10-fold,[220] which explains

why these drugs augment brain allopregnanolone concentrations and perhaps contribute to their antidepressant activity. In addition, x-ray crystallography has shown that the β subunit of the mammalian voltage-gated potassium channel is a tetrameric structure[221] in which each subunit closely resembles the rat liver 3α-HSD (AKR1C9)[222] and even contains bound NADP+ with high occupancy. Although the broader implications of this work are not yet known, these studies suggest a role of HSDs in coupling intracellular redox state to membrane excitation.

The 3α-HSDs differ from the 11β-HSDs, 3β-HSDs, and 17β-HSDs types 1 to 4 in several respects, because all reductive 3α-HSDs are AKR enzymes rather than SDR enzymes. As AKR enzymes, they function as monomers with a TIM-barrel structure; they bind cofactor with the nicotinamide ring draped across the mouth of the "barrel" rather than lying on a Rossman fold; and their kinetic mechanisms are highly ordered, with cofactor dissociation the final and rate-limiting step.[223] Tight NADP(H) binding derives from interaction of Arg276 with the 2′-phosphate, and mutation of Arg276 eliminates a conformational change associated with tight binding[224] and attenuates or reverses the preference for ketosteroid reduction in intact cells.[6] As shown in the structure of AKR1C9,[222] their active sites also contain tyrosine and lysine residues to facilitate proton transfer during catalysis, but these residues are distantly located in linear sequence rather than confined to the Tyr-X-X-X-Lys motif as in SDR enzymes.

In contrast to the reductive 3α-HSDs, the oxidative 3α-HSDs belong to the SDR family and show greatest similarity to the retinol dehydrogenase or cis-retinol/androgen dehydrogenase (RoDH/CRAD) subfamily.[225] Although several of these RoDH/CRAD enzymes show some 3α-HSD activity, the most active enzyme appears to be RODH, the microsomal 3α-HSD, 3 (α→β)-hydroxysteroid epimerase, or formally, 17β-HSD6, whose cDNA was first cloned from prostate.[226] This enzyme converts the inactive C_{19} steroid 5α-androstane-3α,17β-diol to DHT and thus may execute the final step in the backdoor pathway from 17α-hydroxyprogesterone to DHT via androsterone. However, prolonged incubation of 3α-hydroxysteroids with cells transfected with the cDNA for 17β-HSD6 or with microsomes containing the recombinant enzyme yields subsequent 3-ketosteroid metabolites, including both 3α- and 3β-hydroxysteroids and 17β-hydroxysteroids.[227] Hence, this enzyme has complex catalytic flexibility and may serve a variety of biological functions.

11β-HYDROXYSTEROID DEHYDROGENASES

The 11β-hydroxysteroid dehydrogenases (11β-HSDs) regulate the bioactivity of endogenous and synthetic glucocorticoids, and a comparison of the types 1 and 2 enzymes exemplifies some key principles of HSD enzymology (Table 1-3). Both enzymes are hydrophobic, membrane-bound proteins that bind cortisol/cortisone and corticosterone/11-dehydrocorticosterone, but otherwise their properties and physiologic roles differ substantially[228] (see Table 1-3). The type 2 enzyme shares only 21% sequence identity with 11β-HSD1, whereas 11β-HSD2 and 17β-HSD2 share 37% identity and favor steroid oxidation in vivo. Thus, 11β-HSD1 and 2 are only distantly related members of the SDR family, yet they perform opposite functions in specific tissues in human physiology and pharmacology.

The 34-kD type 1 enzyme (11β-HSD1)[229] is expressed in the liver, testis, lung, fat, and proximal convoluted tubule. The type 1 enzyme catalyzes both the oxidation of cortisol, using NADP+ as cofactor (K_m 1 to 2 µM), and the reduction of cortisone, using

Table 1-3. Comparison of 11β-Hydroxysteroid Dehydrogenases Types 1 and 2

Property	Type I	Type 2
Size	34 kD	41 kD
Orientation in ER	Luminal	Cytoplasmic
Expression	Liver, decidua, lung, gonad, pituitary, brain, fat, bone	Kidney, placenta, colon, salivary gland
Principal reaction	Reduction	Oxidation
Cofactor preference	NADPH via H6PDH	Cytoplasmic NAD$^+$
Substrate binding	Low affinity (K_m 0.1-1 μM)	High affinity (K_m 0.01-0.1 μM)
Inhibition by carbenoxolone	Moderate	Strong
Deficiency state	CRD (with H6PDH)	AME

AME, Apparent mineralocorticoid excess; *CRD,* cortisone reductase deficiency; *ER,* endoplasmic reticulum; *H6PDH,* hexose-6-phosphate dehydrogenase; *NAD$^+$,* nicotinamide adenine dinucleotide, oxidized form; *NADPH,* nicotinamide adenine dinucleotide phosphate, reduced form.

NADPH cofactor (K_m 0.1-1 μM), with cortisone reduction being the dominant reaction in transfected cells.[230,231] Many synthetic glucocorticoids (e.g., prednisone and cortisone) are 11-ketosteroids that must be reduced to their 11β-hydroxy derivatives to attain biological activity, and these transformations are performed mainly in the liver by 11β-HSD1. In contrast, when recombinant 11β-HSD1 is studied in vitro, cortisol oxidation with NADP$^+$ is most efficient, and cortisone reduction is only achieved if NADP$^+$ is scrupulously removed with an enzymatic NADPH regeneration system.[232,233] The net flux of steroid driven by 11β-HSD1 depends on the relative concentrations of available NADPH and NADP$^+$, which usually favors reduction in cells, especially given the high K_m of the enzyme for cortisol.[233]

The mechanism for the discrepancy between the prominent oxidative preference in vitro and the reductive dominance in vivo, however, is more complex and derives from the localization of 11β-HSD1 in the lumen of the endoplasmic reticulum.[234] In this compartment, the ratio of NADPH to NADP$^+$ is not maintained by the cytoplasmic NADP$^+$-coupled dehydrogenases (mainly glucose-6-phosphate dehydrogenase) but by hexose-6-phosphate dehydrogenase (H6PDH). Indeed, the disorder cortisone reductase deficiency (CRD), which is characterized by high ratios of cortisone to cortisol and of their respective metabolites in blood and urine,[235] is not caused by mutations in the coding regions of *HSD11B1*. Instead, CRD subjects most commonly harbor inactivating mutations in *H6PDH*[236] which impair NADPH regeneration within the endoplasmic reticulum, where 11β-HSD1 resides. The genetics and pathophysiology of CRD provide an excellent example of the critical role of nicotinamide cofactors in HSD function and biology.

In contrast, the 41-kD type 2 enzyme[237] catalyzes the oxidation of cortisol and corticosterone using NAD$^+$, and although this enzyme has a high affinity for its steroid substrates (K_m 0.01 to 0.1 μM),[238] catalysis of the reductive reactions by 11β-HSD2 has not been conclusively demonstrated. Cortisol is a potent agonist at the mineralocorticoid (glucocorticoid type 2) receptor in the distal nephron, but its oxidized 11-keto derivative, cortisone, is not a mineralocorticoid. The reason cortisol does not act as a mineralocorticoid in vivo, even though cortisol concentrations can exceed aldosterone concentrations by three orders of magnitude, is because cortisol is enzymatically converted to cortisone in the cells lining the cortical and medullary collecting ducts. The type 2 enzyme inactivates the mineralocorticoid activity of cortisol in the kidney tubule,[239] and inactivating mutations in the

type 2 enzyme cause a syndrome of apparent mineralocorticoid excess[240] (see also Chapter 13). The presence of the type 2 enzyme in the placenta[241] also inactivates endogenous and synthetic corticosteroids such as prednisolone, allowing the use of these agents during pregnancy without affecting the fetus. In contrast, 9-fluorinated steroids such as dexamethasone are minimally inactivated by the type 2 enzyme, primarily because of a shift in the oxidation/reduction preference rather than a reduction in affinity for the enzyme.[242] It is this resistance to inactivation by placental 11β-HSD2 that is essential for synthetic glucocorticoids to "cross the placenta" and to exert a pharmacologic effect on the fetus. Furthermore, the relatively high placental concentrations of NADP$^+$ may also favor the oxidative action of 11β-HSD1, so that both placental enzymes protect the fetus from the high maternal concentrations of cortisol that occur during pregnancy.[228]

Pathways

ADRENAL STEROIDOGENIC PATHWAYS

Diagrams of steroidogenic pathways, such as that shown in Fig. 1-2, typically combine the pathways from multiple cell types to give a comprehensive and inclusive illustration; however, such diagrams may be misleading, since dominant pathways by which specific steroids are synthesized differ in each steroidogenic cell type. The three major pathways of steroidogenesis in the human adrenal are shown in Fig. 1-6. The adrenal *zona glomerulosa* (ZG) is characterized by three features: its expression of AII receptors, its unique expression of P450c11AS, and its inability to express P450c17. This combination of factors permits the ZG to produce aldosterone under regulation by the renin/angiotensin system. By contrast, the adrenal *zona fasciculata* (ZF) does not express AII receptors or P450c11AS but instead expresses the melanocortin type 2 receptor (MC2R, the receptor for ACTH) and P450c11β, which *cannot* convert 18-hydroxycorticosterone to aldosterone and has minimal capacity to convert corticosterone to 18-hydroxycorticosterone.[243] Both the ZG and ZF express P450c21, but the ZF also expresses P450c17, which allows aldosterone and cortisol synthesis, respectively, in these zones. The ZF, however, expresses very little cytochrome b_5[86]; consequently, P450c17 in the ZF catalyzes 17α-hydroxylation but very little 17,20 lyase activity. Thus the ZF produces two glucocorticoids, mainly cortisol and smaller amounts of corticosterone, under the influence of ACTH. Patients with severe mutations in P450c17 cannot synthesize cortisol but instead increase corticosterone production[244] (as do rodent adrenals, which lack P450c17), explaining why they are not glucocorticoid deficient, despite the lack of cortisol (see Fig. 1-6). The adrenal *zona reticularis* (ZR) also expresses MC2R but very little P450c21 or P450c11β, and as a result, the ZR produces minimal amounts of cortisol. By contrast, the ZR expresses large amounts of cytochrome b_5,[86] maximizing the 17,20 lyase activity of P450c17,[64] so that DHEA is produced and sulfated by SULT2A1 to DHEAS.[245] The ZR expresses relatively little 3βHSD2, and the K_m of 3βHSD2 is ~5 μM for pregnenolone and 17-hydroxypregnenolone,[68] whereas the K_m for both activities of P450c17 is ~1 μM,[64] so that abundant DHEA is produced. As DHEA accumulates, small amounts are converted to androstenedione, and very small amounts of this androstenedione are converted to testosterone, probably by AKR1C3/17βHSD5. The pattern of steroid products secreted by each adrenal zone is determined by the enzymes produced in

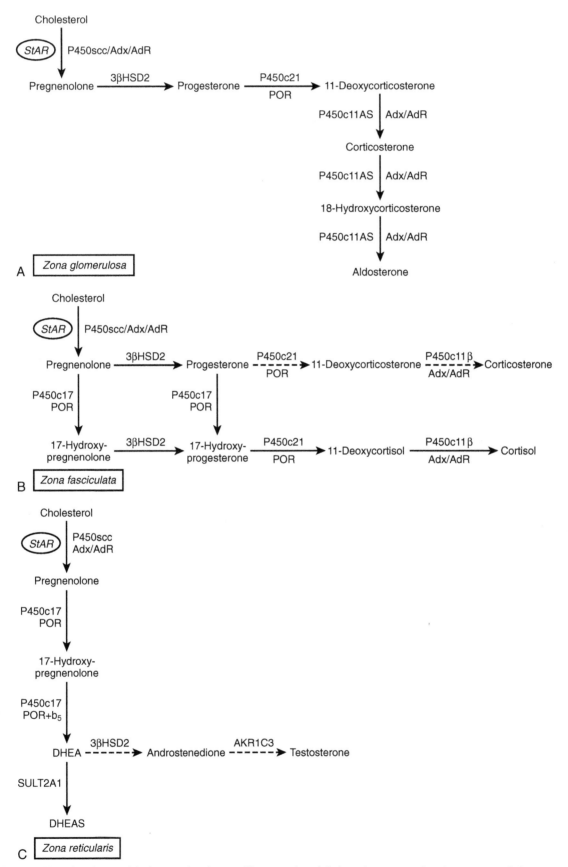

FIGURE I-6. Major steroidogenic pathways of the human adrenal cortex. The conversion of cholesterol to pregnenolone is common to all three zones. **A,** In the zona glomerulosa, 3βHSD2 converts pregnenolone to progesterone. P450c17 is absent, but P450c21 produces 11-deoxycorticosterone, which is a substrate for P450c11AS (aldosterone synthase), the enzyme catalyzing 11-hydroxylation and two 18-oxygenations to complete aldosterone synthesis. **B,** The zona fasciculata expresses P450c17 but little cytochrome b_5, so pregnenolone is hydroxylated to 17α-hydroxypregnenolone but not cleaved to DHEA. Instead, 3βHSD2 yields 17α-hydroxyprogesterone, the preferred substrate for P450c21, which produces 11-deoxycortisol. P450c11β, which is unique to the zona fasciculata, completes the synthesis of cortisol. Corticosterone is normally a minor product *(dashed arrows)* derived from a parallel pathway without the action of P450c17. **C,** The zona reticularis has high P450c17 and cytochrome b_5 but low 3βHSD2, so pregnenolone is sequentially oxidized to 17α-hydroxypregnenolone and then DHEA. SULT2A1 sulfates DHEA, and DHEAS is exported to the circulation.

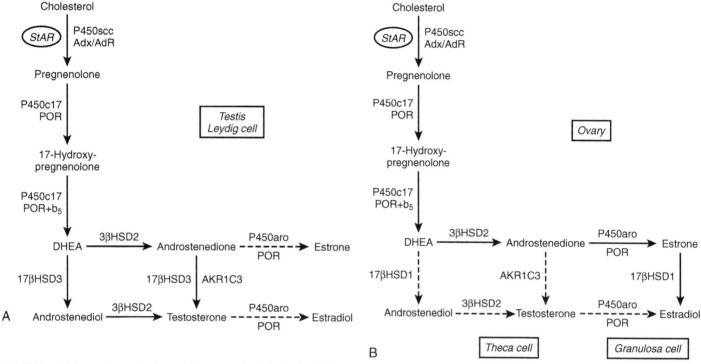

FIGURE I-7. Major steroidogenic pathways of the gonads. Both the Leydig cell of the testis and the theca cell of the ovary convert cholesterol to DHEA and have the capacity to synthesize androstenedione and testosterone. The major difference is their enzymatic machinery is abundant 17βHSD3 in the Leydig cells **(A),** which efficiently completes testosterone synthesis in the testis, whereas androstenedione is the major C19 product of the theca cell **(B).** The granulosa cells of the ovary contain abundant aromatase and 17βHSD1, which complete the biosynthesis of estradiol. Minor pathways are shown with *dashed arrows.*

that zone and may be logically deduced from an understanding of their specific enzymatic properties.[245]

GONADAL STEROIDOGENIC PATHWAYS

Testicular synthesis of testosterone follows a pathway that is similar to C_{19} steroid production in the adrenal zona reticularis, with the notable exceptions that Leydig cells express abundant 3βHSD2 and 17βHSD3 but no SULT2A1, and the stimulus for steroidogenesis is transduced by the luteinizing hormone (LH) receptor rather than MC2R. Consequently, DHEA produced under LH stimulation is not sulfated but readily converted to androstenediol and androstenedione and then testosterone (Fig. 1-7). As in the adrenal, the principal pathway to C_{19} steroids is via Δ^5 steroids to DHEA; the Δ^4 pathway from 17OHP to androstenedione makes a minimal contribution.[67,96] By contrast, ovarian steroidogenesis is more complex, as the enzymatic steps are partitioned between the granulosa and theca cells, which

surround the oocyte and form a follicle. In addition, the patterns of steroidogenesis vary during the cycle, directed mainly to estradiol in the follicular phase and to progesterone in the luteal phase (see Fig. 1-7). The key point in ovarian steroidogenesis is that granulosa cells do not express P450c17. Thus, in general, steroidogenesis is initiated in granulosa cells under the influence of LH, which, via cAMP, stimulates the expression of P450scc.[28] Pregnenolone and progesterone from granulosa cells diffuse into adjacent theca cells, where they can be acted upon by P450c17 and 3βHSD2 to produce androstenedione. Small amounts of this androstenedione are secreted or converted to testosterone (probably by AKR1C3/17βHSD5), but most androstenedione returns to the granulosa cells, where it is converted to estrone and then to estradiol by P450aro and 17βHSD1, respectively. As with the three zones of the adrenal, the patterns of gonadal steroidogenesis are dictated by the cell-specific expression of specific steroidogenic enzymes.

REFERENCES

1. Hall PF: Cytochromes P450 and the regulation of steroid synthesis, Steroids 48:133–196, 1986.
2. Agarwal AK, Auchus RJ: Minireview: cellular redox state regulates hydroxysteroid dehydrogenase activity and intracellular hormone potency, Endocrinology 146:2531–2538, 2005.
3. Miller WL: Regulation of steroidogenesis by electron transfer, Endocrinology 146:2544–2550, 2005.
4. Penning TM: Molecular endocrinology of hydroxysteroid dehydrogenases, Endocr Rev 18:281–305, 1997.
5. Sherbet DP, Papari-Zareei M, Khan N, et al: Cofactors, redox state, and directional preferences of hydroxysteroid dehydrogenases, Mol Cell Endocrinol 265–266:83–88, 2007.
6. Papari-Zareei M, Brandmaier A, Auchus RJ: Arginine 276 controls the directional preference of AKR1C9 (rat

liver 3α-hydroxysteroid dehydrogenase) in human embryonic kidney 293 cells, Endocrinology 147:100–107, 2006.
7. Voutilainen R, Miller WL: Coordinate tropic hormone regulation of mRNAs for insulin-like growth factor II and the cholesterol side-chain cleavage enzyme, P450scc, in human steroidogenic tissues, Proc Natl Acad Sci USA 84:1590–1594, 1987.
8. Mesiano S, Mellon SH, Jaffe RB: Mitogenic action, regulation, and localization of insulin-like growth factors in the human fetal adrenal gland, J Clin Endocrinol Metab 76:968–976, 1993.
9. Mesiano S, Mellon SH, Gospodarowicz D, et al: Basic fibroblast growth factor expression is regulated by corticotropin in the human fetal adrenal: a model for adrenal growth regulation, Proc Natl Acad Sci USA 88:5428–5432, 1991.

10. Coulter CL, Read LC, Carr BR, et al: A role for epidermal growth factor in the morphological and functional maturation of the adrenal gland in the fetal rhesus monkey in vivo, J Clin Endocrinol Metab 81:1254–1260, 1996.
11. Stocco DM, Clark BJ: Regulation of the acute production of steroids in steroidogenic cells, Endocr Rev 17:221–244, 1996.
12. Clark BJ, Wells J, King SR, et al: The purification, cloning and expression of a novel luteinizing hormone-induced mitochondrial protein in MA-10 mouse Leydig tumor cells. Characterization of the steroidogenic acute regulatory protein (StAR), J Biol Chem 269:28314–28322, 1994.
13. Lin D, Sugawara T, Strauss JF III, et al: Role of steroidogenic acute regulatory protein in adrenal and gonadal steroidogenesis, Science 267:1828–1831, 1995.

14. Bose HS, Sugawara T, Strauss JF III, et al: The pathophysiology and genetics of congenital lipoid adrenal hyperplasia, N Engl J Med 335:1870–1878, 1996.

15. Caron K, Soo S-C, Wetsel W, et al: Targeted disruption of the mouse gene encoding steroidogenic acute regulatory protein provides insights into congenital lipoid adrenal hyperplasia, Proc Natl Acad Sci USA 94:11540–11545, 1997.

16. Miller WL: StAR search: What we know about how the steroidogenic acute regulatory protein mediates mitochondrial cholesterol import, Mol Endocrinol 21:589–601, 2007.

17. Arakane F, Sugawara T, Nishino H, et al: Steroidogenic acute regulatory protein (StAR) retains activity in the absence of its mitochondrial targeting sequence: implications for the mechanism of StAR action, Proc Natl Acad Sci USA 93:13731–13736, 1996.

18. Bose H, Lingappa VR, Miller WL: Rapid regulation of steroidogenesis by mitochondrial protein import, Nature 417:87–91, 2002.

19. Tsujishita Y, Hurley JH: Structure and lipid transport mechanism of a StAR-related domain, Nat Struct Biol 7:408–414, 2000.

20. Bose HS, Whittal RM, Baldwin MA, et al: The active form of the steroidogenic acute regulatory protein, StAR, appears to be a molten globule, Proc Natl Acad Sci U S A 96:7250–7255, 1999.

21. Baker BY, Yaworsky DC, Miller WL: A pH-dependent molten globule transition is required for activity of the steroidogenic acute regulatory protein, StAR, J Biol Chem 280:41753–41760, 2005.

22. Tuckey RC, Headlam MJ, Bose HS, et al: Transfer of cholesterol between phospholipid vesicles mediated by the steroidogenic acute regulatory protein (StAR), J Biol Chem 277:47123–47128, 2002.

23. Baker BY, Epand RF, Epand RM, et al: Cholesterol binding does not predict activity of the steroidogenic acute regulatory protein, StAR, J Biol Chem 282:10223–10232, 2007.

24. Hauet T, Yao ZX, Bose HS, et al: Peripheral-type benzodiazepine receptor-mediated action of steroidogenic acute regulatory protein on cholesterol entry into Leydig cell mitochondria, Mol Endocrinol 19:540–554, 2005.

25. Bose M, Whittal RM, Miller WL, et al: Steroidogenic activity of StAR requires contact with mitochondrial VDAC1 and phosphate carrier protein, J Biol Chem 283:8837–8845, 2008.

26. Artemenko IP, Zhao D, Hales DB, et al: Mitochondrial processing of newly synthesized steroidogenic acute regulatory protein (StAR), but not total StAR, mediates cholesterol transfer to cytochrome P450 side chain cleavage enzyme in adrenal cells, J Biol Chem 276:46583–46596, 2001.

27. Miller WL, Strauss JF III: Molecular pathology and mechanism of action of the steroidogenic acute regulatory protein, StAR, J Steroid Biochem Mol Biol 69:131–141, 1999.

28. Voutilainen R, Tapanainen J, Chung B, et al: Hormonal regulation of P450scc (20,22-desmolase) and P450c17 (17α-hydroxylase/17,20-lyase) in cultured human granulosa cells, J Clin Endocrinol Metab 63:202–207, 1986.

29. Tsigos C, Arai K, Hung W, et al: Hereditary isolated glucocorticoid deficiency is associated with abnormalities of the adrenocorticotropin receptor gene, J Clin Invest 92:2458–2461, 1993.

30. Martens JWM, Verhoef-Post M, Abelin N, et al: A homozygous mutation in the luteinizing hormone receptor causes partial Leydig cell hypoplasia: correlation between receptor activity and phenotype, Mol Endocrinol 12:775–784, 1998.

31. Shenker A: G protein-coupled receptor structure and function: the impact of disease-causing mutations, Baillieres Clin Endocrinol Metab 9:427–451, 1995.

32. Parker KL, Schimmer BP: Steroidogenic factor 1:A key determinant of endocrine development and function, Endocr Rev 18:361–377, 1997.

33. Zhang P, Rodriguez H, Mellon SH: Transcriptional regulation of P450scc gene expression in neural and in steroidogenic cells: implications for regulation of neurosteroidogenesis, Mol Endocrinol 9:1571–1582, 1995.

34. Huang N, Miller WL: Cloning of factors related to HIV-inducible LBP proteins that regulate steroidogenic factor-1-independent human placental transcription of the cholesterol side-chain cleavage enzyme, P450scc, J Biol Chem 275:2852–2858, 2000.

35. Henderson YC, Frederick MJ, Wang MT, et al: LBP-1b, LBP-9, and LBP-32/MGR detected in syncytiotrophoblasts from first-trimester human placental tissue and their transcriptional regulation, DNA Cell Biol 27:71–79, 2008.

36. Luo X, Ikeda Y, Parker KL: A cell-specific nuclear receptor is essential for adrenal and gonadal development and sexual differentiation, Cell 77:481–490, 1994.

37. Nachtigal MW, Hirokawa Y, Enyeart-VanHouten DL, et al: Wilms' tumor 1 and Dax-1 modulate the orphan nuclear receptor SF-1 in sex-specific gene expression, Cell 93:445–454, 1998.

38. Hammer GD, Krylova I, Zhang Y, et al: Phosphorylation of the nuclear receptor SF-1 modulates cofactor recruitment: integration of hormone signaling in reproduction and stress, Mol Cell 3:521–526, 1999.

39. Simpson ER, Zhao Y, Agarwal VR, et al: Aromatase expression in health and disease, Recent Prog Horm Res 52:185–214, 1997.

40. Labrie Y, Durocher F, Lachance Y, et al: The human type II 17β-hydroxysteroid dehydrogenase gene encodes two alternatively spliced mRNA species, DNA Cell Biol 14:849–861, 1995.

41. Tuckey RC, Cameron KJ: Catalytic properties of cytochrome P-450scc purified from the human placenta: comparison to bovine cytochrome P-450scc, Arch Biochem Biophys 1163:185–194, 1993.

42. Guryev O, Carvalho RA, Usanov S, et al: A pathway for the metabolism of vitamin D₃:unique hydroxylated metabolites formed during catalysis with cytochrome P450scc (CYP11A1), Proc Natl Acad Sci U S A 100:14754–14759, 2003.

43. Morohashi K, Sogawa K, Omura T, et al: Gene structure of human cytochrome P-450(scc), cholesterol desmolase, J Biochem 101:879–887, 1987.

44. Chung B, Matteson KJ, Voutilainen R, et al: Human cholesterol side-chain cleavage enzyme, P450scc: cDNA cloning, assignment of the gene to chromosome 15, and expression in the placenta, Proc Natl Acad Sci USA 83:8962–8966, 1986.

45. Black SM, Harikrishna JA, Szklarz GD, et al: The mitochondrial environment is required for activity of the cholesterol side-chain cleavage enzyme, cytochrome P450scc, Proc Natl Acad Sci USA 91:7247–7251, 1994.

46. John ME, John MC, Boggaram V, et al: Transcriptional regulation of steroid hydroxylase genes by corticotropin, Proc Natl Acad Sci USA 83:4715–4719, 1986.

47. Mellon SH, Vaisse C: cAMP regulates P450scc gene expression by a cycloheximide-insensitive mechanism in cultured mouse Leydig MA-10 cells, Proc Natl Acad Sci USA 86:7775–7779, 1989.

48. Barrett PQ, Bollag WB, Isales CM, et al: The role of calcium in angiotensin II-mediated aldosterone secretion, Endocr Rev 10:496–518, 1989.

49. Moore CCD, Brentano ST, Miller WL: Human P450scc gene transcription is induced by cyclic AMP and repressed by 12-O-tetradecanolyphorbol-13-acetate and A23187 by independent cis-elements, Mol Cell Biol 10:6013–6023, 1990.

50. Moore CCD, Hum DW, Miller WL: Identification of positive and negative placental-specific basal elements, a transcriptional repressor, and a cAMP response element in the human gene for P450scc, Mol Endocrinol 6:2045–2058, 1992.

51. Huang N, Miller WL: LBP proteins modulate SF1-independent expression of P450scc in human placental JEG-3 cells, Mol Endocrinol 19:409–420, 2005.

52. Baulieu EE: Neurosteroids: of the nervous system, by the nervous system, for the nervous system, Recent Prog Horm Res 52:1–32, 1997.

53. Yang X, Iwamoto K, Wang M, et al: Inherited congenital adrenal hyperplasia in the rabbit is caused by a deletion in the gene encoding cytochrome P450 cholesterol side-chain cleavage enzyme, Endocrinology 132:1977–1982, 1993.

54. Hu MC, Hsu NC, El Hadj NB, et al: Steroid deficiency syndromes in mice with targeted disruption of Cyp11a1, Mol Endocrinol 16:1943–1950, 2002.

55. Tajima T, Fujieda K, Kouda N, et al: Heterozygous mutation in the cholesterol side chain cleavage enzyme (P450scc) gene in a patient with 46,XY sex reversal and adrenal insufficiency, J Clin Endocrinol Metab 86:3820–3825, 2001.

56. Kim CJ, Lin L, Huang N, et al: Severe combined adrenal and gonadal deficiency caused by novel mutations in the cholesterol side chain cleavage enzyme, P450scc, J Clin Endocrinol Metab 93:696–702, 2008.

57. Apter D, Pakarinen A, Hammond GL, et al: Adrenocortical function in puberty, Acta Paediatr Scand 68:599–604, 1979.

58. Orentreich N, Brind JL, Rizer RL, et al: Age changes and sex differences in serum dehydroepiandrosterone sulfate concentrations throughout adulthood, J Clin Endocrinol Metab 59:551–555, 1984.

59. Nakajin S, Shively JE, Yuan P, et al: Microsomal cytochrome P450 from neonatal pig testis: two enzymatic activities (17α-hydroxylase and C17,20-lyase) associated with one protein, Biochemistry 20:4037–4042, 1981.

60. Zuber MX, Simpson ER, Waterman MR: Expression of bovine 17α-hydroxylase cytochrome P450 cDNA in non-steroidogenic (COS-1) cells, Science 234:1258–1261, 1986.

61. Picado-Leonard J, Miller WL: Cloning and sequence of the human gene encoding P450c17 (steroid 17α-hydroxylase/17,20 lyase): Similarity to the gene for P450c21, DNA 6:439–448, 1987.

62. Chung BC, Picado-Leonard J, Haniu M, et al: Cytochrome P450c17 (steroid 17α-hydroxylase/17,20 lyase): cloning of human adrenal and testis cDNAs indicates the same gene is expressed in both tissues, Proc Natl Acad Sci U S A 84:407–411, 1987.

63. Lee-Robichaud P, Wright JN, Akhtar ME, et al: Modulation of the activity of human 17α-hydroxylase-17,20-lyase (CYP17) by cytochrome b₅:endocrinological and mechanistic implications, Biochem J 308:901–908, 1995.

64. Auchus RJ, Lee TC, Miller WL: Cytochrome b₅ augments the 17,20 lyase activity of human P450c17 without direct electron transfer, J Biol Chem 273:3158–3165, 1998.

65. Katagiri M, Kagawa N, Waterman MR: The role of cytochrome b₅ in the biosynthesis of androgens by human P450c17, Arch Biochem Biophys 317:343–347, 1995.

66. Lin D, Black SM, Nagahama Y, et al: Steroid 17α-hydroxylase and 17,20 lyase activities of P450c17: contributions of serine106 and P450 reductase, Endocrinology 132:2498–2506, 1993.

67. Flück CE, Miller WL, Auchus RJ: The 17,20-lyase activity of cytochrome P450c17 from human fetal testis favors the Δ⁵ steroidogenic pathway, J Clin Endocrinol Metab 88:3762–3766, 2003.

68. Lee TC, Miller WL, Auchus RJ: Medroxyprogesterone acetate and dexamethasone are competitive inhibitors of different human steroidogenic enzymes, J Clin Endocrinol Metab 84:2104–2110, 1999.

69. Auchus RJ, Kumar AS, Boswell CA, et al: The enantiomer of progesterone (ent-progesterone) is a competitive inhibitor of human cytochromes P450c17 and P450c21, Arch Biochem Biophys 409:134–144, 2003.

70. Arlt W, Auchus RJ, Miller WL: Thiazolidinediones but not metformin directly inhibit the steroidogenic enzymes P450c17 and 3β-hydroxysteroid dehydrogenase, J Biol Chem 276:16767–16771, 2001.

71. Gupta MK, Guryev OL, Auchus RJ: 5α-reduced C₂₁ steroids are substrates for human cytochrome P450c17, Arch Biochem Biophys 418:151–160, 2003.

72. Wilson JD, Auchus RJ, Leihy MW, et al: 5α-androstane-3α,17β-diol is formed in tammar wallaby pouch young testes by a pathway involving 5α-pregnane-3α,17α-diol-20-one as a key intermediate, Endocrinology 144:575–580, 2003.

73. Auchus RJ: The backdoor pathway to dihydrotestosterone, Trends Endocrinol Metab 15:432–438, 2004.

74. Milewich L, Mendonca BB, Arnhold I, et al: Women with steroid 5α-reductase 2 deficiency have normal concentrations of plasma 5α-dihydroprogesterone during the luteal phase, J Clin Endocrinol Metab 80:3136–3139, 1995.

75. Moisan AM, Ricketts ML, Tardy V, et al: New insight into the molecular basis of 3β-hydroxysteroid dehydrogenase deficiency: identification of eight mutations in the HSD3B2 gene in eleven patients from seven new families and comparison of the functional properties of twenty-five mutant enzymes, J Clin Endocrinol Metab 84:4410–4425, 1999.

76. Hanley NA, Arlt W: The human fetal adrenal cortex and the window of sexual differentiation, Trends Endocrinol Metab 17:391–397, 2006.
77. Ortiz de Montellano PR: Oxygen activation and reactivity. In Ortiz de Montellano PR, editor: Cytochrome P-450:Structure, Mechanism, and Biochemistry, ed 2, New York, 1995, Plenum, pp 245–303.
78. Auchus RJ, Miller WL: Molecular modeling of human P450c17 (17α-hydroxylase/17,20-lyase): insights into reaction mechanisms and effects of mutations, Mol Endocrinol 13:1169–1182, 1999.
79. Cutler GB, Glenn M, Bush M, et al: Adrenarche: a survey of rodents, domestic animals and primates, Endocrinology 103:2112–2118, 1978.
80. Arlt W, Martens JW, Song M, et al: Molecular evolution of adrenarche: structural and functional analysis of P450c17 from four primate species, Endocrinology 143:4665–4672, 2002.
81. Zhang L, Rodriguez H, Ohno S, et al: Serine phosphorylation of human P450c17 increases 17,20 lyase activity: implications for adrenarche and for the polycystic ovary syndrome, Proc Natl Acad Sci USA 92:10619–10623, 1995.
82. Pandey AV, Miller WL: Regulation of 17,20 lyase activity by cytochrome b_5 and by serine phosphorylation of P450c17, J Biol Chem 280:13265–13271, 2005.
83. Bremer AA, Miller WL: The serine phosphorylation hypothesis of polycystic ovary syndrome: a unifying mechanism for hyperandrogenemia and insulin resistance, Fertil Steril 89:1039–1048, 2008.
84. Pandey AV, Mellon SH, Miller WL: Protein phosphatase 2A and phosphoprotein SET regulate androgen production by P450c17, J Biol Chem 278:2837–2844, 2003.
85. Nguyen AD, Mapes SM, Corbin CJ, et al: Morphological adrenarche in rhesus macaques: development of the zona reticularis is concurrent with fetal zone regression in the early neonatal period, J Endocrinol 199:367–378, 2008.
86. Suzuki T, Sasano H, Takeyama J, et al: Developmental changes in steroidogenic enzymes in human postnatal adrenal cortex: immunohistochemical studies, Clin Endocrinol (Oxf) 53:739–747, 2000.
87. Huang N, Miller WL: Regulation of cytochrome b_5 gene transcription by Sp3, GATA-6, and steroidogenic factor 1 in human adrenal NCI-H295A cells, Mol Endocrinol 19:2020–2034, 2005.
88. Gell JS, Carr BR, Sasano H, et al: Adrenarche results from development of a 3β-hydroxysteroid dehydrogenase-deficient adrenal reticularis, J Clin Endocrinol Metab 83:3695–3701, 1998.
89. Biglieri EG, Herron MA, Brust N: 17-hydroxylation deficiency in man, J Clin Invest 45:1946–1954, 1966.
90. Auchus RJ: The genetics, pathophysiology, and management of human deficiencies of P450c17, Endocrinol Metab Clin North Am 30:101–119, 2001.
91. Costa-Santos M, Kater CE, Auchus RJ: Two prevalent CYP17 mutations and genotype/phenotype correlations in 24 Brazilian patients with 17-hydroxylase deficiency, J Clin Endocrinol Metab 89:49–60, 2004.
92. Gupta MK, Geller DH, Auchus RJ: Pitfalls in characterizing P450c17 mutations associated with isolated 17,20-lyase deficiency, J Clin Endocrinol Metab 86:4416–4423, 2001.
93. Geller DH, Auchus RJ, Mendonça BB, et al: The genetic and functional basis of isolated 17,20 lyase deficiency, Nature Genet 17:201–205, 1997.
94. Van Den Akker EL, Koper JW, Boehmer AL, et al: Differential inhibition of 17α-hydroxylase and 17,20-lyase activities by three novel missense CYP17 mutations identified in patients with P450c17 deficiency, J Clin Endocrinol Metab 87:5714–5721, 2002.
95. Geller DH, Auchus RJ, Miller WL: P450c17 mutations R347H and R358Q selectively disrupt 17,20-lyase activity by disrupting interactions with P450 oxidoreductase and cytochrome b_5, Mol Endocrinol 13:167–175, 1999.
96. Sherbet DP, Tiosano D, Kwist KM, et al: CYP17 mutation E305G causes isolated 17,20-lyase deficiency by selectively altering substrate binding, J Biol Chem 278:48563–48569, 2003.
97. Hershkovitz E, Parvari R, Wudy SA, et al: Homozygous mutation G539R in the gene for P450 oxidoreductase in a family previously diagnosed as having 17,20-lyase deficiency, J Clin Endocrinol Metab 93:3584–3588, 2008.
98. Winkel CA, Casey ML, Worley RJ, et al: Extraadrenal steroid 21-hydroxylase activity in a woman with congenital adrenal hyperplasia due to steroid 21-hydroxylase deficiency, J Clin Endocrinol Metab 56:104–107, 1983.
99. Mellon SH, Miller WL: Extra-adrenal steroid 21-hydroxylation is not mediated by P450c21, J Clin Invest 84:1497–1502, 1989.
100. Yamazaki H, Shimada T: Progesterone and testosterone hydroxylation by cytochromes P450 2C19, 2C9, and 3A4 in human liver microsomes, Arch Biochem Biophys 346:161–169, 1997.
101. Gomes LG, Huang N, Agrawal V, et al: Extraadrenal 21-hydroxylation by CYP2C19 and CYP3A4:Effect on 21-hydroxylase deficiency, J Clin Endocrinol Metab 94:89–95, 2009.
102. White PC, Speiser PW: Congenital adrenal hyperplasia due to 21-hydroxylase deficiency, Endocr Rev 21:245–291, 2000.
103. Bristow J, Tee MK, Gitelman SE, et al: Tenascin-X. A novel extracellular matrix protein encoded by the human *XB* gene overlapping P450c21B, J Cell Biol 122:265–278, 1993.
104. Schalkwijk J, Zweers MC, Steijlen PM, et al: A recessive form of the Ehlers-Danlos syndrome caused by tenascin-X deficiency, N Engl J Med 345:1167–1175, 2001.
105. Burch GH, Gong Y, Liu W, et al: Tenascin-X deficiency is associated with Ehlers-Danlos syndrome, Nature Genet 17:104–108, 1997.
106. Helmburg A, Tusie-Luna M, Tabarelli M, et al: R339H and P453S: CYP21 mutations associated with nonclassic steroid 21-hydroxylase deficiency that are not apparent gene conversion, Mol Endocrinol 6:1318–1322, 1992.
107. Ulick S: Diagnosis and nomenclature of the disorders of the terminal portion of aldosterone biosynthetic pathway, J Clin Endocrinol Metab 43:92–96, 1976.
108. Veldhuis JD, Kulin HE, Santen RJ, et al: Inborn error in the terminal step of aldosterone biosynthesis: corticosterone methyl oxidase type II deficiency in a North American pedigree, N Engl J Med 303:118–121, 1980.
109. Yanagibashi K, Haniu M, Shively JE, et al: The synthesis of aldosterone by the adrenal cortex: two zones (fasciculata and glomerulosa) possess one enzyme for 11-, 18-hydroxylation, and aldehyde synthesis, J Biol Chem 261:3556–3562, 1986.
110. Morohashi K, Yoshioka H, Gotoh O, et al: Molecular cloning and nucleotide sequence of DNA of mitochondrial P-450(11) of bovine adrenal cortex, J Biochem 102:559–568, 1987.
111. Mornet E, Dupont J, Vitek A, et al: Characterization of two genes encoding human steroid 11β-hydroxylase (P45011β), J Biol Chem 264:20961–20967, 1989.
112. Mellon SH, Bair SR, Monis H: P450c11B3 mRNA, transcribed from a third P450c11 gene, is expressed in a tissue-specific, developmentally and hormonally regulated fashion in the rodent adrenal, and encodes a protein with both 11-hydroxylase and 18-hydroxylase activities, J Biol Chem 270:1643–1649, 1995.
113. Carnow KM, Tusie-Lung M, Pascoe L, et al: The product of the *CYP11B2* gene is required for aldosterone biosynthesis in the human adrenal cortex, Mol Endocrinol 5:1513–1522, 1991.
114. Kawamoto T, Mitsuuchi Y, Toda K, et al: Role of steroid 11β-hydroxylase and 18-hydroxylase in the biosynthesis of glucocorticoids and mineralocorticoids in humans, Proc Natl Acad Sci USA 89:1458–1462, 1992.
115. White PC, Dupont J, New MI, et al: A mutation in CYP11B1 (Arg 448→His) associated with steroid 11β-hydroxylase deficiency in Jews of Moroccan origin, J Clin Invest 87:1664–1667, 1991.
116. White PC, Curnow KM, Pascoe L: Disorders of steroid 11β-hydroxylase isozymes, Endocr Rev 15:421–438, 1994.
117. Pascoe L, Curnow K, Slutsker L, et al: Mutations in the human *CYP11B2* (aldosterone synthase) gene causing corticosterone methyloxidase II deficiency, Proc Natl Acad Sci USA 89:4996–5000, 1992.
118. Fu GK, Portale AA, Miller WL: Complete structure of the human gene for the vitamin D 1α-hydroxyase, P450c1α DNA Cell Biol 16:1499–1507, 1997.
119. Clyne CD, Zhang Y, Slutsker L, et al: Angiotensin II and potassium regulate human CYP11B2 transcription through common *cis*-elements, Mol Endocrinol 11: 638–649, 1997.
120. Fardella CE, Hum DW, Rodriguez H, et al: Gene conversion in the *CYP11B2* gene encoding aldosterone synthase (P450c11AS) is associated with, but does not cause, the syndrome of corticosterone methyl oxidase II deficiency, J Clin Endocrinol Metab 81:321–326, 1996.
121. Lifton R, Dluhy RG, Powers M, et al: A chimaeric 11β-hydroxylase/aldosterone synthase gene causes glucocorticoid-remediable aldosteronism and human hypertension, Nature 335:262–265, 1992.
122. Pascoe L, Curnow K, Slutsker L, et al: Glucocorticoid-suppressible hyperaldosteronism results from hybrid genes created by unequal crossover between CYP11B1 and CYP11B2, Proc Natl Acad Sci USA 89:8327–8331, 1992.
123. Litchfield WR, New MI, Coolidge C, et al: Evaluation of the dexamethasone suppression test for the diagnosis of glucocorticoid-remediable aldosteronism, J Clin Endocrinol Metab 82:3570–3573, 1997.
124. Fardella CE, Mosso L, Gómez-Sánchez C, et al: Primary hyperaldosteronism in essential hypertensives: prevalence, biochemical profile, and molecular biology, J Clin Endocrinol Metab 85:1863–1867, 2000.
125. Bottner B, Denner K, Bernhardt R: Conferring aldosterone synthesis to human CYP11B1 by replacing key amino acid residues with CYP11B2-specific ones, Eur J Biochem 252:458–466, 1998.
126. Curnow KM, Mulatero P, Emeric-Blanchouin N, et al: The amino acid substitutions Ser288Gly and Val320Ala convert the cortisol producing enzyme, CYP11B1, into an aldosterone producing enzyme [letter], Nat Struct Biol 4:32–35, 1997.
127. Simpson ER, Mahendroo MS, Means GD, et al: Aromatase cytochrome P450, the enzyme responsible for estrogen biosynthesis, Endocr Rev 15:342–355, 1994.
128. Beusen DD, Carrell HL, Covey DF: Metabolism of 19-methyl-substituted steroids by human placental aromatase, Biochemistry 26:7833–7841, 1987.
129. Mahendroo MS, Means GD, Mendelson CR, et al: Tissue-specific expression of human P450 arom: the promoter responsible in adipose tissue is different from that utilized in placenta, J Biol Chem 266:11276, 1991.
130. Simpson ER, Mahendroo MS, Means GD, et al: Tissue-specific promoters regulate aromatase cytochrome P450 expression, Clin Chem 39:317, 1993.
131. Conte FA, Grumbach MM, Ito Y, et al: A syndrome of female pseudohermaphrodism, hypergonadotropic hypogonadism, and multicystic ovaries associated with missense mutations in the gene encoding aromatase (P450arom), J Clin Endocrinol Metab 78:1287–1292, 1994.
132. Grumbach MM, Auchus RJ: Estrogen: consequences and implications of human mutations in synthesis and action, J Clin Endocrinol Metab 84:4677–4694, 1999.
133. Fisher CR, Graves KH, Parlow AF, et al: Characterization of mice deficient in aromatase (ArKO) because of targeted disruption of the *cyp19* gene, Proc Natl Acad Sci U S A 95:6965–6970, 1998.
134. Voutilainen R, Miller WL: Developmental expression of genes for the steroidogenic enzymes P450scc (20,22 desmolase), P450c17 (17α-hydroxylase/17,20 lyase) and P450c21 (21-hydroxylase) in the human fetus, J Clin Endocrinol Metab 63:1145–1150, 1986.
135. Miller WL: Steroid hormone biosynthesis and actions in the materno-feto-placental unit, Clin Perinatol 25:799–817, 1998.
136. Lo JC, Schwitzgebel VM, Tyrrell JB, et al: Normal female infants born of mothers with classic congenital adrenal hyperplasia due to 21-hydroxylase deficiency, J Clin Endocrinol Metab 84:930–936, 1999.
137. Morishima A, Grumbach MM, Simpson ER, et al: Aromatase deficiency in male and female siblings caused by a novel mutation and the physiological role of estrogens, J Clin Endocrinol Metab 80:3689–3698, 1995.
138. Hanukoglu I, Suh BS, Himmelhoch S, et al: Induction and mitochondrial localization of cytochrome P450scc system enzymes in normal and transformed ovarian granulosa cells, J Cell Biol 111:1373–1381, 1990.
139. Voutilainen R, Picado-Leonard J, DiBlasio AM, et al: Hormonal and developmental regulation of human adrenodoxin mRNA in steroidogenic tissues, J Clin Endocrinol Metab 66:383–388, 1988.
140. Müller A, Müller JJ, Müller YA, et al: New aspects of electron transfer revealed by the crystal structure of a truncated bovine adrenodoxin, Adx(4-108), Structure 6:269–280, 1998.

141. Coghlan VM, Vickery LE: Site-specific mutations in human ferredoxin that affect binding to ferredoxin reductase and cytochrome P450scc, J Biol Chem 266:18606–18612, 1991.
142. Vickery LE: Molecular recognition and electron transfer in mitochondrial steroid hydroxylase systems, Steroids 62:124–127, 1997.
143. Wada A, Waterman MR: Identification by site-directed mutagenesis of two lysine residues in cholesterol side chain cleavage cytochrome P450 that are essential for adrenodoxin binding, J Biol Chem 267:22877–22882, 1992.
144. Brentano ST, Black SM, Lin D, et al: cAMP post-transcriptionally diminishes the abundance of adrenodoxin reductase mRNA, Proc Natl Acad Sci USA 89:4099–4103, 1992.
145. Lin D, Shi Y, Miller WL: Cloning and sequence of the human adrenodoxin reductase gene, Proc Natl Acad Sci USA 87:8516–8520, 1990.
146. Sparkes RS, Klisak I, Miller WL: Regional mapping of genes encoding human steroidogenic enzymes: P450scc to 15q23-q24, adrenodoxin to 11q22; adrenodoxin reductase to 17q24-q25; and P450c17 to 10q24-q25, DNA Cell Biol 10:359–365, 1991.
147. Solish SB, Picado-Leonard J, Morel Y, et al: Human adrenodoxin reductase: two mRNAs encoded by a single gene of chromosome 17cen→q25 are expressed in steroidogenic tissues, Proc Natl Acad Sci USA 71:7104–7108, 1988.
148. Brandt ME, Vickery LE: Expression and characterization of human mitochondrial ferredoxin reductase in *Escherichia coli*, Arch Biochem Biophys 294:735–740, 1992.
149. Freeman MR, Dobritsa A, Gaines P, et al: The *dare* gene: steroid hormone production, olfactory behavior, and neural degeneration in *Drosophila*, Development 126:4591–4602, 1999.
150. Ziegler GA, Vonrhein C, Hanukoglu I, et al: The structure of adrenodoxin reductase of mitochondrial P450 systems: electron transfer for steroid biosynthesis, J Mol Biol 289:981–990, 1999.
151. Brandt ME, Vickery LE: Charge pair interactions stabilizing ferredoxin-ferredoxin reductase complexes. Identification by complementary site-specific mutations, J Biol Chem 268:17126–17130, 1993.
152. Wang M, Roberts DL, Paschke R, et al: Three-dimensional structure of NADPH-cytochrome P450 reductase: prototype for FMN- and FAD-containing enzymes, Proc Natl Acad Sci USA 94:8411–8416, 1997.
153. Sevrioukova I, Huiying L, Zhong H, et al: Structure of a cytochrome P450-redox partner electron-transfer complex, Proceedings of the National Academy of Sciences (USA) 96:1863–1868, 1999.
154. Hasemann CA, Kurumbail RG, Boddupalli SS, et al: Structure and function of cytochromes P450: a comparative analysis of three crystal structures, Structure 2:41–62, 1995.
155. Peterson RE, Imperato-McGinley J, Gautier T, et al: Male pseudohermaphroditism due to multiple defects in steroid-biosynthetic microsomal mixed-function oxidases. A new variant of congenital adrenal hyperplasia, N Engl J Med 313:1182–1191, 1985.
156. Shackleton C, Malunowicz E: Apparent pregnene hydroxylation deficiency (APHD): seeking the parentage of an orphan metabolome, Steroids 68:707–717, 2003.
157. Reardon W, Smith A, Honour JW, et al: Evidence for digenic inheritance in some cases of Antley-Bixler syndrome? J Med Genet 37:26–32, 2000.
158. Flück CE, Tajima T, Pandey AV, et al: Mutant P450 oxidoreductase causes disordered steroidogenesis with and without Antley-Bixler syndrome, Nat Genet 36: 228–230, 2004.
159. Huang N, Pandey AV, Agrawal V, et al: Diversity and function of mutations in P450 oxidoreductase in patients with Antley-Bixler syndrome and disordered steroidogenesis, Am J Hum Genet 76:729–749, 2005.
160. Scott RR, Miller WL: Genetic and clinical features of P450 oxidoreductase deficiency, Horm Res 69:266–275, 2008.
161. Shen AL, O'Leary KA, Kasper CB: Association of multiple developmental defects and embryonic lethality with loss of microsomal NADPH-cytochrome P450 oxidoreductase, J Biol Chem 277:6536–6541, 2002.
162. Otto DM, Henderson CJ, Carrie D, et al: Identification of novel roles of the cytochrome P450 system in early embryogenesis: effects on vasculogenesis and retinoic acid homeostasis, Mol Cell Biol 23:6103–6116, 2003.
163. Henderson CJ, Otto DM, Carrie D, et al: Inactivation of the hepatic cytochrome P450 system by conditional deletion of hepatic cytochrome P450 reductase, J Biol Chem 278:13480–13486, 2003.
164. Gu J, Weng Y, Zhang QY, et al: Liver-specific deletion of the NADPH-cytochrome P450 reductase gene: impact on plasma cholesterol homeostasis and the function and regulation of microsomal cytochrome P450 and heme oxygenase, J Biol Chem 278:25895–25901, 2003.
165. Scott RR, Gomes LG, Huang N, et al: Apparent manifesting heterozygosity in P450 oxidoreductase deficiency and its effect on coexisting 21-hydroxylase deficiency, J Clin Endocrinol Metab 92:2318–2322, 2007.
166. Huang N, Agrawal V, Giacomini KM, et al: Genetics of P450 oxidoreductase: sequence variation in 842 individuals of four ethnicities and activities of 15 missense mutations, Proc Natl Acad Sci U S A 105:1733–1738, 2008.
167. Gomes LG, Huang N, Agrawal V, et al: The common P450 oxidoreductase variant A503V is not a modifier gene for 21-hydroxylase deficiency, J Clin Endocrinol Metab 93:2913–2916, 2008.
168. Agrawal V, Huang N, Miller WL: Pharmacogenetics of P450 oxidoreductase: effect of sequence variants on activities of CYP1A2 and CYP2C19, Pharmacogenet Genomics 18:569–576, 2008.
169. Bridges A, Gruenke L, Chang YT, et al: Identification of the binding site on cytochrome P450 2B4 for cytochrome b_5 and cytochrome P450 reductase, J Biol Chem 273:17036–17049, 1998.
170. Yamazaki H, Johnson WW, Ueng YF, et al: Lack of electron transfer from cytochrome b_5 in stimulation of catalytic activities of cytochrome P450 3A4. Characterization of a reconstituted cytochrome P450 3A4/NADPH-cytochrome P450 reductase system and studies with apo-cytochrome b_5, J Biol Chem 271: 27438–27444, 1996.
171. Muskett FW, Kelly GP, Whitford D: The solution structure of bovine ferricytochrome b_5 determined using heteronuclear NMR methods, J Mol Biol 258:172–189, 1996.
172. Falzone CJ, Mayer MR, Whiteman EL, et al: Design challenges for hemoproteins: the solution structure of apocytochrome b_5, Biochemistry 35:6519–6526, 1996.
173. Lee-Robichaud P, Kaderbhai MA, Kaderbhai N, et al: Interaction of human CYP17 (P-$450_{17\alpha}$, 17α-hydroxylase-17,20-lyase) with cytochrome b_5: importance of the orientation of the hydrophobic domain of cytochrome b_5, Biochem J 321:857–863, 1997.
174. Naffin-Olivos JL, Auchus RJ: Human cytochrome b_5 requires residues E48 and E49 to stimulate the 17, 20-lyase activity of cytochrome P450c17, Biochemistry 46:100–108, 2006.
175. Thomas JL, Frieden C, Nash WE, et al: An NADH-induced conformational change that mediates the sequential 3β-hydroxysteroid dehydrogenase/isomerase activities is supported by affinity labeling and the time-dependent activation of isomerase, J Biol Chem 270:21003–21008, 1995.
176. Thomas JL, Myers RP, Strickler RC: Human placental 3β-hydroxy-5-ene-steroid dehydrogenase and steroid 5/4-ene-isomerase: purification from mitochondria and kinetic profiles, biophysical characterization of the purified mitochondrial and microsomal enzymes, J Steroid Biochem 33:209–217, 1989.
177. Luu-The V, Lechance Y, Labrie C, et al: Full length cDNA structure and deduced amino acid sequence of human 3β-hydroxy-5-ene steroid dehydrogenase, Mol Endocrinol 3:1310–1312, 1989.
178. Rhéaume E, Lachance Y, Zhao HL, et al: Structure and expression of a new complementary DNA encoding the almost exclusive 3β-hydroxysteroid dehydrogenase/Δ^5-Δ^4-isomerase in human adrenals and gonads, Mol Endocrinol 5:1147–1157, 1991.
179. Thomas JL, Berko EA, Faustino A, et al: Human placental 3β-hydroxy-5-ene-steroid dehydrogenase and steroid 5/4-ene-isomerase: purification from microsomes, substrate kinetics, and inhibition by product steroids, J Steroid Biochem 31:785–793, 1988.
180. Cherradi N, Rossier MF, Vallotton MB, et al: Submitochondrial distribution of three key steroidogenic proteins (steroidogenic acute regulatory protein and cytochrome P450scc and 3β-hydroxysteroid dehydrogenase isomerase enzymes) upon stimulation by intracellular calcium in adrenal glomerulosa cells, J Biol Chem 272:7899–7907, 1997.
181. Mesiano S, Coulter CL, Jaffe RB: Localization of cytochrome P450 cholesterol side-chain cleavage, cytochrome P450 17α-hydroxylase/17,20 lyase, and 3β-hydroxysteroid dehydrogenase-isomerase steroidogenic enzymes in human and rhesus monkey fetal adrenal glands: reappraisal of functional zonation, J Clin Endocrinol Metab 77:1184–1189, 1993.
182. Endoh A, Kristiansen SB, Casson PR, et al: The zona reticularis is the site of biosynthesis of dehydroepiandrosterone and dehydroepiandrosterone sulfate in the adult human adrenal cortex resulting from its low expression of 3β-hydroxysteroid dehydrogenase, J Clin Endocrinol Metab 81:3558–3565, 1996.
183. Remer T, Boye KR, Hartmann MF, et al: Urinary markers of adrenarche: reference values in healthy subjects, aged 3–18 years, J Clin Endocrinol Metab 90:2015–2021, 2005.
184. Peltoketo H, Luu-The V, Simard J, et al: 17β-hydroxysteroid dehydrogenase (HSD)/17-ketosteroid reductase (KSR) family; nomenclature and main characteristics of the 17HSD/KSR enzymes, J Mol Endocrinol 23:1–11, 1999.
185. Peltoketo H, Isomaa V, Mäenlavsta O, et al: Complete amino acid sequence of human placental 17β-hydroxysteroid dehydrogenase deduced from cDNA, FEBS Lett 239:73–77, 1988.
186. Tremblay Y, Ringler GE, Morel Y, et al: Regulation of the gene for estrogenic 17-ketosteroid reductase lying on chromosome 17cen→q25, J Biol Chem 264:20458–20462, 1989.
187. Luu-The V, Labrie C, Simard J, et al: Structure of two in tandem human 17β-hydroxysteroid dehydrogenase genes, Mol Endocrinol 4:268–275, 1990.
188. Luu-The V, Zhang Y, Poirier D, et al: Characteristics of human types 1, 2 and 3 17β-hydroxysteroid dehydrogenase activities: oxidation/reduction and inhibition, J Steroid Biochem Mol Biol 55:581–587, 1995.
189. Auchus RJ, Covey DF, Bork V, et al: Solid-state NMR observation of cysteine and lysine Michael adducts of inactivated estradiol dehydrogenase, J Biol Chem 263:11640–11645, 1988.
190. Ghosh D, Pletnev VZ, Zhu DW, et al: Structure of human estrogenic 17β-hydroxysteroid dehydrogenase at 2.20 Å resolution, Structure 3:503–513, 1995.
191. Sasano H, Frost AR, Saitoh R, et al: Aromatase and 17β-hydroxysteroid dehydrogenase type 1 in human breast carcinoma, J Clin Endocrinol Metab 81:4042–4046, 1996.
192. Wu L, Einstein M, Geissler WM, et al: Expression cloning and characterization of human 17β–hydrosteroid dehydrogenase Type 2, a microsomal enzyme possessing 20α-hydroxysteroid dehydrogenase activity, J Biol Chem 268:12964–12969, 1993.
193. Casey ML, MacDonald PC, Andersson S: 17β-Hydroxysteroid dehydrogenase type 2:chromosomal assignment and progestin regulation of gene expression in human endometrium, Journal of Clinical Investigation 94:2135–2141, 1994.
194. Saez JM, De Peretti E, Morera AM, et al: Familial male pseudohermaphroditism with gynecomastia due to a testicular 17-ketosteroid reductase defect. I. Studies in vivo, J Clin Endocrinol Metab 32:604–610, 1971.
195. Geissler WM, Davis DL, Wu L, et al: Male pseudohermaphroditism caused by mutations of testicular 17β-hydroxysteroid dehydrogenase 3, Nature Genet 7:34–39, 1994.
196. Moghrabi N, Hughes IA, Dunaif A, et al: Deleterious missense mutations and silent polymorphism in the human 17β-hydroxysteroid dehydrogenase 3 gene (HSD17B3), J Clin Endocrinol Metab 83:2855–2860, 1998.
197. Mendonca BB, Arnhold IJ, Bloise W, et al: 17β-hydroxysteroid dehydrogenase 3 deficiency in women, J Clin Endocrinol Metab 84:802–804, 1999.
198. Adamski J, Normand T, Leenders F, et al: Molecular cloning of a novel widely expressed human 80 kDa 17β-hydroxysteroid dehydrogenase IV, Biochemical Journal 311:437–443, 1995.
199. Qin YM, Poutanen MH, Helander HM, et al: Peroxisomal multifunctional enzyme of beta-oxidation

metabolizing D-3-hydroxyacyl-CoA esters in rat liver: molecular cloning, expression and characterization, Biochem J 321:21–28, 1997.

200. van Grunsven EG, van Berkel E, Ijlst L, et al: Peroxisomal D-hydroxyacyl-CoA dehydrogenase deficiency: resolution of the enzyme defect and its molecular basis in bifunctional protein deficiency, Proc Natl Acad Sci U S A 95:2128–2133, 1998.

201. Lin HK, Jez JM, Schlegel BP, et al: Expression and characterization of recombinant type 2 3α-hydroxysteroid dehydrogenase (HSD) from human prostate: demonstration of bifunctional 3α/17β-HSD activity and cellular distribution, Molecular Endocrinology 11:1971–1984, 1997.

202. Deyashiki Y, Ogasawara A, Nakayama T, et al: Molecular cloning of two human liver 3α-hydroxysteroid/dihydrodiol dehydrogenase isoenzymes that are identical with chlordecone reductase and bile-acid binder, Biochem J 299:545–552, 1994.

203. El-Alfy M, Luu-The V, Huang XF, et al: Localization of type 5 17β-hydroxysteroid dehydrogenase, 3beta-hydroxysteroid dehydrogenase, and androgen receptor in the human prostate by in situ hybridization and immunocytochemistry, Endocrinology 140:1481–1491, 1999.

204. Penning TM, Burczynski ME, Jez JM, et al: Human 3α-hydroxysteroid dehydrogenase isoforms (AKR1C1-AKR1C4) of the aldo-keto reductase superfamily: functional plasticity and tissue distribution reveals roles in the inactivation and formation of male and female sex hormones, Biochem J 351:67–77, 2000.

205. Sharma KK, Lindqvist A, Zhou XJ, et al: Deoxycorticosterone inactivation by AKR1C3 in human mineralocorticoid target tissues, Mol Cell Endocrinol 248:79–86, 2006.

206. Byrns MC, Steckelbroeck S, Penning TM: An indomethacin analogue, N-(4-chlorobenzoyl)-melatonin, is a selective inhibitor of aldo-keto reductase 1C3 (type 2 3α-HSD, type 5 17β-HSD, and prostaglandin F synthase), a potential target for the treatment of hormone dependent and hormone independent malignancies, Biochem Pharmacol 75:484–493, 2008.

207. Goto M, Piper Hanley K, Marcos J, et al: In humans, early cortisol biosynthesis provides a mechanism to safeguard female sexual development, J Clin Invest 116:953–960, 2006.

208. Bruchovsky N, Wilson JD: The intranuclear binding of testosterone and 5α-androstan-17β-ol-3-one by rat prostate, J Biol Chem 243:5953–5960, 1968.

209. Moore RJ, Wilson JD: Steroid 5α-reductase in cultured human fibroblasts. Biochemical and genetic evidence for two distinct enzyme activities, J Biol Chem 251:5895–5900, 1976.

210. Jenkins EP, Andersson S, Imperato-McGinley J, et al: Genetic and pharmacologic evidence for more than one human steroid 5α-reductase, J Clin Invest 89:293–300, 1992.

211. Andersson S, Berman DM, Jenkins EP, et al: Deletion of a steroid 5α-reductase 2 gene in male pseudohermaphroditism, Nature 354:159–161, 1991.

212. Thigpen AE, Silver RI, Guileyardo JM, et al: Tissue distribution and ontogeny of steroid 5α-reductase isozyme expression, J Clin Invest 92:903–910, 1993.

213. Frederiksen DW, Wilson JD: Partial characterization of the nuclear reduced nicotinamide adenine dinucleotide phosphate: Δ⁴-3-ketosteroid 5α-oxidoreductase of rat prostate, J Biol Chem 246:2584–2593, 1971.

214. McConnell JD, Bruskewitz R, Walsh P, et al: The effect of finasteride on the risk of acute urinary retention and the need for surgical treatment among men with benign prostatic hyperplasia. Finasteride Long-Term Efficacy and Safety Study Group, N Engl J Med 338:557–563, 1998.

215. Mahendroo MS, Cala KM, Russell DW: 5α-reduced androgens play a key role in murine parturition, Mol Endocrinol 10:380–392, 1996.

216. Mahendroo MS, Wilson JD, Richardson JA, et al: Steroid 5α-reductase 1 promotes 5α-androstane-3α,17β-diol synthesis in immature mouse testes by two pathways, Mol Cell Endocrinol 222:113–120, 2004.

217. Khanna M, Qin KN, Wang RW, et al: Substrate specificity, gene structure and tissue-specific distribution of multiple human 3α-hydroxysteroid dehydrogenases, J Biol Chem 270:20162–20168, 1995.

218. Nishizawa M, Nakajima T, Yasuda K, et al: Close kinship of human 20α-hydroxysteroid dehydrogenase gene with three aldo-keto reductase genes, Genes Cells 5:111–125, 2000.

219. Rupprecht R, Hauser CA, Trapp T, et al: Neurosteroids: molecular mechanisms of action and psychopharmacological significance, J Steroid Biochem Mol Biol 56:163–168, 1996.

220. Griffin LD, Mellon SH: Selective serotonin reuptake inhibitors directly alter activity of neurosteroidogenic enzymes, Proc Natl Acad Sci U S A 96:13512–13517, 1999.

221. Gulbis JM, Mann S, MacKinnon R: Structure of a voltage-dependent K⁺ channel beta subunit, Cell 97:943–952, 1999.

222. Hoog SS, Pawlowski JE, Alzari PM, et al: Three-dimensional structure of rat liver 3α-hydroxysteroid/dihydrodiol dehydrogenase: a member of the aldo-keto reductase superfamily, Proc Natl Acad Sci U S A 91:2517–2521, 1994.

223. Cooper WC, Jin Y, Penning TM: Elucidation of a complete kinetic mechanism for a mammalian hydroxysteroid dehydrogenase (HSD) and identification of all enzyme forms on the reaction coordinate: the example of rat liver 3α-HSD (AKR1C9), J Biol Chem 282:33484–33493, 2007.

224. Ratnam K, Ma H, Penning TM: The arginine 276 anchor for NADP(H) dictates fluorescence kinetic transients in 3α-hydroxysteroid dehydrogenase, a representative aldo-keto reductase, Biochemistry 38:7856–7864, 1999.

225. Napoli JL: 17β-Hydroxysteroid dehydrogenase type 9 and other short-chain dehydrogenases/reductases that catalyze retinoid, 17β- and 3α-hydroxysteroid metabolism, Mol Cell Endocrinol 171:103–109, 2001.

226. Biswas MG, Russell DW: Expression cloning and characterization of oxidative 17β- and 3α-hydroxysteroid dehydrogenases from rat and human prostate, J Biol Chem 272:15959–15966, 1997.

227. Chetyrkin SV, Hu J, Gough WH, et al: Further characterization of human microsomal 3α-hydroxysteroid dehydrogenase, Arch Biochem Biophys 386:1–10, 2001.

228. White PC, Mune T, Agarwal AK: 11β-hydroxysteroid dehydrogenase and the syndrome of apparent mineralocorticoid excess, Endocr Rev 18:135–156, 1997.

229. Tannin GM, Agarwal AK, Monder C, et al: The human gene for 11β-hydroxysteroid dehydrogenase. Structure, tissue distribution, and chromosomal localization, J Biol Chem 266:16653–16658, 1991.

230. Agarwal AK, Monder C, Eckstein B, et al: Cloning and expression of rat cDNA encoding corticosteroid 11β-dehydrogenase, J Biol Chem 264:18939–18943, 1989.

231. Moore CCD, Mellon SH, Murai J, et al: Structure and function of the hepatic form of 11β-hydroxysteroid dehydrogenase in the squirrel monkey, an animal model of glucocorticoid resistance, Endocrinology 133:368–375, 1993.

232. Agarwal AK, Tusie-Luna M-T, Monder C, et al: Expression of 11β-hydroxysteroid dehydrogenase using recombinant vaccinia virus, Mol Endocrinol 4:1827–1832, 1990.

233. Walker EA, Clark AM, Hewison M, et al: Functional expression, characterization, and purification of the catalytic domain of human 11β-hydroxysteroid dehydrogenase type 1, J Biol Chem 276:21343–21350, 2001.

234. Odermatt A, Arnold P, Stauffer A, et al: The N-terminal anchor sequences of 11β-hydroxysteroid dehydrogenases determine their orientation in the endoplasmic reticulum membrane, J Biol Chem 274:28762–28770, 1999.

235. Jamieson A, Wallace AM, Andrew R, et al: Apparent cortisone reductase deficiency: a functional defect in 11β-hydroxysteroid dehydrogenase type 1, J Clin Endocrinol Metab 84:3570–3574, 1999.

236. Lavery GG, Walker EA, Tiganescu A, et al: Steroid biomarkers and genetic studies reveal inactivating mutations in hexose-6-phosphate dehydrogenase in patients with cortisone reductase deficiency, J Clin Endocrinol Metab 93:3827–3832, 2008.

237. Albiston AL, Obeyesekere VR, Smith RE, et al: Cloning and tissue distribution of the human 11β-hydroxysteroid dehydrogenase Type II enzyme, Mol Cell Endocrinol 105:R11–R17, 1994.

238. Brown RW, Chapman KE, Edwards CRW, et al: Human placental 11β-hydroxysteroid dehydrogenase: evidence for and partial purification of a distinct NAD⁺-dependent isoform, Endocrinology 132:2614–2621, 1993.

239. Funder JW, Pearce PT, Smith R, et al: Mineralocorticoid action: target tissue specificity is enzyme, not receptor, mediated, Science 242:583–585, 1988.

240. Mune T, Rogerson FM, Nikkila H, et al: Human hypertension caused by mutations in the kidney isozyme of 11β-hydroxysteroid dehydrogenase, Nature Genet 10:394–399, 1995.

241. Krozowski Z, MaGuire JA, Stein-Oakley AN, et al: Immunohistochemical localization of the 11β-hydroxysteroid dehydrogenase type II enzyme in human kidney and placenta, J Clin Endocrinol Metab 80:2203–2209, 1995.

242. Li KX, Obeyesekere VR, Krozowski ZS, et al: Oxoreductase and dehydrogenase activities of the human and rat 11β-hydroxysteroid dehydrogenase type 2 enzyme, Endocrinology 138:2948–2952, 1997.

243. Mulatero P, Curnow KM, Aupetit-Faisant B, et al: Recombinant CYP11B genes encode enzymes that can catalyze conversion of 11-deoxycortisol to cortisol, 18-hydroxycortisol, and 18-oxocortisol, J Clin Endocrinol Metab 83:3996–4001, 1998.

244. Kater CE, Biglieri EG: Disorders of steroid 17α-hydroxylase deficiency, Endocrinol Metab Clin North Am 23:341–357, 1994.

245. Auchus RJ, Rainey WE: Adrenarche: physiology, biochemistry and human disease, Clin Endocrinol (Oxf) 60:288–296, 2004.

Chapter 2

GLUCOCORTICOID ACTION:
Physiology

ALLAN U. MUNCK and ANIKÓ NÁRAY-FEJES-TÓTH

Historical Developments and Background

Glucocorticoid physiology at times has occupied the mainstream of endocrinology, at others, a backwater. We begin by describing some of those ebbs and flows up to the dramatic announcement in 1949 that glucocorticoids have powerful antiinflammatory activity, a discovery that for decades isolated glucocorticoid physiology from the major clinical applications of those newly uncovered "miracle drugs."

THE ADRENAL CORTEX, SURVIVAL, AND THE ROLE OF GLUCOCORTICOIDS AND MINERALOCORTICOIDS

Thomas Addison's discovery in the mid-1800s that the adrenal cortex was essential for survival[1,2] preceded by nearly a century the demonstration that this gland produced at least two distinct hormones—eventually called glucocorticoids and mineralocorticoids[3]—each essential for normal life.[4] During that century, many of the actions on glucose metabolism that would characterize glucocorticoids, and on salt and water balance that would characterize mineralocorticoids, were foreshadowed in the symptoms of Addisonian patients[2] and adrenalectomized animals, and in the effects of lipid extracts from the adrenal cortex. By 1940, studies with pure glucocorticoids and mineralocorticoids showed that both were essential for survival, mineralocorticoids clearly sustaining life by maintaining electrolyte balance. How glucocorticoids sustained life, however, remained a mystery for decades.

CARBOHYDRATE METABOLISM

Glucocorticoids were named for their hyperglycemic effect.[3] Low blood glucose in Addisonian patients and adrenalectomized animals and low liver glycogen in the latter were described in the early 1900s. The 1930s saw the use of adrenal extracts to restore normal glucose levels, as well as the striking discovery that adrenalectomy,[5] like hypophysectomy,[6] ameliorated symptoms of diabetes. A landmark paper by Long, Katzin, and Fry,[7] in 1940, demonstrated that glucocorticoids stimulate gluconeogenesis from amino acids derived from protein catabolism, decrease glucose oxidation, and can elicit steroid diabetes. Ingle showed that glucocorticoids decrease glucose utilization[8] and cause insulin resistance.[9] These papers set the stage for most later work in this area.

GLUCOCORTICOID-INDUCED APOPTOSIS OF LYMPHOCYTES

Lymphoid tissue as a target for glucocorticoids was perhaps first noted by Addison, who observed "a considerable excess of white corpuscles" in the blood of one of his patients.[2] By 1900, thymus enlargement had been described in Addisonian and adrenalecto-mized rats. Around then, pathologists, unaware that they were dealing with atrophic tissues, used specimens from victims of prolonged illness as standards for normal lymphoid organs. In cases of sudden death in which they judged the thymus and other lymphoid tissues to be enlarged, they pronounced the resounding diagnosis of "status thymico-lymphaticus."[10] Eventually, Selye showed that via the adrenals, any illness or other source of stress can atrophy the thymus.[11] These effects on lymphoid tissues were later reproduced with adrenal extracts and pure glucocorticoids, which are now recognized to induce lymphocytolysis by apoptosis.[12]

REGULATORY AND PERMISSIVE GLUCOCORTICOID ACTIONS IN STRESS

Intimate connections between stress and adrenocortical hormones were revealed in the 1930s by observations that stress stimulates adrenocortical secretion and adrenal extracts protect against stress.[11,13] Protection was traced to glucocorticoids,[13] which remain prominent among stress hormones. Selye, who pioneered and popularized the subject of stress, demonstrated that innumerable stimuli activate the adrenal cortex.[11] His unified theory of stress introduced such concepts as the "alarm reaction" and the "general adaptation syndrome," along with the much disputed claim that by raising levels of adrenocortical hormones, stress caused "diseases of adaptation," which included arthritis and allergy.[14] As to how glucocorticoids protect against stress, White and Dougherty proposed that they enhance immune responses through lymphocytolysis by releasing preformed antibodies, and Selye suggested that they satisfy an increased demand for glucose.[14] Neither of these ideas gained experimental support.

Ingle[15,16] described a protective role for glucocorticoids distinct from the "regulatory" one of high, stress-induced hormone levels. Observing that adrenalectomized animals respond normally to certain forms of stress when administered glucocorticoids at basal levels, he proposed that basal levels exert "permissive" effects that maintain the capacity of some homeostatic functions to respond to moderate stress. He recognized, though, that glucocorticoids are required at stress-induced levels to maintain homeostasis in severe stress.[15]

FEEDBACK REGULATION

Addison[2] remarked on "a peculiar change of colour of the skin, occurring in connection with a diseased condition of the suprarenal capsules," a manifestation of negative feedback linking glucocorticoids to anterior pituitary hormones. This link was explored by Smith, who in 1930 reported that hypophysectomy of rats caused adrenocortical atrophy that was reversed by implanting pituitaries. Pituitaries eventually yielded ACTH, the adrenocorticotropic hormone. Negative feedback control of ACTH by an adrenocortical hormone was described in a remarkable half-page article by Ingle and Kendall,[17] which showed that administration of adrenal extracts to rats caused atrophy of the adrenal cortex that was countered by simultaneous administration of a pituitary extract. Stress, furthermore, caused hypertrophy of the adrenal cortex in normal but not hypophysectomized animals, implying that stress stimulated secretion of ACTH.[18] Harris's 1937 proposal that control of secretion of ACTH resides in the hypothalamus,[19] followed by evidence that this control is mediated by a hormone via the hypophyseal portal vessels,[20] led to identification of CRH, the corticotropin-releasing hormone. Thus arose the concept of the hypothalamo-pituitary-adrenal, or HPA, axis.

ANTIINFLAMMATORY ACTIONS AND THEIR REPERCUSSIONS ON GLUCOCORTICOID PHYSIOLOGY

By the late 1940s, the main outlines of glucocorticoid physiology appeared to be firmly drawn. Then 1949 brought a watershed event that was to cast a long shadow over this discipline. Hench, Kendall, Slocumb, and Polley[21] reported that cortisone in high doses and ACTH exerted powerful anti-inflammatory activity that dramatically improved the condition of patients with rheumatoid arthritis.[22] This totally unexpected discovery was celebrated by clinicians and their patients but caused turmoil among glucocorticoid physiologists, who could offer no physiologic explanation for actions wholly inconsistent with their belief that stress-induced levels of glucocorticoids protected against stress by enhancing—not suppressing—defense mechanisms.[23] These actions were also at odds with Selye's idea of diseases of adaptation.[13,22] Despite a rare voice to the contrary,[23] physiologists concluded that the antiinflammatory and closely linked immunosuppressive actions were pharmacologic rather than physiologic in nature.[13]

That view persisted for longer than three decades. For example, neither a 1952 review by Ingle[15] nor a 1971 review by Hoffman[24] on the role of the adrenal cortex in homeostasis even mention the antiinflammatory actions. Consequently, the spectacular rise in therapeutic applications of these hormones, the "miracle drugs" of the 1950s, and the development of synthetic glucocorticoid analogues such as prednisolone, dexamethasone, and countless others proceeded largely without ties to physiology—a situation probably unique in endocrinology.

A central but unrealized goal in the development of those synthetic analogues was to separate antiinflammatory activity from such "side effects" as increased blood glucose and feedback suppression. As we now know, antiinflammatory actions are in fact quintessentially physiologic,[25,26] and glucocorticoids administered to produce one physiologic effect generally produce others. Recent progress in circumventing that problem by separating physiologic effects on the basis of their molecular mechanisms is described below.

Background to Modern Glucocorticoid Physiology

Antiinflammatory and immunosuppressive actions today are embedded in the foundations of glucocorticoid physiology, where they belonged all along. Such suppressive actions, along with permissive actions, protect the organism from stress. Glucocorticoid researchers are using cell and molecular biological techniques to unravel the mechanisms of these and many other actions.

The discovery of the glucocorticoid receptor (GR) in the 1960s opened new avenues to physiology. Most cells have GRs, through which they respond in some way to glucocorticoids. Cloning of GRs and other receptors in the 1980s revealed close structural homologies between receptors for steroid hormones, thyroid hormones, and retinoids. All are ligand-dependent regulators of gene transcription, inducing effects that generally take hours or days to appear in the whole organism.

Cortisone, for years considered the prototypical glucocorticoid, hardly binds to GRs and is inactive until converted to cortisol by 11β-hydroxysteroid dehydrogenase type 1 (11β-

HSD1). Quite unexpectedly, cortisol and corticosterone, the natural glucocorticoids, were found to bind to mineralocorticoid receptors (MRs) with much higher affinity than to GRs. Those steroids normally circulate at concentrations that saturate MRs, immediately raising the question of why they do not block binding to MRs in mineralocorticoid target cells by aldosterone, which is present at much lower concentrations. The answer unveiled a fascinating enzyme, 11β-HSD2, which "protects" MRs in target cells by rapidly converting cortisol to cortisone and corticosterone to its inactive 11-keto form.

The GR is a protein that on binding hormone translocates to nuclear sites, where it regulates transcription of certain genes. It accounts so far for most glucocorticoid actions and sometimes is called GRα to distinguish it from an isoform, GRβ, which cannot bind hormone but acts as an antagonist. Several naturally occurring mutants of the human GR can cause generalized glucocorticoid resistance. Some evidence indicates that receptor-like proteins found in cell membranes may initiate rapid glucocorticoid effects through nongenomic mechanisms (see also Chapter 4).

The development of transgenic mice with modified GRs, MRs, 11β-HSDs, and other proteins, sometimes targeted to specific tissues,[27] is bringing new insights to glucocorticoid physiology, some of which will be described below.

General Molecular Aspects of Glucocorticoid Physiology

GRs date back hundreds of millions of years, having evolved along with mineralocorticoid receptors from an ancestral estrogen receptor that appeared almost a billion years ago.[28] Originally identified in rat thymocytes,[29] GRs are found in almost all nucleated cells, where they initiate hormonal activity by regulating transcription of specific genes in a ligand-dependent and cell-specific manner. When unliganded, they are predominantly cytoplasmic. After binding a ligand (cortisol, corticosterone, or powerful synthetic analogues like dexamethasone), they become activated and translocate to the nucleus.[30] There they regulate target genes in several ways.[31,32]

By binding as dimers to glucocorticoid response elements (GREs), which are short palindromic sequences of nucleotides associated with the target gene promoter, liganded GRs activate transcription when appropriate transcription factors and co-activators are present. Similarly, they repress transcription by binding as dimers to negative GREs (nGREs), or to composite GREs consisting of a GRE and a contiguous site for transcription factors such as AP-1 proteins (cJun/cFos).

Liganded GRs also regulate transcription through a mechanism of transcriptional cross-talk that does not require dimerization, DNA binding, or GREs in the regulated gene. Through protein-protein interactions, they bind as monomers to transcription factors like nuclear factor-κB (NF-κB), AP-1, cyclic AMP response element binding protein (CREB), and others, generally repressing transcription of the associated genes.[33] This cross-talk probably mediates most anti-inflammatory glucocorticoid actions, which are unimpaired in transgenic mice carrying mutated GRs that cannot dimerize.[34] In immortalized fibroblasts from these mice, glucocorticoids suppress the phorbol ester–activated collagenase-3 gene, known to be mediated through AP-1, but barely activate a transfected reporter under control of

the mouse mammary tumor virus (MMTV) promoter, which requires GR binding to GREs.[35] However, results with dimerization-deficient GRs show no sharp functional separation between these two mechanisms,[36] so it may not be possible to separate immunosuppressive from other glucocorticoid effects using "designer" GR ligands that favor gene repression over activation.[37,38] Of possible physiologic relevance are observations that, within a cell, translation of GR mRNA can produce several isoforms with different transcriptional specificities.[32]

Since the discovery that cortisol and corticosterone have much higher affinity for MRs than GRs, it has become clear that under physiologic conditions, some glucocorticoid effects, notably in the hippocampus, are mediated through MRs. Whereas MRs in mineralocorticoid target tissues are protected from high glucocorticoid levels by 11β-HSD2, which oxidizes cortisol to cortisone and corticosterone to 11-dehydrocorticosterone,[39-41] that enzyme is absent in the hippocampus.[42] In male and female reproductive tracts, 11β-HSD2 may protect GRs from excessive glucocorticoid levels. In pregnancy, it appears to protect the fetus from stress level maternal glucocorticoids, which can cause growth, low birth weight, and permanent postnatal pathologies such as hypertension and impaired HPA function.[43,44]

In contrast, 11β-HSD1, which is found in many tissues, functions primarily (not exclusively) as a reductase, activating cortisone to cortisol and 11-dehydrocorticosterone to corticosterone: it thereby amplifies local glucocorticoid activity in several tissues[45] and may cause what has been called tissue-specific Cushing's syndrome.[46] The importance of 11β-HSD1 for glucocorticoid action has been demonstrated with transgenic mice. Knockout mice that lack 11β-HSD1 have weakened stress-induced glucocorticoid responses. Mice with 11β-HSD1 locally overexpressed in adipose tissue develop the metabolic syndrome.[47] Adipose tissue 11β-HSD1 is regulated by both insulin and glucocorticoids.[48] Levels of 11β-HSD1 and 11β-HSD2 differ in fetal and adult tissues, and this may have a role in development.[49]

Because of their higher affinity for MRs than GRs, at low basal levels the natural glucocorticoids occupy mainly unprotected MRs. As levels increase during the circadian cycle, MRs approach saturation and GRs become occupied. With stress, glucocorticoid levels may rise sufficiently to nearly saturate GRs.[42]

GRβ, an alternative splice isoform of GRα, lacks a hormone-binding domain. Although it cannot bind hormone, it acts as a dominant-negative antagonist to GRα. Its presence at high constitutive levels accounts for the ability of human neutrophils to escape glucocorticoid-induced cell death.[50] Increased levels of GRβ may be associated with incidence of rheumatoid arthritis. Levels and functions of both GRα and GRβ are influenced by cytokines.

Glucocorticoid resistance, a significant clinical problem, arises through numerous mechanisms. These include downregulation and altered binding characteristics of GRs in the course of glucocorticoid therapy or disease,[51] inactivating mutations and polymorphisms of GRs,[52] overexpression of GRβ,[53] efflux transporters that remove certain steroids from lymphocytes or the brain,[54] and interactions with transcription factors such as AP-1 proteins and NF-κB.[55]

Membrane receptors for glucocorticoids and rapid actions through nongenomic mechanisms have been reported for many cells and tissues,[56,57] but their functional significance is unclear.

Feedback Regulation of Glucocorticoid Production

Although glucocorticoids are essential for the response to stress and for survival, they normally exert *major* control over few physiologic processes other than their own feedback mechanisms. For example, they influence blood glucose, but the dominant regulators are insulin and glucagon. Reflecting this role and contrasting with hormones like insulin and aldosterone, glucocorticoids control their plasma levels directly by negative feedback via GRs and MRs rather than via a physiologic effect. Such a design is common to hormones with wide-ranging homeostatic functions. This scheme, outlined in Fig. 2-1, emphasizes a central theme of this chapter, namely, the physiologic function of glucocorticoids to protect the organism against stress.[58]

Normal glucocorticoid levels are regulated in a range and time course that reflect varying physiologic needs as well as the vulnerability of the organism, particularly the brain,[59] to harm from excessive exposure. Basal hormone levels follow a circadian rhythm and reach peak values before the period of daily activity.[60] Their actions maintain or permissively "prime" homeostatic mechanisms and protect against moderate stress. Stress-induced levels, which can far exceed peak basal levels, appear necessary to cope with severe stress. Peak basal levels cause Cushing's syndrome if maintained indefinitely, so circadian lowering of glucocorticoid concentrations is physiologically necessary.

Synthesis and secretion of glucocorticoids is controlled by neural and humoral signals that change throughout the day and respond to stress and negative feedback.[60] The main components of this system (see Fig. 2-1) are the adrenal cortex, where glucocorticoid secretion is stimulated by ACTH; the anterior pituitary, where ACTH secretion is stimulated by CRH, vasopressin (VP), and other secretagogues, and are inhibited by glucocorticoids; and the central nervous system, where CRH and VP synthesis in the hypothalamus is stimulated by stress and other influences, and is inhibited by glucocorticoids. Paradoxically, chronic actions of glucocorticoids on the brain exerted over days can be excitatory.[61]

Glucocorticoids exert feedback control on pituitary corticotrophs, the paraventricular nucleus (PVN) of the hypothalamus, and probably the hippocampus.[42] Synthetic analogues like dexamethasone and prednisolone are exported from the brain by a multidrug resistance efflux transporter P-glycoprotein in the blood-brain barrier, which acts predominantly on the pituitary.[42,54] Glucocorticoid regulation appears to be mediated both by GRs, which are found throughout the brain with high concentrations in the PVN, and by MRs, which are located mainly in the hippocampus and lateral septum. Actions on the brain via MRs can be considered to permissively control sensitivity to rapid CRH responses via CRH-1 receptors, maintaining the capacity of the HPA axis to respond to stress and maintain homeostasis; actions through GRs restrain stress-induced responses and facilitate learning and recovery of homeostasis.[58]

Studies on transgenic mice with altered GRs extend these conclusions.[62,63] Mice with low levels of GRs have increased levels of CRH (not VP), ACTH, and corticosterone, as well as hypertrophy of the adrenal cortex. Overexpressed GRs reverse this picture. Mice with GRs that cannot dimerize have normal CRH and ACTH, showing that feedback via GRs probably is provided through genes controlled by protein-protein cross-talk. However, the gene for pro-opiomelanocortin (POMC), the ACTH precursor, is upregulated, implying control by GR dimers, which probably bind to nGREs, as noted below.

Inactivation of GRs in the nervous system[64] leads to higher levels of corticosterone with Cushing's-like symptoms. CRH is elevated, as is ACTH in pituitary corticotrophs, but circulating ACTH levels are slightly reduced—a divergence between ACTH and corticosterone reminiscent of that seen in clinically depressed patients.

Fig. 2-1 also illustrates one side of the reciprocal relation between the immune and neuroendocrine systems.[65] Cytokines like interleukin 1 (IL-1), IL-6, and tumor necrosis factor (TNF)-α, which are produced mainly in the immune system but also by brain cells, stimulate the HPA axis. IL-1, IL-6, and TNF-α are proinflammatory cytokines, so stimulation of glucocorticoid secretion limits their activity throughout the organism. The importance of IL-1, for example, is revealed in knockout mice lacking IL-1 receptors and in mice overexpressing IL-1 antagonist in the brain[66]: they have reduced stress responses and fail to hypersecrete ACTH after adrenalectomy. Another regulator of the HPA axis may be leptin.[67] A remarkable observation is that sucrose ingestion, like glucocorticoid replacement, can restore to normal most of the consequences of adrenalectomy on feeding and metabolism, and on the HPA axis, including ACTH levels, which presumably mimic signals from the metabolic effects of glucocorticoids.[68]

Each stage of the HPA feedback loop will now be considered.

ADRENAL CORTEX: GLUCOCORTICOIDS

Synthesis of glucocorticoids, generally ascribed solely to the adrenal cortex, has been reported to occur in the thymus.[69] It also occurs in the intestinal mucosa, where it influences local immune responses.[70] In the adrenal cortex, glucocorticoid synthesis is closely tied to plasma levels of ACTH, which exhibit episodic peaks and circadian rhythm similar to plasma levels of glucocorticoids. ACTH stimulates steroidogenesis by binding to membrane receptors on adrenal cells, which activates adenylate cyclase and also causes hypertrophy and hyperplasia of the adrenal cortex. Leptin inhibits ACTH stimulation of cortisol secretion by adrenal cells.[67]

PITUITARY: ACTH

The synthesis and secretion of ACTH in anterior pituitary corticotrophs are stimulated by CRH and VP, modulated by catechol-

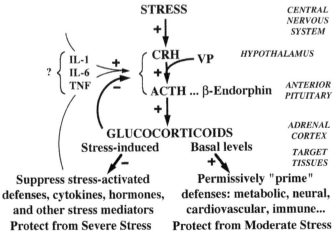

FIGURE 2-1. Outline of regulation and actions of glucocorticoids. See text for details.

amines, and inhibited by glucocorticoids. CRH binds to receptors on pituitary cell membranes and activates adenylate cyclase; cAMP then stimulates both secretion and synthesis of ACTH. Activity of CRH is strongly potentiated by VP. Whereas CRH increases the amount of ACTH secreted from each responsive corticotroph, VP, probably through the phosphoinositide pathway, increases the number of CRH-responsive corticotrophs. Nonetheless, knockout mice defective in type 1 CRH receptor (CRH-R1) respond to inflammatory stress with pronounced increases in ACTH and corticosterone that do not depend critically on CRH or VP.[71]

Glucocorticoids inhibit ACTH secretion directly by suppressing POMC expression in pituitary corticotrophs, and indirectly by inhibiting secretion of CRH and VP.[60] After adrenalectomy, ACTH secretion rises, retaining its circadian rhythm. CRH and VP levels in the PVN also rise. These and other changes are reversed by glucocorticoids. Annexin 1 (lipocortin 1), a glucocorticoid-induced protein, mediates glucocorticoid inhibition of secretion of ACTH from the pituitary, apparently through a nongenomic mechanism.

Feedback has been classified according to how rapidly it inhibits ACTH secretion[60]: fast (within 30 minutes of hormone administration), delayed (minutes to hours), and slow (hours to days). The first two are believed to operate after moderate or intermittent stress; the third, in pathologic conditions or therapy with high glucocorticoid levels sustained for days.

Sensitivity to feedback depends on many factors, including the time of day. Basal ACTH release is less sensitive than stimulated release. Furthermore, a stressful stimulus in some way facilitates the ACTH response to a subsequent stress, overcoming the feedback inhibition due to the elevated glucocorticoid levels produced by the first stress. Some feedback can be seen as facilitative or permissive.[72]

Regulation of basal activity of the HPA axis requires glucocorticoid binding to both MRs and GRs. Inhibition of basal secretion of ACTH by corticosterone in rats at the low point of diurnal HPA activity (the morning) appears to occur through MRs, whereas inhibition at peak activity (evening) occurs through GRs potentiated by MRs.[73] Suppression of stimulated ACTH secretion, which prevents overactivity in the stress-induced HPA axis, occurs through binding to GRs in pituitary corticotrophs and hypothalamic CRH neurons.

ACTH is produced as part of the larger precursor protein, POMC, which is also the progenitor of the melanocyte-stimulating hormones α- and β-MSH, β-endorphin, and the lipoproteins. Increased MSH activity associated with increased ACTH appears to be responsible for the changed skin color of Addisonian patients, as originally noted by Addison.[2] Synthesis of POMC in pituitary corticotrophs is stimulated by CRH and is inhibited by glucocorticoids, at least partly at the level of transcription of the POMC gene. Direct repression by glucocorticoids occurs through nGREs, which may repress by disrupting interactions that maintain basal transcription. Indirect repression occurs via the hypothalamus.

Corticotrophs are also directly influenced by other hormones, including angiotensin II, paracrine secretions from neighboring pituitary cells, and cytokines such as TNF-α, IL-1, and IL-6.

HYPOTHALAMUS: CRH AND VP

Secretion of CRH and VP from the paraventricular nuclei, along with other ACTH secretagogues, is subject to both humoral and neural regulation. Secretion increases following adrenalectomy, is stimulated in a stress-specific manner by hemorrhage, injury, hypoglycemia, hypoxia, pain, fear, and other kinds of stress, and generally is inhibited by glucocorticoids[74] (see Fig. 2-1). Some inhibition by glucocorticoids may occur via a nongenomic path involving rapid endocannabinoid release in the PVN.[75] CRH output can be modulated by catecholamines, leptin, and several cytokines.[76] Acute hemorrhage raises levels in hypothalamic neurons of mRNA for CRH but not VP. CRH, via CRH-1 receptors, is thought to orchestrate the immediate behavioral, sympathetic, and HPA axis responses to stress, whereas the CRH-related neuropeptides stresscopin and urocortins, which bind to CRH-2 receptors, may assist slower stress responses.[58]

In normal rats, stress activates CRH gene expression in the PVN, which is suppressed by glucocorticoids at high levels. In adrenalectomized rats, stress does not activate *CRH* gene expression unless the animals are first treated with glucocorticoids at low levels.[77] The low, facilitative, or permissive levels are thought to act through MRs, and the high, suppressive levels through GRs.[77]

CRH knockouts homozygous for the defective gene are viable as long as they receive glucocorticoids during the period from a week before birth until 2 weeks after birth. Without glucocorticoids, they die within 12 hours of gestation owing to severe lung abnormalities, including low surfactant mRNA. Glucocorticoids are known to be important for lung development, particularly for synthesis of surfactant.[78] Compared with normal mice, the CRH knockouts exhibited a drastically diminished rise in corticosterone levels in response to stress.[79]

In addition to controlling ACTH secretion, CRH has numerous actions within and outside the brain. When secreted by peripheral nerves, it acts as a proinflammatory agent: mRNAs for CRH-R1 and CRH-R2 are expressed in adipose tissue, whereas CRH downregulates 11β-HSD1.[47,80] Stresscopin and urocortins, via CRH-2 receptors, reduce appetite and may participate in delayed stress responses.[58]

CYTOKINE FEEDBACK

As first proposed by Besedovsky and Sorkin,[81] cytokines communicate between the immune system and the HPA axis. IL-1 has been shown to mediate HPA stimulation by endotoxin. IL-1α, IL-1β, IL-6, and TNF-α administered peripherally increase HPA activity with increased levels of glucocorticoids, ACTH, or POMC mRNA, and CRH or CRH mRNA. IL-1 causes release of both CRH and VP from neurosecretory cells.[76] The brain has receptors for IL-1, IL-2, IL-6, and other cytokines, and it produces IL-1.[82] (In Fig. 2-1, the question mark indicates uncertainty about which cytokines are most important and how their message is conveyed.)

Transgenic mice reveal the central role of IL-1 in feedback control and stress activation of the HPA axis. Mice lacking IL-1β fail to respond with increased plasma corticosterone to inflammatory stress, whereas mice lacking IL-1α respond normally, suggesting that IL-1β is crucial to the neuro-immuno-endocrine response.[83] Mice lacking IL-1 receptor type 1 have diminished corticosterone responses to psychological, metabolic, and restraint stresses. These mice and mice with overexpressed IL-1 receptor antagonist targeted to the brain do not hypersecrete ACTH after adrenalectomy.[66]

Whether peripherally released cytokines like IL-1 enter the brain in physiologically significant amounts, and if not how their message reaches the hypothalamus, are unsettled issues. Among hypotheses that have been proposed are that cytokine messages are transmitted via the vagus or through specialized brain regions like the organum vascularis laminae terminalis (OVLT), or via mediators like eicosanoids, catecholamines, nitric oxide, or cytokines generated in the brain.

Physiologic Actions of Glucocorticoids

METABOLISM

Control of Blood Glucose

Glucocorticoids act in concert with other hormones to maintain or raise blood glucose levels by (1) stimulating hepatic gluconeogenesis, (2) mobilizing gluconeogenic substrates from peripheral tissues, (3) permissively enhancing and prolonging the effects of glucagon and epinephrine on gluconeogenesis and glycogenolysis, (4) inhibiting peripheral glucose utilization, and (5) promoting liver glycogen synthesis to store substrate in preparation for acute responses to glycogenolytic agents such as glucagon and epinephrine.[45]

From an evolutionary standpoint, glucocorticoids in this way support stress responses that require glucose for rapid and intense exertion, such as an encounter of prey with predator.[26] From a physiologic and clinical standpoint, glucocorticoids are counterregulatory hormones that protect the body from insulin-induced hypoglycemia. Both of these roles, in which glucocorticoid effects develop over the course of hours, are shared with the rapidly acting glucagon and epinephrine and to some extent with growth hormone.[84]

Glucocorticoid actions interact with those of insulin during feeding and fasting in complex ways that not only maintain blood glucose but influence appetite, feeding patterns, disposal of foodstuffs, and body composition.[26,85] Antagonism with insulin in both glucose synthesis and utilization accounts at least partly for the diabetogenic actions of excessive glucocorticoids.[45,86] Studies with transgenic mice show that expression of hepatic peroxisome-proliferator–activated receptor-α (PPAR-α) may be one mechanism underlying glucocorticoid-induced hypertension and insulin resistance.[87]

Gluconeogenesis

Hepatic gluconeogenesis is stimulated by glucocorticoids, mainly through the increased activities of phosphoenolpyruvate carboxykinase (PEPCK) and glucose-6-phosphatase. These enzymes catalyze the conversion of oxaloacetate to phosphoenolpyruvate and of glucose-6-phosphate to glucose—both rate-limiting steps in gluconeogenesis.[45,88] Glucocorticoids also regulate expression of 6-phosphofructo-2-kinase/fructose 2,6-biphosphatase, a bifunctional enzyme that controls the level of fructose-2,6-biphosphate. Fructose-2,6-biphosphate is an allosteric regulator of gluconeogenic and glycolytic enzymes. PEPCK and 6-phosphofructo-2-kinase/fructose 2,6-biphosphatase activities are controlled principally through synthesis of the enzymes.[88] On starvation, 11β-HSD1 knockout mice have diminished activation of PEPCK and glucose-6-phosphatase.[89]

Control of PEPCK gene expression reflects the complexity of regulation of gluconeogenesis in the body, involving glucocorticoids, insulin, glucagon, catecholamines, cyclic adenosine monophosphate (cAMP), and retinoic acid.[88,90] In particular, glucocorticoids and insulin, by respectively promoting and indirectly disrupting association of CBP (CREB-binding protein) and RNA polymerase II with the PEPCK promoter, reciprocally regulate PEPCK gene expression. The *PEPCK* gene has a glucocorticoid response unit (GRU) that spans 110 base pairs. There are two GR-binding sites and four accessory factor elements, all of

which are required for glucocorticoid regulation, and within the GRU are insulin-responsive and retinoic acid–responsive sequences.[88,91] The *6-phosphofructo-2-kinase/fructose 2,6-biphosphatase* gene has a complex glucocorticoid response element that resembles the GRU of the *PEPCK* gene. Hepatocyte nuclear factor-6 (HNF-6) inhibits glucocorticoid activation of both these genes by binding to DNA and GRs. As would be expected, treatment with glucocorticoids of transgenic mice with dimerization-deficient GRs (i.e., GRs that cannot bind to GREs) failed to induce PEPCK.[35]

Substrates for gluconeogenesis are generated by glucocorticoids through release of amino acids from muscle and other peripheral tissues and release of glycerol along with lipolysis.

Permissive actions of glucocorticoids on gluconeogenesis by glucagon and epinephrine, possibly due to enhanced responsiveness to cAMP or other intracellular mediators, are evidenced by the impairment of gluconeogenesis caused by adrenalectomy and its normalization by glucocorticoids.

Glucose Utilization

Glucocorticoid inhibition of peripheral glucose utilization can be demonstrated both in intact organisms and with isolated cells.[92] It probably accounts for significant insulin antagonism and for the early rise in blood glucose seen after glucocorticoid treatment, and it may play a role in the release of gluconeogenic substrates from peripheral tissues. Glucose uptake is inhibited by direct glucocorticoid actions on normal skin, fibroblast, adipose tissue, adipocytes, lymphoid cells, and polymorphonuclear leukocytes. This inhibition, which requires RNA and protein synthesis, has been postulated to be mediated by a glucocorticoid-induced protein. It results mainly from translocation of glucose transporters from the plasma membrane to intracellular sites.[93,94] Glucose uptake by muscle is inhibited in intact organisms treated with glucocorticoids. This action may be indirect.

Glycogen Synthesis and Breakdown

Stimulation of glycogen synthesis by glucocorticoids takes place in the fetus and in the adult. It depends on increased synthesis of hepatic glycogen synthase and activation by dephosphorylation of its inactive form, as well as on inactivation by dephosphorylation of phosphorylase *a*. Some of these changes can be accounted for by increases in glycogen-bound phosphatase activity.

Stimulation of liver glycogen synthesis by stress-induced glucocorticoids can be interpreted as preparation for a subsequent challenge in which glycogen will be used for rapid conversion to glucose by glycogenolysis.[26] Furthermore, glucocorticoids at basal levels are required to permissively maintain epinephrine-induced glycogenolysis, which is impaired by adrenalectomy.

Fat Metabolism

Glucocorticoids, in opposition to insulin, inhibit glucose transport by adipose cells and stimulate free fatty acid release, which in humans results in an increase in plasma free fatty acids within 1 to 2 hours of administration of hormone.[95] Increased release of fatty acids also occurs after incubation of adipose tissue with glucocorticoids, an effect that is due in part to decreased reesterification resulting from the decrease in glucose uptake, and in part to increased lipolysis. Stimulation of lipolysis is largely a permissive effect seen in the presence of growth hormone and other lipolytic agents.[95] Glucocorticoids also inhibit the action of leptin and are permissive for the obesity syndrome in mutant rodents, which is ameliorated by adrenalectomy. A curious observation is that mice expressing a GR antisense construct that lowers their GR levels have as their most striking abnormality an increase in fat deposition, which can double their weight compared with normal mice. Because these mice eat less than normal, they are presumed to have increased energy efficiency.[96]

Chronic stress, which increases low diurnal concentrations of glucocorticoids, has been linked to central obesity and the metabolic syndrome, a disorder that combines diabetes, insulin resistance, dyslipidemia, and hypertension.[61] 11β-HSD1 knockout mice have weakened glucocorticoid-induced responses and resist hyperglycemia provoked by obesity or stress.[89] The critical importance of local glucocorticoid levels has been demonstrated with transgenic mice that overexpress 11β-HSD1 in fat cells: those mice develop central obesity and the metabolic syndrome.[45,47]

Catabolic Effects

Chronic high levels of glucocorticoids lead to massive catabolic effects on proteins and other components of peripheral tissues, causing muscle wasting[97] and lipolysis with redistribution of fat. These pathologic changes are probably magnified expressions of physiologic mechanisms for generating gluconeogenic substrates and may result from interactions with insulin and other hormones.[45]

BONE

Glucocorticoids act on bone and cartilage during development and adulthood. When present in excess, they cause osteoporosis and impair skeletal growth, inhibiting bone formation by decreasing the number of osteoblasts and their function, increasing collagenase expression, and inhibiting collagen synthesis.[98] On osteoblasts, they exert both permissive and suppressive effects.[99] At basal levels, they mobilize neutrophils from bone marrow to blood and other tissues[100]: possible molecular mechanisms of these glucocorticoid actions include decreased expression of insulin-like growth factor-1 (IGF-1), IGF-binding protein, IGF-1 and growth hormone receptors, and interactions with thyroid hormones. Glucocorticoids and cytokines in bone cells influence each other in complex ways, glucocorticoids generally suppressing cytokines and cytokines upregulating or downregulating GRs.[101] Levels of glucocorticoids in bone appear to depend on local 11β-HSD1. CRH, through direct peripheral inflammatory effects rather than through glucocorticoids, induces in rats degeneration of cartilage and bone.[102]

IMMUNE AND INFLAMMATORY REACTIONS

Antiinflammatory and Immunosuppressive Actions

Among the major clinical applications of hormones is the use of glucocorticoids for suppression of inflammatory and immune reactions and for treatment of patients with cancers of the lymphoid system. (Evolution anticipated such a use with vaccinia virus, which encodes an enzyme, 3β-hydroxysteroid dehydrogenase, which in infected organisms enhances glucocorticoid production, suppressing the inflammatory response and increasing virulence.[103])

As already described, for years glucocorticoid suppression of inflammatory and immune reactions was believed to result from pharmacologic actions with no physiologic significance. Strong evidence, however, points to their physiologic nature. They are elicited through the same receptor-mediated genomic mechanisms as physiologic effects. Adrenalectomy or administration

of the glucocorticoid antagonist mifepristone (RU486) enhance responses to inflammatory agents, showing that endogenous glucocorticoids normally control inflammation and similarly control autoimmune reactions. A striking example is the high susceptibility to arthritis of Lewis rats compared to the largely histocompatible Fischer rats after challenge with streptococcal cell wall polysaccharide (SCW).[104] This difference is due to a defect in biosynthesis of CRH that limits the glucocorticoid response of Lewis rats to a challenge. Lewis rats can be protected from SCW with dexamethasone, whereas Fischer rats become susceptible to SCW when pretreated with RU486. Defective HPA function may have an etiologic role in rheumatoid arthritis.[105] In transgenic mice with GRs that cannot dimerize and therefore cannot transactivate genes through binding to palindromic GREs, most anti-inflammatory and immunosuppressive actions of glucocorticoids remain intact, indicating that they are mediated through binding of GRs to factors such as AP-1 and NF-κB.[34]

Glucocorticoids also exert permissive actions on the immune system, as will be described below. Stimulation of the HPA axis may mobilize immunoregulatory agents other than glucocorticoids. One already mentioned is CRH, which peripherally has proinflammatory activity.[104] Whether such agents normally participate in immune responses to stress is uncertain.

Effects on Leukocytes

Glucocorticoids influence most cells responsible for immune and inflammatory reactions, including lymphocytes, natural killer (NK) cells, monocytes and macrophages, dendritic cells, eosinophils, neutrophils, mast cells, and basophils. Accumulation of most of these cells is decreased at inflammatory sites, an effect that can be induced by local application of hormones, but they mobilize neutrophils from bone marrow to blood.[100,106] Glucocorticoids may have both beneficial and detrimental effects on wound healing.[107] Blood counts of lymphocytes, monocytes, eosinophils, and basophils drop within 1 to 3 hours of glucocorticoid administration, generally recovering in 12 to 48 hours. NK cells are unaffected, and neutrophil counts rise. CD4 or helper T cells are more sensitive to lymphopenia than are B cells, and CD8 or cytotoxic T cells are relatively insensitive. Increased neutrophil number is thought to reflect increased release of marginated cells to the circulation and increased half-life. These alterations in cell traffic probably depend on inhibiting expression of surface molecules such as endothelial leukocyte adhesion molecule (ELAM)-1 and intercellular adhesion molecule (ICAM)-1,[104,108] thus decreasing adhesion of leukocytes to endothelial and other cells.

Glucocorticoid administration usually reduces antigen- or lectin-induced mitogenesis measured with peripheral lymphocytes, an effect also observed with lymphocytes in culture. T cells are more sensitive than B cells, and helper more sensitive than cytotoxic T cells. Glucocorticoids also directly inhibit T and B cell proliferation, early B cell differentiation, NK activity, and the differentiation and function of macrophages. They inhibit antigen presentation by monocytes and by dendritic cells (the most potent antigen-presenting cells) and shift responses from T helper 1 (Th1) cells to Th2 cells[109] Although glucocorticoids have stimulatory effects on immunoglobulin synthesis in cell culture, in whole organisms glucocorticoids usually inhibit B cell function.

Permissive glucocorticoid actions on T cell function have been observed in human volunteers treated with lipopolysaccharide (LPS), a mediator of septic shock: when administered within 6 hours of LPS, cortisol hemisuccinate suppressed the LPS-induced increase in TNF, but when given 12 to 144 hours before LPS, it magnified the TNF response.[110] Both in rats and in cultured splenic lymphocytes, glucocorticoids at low concentrations, presumably acting through MRs, can enhance T cell responses to concanavalin A, whereas at higher concentrations, through GRs, they suppress.[111] Hormone concentration and timing appear to be important for these actions to be displayed separately from the usually predominant suppressive effects.[112] Delayed-type hypersensitivity (DTH) reactions to cutaneous antigen exposure are enhanced by acute physiologic increases in glucocorticoid levels (and eliminated by adrenalectomy), but they are suppressed by chronic exposure to glucocorticoids.[113] In treatment for contact hypersensitivity, the therapeutic action of glucocorticoids is exerted through macrophages and neutrophils and requires GR dimerization.[114] The value of glucocorticoids in treatment for septic shock is controversial[108].

Important effects of glucocorticoids are exerted through the innate immune system. This ancient defense system uses about 10 invariant germline-encoded toll-like receptors (TLRs) on monocytes, macrophages, and dendritic and other cells to respond to infectious molecules of microbial origin by inducing antimicrobial genes along with inflammatory cytokines and chemokines, thus stimulating leukocyte migration and triggering adaptive immune responses.[115] LPS, the best-known stimulator of the innate system, provokes a rapid increase in glucocorticoid levels, which, in turn, protects the organism from potentially lethal effects of LPS.[108,116] The HPA response and other effects of LPS are mediated in part by the proinflammatory cytokines TNF-α, IL-1, and IL-6. In the airway epithelium, glucocorticoids may enhance innate immunity.[117,118] Glucocorticoid treatment of myeloid progenitors also enhances TLR signaling in macrophages to which they differentiate.[119] In other circumstances, glucocorticoids inhibit TLR signaling.[120]

Glucocorticoids protect against overactivity of immune reactions through several mechanisms, including suppression of production or potentially toxic activity of proinflammatory cytokines, histamine, adhesion molecules, inducible cyclooxygenase, and inducible nitric oxide synthase. Glucocorticoids also suppress expression and release of the LPS receptor CD-14. Overexpression of GRs increases resistance to LPS, thereby reducing production of IL-6.[121]

The anti-inflammatory cytokine IL-10 may play an important role in controlling LPS effects. Neutralization of IL-10 enhances the lethality of LPS in mice, whereas IL-10 administration reduces lethality.[122] Optimal IL-10 production during cardiac surgery requires a surge in glucocorticoid levels.[123] In experimental human endotoxemia, even high doses of glucocorticoids enhance IL-10 production.[124]

During development, LPS may affect the HPA axis and have long-lasting effects on immune regulation. Exposure of neonatal rats to LPS raises their adult corticosterone levels and protects the adults from adjuvant-induced arthritis.[125]

Apoptosis

Glucocorticoid-induced apoptosis of thymocytes and other lymphocytes is among the most striking effects of these hormones,[12,126,127] and the underlying mechanisms of this effect are being revealed gradually.[31] Apoptosis is directly linked to control of T cell pools in vivo, as is demonstrated with transgenic mice. Mice with increased GR expression have increased sensitivity to glucocorticoid-induced apoptosis,[121] and mice with higher or lower GR levels targeted to lymphocytes have, respectively,

smaller or larger T cell pools.[128] Glucocorticoid-induced apoptosis has been demonstrated with most hematologic cells, as well as with other cells such as epithelial and carcinoma cells and osteoblasts.[129,130] In some circumstances, glucocorticoids protect thymocytes from apoptosis[69]; such antiapoptosis is also found with neural and other cells.[129-133]

The physiologic significance of these effects is uncertain. Glucocorticoid-induced apoptosis has been invoked to account for immunosuppression, which, at least for short-term effects (hours or days), is better explained by actions on cytokines as described below. Apoptosis might serve to eliminate toxic or otherwise dangerous activated lymphocytes.[134] Several plausible ideas have been proposed for glucocorticoid involvement in positive or negative thymic selection of the T cell repertoire.[69] Thymocyte apoptosis, in contrast to many antiinflammatory and immunosuppressive reactions of glucocorticoids, requires GRs that dimerize (i.e., it is mediated by transactivation of genes through palindromic GREs).[34]

Effects via Cytokines and Other Mediators, and via Their Receptors

Many suppressive effects of glucocorticoids on immune and inflammatory reactions appear to be due to inhibition of production or activity of cytokines, chemokines, inflammatory agents, certain hormones and neurotransmitters, and other mediators that are released during responses to LPS and other forms of stress.[108,135,136] Although many of these results were originally obtained with cell cultures, most have been observed in intact organisms.[26]

These mediators form communication networks for defense mechanisms that respond to stress-induced challenges to homeostasis: cytokines and chemokines respond to infection, inflammatory agents to tissue damage, neurotransmitters to "fight or flight" encounters, and so forth. By blocking communication, glucocorticoids limit the stress response, preventing it from overshooting and damaging the organism. Most mediators in excess can be toxic, even lethal. Glucocorticoids limit not only production of mediators but sometimes their effects, such as TNF-α toxicity and responses of lymphocytes to IL-2 and of eosinophils to IL-3, IL-5, interferon (IFN)-γ, and granulocyte-macrophage colony-stimulating factor (GM-CSF).[137]

Chemokines or chemotactic cytokines are produced locally in tissues, thus influencing traffic and homing of leukocytes by binding to G protein–coupled cell-surface receptors. Their secretion, probably stimulated by such cytokines as IL-1 and TNF-α, is dramatically increased during inflammation, resulting in recruitment of leukocytes to the inflamed site. Significant glucocorticoid effects on cell traffic are due to inhibition of chemokine secretion and cell adhesion molecules.

Not all mediators are suppressed by glucocorticoids. Annexin 1 (lipocortin 1) is induced by glucocorticoids.[138] It is antiinflammatory in several systems and may mediate inhibitory effects of glucocorticoids on release of ACTH from the pituitary.[139] Macrophage migration inhibitory factor (MIF) represents a special case because it *antagonizes* glucocorticoid actions.[140] In vivo, glucocorticoids raise MIF levels in plasma and in thymus, spleen, and other cells, and MIF in turn counteracts glucocorticoid effects.[136,141] Some mediators, like IL-10, are stimulated under some conditions and are suppressed under others. In the acute phase response, which involves the proinflammatory cytokines IL-1, IL-6, and TNF-α, glucocorticoids both potentiate induction by cytokines of certain acute phase proteins and suppress production of the cytokines.[142]

Several mediators that are suppressed by glucocorticoids have receptors that, paradoxically, are induced by glucocorticoids. As discussed below, glucocorticoid induction of mediator receptors is a possible mechanism for some permissive effects.

Molecular mechanisms by which glucocorticoids control mediator production vary.[108,143] IL-1 production is blocked at the levels of transcription, translation, and secretion. TNF-α and GM-CSF appear to be blocked through increased degradation of their mRNAs. IL-2, IL-3, and possibly IFN-γ are blocked at the transcriptional level. Some, like prostaglandins and nitric oxide, may be suppressed because induction of the enzyme that synthesizes them is inhibited. Underlying many of these effects may be GR protein-protein cross-talk with NF-κB, AP-1, and other transcription factors,[143] which is consistent with the fact that most antiinflammatory actions are unaffected in transgenic mice with GRs that cannot dimerize.[34] Mitogen-activated protein kinase (MAPK) phosphatase 1 (MKP-1) is involved in MIF-glucocorticoid cross-talk.[141] Numerous other mechanisms are being investigated.

Not only do glucocorticoids influence cytokines, but glucocorticoid actions are regulated by such cytokines as MIF, which was already mentioned, and IL-1, IL-2, TNF-α, IL-10, and IL-11.

CARDIOVASCULAR SYSTEM

Glucocorticoids have complex—sometimes opposing—effects on the cardiovascular system and on electrolyte balance. The most significant of these is the regulation of vascular reactivity and blood pressure. Glucocorticoid effects are exerted on a number of target cells (epithelia, vascular smooth muscle and endothelium, cardiocytes) and can be both direct and indirect.

Under normal physiologic conditions, perhaps the most important cardiovascular action of glucocorticoids is permissive enhancement of vascular reactivity to other vasoactive agents (angiotensin II, norepinephrine), which contributes to maintenance of normal blood pressure. This action is best appreciated in patients with glucocorticoid deficiency or in adrenalectomized animals, which generally are hypotensive and exhibit reduced reactivity to vasoconstrictors.[108] In normal rats, the GR antagonist RU486 blunts vascular reactivity to norepinephrine and angiotensin II. The loss of permissive effects can contribute to cardiovascular collapse in Addisonian patients. Glucocorticoids at basal levels, possible acting via brain MRs, are necessary for the cardiovascular response of rats to mild stress.[144]

Although the exact mechanisms of these permissive actions remain to be determined, increased numbers of receptors for vasoactive hormones may play a significant role. Glucocorticoids induce transcription and expression of α_{1B} and β_2 receptors in smooth muscle cells.[145] They also have direct effects on the heart, such as induction of Na/K-ATPase in cardiocytes and enhanced cardiac epinephrine synthesis.[146] These effects could be responsible for the positive inotropic effect of glucocorticoids, which leads to increased cardiac output. Increased uptake of Ca^{2+} due to induction of voltage-dependent Ca^{2+} channels is observed in isolated vascular smooth muscle cells and might also contribute to increased vascular contractility.[147]

High levels of glucocorticoids are important for surviving hemorrhagic shock. Among adrenalectomized rats treated with corticosterone and subjected to the stress of hemorrhage, those that succumbed had much higher plasma levels of VP and norepinephrine than did those that survived. Untreated adrenalectomized rats had the highest levels and control rats (sham adrenalectomized) the lowest, suggesting that glucocorticoids protected by restraining the pressor response to hemorrhage transmitted by VP and norepinephrine.[148] Catecholamine synthesis and release during immobilization stress of rats is inhibited by glucocorticoids.[149] As already noted, optimal IL-10 production during cardiac surgery requires a surge in glucocorticoids.[123]

Chronic exposure to high levels of glucocorticoids (as occurs in Cushing's syndrome) frequently leads to hypertension. The mechanism of glucocorticoid-induced hypertension, as well as whether it is mediated through GRs or MRs, is unclear. Elevated blood pressure in glucocorticoid excess is probably due to several factors. When endogenous glucocorticoids are not inactivated by 11β-HSD2 in mineralocorticoid target cells in the kidney, severe hypertension develops as the result of mineralocorticoid-like effects of glucocorticoids.[150,151] Chronically elevated levels of glucocorticoids are also likely to have direct effects on the heart and on vascular smooth muscle cells, and may increase responses to vasoconstrictor agents through their permissive action.[152] The renin-angiotensin system is probably not of major significance in glucocorticoid-induced hypertension, as plasma renin activity is often normal or low in Cushing's syndrome.[153] Furthermore, although glucocorticoids induce angiotensinogen (i.e., renin substrate) production by the liver,[153] this action is unlikely to affect blood pressure, because the only rate-limiting step in the activity of the renin-angiotensin system is renin release. Atrial natriuretic factor (ANF) is also unlikely to play a role, as its synthesis is increased by glucocorticoids (see below), which would decrease rather than increase blood pressure. On the other hand, glucocorticoids coordinately inhibit the expression of both cyclooxygenase-2[154] and inducible nitric oxide synthetase.[155] Because prostaglandins and nitric oxide are powerful vasodilators, inhibition of their synthesis could be responsible for part of the hypertensive effect. Finally, the central nervous system (CNS) may have a role because intraventricular administration of glucocorticoids causes hypertension.[156] In summary, glucocorticoid-induced hypertension is probably due to complex interactions at peripheral (kidney, vasculature) and central (CNS) levels.

Transgenic mice overexpressing 11β-HSD2 in cardiomyocytes are normotensive but spontaneously develop cardiac hypertrophy, fibrosis, and heart failure, and die prematurely on a normal salt diet.[157] A selective MR inhibitor, eplerenone, ameliorates this condition, demonstrating the negative effects of inappropriate activation of cardiomyocyte MRs by aldosterone, and revealing that under normal physiologic conditions, tonic inhibition by glucocorticoids prevents such effects.[158] Local glucocorticoid excess in vascular smooth muscle cells may play a direct role in coronary vascular inflammatory responses under circumstances of a high salt intake.[159] Already mentioned is that glucocorticoids, apparently through PPAR-α,[87] promote the metabolic syndrome with diabetes and hypertension. This role is exacerbated in mice overexpressing 11β-HSD1 in fat cells.[46,47]

ELECTROLYTE HOMEOSTASIS
Direct Epithelial Effects

Through GRs, glucocorticoids directly increase epithelial Na^+ absorption and K^+ secretion, both in cultured collecting duct cells[160] and in the colon.[161,162] The genes that mediate the early effects of glucocorticoids are not all known, but serum and glucocorticoid-induced kinase (SGK) has been identified as a potential mediator of steroid hormone–stimulated Na reabsorption. SGK, both in oocytes and in mammalian kidney cells, increases activity of the epithelial sodium channel[163-165] and several other ion transporters.[166-169] In addition, SGK1 knockout mice are unable to conserve Na when challenged with a low-sodium diet.[170]

Cortisol and corticosterone can also induce salt retention via MRs, but these effects are rarely observed under physiologic conditions because these steroids are rapidly inactivated by 11β-HSD2 in aldosterone target cells.[39-41] If the enzyme is congenitally defective, however, as in the syndrome of apparent mineralocorticoid excess,[150,171] or is inhibited by licorice consumption,[151] cortisol can occupy both renal MRs and GRs and can induce salt retention and hypertension. Cortisol can also bind to MRs if the capacity of 11β-HSD2 is overwhelmed by high concentrations of glucocorticoids, as might occur in Cushing's disease (especially the high levels seen in the ectopic ACTH syndrome). Inhibition of 11β-HSD2 in pregnant rats produces elevated blood pressure in the adult offspring, suggesting that excessive exposure of the fetus to maternal glucocorticoids programs subsequent hypertension.[172]

Glucocorticoids increase renal tubular acid secretion, probably through increased activity of Na/H exchanger in the proximal tubule.[173] SGK mediates this effect.[174] Glucocorticoids can also induce phosphaturia by inhibiting Na-dependent phosphate uptake in brush border membrane vesicles.[173]

Indirect Effects

Glucocorticoid deficiency is associated with a decreased ability to excrete water, which appears to be due to decreased glomerular filtration rate (GFR) and increased synthesis of VP. Administration of glucocorticoids increases GFR and thus urine flow in both humans and experimental animals,[175] and it produces kaliuresis and natriuresis.[176-178] The mechanism of the diuretic and natriuretic action of glucocorticoids is still unknown, but probably involves ANF. Glucocorticoids increase the rate of transcription of ANF mRNA in cardiocytes,[179,180] stimulate ANF secretion,[181-183] and upregulate ANF receptors on endothelial cells.[184] Plasma concentrations of ANF were found to be elevated in patients with Cushing's disease,[185] and exogenous glucocorticoids seem to have a permissive effect on ANF-mediated natriuresis and diuresis in patients with adrenocortical insufficiency.[186]

Suppression of synthesis of VP[187] by glucocorticoids, which is part of the negative feedback mechanism by which glucocorticoids regulate their own concentration (see Fig. 2-1), leads to increased free water clearance. Patients with adrenal insufficiency have reduced free water clearance and increased plasma VP levels, probably due to increased rate of transcription of VP mRNAs.[188]

GLUCOCORTICOIDS AND THE CENTRAL NERVOUS SYSTEM

Glucocorticoids influence behavior, mood, excitability, and electrical activity of neurons. Behavioral changes are frequently observed with both excess and deficit of glucocorticoids,[58,62] and sleep disorders are a common feature of glucocorticoid therapy. High HPA activity and plasma cortisol levels are found in many patients with depression.[42] Extensive use is being made of genetically modified mice to enhance understanding of glucocorticoid functions in the brain.[27,63]

Both GRs and MRs are present in the brain and in other parts of the CNS, including the spinal cord.[42] MRs are abundant in the dentate gyrus and pyramidal cells of the hippocampus and in other regions of the limbic system, whereas GRs are widely dispersed in neurons and glial cells. MRs that are protected from glucocorticoids by 11β-HSD2 are present only in the anterior hypothalamus and circumventricular organs. No 11β-HSD2 is detectable in the hippocampus, but 11β-HSD1 can be found.[42] Other MRs in limbic structures are unprotected and thus respond to glucocorticoids.

Stress and glucocorticoids impair retrieval of long-term memory,[62,189] and impair or facilitate hippocampal long-term potentiation through GRs and MRs, respectively.[190] Either glucocorticoid excess or deficiency can damage hippocampal neurons: adrenalectomy leads to loss of neurons of the dentate gyrus and pyramidal neurons; extremely high levels of glucocorticoids cause death of CA3 neurons and potentiate neuronal death evoked by toxic substances.[59] Studies with GR and MR knockout mice show that cells in the dentate gyrus are dependent for survival on MRs but not on GRs.[62] Glucocorticoids can prevent apoptosis of mature neurons in the hippocampus.[131]

Electrophysiologic studies with isolated hippocampal tissue from adrenalectomized rats demonstrate that low concentrations of corticosterone, which mainly activate MRs, diminish afterhyperpolarization of neuronal membranes and enhance neuronal excitability. High concentrations of corticosterone, which activate GRs, suppress hippocampal excitability.[42] Thus, glucocorticoids at basal levels maintain neuronal excitability via MRs, and at stress-induced levels suppress stimulated neuronal activity via GRs.[42] CRH, through CRH-1 receptors and MRs, has been suggested to mediate rapid stress responses, whereas urocortin, through CRH-2 receptors and GRs, has been suggested to mediate slower adaptation to stress.[58,191] Transgenic mice with dimerization-deficient GRs fail to show various hippocampal responses to glucocorticoids, indicating that those responses require GR dimerization and binding to GREs.[192]

Several enzymes and transport processes in the CNS are influenced by glucocorticoids, with physiologic consequences that are not yet clear. Glucocorticoids induce glycerophosphate dehydrogenase and glutamine synthetase in cultured astrocytes, K channels in pituitary cells, and Na,K-ATPase subunit mRNA in the spinal cord. They inhibit glucose transport in hippocampal neurons and glia.[193] A large number of studies, some already mentioned, demonstrate that in neural systems glucocorticoids can exert rapid effects via nongenomic pathways.[56,57,75] The physiologic role of these effects remains uncertain.

Glucocorticoid Physiology in Relation to Stress

STRESS AND THE HPA AXIS

The intimate association between stress and glucocorticoids is manifested in many ways. Stress from diverse sources—fear, pain, trauma, hemorrhage, cold, infection, hypoglycemia, emotional distress, inflammatory agents, heavy exercise, and other challenges to homeostasis—stimulates the HPA axis with increased secretion of glucocorticoids. Untreated Addisonians and adrenalectomized animals can succumb to even mild stress but are protected by glucocorticoids. Organisms with basal levels of glucocorticoids that cannot increase their levels in response to stress—patients and animals with suppressed or otherwise compromised HPA functions—may tolerate mild stress but succumb to severe stress. The question of what levels of glucocorticoids are needed for protection is still open. As Ingle suggested,[15] a graded response seems likely, with basal levels sufficing for mild stress but progressively higher levels being required for more severe stress.[148]

Studies with transgenic mice designed to understand how glucocorticoids protect against stress and promote survival are still limited.[62] Regarding survival, CRE knockout mice, as already mentioned, show that glucocorticoids are essential because offspring fail to develop normal lungs and do not live much beyond birth.[194] They also have diminished stress-induced increases in corticosterone levels and impaired release of epinephrine.[194] Homozygous GR knockouts similarly fail to develop normal lungs. They have enlarged and disorganized adrenal cortexes, atrophied adrenal medullas lacking phenylethanolamine N-methyl transferase (PNMT), which methylates norepinephrine to epinephrine, and impaired activation of genes for hepatic gluconeogenic enzymes like PEPCK. Their ACTH and corticosterone levels are high.[195]

Homozygous offspring of transgenic mice with dimerization-defective GRs are viable, indicating that lung development probably depends on protein-protein cross-talk between GRs and transcription factors. They have normal adrenal medullas and PNMT levels and can suppress inflammatory and immune responses, but they cannot activate PEPCK.[34,35]

11β-HSD1 knockout mice, despite compensatory adrenal hyperplasia and increased adrenal secretion of corticosterone, have weakened stress-induced glucocorticoid responses. On starvation, they have diminished activation of glucose-6-phosphatase and PEPCK, and they resist hyperglycemia provoked by stress or obesity.[89]

Failure of lung development is the only fatal defect reported so far in transgenic mice with drastically impaired function of the HPA axis. Mice are viable after overcoming this hurdle, despite lack of glucocorticoid functions. This is not surprising, because under laboratory conditions, adrenalectomized rats and mice thrive without glucocorticoids, as long as they receive salt to compensate for lack of aldosterone and are not stressed.

Physiologic Mechanisms of Glucocorticoid Protection from Stress: Permissive and Suppressive Actions

General mechanisms by which glucocorticoids protect against stress can be traced to two common threads linking many otherwise disparate hormone effects.[25,152] One is the need for permissive (i.e., enhancing or sensitizing) effects of glucocorticoids to maintain or "prime" many homeostatic defense mechanisms, so that they can be called into action when necessary. In preceding sections, we have described permissive actions on gluconeogenesis, glycogenolysis, lipolysis, immune reactions, bone, pressor activities of vasoactive agents, other cardiovascular responses, hypothalamic responses to stress, pituitary responses to CRH, and neural processes. Glucocorticoids also help cells adapt to hypoxic stress.[196] Without glucocorticoids at basal levels, those defense mechanisms cannot respond adequately to a challenge.

The second thread is the need for glucocorticoids—usually at higher, stress-induced levels—to suppress activated defense mechanisms, thereby preventing them from overshooting and damaging or killing the organism. Among the most striking examples is suppression of production or activity of mediators that are secreted as a first line of defense against challenges to homeostasis.

Glucocorticoids therefore can be viewed as sustaining life through two actions: they are required on the one hand to permissively maintain many homeostatic defense mechanisms, on the other to prevent those mechanisms from overshooting. In the course of normal diurnal variation, glucocorticoids probably exert both actions to varying degrees; under stress, the second may predominate. If glucocorticoid regulation is defective, an organism may succumb either because its defense mechanisms cannot react, or because they may overreact. Not all defense mechanisms are under such dual glucocorticoid control. Inflammation, for example, does not appear to require permissive actions, because it usually is exacerbated by lack of glucocorticoids.

Permissive actions protect against stress, much as originally envisioned by Ingle.[15,16] That suppressive actions protect against overshooting of defense mechanisms was suggested in germinal form by Tausk in 1951,[23] soon after the discovery of antiinflammatory effects. Physiologists, however, at that time were convinced that anti-inflammatory effects were not physiologic, and Tausk's idea, published in a pharmaceutical company handout, never penetrated the regular endocrine literature. It was independently proposed in 1984 in a physiologic context,[25] as we have presented it here.

Fig. 2-2 illustrates with a simple model[152] how apparently opposing permissive and suppressive glucocorticoid actions, which may occur in the same tissues or cells,[197] can complement each other. For several mediators (e.g., IFN-γ, IL-6), glucocorticoids permissively enhance their activity by inducing their receptors on target cells, and they suppress their activity by inhibiting their synthesis. The outcomes predicted from the model are shown in Fig. 2-2 for two circumstances. In one (solid lines), both permissive and suppressive actions are assumed to be exerted via GRs, with identical dose response relationships; in

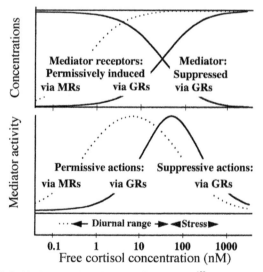

FIGURE 2-2. Model cortisol-regulated mediator system.[152] *Upper panel* (arbitrary linear vertical scale): Cortisol is assumed to permissively increase the concentration of mediator receptors and to suppress the concentration of the mediator. *Solid curves* depict effects of cortisol binding to glucocorticoid receptors (GRs) with dissociation constant K_d = 30 nM, the effects being proportional to the concentration of the cortisol/GR complex. The *dotted curve* depicts the effect on mediator receptors of cortisol binding to mineralocorticoid receptors (MRs) with K_d = 0.5 nM, the effect being proportional to the concentration of the cortisol/MR complex. *Lower panel* (arbitrary linear vertical scale): Mediator activity for each cortisol concentration is calculated to be proportional to the concentration of the mediator/receptor complex formed by binding of mediator to mediator receptor, using the concentrations of mediator and mediator receptor in the *upper panel*. The solid bell-shaped curve shows how mediator activity varies with cortisol concentration when mediator receptors are permissively induced via GRs and mediator is suppressed via GRs. The *dotted curve* shows mediator activity when mediator receptors are induced via MRs and mediator is suppressed via GRs. See text for further details.

the other (dotted lines), permissive actions are assumed to occur via MRs and suppressive actions via GRs, as may be noted in several of the cases described earlier. Because the affinity of cortisol for MRs is much higher than for GRs, the dotted dose response curves are shifted toward lower cortisol concentrations.

In the upper panel of Fig. 2-2, dose response curves for concentrations of mediator and mediator receptor are plotted over a range of cortisol concentrations. The bell-shaped curves in the lower panel of Fig. 2-2 represent "mediator activity"—for instance, the activity with which IL-2 at some concentration acts on a T cell with a certain level of IL-2 receptors—assumed proportional to the concentration of mediator-receptor complexes formed at each cortisol concentration. Mediator activity can be thought of as activity of any defense mechanism that is regulated through permissive and suppressive actions. As cortisol concentrations increase from low levels, mediator activity increases permissively because receptor concentrations rise. Activity reaches a peak value and then drops when increasing cortisol levels suppress mediator. Similar bell-shaped curves would be generated by almost any such combination of permissive and suppressive actions, regardless of their specific mechanisms, and have been found with several systems.[112,198]

Under normal unstressed conditions, basal levels of free glucocorticoids vary diurnally over a range (indicated roughly below the lower panel of Fig. 2-2) that corresponds to what might be called the "permissive" left slope of the solid bell-shaped curve, up to about the peak. Stress-induced levels (also shown in Fig. 2-2) can increase well beyond the peak, to the suppressive slope on the right. Thus, basal glucocorticoid levels can be viewed as varying diurnally in such a way as to permissively "prime" homeostatic defenses to a state of peak readiness for the activities of the day. Even at basal levels, however, as seen in the upper panel, glucocorticoids exert suppressive activity and can control responses to moderate stress. Stress-induced levels, on the other hand, are summoned for emergencies to prevent activated defense mechanisms from overshooting. In this emergency mode, they also suppress reproductive functions[26,199-201] in favor of more urgent needs, and, as described earlier, they help provide glucose for rapid and intense exertion.[26] These interpretations correspond well with the physiologic roles of glucocorticoids as sketched earlier.

REFERENCES

1. Addison T: Anaemia—disease of the supra-renal capsules, London Medical Gazette 43:517–518, 1849.
2. Addison T: On the constitutional and local effects of disease of the suprarenal capsules, London, 1855, Highley.
3. Selye H: Textbook of Endocrinology, Montreal, 1947, Acta Endocrinologica.
4. Wells BB, Kendall EC: A qualitative difference in the effect of compounds separated from the adrenal cortex on distribution of electrolytes and on atrophy of the adrenal and thymus glands of rats, Proc Mayo Clinic 15:133–139, 1940.
5. Long CNH, Lukens FDW: The effects of adrenalectomy and hypophysectomy upon experimental diabetes in the cat, J Exp Med 63:465–490, 1936.
6. Houssay BA, Biasotti A: The hypophysis, carbohydrate metabolism and diabetes, Endocrinology 15:511–523, 1931.
7. Long CNH, Katzin B, Fry EG: The adrenal cortex and carbohydrate metabolism, Endocrinology 26:309–344, 1940.
8. Ingle DJ: The production of glycosuria in the normal rat by means of 17-hydroxy-11-dehydrocorticosterone, Endocrinology 29:649–652, 1941.
9. Ingle DJ, Sheppard R, Evans JS, et al: A comparison of adrenal steroid diabetes and pancreatic diabetes in the rat, Endocrinology 37:341–356, 1945.
10. Greenwood M, Woods HM: "Status thymico-lymphaticus" considered in the light of recent work on the thymus, J Hyg (Lond) 26:305–326, 1927.
11. Selye H: Thymus and adrenals in the response of the organism to injuries and intoxications, Br J Exp Path 17:234–248, 1936.
12. Wyllie AH: Glucocorticoid-induced thymocyte apoptosis is associated with endogenous endonuclease activation, Nature 284:555–556, 1980.
13. Sayers G: The adrenal cortex and homeostasis, Physiol Rev 30:241–320, 1950.
14. Selye H: The general adaptation syndrome and the diseases of adaptation, J Clin Endocrinol Metab 6:117–230, 1946.
15. Ingle DJ: The role of the adrenal cortex in homeostasis, J Endocrinol 8:xxiii–xxxvii, 1952.
16. Ingle DJ: Permissibility of hormone action, A review, Acta Endocrinol 17:172–186, 1954.
17. Ingle DJ, Kendall EC: Atrophy of the adrenal cortex of the rat produced by the administration of large amounts of cortin, Science 86:245, 1937.
18. Ingle DJ: The time for the occurrence of cortico-adrenal hypertrophy in rats during continued work, Am J Physiol 124:627–630, 1938.
19. Harris GW: The induction of ovulation in the rabbit, by electrical stimulation of the hypothalamo-hypophysial mechanism, Proc Roy Soc Lond B 122:374–394, 1937.
20. Harris GW: Neural control of the pituitary gland, Physiol Rev 28:139–179, 1948.
21. Hench PS, Kendall EC, Slocumb CH, et al: The effect of a hormone of the adrenal cortex (17-hydroxy-11-dehydrocorticosterone: compound E) and of pituitary adrenocorticotropic hormone on rheumatoid arthritis, Proc Mayo Clinic 24:181–197, 1949.
22. Kendall EC: Cortisone, New York, 1971, Charles Scribner's Sons.
23. Tausk M: Hat die Nebenniere tatsächlich eine Verteidigungsfunktion? Das Hormon (Organon, Holland) 3:1–24, 1951.
24. Hoffman FG: Role of the adrenal cortex in homeostasis and growth. In Christy NP, editor: The human adrenal cortex, New York, 1971, Harper & Row, pp 303–316.
25. Munck A, Guyre PM, Holbrook NJ: Physiological functions of glucocorticoids in stress and their relation to pharmacological actions, Endocr Rev 5:25–44, 1984.
26. Sapolsky RM, Romero LM, Munck A: How do glucocorticoids influence stress-responses? Integrating permissive, suppressive, stimulatory, and preparative actions, Endocr Rev 21:55–89, 2000.
27. Wintermantel TM, Berger S, Greiner EF, et al: Evaluation of steroid receptor function by gene targeting in mice, J Steroid Biochem Mol Biol 93:107–112, 2005.
28. Bridgham JT, Carroll SM, Thornton JW: Evolution of hormone-receptor complexity by molecular exploitation, Science 312:97–101, 2006.
29. Munck A, Brinck-Johnsen T: Specific and nonspecific physicochemical interactions of glucocorticoids and related steroids with rat thymus cells in vitro, J Biol Chem 243:5556–5565, 1968.
30. Pratt WB, Galigniaaa MD, Harrell JM, et al: Role of hsp90 and the hsp90-binding immunophilins in signalling protein movement, Cell Signal 16:857–872, 2004.
31. Tuckermann JP, Kleiman A, McPherson KG, et al: Molecular mechanisms of glucocorticoids in the control of inflammation and lymphocyte apoptosis, Crit Rev Clin Lab Sci 42:71–104, 2005.
32. Duma D, Jewell CM, Cidlowski JA: Multiple glucocorticoid receptor isoforms and mechanisms of post-translational modification, J Steroid Biochem Mol Biol 102:11–21, 2006.
33. Beck IM, Vanden Berghe W, Vermeulen L, et al: Altered subcellular distribution of MSK1 induced by glucocorticoids contributes to NF-κB inhibition, EMBO J 27:1682–1693, 2008.
34. Reichardt HM, Tuckermann JP, Gottlicher M, et al: Repression of inflammatory responses in the absence of DNA binding by the glucocorticoid receptor, EMBO J 20:7168–7173, 2001.
35. Reichardt HM, Kaestner KH, Tuckermann J, et al: DNA binding of the glucocorticoid receptor is not essential for survival, Cell 93:531–541, 1998.
36. Adams M, Meijer OC, Wang J, et al: Homodimerization of the glucocorticoid receptor is not essential for response element binding: activation of the phenylethanolamine N-methyltransferase gene by dimerization-defective mutants, Mol Endocrinol 17:2583–2592, 2003.
37. Schacke H, Schottelius A, Docke WD, et al: Dissociation of transactivation from transrepression by a selective glucocorticoid receptor agonist leads to separation of therapeutic effects from side effects, Proc Natl Acad Sci U S A 101:227–232, 2004.
38. Kleiman A, Tuckermann J: Glucocorticoid receptor action in beneficial and side effects of steroid therapy: lessons from conditional knockout mice, Mol Cell Endocrinol 275:98–108, 2007.
39. Funder JW, Pearce PT, Smith R, et al: Mineralocorticoid action: target tissue specificity is enzyme, not receptor, mediated, Science 242:583–585, 1988.
40. Náray-Fejes-Tóth A, Watlington CO, Fejes-Tóth G: 11β-hydroxysteroid dehydrogenase activity in the renal target cells of aldosterone, Endocrinology 129:17–21, 1991.
41. Rusvai E, Náray-Fejes-Tóth A: A new isoform of 11β-hydroxysteroid dehydrogenase in aldosterone target cells, J Biol Chem 268:10717–10720, 1993.
42. De Kloet ER, Vreugdenhil E, Oitzl MS, et al: Brain corticosteroid receptor balance in health and disease, Endocr Rev 19:269–301, 1998.
43. Seckl J, Holmes M: Mechanisms of disease: glucocorticoids, their placental metabolism and fetal "programming" of adult pathophysiology, Nat Clin Pract Endocrinol Metab 3:479–488, 2007.
44. Drake A, Tang J, Nyirenda M: Mechanisms underlying the role of glucocorticoids in the early life programming of adult disease, Clin Sci (Lond) 113:219–232, 2007.
45. Vegiopoulos A, Herzig S: Glucocorticoids, metabolism and metabolic diseases, Mol Cell Endocrinol 275:43–61, 2007.
46. Stewart PM: Tissue-specific Cushing's syndrome, 11beta-hydroxysteroid dehydrogenases and the redefinition of corticosteroid hormone action, Eur J Endocrinol 149:163–168, 2003.

47. Masuzaki H, Yamamoto H, Kenyon CJ, et al: Transgenic amplification of glucocorticoid action in adipose tissue causes high blood pressure in mice, J Clin Invest 112:83–90, 2003.

48. Balachandran A, Guan H, Sellan M, et al: Insulin and dexamethasone dynamically regulate adipocyte 11beta-hydroxysteroid dehydrogenase type 1, Endocrinology 149:4069–4079, 2008.

49. Rabbitt EH, Gittoes NJ, Stewart PM, et al: 11beta-hydroxysteroid dehydrogenases, cell proliferation and malignancy, J Steroid Biochem Mol Biol 85:415–421, 2003.

50. Strickland I, Kisich K, Hauk PJ, et al: High constitutive glucocorticoid receptor b in human neutrophils enables them to reduce their spontaneous rate of cell death in response to corticosteroids, J Exp Med 193:585–594, 2001.

51. Irusen E, Matthews JG, Takahashi A, et al: p38 Mitogen-activated protein kinase-induced glucocorticoid receptor phosphorylation reduces its activity: role in steroid-insensitive asthma, J Allergy Clin Immunol 109:649–657, 2002.

52. Charmandari E, Kino T, Ichijo T, et al: Generalized glucocorticoid resistance: clinical aspects, molecular mechanisms, and implications of a rare genetic disorder, J Clin Endocrinol Metab 93:1563–1572, 2008.

53. Chikanza IC: Mechanisms of corticosteroid resistance in rheumatoid arthritis: a putative role for the corticosteroid receptor beta isoform, Ann N Y Acad Sci 966:39–48, 2002.

54. Meijer OC, Karssen AM, de Kloet ER: Cell- and tissue-specific effects of corticosteroids in relation to glucocorticoid resistance: examples from the brain, J Endocrinol 178:13–18, 2003.

55. Adcock I, Ford P, Bhavsar P, et al: Steroid resistance in asthma: mechanisms and treatment options, Curr Allergy Asthma Rep 8:171–178, 2008.

56. Makara GB, Haller J: Non-genomic effects of glucocorticoids in the neural system, evidence, mechanisms and implications, Prog Neurobiol 65:367–390, 2001.

57. Tasker J, Di S, Malcher-Lopes R: Minireview: rapid glucocorticoid signaling via membrane-associated receptors, Endocrinology 147:5549–5556, 2006.

58. de Kloet RE: Hormones, brain and stress, Endocr Regul 37:51–68, 2003.

59. Sorrells SF, Sapolsky RM: An inflammatory review of glucocorticoid actions in the CNS. Brain Behav Immun 21:259–272, 2006.

60. Dallman MF, Akana SF, Cascio CS, et al: Regulation of ACTH secretion: variations on a theme of B, Recent Prog Horm Res 43:113–173, 1987.

61. Dallman MF, Pecoraro N, Akana SF, et al: Chronic stress and obesity: a new view of "comfort food," Proc Natl Acad Sci U S A 100:11696–11701, 2003.

62. Kellendonk C, Gass P, Kretz O, et al: Corticosteroid receptors in the brain: gene targeting studies, Brain Res Bull 57:73–83, 2002.

63. Erdmann G, Berger S, Schutz G: Genetic Dissection of glucocorticoid receptor function in the mouse brain, J Neuroendocrinol 20:655–659, 2008.

64. Tronche F, Kellendonk C, Kretz O, et al: Disruption of the glucocorticoid receptor gene in the nervous system results in reduced anxiety, Nat Genet 23:99–103, 1999.

65. Eskandari F, Sternberg EM: Neural-immune interactions in health and disease, Ann N Y Acad Sci 966:20–27, 2002.

66. Goshen I, Yirmiya R, Iverfeldt K, et al: The role of endogenous interleukin-1 in stress-induced adrenal activation and adrenalectomy-induced adrenocorticotropic hormone hypersecretion, Endocrinology 144:4453–4458, 2003.

67. Gaillard RC, Spinedi E, Chautard T, et al: Cytokines, leptin, and the hypothalamo-pituitary-adrenal axis, Ann N Y Acad Sci 917:647–657, 2000.

68. Dallman MF, Akana SF, Laugero KD, et al: A spoonful of sugar: feedback signals of energy stores and corticosterone regulate responses to chronic stress, Physiol Behav 79:3–12, 2003.

69. Ashwell JD, Lu FW, Vacchio MS: Glucocorticoids in T cell development and function, Annu Rev Immunol 18:309–345, 2000.

70. Cima I, Corazza N, Dick B, et al: Intestinal epithelial cells synthesize glucocorticoids and regulate T cell activation, J Exp Med 200:1635–1646, 2004.

71. Turnbull AV, Smith GW, Lee S, et al: CRF type I receptor-deficient mice exhibit a pronounced pituitary-adrenal response to local inflammation, Endocrinology 140:1013–1017, 1999.

72. Akana SF, Dallman MF, Bradbury MJ, et al: Feedback and facilitation in the adrenocortical system: unmasking facilitation by partial inhibition of the glucocorticoid response to prior stress, Endocrinology 131:57–68, 1992.

73. Bradbury MJ, Akana SF, Dallman MF: Role of Type I and Type II corticosteroid receptors in regulation of basal activity in the hypothalamo-pituitary-adrenal axis during the diurnal trough and the peak: evidence for a nonadditive effect of combined receptor occupancy, Endocrinology 134:1286–1296, 1994.

74. Yao M, Denver R: Regulation of vertebrate corticotropin-releasing factor genes, Gen Comp Endocrinol 153:200–216, 2007.

75. Di S, Malcher-Lopes R, Halmos KC, et al: Nongenomic glucocorticoid inhibition via endocannabinoid release in the hypothalamus: a fast feedback mechanism, J Neurosci 23:4850–4857, 2003.

76. Schmidt ED, Aguilera G, Binnekade R, et al: Single administration of interleukin-1 increased corticotropin releasing hormone and corticotropin releasing hormone-receptor mRNA in the hypothalamic paraventricular nucleus which paralleled long-lasting (weeks) sensitization to emotional stressors, Neuroscience 116:275–283, 2003.

77. Tanimura SM, Watts AG: Corticosterone can facilitate as well as inhibit corticotropin-releasing hormone gene expression in the rat hypothalamic paraventricular nucleus, Endocrinology 139:3830–3836, 1998.

78. Wang J, Kuliszewski M, Yee W, et al: Cloning and espression of glucocorticoid-induced genes in fetal rat lung fibroblasts, J Biol Chem 270:2722–2728, 1995.

79. Jeong K-H, Jacobson L, Pacák K, et al: Impaired basal and restraint-induced epinephrine secretion in corticotropin-releasing hormone-deficient mice, Endocrinology 141:1142–1150, 2000.

80. Seres J, Bornstein SR, Seres P, et al: Corticotropin-releasing hormone system in human adipose tissue, J Clin Endocrinol Metab 89:965–970, 2004.

81. Besedovsky H, Sorkin E: Network of immune-neuroendocrine interactions, Clin Exp Immunol 27:1–12, 1977.

82. Besedovsky HO, del Rey A: Immuno-neuro-endocrine interactions: facts and hypotheses, Endocr Rev 17:64–102, 1996.

83. Horai R, Asano M, Sudo K, et al: Production of mice deficient in genes for interleukin Horai, and IL-1 receptor antagonist shows that IL-1b is crucial in turpentine-induced fever development and glucocorticoid secretion, J Exp Med 187:1463–1475, 1998.

84. Service FJ: Hypoglycemic disorders, N Engl J Med 332:1144–1152, 1995.

85. Dallman MF, Strack AM, Akana SF, et al: Feast and famine: critical role of glucocorticoids with insulin in daily energy flow, Front Neuroendocrinol 14:303–347, 1993.

86. Gounarides J, Korach-Andre M, Killary K, et al: Effect of dexamethasone on glucose tolerance and fat metabolism in a diet-induced obesity mouse model, Endocrinology 149:758–766, 2008.

87. Bernal-Mizrachi C, Weng S, Feng C, et al: Dexamethasone induction of hypertension and diabetes is PPAR-alpha dependent in LDL receptor-null mice, Nat Med 9:1069–1075, 2003.

88. Pilkis SJ, Granner DK: Molecular physiology of the regulation of hepatic gluconeogenesis and glycolysis, Annu Rev Physiol 54:885–909, 1992.

89. Kotelevtsev Y, Holmes MC, Burchell A, et al: 11β-Hydroxysteroid dehydrogenase type 1 knockout mice show attenuated glucocorticoid-inducible responses and resist hyperglycemia on obesity or stress, Proc Natl Acad Sci U S A 94:14924–14929, 1997.

90. Waltner-Law M, Duong DT, Daniels MC, et al: Elements of the glucocorticoid and retinoic acid response units are involved in cAMP-mediated expression of the PEPCK gene, J Biol Chem 278:10427–10435, 2003.

91. Stafford JM, Waltner-Law M, Granner DK: Role of accessory factors and steroid receptor coactivator 1 in the regulation of phosphoenolpyruvate carboxykinase gene transcription by glucocorticoids, J Biol Chem 276:3811–3819, 2001.

92. Munck A: Glucocorticoid inhibition of glucose uptake by peripheral tissues: old and new evidence, molecular mechanisms, and physiological significance, Perspect Biol Med 14:265–289, 1971.

93. Carter-Su C, Okamoto K: Effect of glucocorticoids on hexose transport in rat adipocytes: evidence for decreased transporters in the plasma membrane, J Biol Chem 260:11091–11098, 1985.

94. Horner HC, Munck A, Lienhard GE: Dexamethasone causes translocation of glucose transporters from the plasma membrane to an intracellular site in human fibroblasts, J Biol Chem 262:17696–17702, 1987.

95. Fain JN: Inhibition of glucose transport in fat cells and activation of lipolysis by glucocorticoids. In Baxter JD, Rousseau GG, editors: Glucocorticoid Hormone Action, Berlin, 1979, Springer-Verlag, pp 547–560.

96. Richard D, Chapdelaine S, Deshaies Y, et al: Energy balance and lipid metabolism in transgenic mice bearing an antisense CGR construct, Am J Physiol 265:R146–R150, 1993.

97. Menconi M, Fareed M, O'Neal P, et al: Role of glucocorticoids in the molecular regulation of muscle wasting, Crit Care Med 35(9Suppl):S602–S608, 2007.

98. Canalis E, Delany AM: Mechanisms of glucocorticoid action in bone, Ann N Y Acad Sci 966:73–81, 2002.

99. McCarthy TL, Ji C, Chen Y, et al: Time- and dose-related interactions between glucocorticoid and cyclic adenosine 3',5'-monophosphate on CCAAT/enhancer-binding protein-dependent insulin-like growth factor I expression by osteoblasts, Endocrinology 141:127–137, 2000.

100. Cavalcanti D, Lotufo C, Borelli P, et al: Endogenous glucocorticoids control neutrophil mobilization from bone marrow to blood and tissues in non-inflammatory conditions, Br J Pharmacol 152:1291–1300, 2007.

101. Takuma A, Kaneda T, Sato T, et al: Dexamethasone enhances osteoclast formation synergistically with transforming growth factor-beta by stimulating the priming of osteoclast progenitors for differentiation into osteoclasts, J Biol Chem 278:44667–44674, 2003.

102. Webster EL, Barrientos RM, Contoreggi C, et al: Corticotropin releasing hormone (CRH) antagonist attenuates adjuvant induced arthritis: role of CRH in peripheral inflammation, J Rheumatol 29:1252–1261, 2002.

103. Reading PC, Moore JB, Smith GL: Steroid hormone synthesis by vaccinia virus suppresses the inflammatory response to infection, J Exp Med 197:1269–1278, 2003.

104. Webster JI, Tonelli L, Sternberg EM: Neuroendocrine regulation of immunity, Annu Rev Immunol 20:125–163, 2002.

105. Harbuz MS, Chover-Gonzalez AJ, Jessop DS: Hypothalamo-pituitary-adrenal axis and chronic immune activation, Ann N Y Acad Sci 992:99–106, 2003.

106. Umland SP, Schleimer RP, Johnston SL: Review of the molecular and cellular mechanisms of action of glucocorticoids for use in asthma, Pulm Pharmacol Ther 15:35–50, 2002.

107. Stojadinovic O, Lee B, Vouthounis C, et al: Novel genomic effects of glucocorticoids in epidermal keratinocytes: inhibition of apoptosis, interferon-gamma pathway, and wound healing along with promotion of terminal differentiation, J Biol Chem 282:4021–4034, 2007.

108. Annane D, Cavaillon JM: Corticosteroids in sepsis: from bench to bedside? Shock 20:197–207, 2003.

109. Ramirez F, Fowell DJ, Puklavec M, et al: Glucocorticoids promote a TH2 cytokine response by CD4+ T cells in vitro, J Immunol 156:2406–2412, 1996.

110. Barber AE, Coyle SM, Marano MA, et al: Glucocorticoid therapy alters hormonal and cytokine responses to endotoxin in man, J Immunol 150:1999–2006, 1993.

111. Wiegers GJ, Reul JMHM: Induction of cytokine receptors by glucocorticoids: functional and pathological significance, Trends Pharmacol Sci 19:317–321, 1998.

112. Yeager MP, Guyre PM, Munck AU: Glucocorticoid regulation of the inflammatory response to injury, Acta Anaesthesiol Scand 48:799–813, 2004.

113. Dhabhar FS: Stress, leukocyte trafficking, and the augmentation of skin immune function, Ann N Y Acad Sci 992:205–217, 2003.

114. Tuckermann JP, Kleiman A, Moriggl R, et al: Macrophages and neutrophils are the targets for immune

suppression by glucocorticoids in contact allergy, J Clin Invest 117:1381–1390, 2007.

115. Janeway CA Jr, Medzhitov R: Innate immune recognition, Annu Rev Immunol 20:197–216, 2002.

116. Nadeau S, Rivest S: Glucocorticoids play a fundamental role in protecting the brain during innate immune response, J Neurosci 23:5536–5544, 2003.

117. Zhang N, Truong-Tran Q, Tancowny B, et al: Glucocorticoids enhance or spare innate immunity: effects in airway epithelium are mediated by CCAAT/enhancer binding proteins, J Immunol 179:578–589, 2007.

118. Stellato C: Glucocorticoid actions on airway epithelial responses in immunity: functional outcomes and molecular targets, J Allergy Clin Immunol 120:1247–1263, 2007.

119. Zhang T, Daynes R: Glucocorticoid conditioning of myeloid progenitors enhances TLR4 signaling via negative regulation of the phosphatidylinositol 3-kinase-akt pathway, J Immunol 178:2517–2526, 2007.

120. Mogensen T, Berg R, Paludan S, et al: Mechanisms of dexamethasone-mediated inhibition of toll-like receptor signaling induced by *Neisseria meningitidis* and *Streptococcus pneumoniae*, Infect Immun 76:189–197, 2008.

121. Reichardt HM, Umland T, Bauer A, et al: Mice with an increased glucocorticoid receptor gene dosage show enhanced resistance to stress and endotoxic shock, Mol Cell Biol 20:9009–9017, 2000.

122. Standiford TJ, Strieter RM, Lukacs NW, et al: Neutralization of IL-10 increases lethality in endotoxemia. Cooperative effects of macrophage inflammatory protein-2 and tumor necrosis factor, J Immunol 155:2222–2229, 1995.

123. Fillinger MP, Rassias AJ, Guyre PM, et al: Glucocorticoid effects on the inflammatory and clinical responses to cardiac surgery, J Cardiothorac Vasc Anesth 16:163–169, 2002.

124. van der Poll T, Barber AE, Coyle SM, et al: Hypercortisolemia increases plasma interleukin-10 concentrations during human endotoxemia—a clinical research center study, J Clin Endocrinol Metab 81:3604–3606, 1996.

125. Shanks N, Windle RJ, Perks PA, et al: Early-life exposure to endotoxin alters hypothalamic-pituitary-adrenal function and predisposition to inflammation, Proc Natl Acad Sci U S A 97:5645–5650, 2000.

126. Brewer JA, Kanagawa O, Sleckman BP, et al: Thymocyte apoptosis induced by T cell activation is mediated by glucocorticoids *in vivo*, J Immunol 169:1837–1843, 2002.

127. Brewer JA, Sleckman BP, Swat W, et al: Green fluorescent protein-glucocorticoid receptor knockin mice reveal dynamic receptor modulation during thymocyte development, J Immunol 169:1309–1318, 2002.

128. Pazirandeh A, Xue Y, Prestegaard T, et al: Effects of altered glucocorticoid sensitivity in the T cell lineage on thymocyte and T cell homeostasis, FASEB J 16:727–729, 2002.

129. Herr I, Gassler N, Friess H, et al: Regulation of differential pro- and anti-apoptotic signaling by glucocorticoids, Apoptosis 12:271–291, 2007.

130. Espina B, Liang M, Russell R, et al: Regulation of bim in glucocorticoid-mediated osteoblast apoptosis, J Cell Physiol 215:488–496, 2008.

131. Nichols N, Agolley D, Zieba M, et al: Glucocorticoid regulation of glial responses during hippocampal neurodegeneration and regeneration, Brain Res Rev 48:287–301, 2005.

132. Viegas LR, Hoijman E, Beato M, et al: Mechanisms involved in tissue-specific apopotosis regulated by glucocorticoids, Journal Steroid Biochem Mol Biol 109:273–278, 2008.

133. Jeanneteau F, Garabedian M, Chao M: Activation of Trk neurotrophin receptors by glucocorticoids provides a neuroprotective effect, Proc Natl Acad Sci U S A 105:4862–4867, 2008.

134. Abbas AK: Die and let live: eliminating dangerous lymphocytes, Cell 84:655–657, 1996.

135. Refojo D, Liberman AC, Giacomini D, et al: Integrating systemic information at the molecular level: cross-talk between steroid receptors and cytokine signaling on different target cells, Ann N Y Acad Sci 992:196–204, 2003.

136. VanMolle W, Libert C: How glucocorticoids control their own strength and the balance between pro- and anti-inflammatory mediators, Eur J Immunol 35:3396–3399, 2005.

137. Wallen N, Kita H, Weiler D, et al: Glucocorticoids inhibit cytokine-mediated eosinophil survival, J Immunol 147:3490–3495, 1991.

138. Goulding NJ: Corticosteroids—a case of mistaken identity, Br J Rheumatol 37:477–483, 1998.

139. Taylor AD, Christian HC, Morris JF, et al: An antisense oligodeoxynucleotide to lipocortin 1 reverses the inhibitory actions of dexamethasone on the release of adrenocorticotropin from rat pituitary tissue in vitro, Endocrinology 138:2909–2918, 1997.

140. Baugh JA, Donnelly SC: Macrophage migration inhibitory factor: a neuroendocrine modulator of chronic inflammation, J Endocrinol 179:15–23, 2003.

141. Roger T, Chanson A, Knaup-Reymond M, et al: Macrophage migration inhibitory factor promotes innate immune responses by suppressing glucocorticoid-induced expression of mitogen-activated protein kinase phosphatase-1, Eur J Immunol 35:3405–3413, 2005.

142. Thorn CF, Whitehead AS: Differential glucocorticoid enhancement of the cytokine-driven transcriptional activation of the human acute phase serum amyloid A genes, SAA1 and SAA2, J Immunol 169:399–406, 2002.

143. De Bosscher K, Vanden Berghe W, Haegeman G: The interplay between the glucocorticoid receptor and nuclear factor-kappaB or activator protein-1: molecular mechanisms for gene repression, Endocr Rev 24:488–522, 2003.

144. van den Buuse M, van Acker SA, Fluttert MF, et al: Involvement of corticosterone in cardiovascular responses to an open-field novelty stressor in freely moving rats, Physiol Behav 75:207–215, 2002.

145. Sakaue M, Hoffman BB: Glucocorticoids induce transcription and expression of the a1B adrenergic receptor gene in DTT1 MF-2 smooth muscle cells, J Clin Invest 88:385–389, 1991.

146. Kennedy B, Ziegler MG: Cardiac epinephrine synthesis. Regulation by a glucocorticoid, Circulation 84:891–895, 1991.

147. Hayashi T, Nakai T, Miyabo S: Glucocorticoids increase Ca2+ uptake and [3H]dihydropyridine binding in A7r5 vascular smooth muscle cells, Am J Physiol 261:C106–C114, 1991.

148. Darlington DN, Chew G, Ha T, et al: Corticosterone, but not glucose, treatment enables fasted adrenalectomized rats to survive moderate hemorrhage, Endocrinology 127:766–772, 1990.

149. Kvetnansky R, Fukuhara K, Pacák K, et al: Endogenous glucocorticoids restrain catecholamine synthesis and release at rest and during immobilization stress in rats, Endocrinology 133:1411–1419, 1993.

150. Stewart PM, Corrie JET, Shackleton CHL, et al: Syndrome of apparent mineralocorticoid excess: a defect in the cortisol-cortisone shuttle, J Clin Invest 82:340–349, 1988.

151. Stewart PM, Wallace AM, Valentino R, et al: Mineralocorticoid activity of licorice: 11-beta-hydroxysteroid dehydrogenase deficiency comes of age, The Lancet ii:821–824, 1987.

152. Munck A, Náray-Fejes-Tóth A: The ups and downs of glucocorticoid physiology. Permissive and suppressive effects revisited, Mol Cell Endocrinol 90:C1–C4, 1992.

153. Mantero F, Armanini D, Boscaro M, et al: Steroids and hypertension, J Steroid Biochem Mol Biol 40:35–44, 1991.

154. O'Banion MK, Winn VD, Young DA: cDNA cloning and functional activity of a glucocorticoid-regulated inflammatory cyclooxygenase, Proc Natl Acad Sci U S A 89:4888–4892, 1992.

155. Walker G, Pfeilschifter J, Kunz D: Mechanisms of suppression of inducible nitric-oxide synthase (iNOS) expression in interferon (IFN)-gamma-stimulated RAW 264.7 cells by dexamethasone. Evidence for glucocorticoid-induced degradation of iNOS protein by calpain as a key step in post-transcriptional regulation, J Biol Chem 272:16679–16687, 1997.

156. Grünfeld J-P: Glucocorticoids and blood pressure regulation, Horm Res 34:111–113, 1990.

157. Whitworth JA, Mangos GJ, Kelly JJ: Cushing, cortisol, and cardiovascular disease, Hypertension 36:912–916, 2000.

158. Qin W, Rudolph AE, Bond BR, et al: Transgenic model of aldosterone-driven cardiac hypertrophy and heart failure, Circ Res 93:69–76, 2003.

159. Young MJ, Moussa L, Dilley R, et al: Early inflammatory responses in experimental cardiac hypertrophy and fibrosis: effects of 11 beta-hydroxysteroid dehydrogenase inactivation, Endocrinology 144:1121–1125, 2003.

160. Náray-Fejes-Tóth A, Fejes-Tóth G: Glucocorticoid receptors mediate mineralocorticoid-like effects in cultured collecting duct cells, Am J Physiol 259:F672–F678, 1990.

161. Bastl CP, Binder HJ, Hayslett JP: Role of glucocorticoids and aldosterone in maintenance of colonic cation transport, Am J Physiol 238:F181–F186, 1980.

162. Bastl CP: Effect of spironolactone on glucocorticoid-induced colonic cation transport, Am J Physiol 25:F1235–F1242, 1988.

163. Alvarez de la Rosa D, Zhang P, Náray-Fejes-Tóth A, et al: The serum and glucocorticoid kinase sgk increases the abundance of epithelial sodium channels in the plasma membrane of Xenopus oocytes, J Biol Chem 274:37834–37839, 1999.

164. Chen SY, Bhargava A, Mastroberardino L, et al: Epithelial sodium channel regulated by aldosterone-induced protein sgk, Proc Natl Acad Sci U S A 96:2514–2519, 1999.

165. Náray-Fejes-Tóth A, Canessa C, Cleaveland ES, et al: SGK is an aldosterone-induced kinase in the renal collecting duct: effects on epithelial Na+ channels, J Biol Chem 274:16973–16978, 1999.

166. Henke G, Setiawan I, Bohmer C, et al: Activation of Na+/K+-ATPase by the serum and glucocorticoid-dependent kinase isoforms, Kidney Blood Press Res 25:370–374, 2002.

167. Pearce D: SGK1 regulation of epithelial sodium transport, Cell Physiol Biochem 13:13–20, 2003.

168. Palmada M, Embark HM, Yun C, et al: Molecular requirements for the regulation of the renal outer medullary K(+) channel ROMK1 by the serum- and glucocorticoid-inducible kinase SGK1, Biochem Biophys Res Commun 311:629–634, 2003.

169. Boehmer C, Wilhelm V, Palmada M, et al: Serum and glucocorticoid inducible kinases in the regulation of the cardiac sodium channel SCN5A, Cardiovasc Res 57:1079–1084, 2003.

170. Wulff P, Vallon V, Huang DY, et al: Impaired renal Na(+) retention in the sgk1-knockout mouse, J Clin Invest 110:1263–1268, 2002.

171. Edwards CRW, Stewart PM, Burt D, et al: Localization of 11β-hydroxysteroid dehydrogenase–tissue specific protector of the mineralocorticoid receptor, The Lancet ii:986–989, 1988.

172. Lindsay RM, Edwards CR, Seckl JR: Inhibition of 11-beta-hydroxysteroid dehydrogenase in pregnant rats and the programming of blood pressure in the offspring, Hypertension 27:1200–1204, 1996.

173. Freiberg JM, Kinsella J, Sacktor B: Glucocorticoids increase the Na+-H+ exchange and decrease the Na+ gradient-dependent phosphate-uptake systems in renal brush border membrane vesicles, Proc Natl Acad Sci U S A 79:4932–4936, 1982.

174. Yun CC, Chen Y, Lang F: Glucocorticoid activation of Na(+)/H(+) exchanger isoform 3 revisited, the roles of SGK1 and NHERF2, J Biol Chem 277:7676–7683, 2002.

175. Kurokawa K, Fukagawa M, Hayashi M, et al: Renal receptors and cellular mechanisms of hormone action in the kidney. In Seldin DW, Giebisch G, editors: The Kidney, ed 2, New York, 1992, Raven Press, pp 1339–1372.

176. Bia MJ, Tyler K, DeFronzo RA: The effect of dexamethasone on renal electrolyte excretion in the adrenalectomized rat, Endocrinology 111:882–888, 1982.

177. Campen TJ, Vaughn DA, Fanestil DD: Mineralo- and glucocorticoid effects on renal excretion of electrolytes, Pfluegers Arch 399:93–101, 1983.

178. Clore JN, Estep H, Ross-Clunis H, et al: Adrenocorticotropin and cortisol-induced changes in urinary sodium and potassium excretion in man: effects of spironolactone and RU 486, J Clin Endocrinol Metab 67:824–831, 1988.

179. Gardner DG, Gertz BJ, Deschepper CF, et al: Gene for the atrial natriuretic peptide is regulated by glucocorticoids *in vitro*, J Clin Invest 82:1275–1281, 1988.

180. Argentin S, Sun YL, Lihrmann I, et al: Distal cis-acting promotor sequences mediate glucocorticoid stimulation of cardiac atrial natriuretic factor gene transcription, J Biol Chem 266:23315–23322, 1991.

181. Shields PP, Dixon JE, Glembotski CC: The secretion of atrial natriuretic factor-(99–126) by cultured cardiac myocytes is regulated by glucocorticoids, J Biol Chem 263:12619–12628, 1988.

182. Fullerton MJ, Krozowski ZS, Funder JW: Adrenalectomy and dexamethasone administration: effect on atrial natriuretic peptide synthesis and circulating forms, Mol Cell Endocrinol 82:33–40, 1991.

183. Weidmann P, Matter DR, Matter EE, et al: Glucocorticoid and mineralocorticoid stimulation of atrial natriuretic peptide release in man, J Clin Endocrinol Metab 66:1233–1239, 1988.

184. Lanier-Smith KL, Currie MG: Glucocorticoid regulation of atrial natriuretic peptide receptors on cultured endothelial cells, Endocrinology 129:2311–2317, 1991.

185. Yamaji T, Ishibashi M, Yamada A, et al: Plasma levels of atrial natriuretic hormone in Cushing's syndrome, J Clin Endocrinol Metab 67:348–352, 1988.

186. Damjancic P, Vierhapper H: Permissive action of glucocorticoid substitution therapy on the effects of atrial natriuretic peptide (hANP) in patients with adrenocortical insuffiency, Exp Clin Endocrinol 95:315–321, 1990.

187. Raff H: Glucocorticoid inhibition of neurohypophysial vasopressin secretion, Am J Physiol 252:R635–R644, 1987.

188. Davies LG, Arentzen R, Reid JM, et al: Glucocorticoid sensitivity of vasopressin mRNA levels in the paraventricular nucleus of the rat, Proc Natl Acad Sci U S A 83:1145–1149, 1986.

189. Roozendaal B, Phillips RG, Power AE, et al: Memory retrieval impairment induced by hippocampal CA3 lesions is blocked by adrenocortical suppression, Nat Neurosci 4:1169–1171, 2001.

190. Korz V, Frey JU: Stress-related modulation of hippocampal long-term potentiation in rats: involvement of adrenal steroid receptors, J Neurosci 23:7281–7287, 2003.

191. Hsu SY, Hsueh AJ: Human stresscopin and stresscopin-related peptide are selective ligands for the type 2 corticotropin-releasing hormone receptor, Nat Med 7:605–611, 2001.

192. Karst H, Karten YJ, Reichardt HM, et al: Corticosteroid actions in hippocampus require DNA binding of glucocorticoid receptor homodimers, Nat Neurosci 3:977–978, 2000.

193. Horner HC, Packan DR, Sapolsky RM: Glucocorticoids inhibit glucose transport in cultured hippocampal neurons and glia, Neuroendocrinology 52:57–64, 1990.

194. Muglia L, Jacobson L, Dikkes P, et al: Corticotropin-releasing hormone deficiency reveals major fetal but not adult glucocorticoid need, Nature 373:427–432, 1995.

195. Cole TJ, Blendy JA, Monaghan AP, et al: Targeted disruption of the glucocorticoid receptor gene blocks adrenergic chromaffin development and severely retards lung maturation, Genes Dev 9:1608–1625, 1995.

196. Kodama T, Shimizu N, Yoshikawa N, et al: Role of the glucocorticoid receptor for regulation of hypoxia-dependent gene expression, J Biol Chem 278:33384–33391, 2003.

197. Galon J, Franchimont D, Hiroi N, et al: Gene profiling reveals unknown enhancing and suppressive actions of glucocorticoids on immune cells, FASEB J 16:61–71, 2002.

198. Lim H-Y, Muller N, Herold MJ, et al: Glucocorticoids exert opposing effects on macrophage function dependent on their concentration, Immunology 122:47–53, 2007.

199. Gore A, Attardi B, DeFranco D: Glucocorticoid repression of the reproductive axis: effects on GnRH and gonadotropin subunit mRNA levels, Mol Cell Endocrinol 256:40–48, 2006.

200. Hu G, Lian Q, Lin H, et al: Rapid mechanisms of glucocorticoid signaling in the Leydig cell, Steroids 73:1018–1024, 2007.

201. Martin L, Tremblay J: Glucocorticoids antagonize cAMP-induced StAR transcription in Leydig cells through the orphan nuclear receptor NUR77, J Mol Endocrinol 41:165–175, 2008.

Chapter 3

GLUCOCORTICOID RECEPTORS:
Their Mechanisms of Action and Glucocorticoid Resistance

ROBERT H. OAKLEY, LAURA J. LEWIS-TUFFIN, CARL D. MALCHOFF, DIANA MARK MALCHOFF, and JOHN A. CIDLOWSKI

GLUCOCORTICOID RECEPTORS*

Glucocorticoids are a class of endogenous and synthetic steroid hormones that affect virtually every aspect of human physiology. Currently they are one of the most commonly prescribed classes of drugs.[1] The physiologic actions of glucocorticoids include highly effective antiinflammatory and immunomodulatory actions that are exploited for the treatment of diseases such as asthma, arthritis, allergic rhinitis, and leukemia/lymphoma.[2,3] In addition, glucocorticoids have important roles in development of the lung and nervous systems, skeletal growth, behavior, reproduction, and intermediary metabolism. Ultimately, glucocorticoids act to maintain homeostasis in the face of stressful stimuli. The broad actions of glucocorticoids account for the serious side effects commonly experienced with chronic glucocorticoid treatment. These include the development of glucocorticoid resistance in diseased tissues, osteoporosis, growth retardation in children, muscle atrophy, and signs of the metabolic syndrome.[1,4,5] The physiologic and pharmacologic actions of glucocorticoids are mediated by the glucocorticoid receptor (GR), a member of the nuclear receptor superfamily of proteins that regulate gene transcription in a ligand-dependent manner.[6] In this section, we review the basic mechanisms of glucocorticoid action with an emphasis on how these mechanisms contribute to the antiinflammatory and immunomodulatory effects of glucocorticoids.

The Glucocorticoid Receptor

Like other members of the nuclear receptor superfamily, GR is a modular protein comprising an amino-terminal transactivation domain (NTD); a central, two-zinc-finger DNA-binding domain (DBD); and a carboxyl-terminal ligand-binding domain (LBD) (Fig. 3-1A).[7] Separating the DBD and LBD is a flexible region of the molecule termed the *hinge region*. The receptor contains two regions involved in activating transcription, one in the NTD (AF1) which can act independently of ligand binding, and a second in the LBD (AF2) whose function is dependent on glucocorticoid binding. The LBD also possesses a nuclear localization signal and sites for interaction with other transcription factors, coregulators, and protein chaperones. An additional nuclear localization signal spans the junction of the DBD and hinge region. The GR protein is also a substrate for various types of posttranslational modifications including phosphorylation, ubiquitination, sumoylation, and acetylation that regulate GR signaling by modulating the expression level and/or transcriptional activity of the receptor.[8]

---

*The section titled "Glucocorticoid Receptors" was written by Robert H. Oakley, Laura J. Lewis-Tuffin, and John A. Cidlowski.

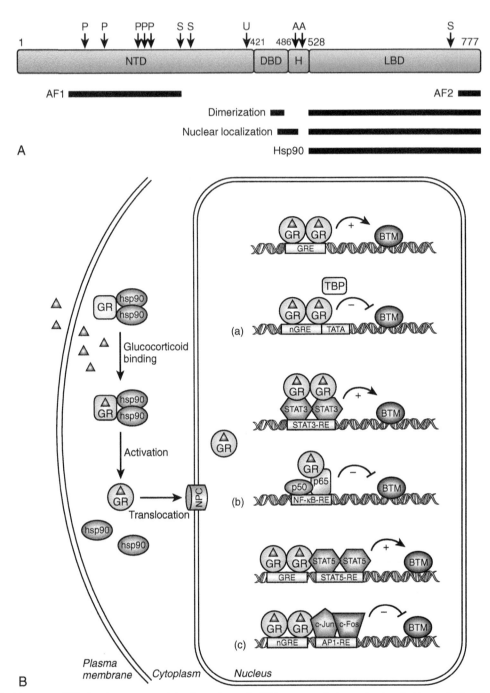

FIGURE 3-1. Glucocorticoid receptor (GR) domain structure and signaling pathway. **A,** GR is composed of an amino-terminal transactivation domain (NTD), DNA-binding domain (DBD), hinge region (H), and ligand-binding domain (LBD). Regions involved in transactivation (AF1 and AF2), dimerization, nuclear localization, and hsp90 binding are indicated. The location of residues posttranslationally modified by phosphorylation (P) (Ser-113, Ser-141, Ser-203, Ser-211, and Ser-226); ubiquitination (U) (Lys-419); sumoylation (S) (Lys-277, Lys-293, and Lys-703); and acetylation (A) (Lys-494 and Lys-495) are also depicted. Numbers are for the human glucocorticoid receptor. **B,** The unliganded GR resides in the cytoplasm of cells in a complex with chaperone proteins. Upon binding glucocorticoids (▲), the receptor undergoes a change in conformation, dissociates from accessory proteins, and translocates into nucleus via the nuclear pore complex (NPC). Nuclear GR regulates gene expression in three primary ways: (a) GR binds directly to DNA and enhances or inhibits transcription of target genes. (b) GR interacts with DNA-bound transcription factors without itself binding to DNA and enhances or inhibits transcription of target genes. (c) GR binds directly to DNA and interacts with transcription factors bound to neighboring sites and enhances or inhibits transcription of target genes. BTM, Basal transcription machinery; TBP, TATA-box binding protein.

GR Regulation of Transcription via Direct Binding to DNA

Unliganded GR is located in the cytoplasm of cells as part of a multiprotein complex that includes two molecules of heat shock protein 90 (hsp90) (see Fig. 3-1B).[9] These chaperone proteins maintain the receptor in a transcriptionally inactive state that favors high-affinity ligand binding. Upon binding glucocorticoids, GR undergoes a conformational change resulting in the dissociation of hsp90, exposure of the nuclear localization signals, and translocation of the receptor into the nucleus via the nuclear pore. The receptor then regulates gene transcription by binding directly to specific DNA sequences known as *glucocorticoid response elements* (GREs) and/or by binding other transcription factors and modulating their activity. Global gene expression analyses indicate that up to 20% of the genome is induced or repressed by glucocorticoids.[5,10]

The consensus GRE is an imperfect palindrome, GGTA-CAnnnTGTTCT, that is usually found in the promoter region of target genes.[11,12] The interaction of ligand-bound GR with the GRE stimulates the transcription of numerous genes, including the metabolic enzymes tyrosine amino transferase, phosphoenolpyruvate carboxykinase, and glucose-6-phosphatase (see Fig. 3-1B[a], upper scheme). High-affinity GRE binding requires receptor dimerization and is short lived because the receptor rapidly cycles on and off target sites every few seconds.[13,14] Upon binding DNA, GR undergoes a conformational change that results in the coordinated recruitment of three general types of coactivators necessary for stimulating transcription of the target gene: the ATP-dependent complex BRG1 (SWI/SNF) that mediates large noncovalent disruptions in chromatin structure; CBP, p300, and members of the SRC/p160 family of proteins that modify chromatin structure locally through their intrinsic histone acetyltransferase activity; and components of the DRIP/TRAP complex that assist in the recruitment of the basal transcription machinery.[15] The alterations in chromatin structure result in DNA unwinding, thereby permitting promoter access to transcription factors and cofactors that enhance target gene expression. The specific coactivators recruited by GR determine the gene induction profile, and this assembly is dependent on the promoter context, the bound glucocorticoid, and the availability and activity of the coactivators themselves.

Negative GREs (nGREs) are the transcription-repressing counterpart of positive GREs.[16] These response elements bear little resemblance to positive GREs, are highly variable, and a consensus sequence has not been determined. How ligand-bound GR represses transcription via nGREs is unclear and likely involves multiple mechanisms dependent upon the promoter context. For some genes, such as osteocalcin, DNA-bound GR may sterically interfere with binding of positively acting transcription factors to elements that overlap the nGRE (see Fig. 3-1B[a], lower scheme).[17] The situation is more complex for other repressed genes, since both binding to DNA and interacting with neighboring transcription factors appear to be required of the receptor (see Fig. 3-1B[c], lower scheme). Referred to as a *composite GRE*, nGREs of this nature are found in the promoters of the proliferin and corticotropin-releasing hormone (CRH) genes. Here, DNA-bound GR interacts with the activator protein-1 (AP-1) transcription factor occupying an adjacent site to repress transcription.[18,19] Finally, since nGREs correspond poorly to the GRE consensus sequence, negative regulation may be achieved at some target genes by GR interacting with DNA-bound positive transcription factors without itself binding to the promoter. This "tethering" mechanism of repression (described in more detail later) appears to mediate the glucocorticoid-dependent inhibition of gonadotropin-releasing hormone receptor and pro-opiomelanocortin expression via the interaction of GR with the promoter-bound Oct1 and Nur77 transcription factors, respectively.[20,21]

GR Regulation of Transcription via Protein-Protein Interactions

In addition to transcriptional regulation by direct binding to DNA, ligand-bound GR can also interact with other transcription factors and modulate their activity on glucocorticoid-responsive

promoters without itself binding to DNA. The two most studied examples of this form of regulation involve the transcription factors AP-1 and nuclear factor κB (NF-κB). These two proteins are central mediators of the inflammatory and immune responses, and their inhibition by GR is thought to underlie the major antiinflammatory and immunosuppressive actions of glucocorticoids.[22,23] When activated by stress signals such as proinflammatory cytokines, bacterial and viral infectious agents, or pro-apoptotic stimuli, AP-1 and NF-κB bind their cognate response elements and induce the expression of many proinflammatory genes, including cytokines, cell adhesion molecules, and enzymes involved in tissue destruction. Glucocorticoids indirectly antagonize the actions of AP-1 and NF-κB at multiple levels by inducing the expression of other regulatory proteins. Activated GR stimulates expression of the IκB protein, which sequesters NF-κB in the cytoplasm,[24] MAPK phosphatase 1, which dephosphorylates c-Jun N-terminal kinase to prevent activation of AP-1,[25] and tristetraprolin, which destabilizes the mRNA of many AP-1 and NF-κB-induced genes.[26]

The primary way, however, by which hormone-bound GR represses the activity of AP-1 and NF-κB is through a direct interaction with the c-Jun subunit of AP-1 and the p65 subunit of NF-κB (see Fig. 3-1B[b], lower scheme).[22,23] Interestingly, the antagonism is reciprocal; the association of these proteins with GR represses its activity on target genes. Multiple mechanisms appear to underlie the antagonism, suggesting the mode of action may vary in a promoter, cell-type, and/or signal-dependent manner. In early studies, the receptor was reported to sequester AP-1 and NF-κB in the cytoplasm and/or nucleus and prevent DNA binding. More recent findings, however, suggest the receptor is tethered to DNA-bound AP-1 and NF-κB and alters the subsequent assembly and/or activity of recruited transcriptional proteins. For example, on several toll-like receptor genes, GR represses NF-κB by disrupting the interaction of p65 with the promoter-specific coactivator IRF3 (interferon regulatory factor 3).[27] At the interleukin 8 (IL-8) and intercellular adhesion molecule 1 (ICAM-1) promoters, the association of GR with NF-κB impairs the phosphorylation of the C-terminal domain of RNA polymerase II.[28] GR-mediated repression of the AP-1-responsive collagenase-3 promoter and the NF-κB-responsive IL-8 promoter have both been shown to be potentiated by receptor-dependent recruitment of the coactivator GRIP1, indicating coactivators can actually function as corepressors in the appropriate configuration with GR.[29] Finally, GR has been reported to interact with histone deacetylase 2 (HDAC2) and to repress the histone acetyltransferase activity of NF-κB, suggesting that GR antagonizes NF-κB by effects on chromatin structure.[30]

In contrast to AP-1 and NF-κB, the physical association of GR with the signal transducer and activator of transcription (STAT) family of proteins enhances their activity on target genes.[31] STAT transcription factors are activated by a range of cytokines through induction of the Janus kinase pathway (JAK) and tyrosine phosphorylation. Upon binding their cognate response elements, STATs regulate genes involved in the immune response, differentiation, survival, and apoptosis. GR has been shown to interact with several members of the STAT family, including STAT3 and STAT5, and to synergistically enhance their activity on target genes in a promoter-dependent fashion.[31] The association of GR with STAT3 at the γ-fibrinogen and α$_2$-macroglobulin promoters, which lack identifiable GREs, super-induces their expression (see Fig. 3-1B[b], upper scheme).[32-34] Similarly, the synergistic activation of the β-casein and toll-like receptor-2 genes results from the association of GR with promoter-bound STAT5.[35-38]

However, the observed synergy at these STAT5-responsive genes may also require GR binding to DNA and more accurately reflect a composite GRE (see Fig. 3-1B[c], upper scheme).[37,38] How GR synergistically activates STAT-regulated genes is poorly understood but may involve GR enhancing STAT nuclear localization,[39] prolonging the promoter occupancy of STAT by inhibiting its tyrosine dephosphorylation[32,40] and/or promoting the co-utilization of certain coactivators.[31] Interestingly, the synergism of these two transcription factors is not always mutual, since GR activity is inhibited or stimulated depending on the particular STAT isoform employed.[34,35,41,42]

Multiple GR Isoforms Derived from Single Gene

The human GR gene is located on chromosome 5q31-32 and comprises 9 exons.[43-46] Alternative splicing in exon 9 generates two receptor isoforms, termed GRα and GRβ, that are identical through to amino acid 727 but then diverge at their carboxyl-termini (Fig. 3-2).[45-47] The classic, full-length GRα contains an additional 50 amino acids, whereas GRβ has an additional, non-homologous 15 amino acids. Because of its unique carboxyl-terminus, GRβ does not bind glucocorticoids and resides constitutively in the nucleus of cells.[45,48] GRβ has been shown to

function as a dominant negative inhibitor and repress the transcriptional activity of GRα[45,49-51]; therefore, alterations in GRβ expression may contribute to changes in glucocorticoid responsiveness. Indeed, expression of GRβ is selectively increased over GRα in cells exposed to proinflammatory cytokines and microbial superantigens, leading to reduced sensitivity to glucocorticoids.[52-56] In addition, glucocorticoid-resistant forms of inflammatory diseases (e.g., asthma, rheumatoid arthritis, and ulcerative colitis) have been associated with elevated expression of GRβ.[50] Conversely, methotrexate, an effective drug for treating autoimmune and inflammatory diseases, promotes a selective increase in GRα at the expense of GRβ and improves glucocorticoid sensitivity of lymphocytes.[57]

Elevated GRβ levels also result from a naturally occurring ATTTA to GTTTA polymorphism (A3669G) in the 3' untranslated region of GRβ. This nucleotide substitution disrupts an mRNA destabilization motif and leads to increased stability of the GRβ mRNA and enhanced protein expression.[58,59] The A3669G allele has been associated with reduced central obesity in women and a more favorable lipid profile in men,[60] suggesting the increase in GRβ might antagonize some of the undesirable effects of GRα on fat distribution and lipid metabolism. The A3669G-directed rise in GRβ may also compromise the immunosuppressive actions of GRα. Persons harboring the A3669G allele have an elevated risk of the autoimmune disease rheumatoid arthritis and a reduced risk of bacterial nasal infection.[58,61]

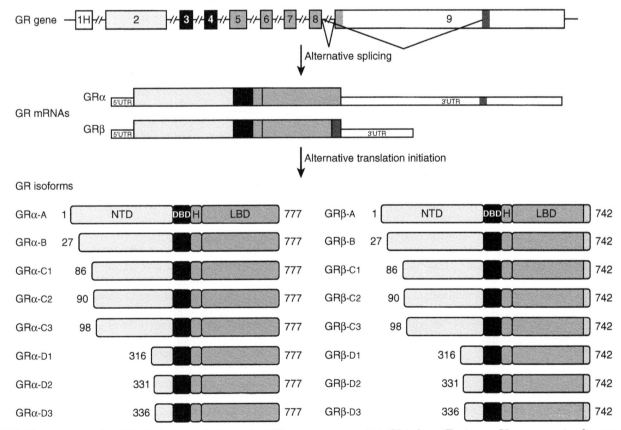

FIGURE 3-2. Alternative processing of the single glucocorticoid receptor (GR) gene generates multiple GR isoforms. The human GR gene comprises 9 exons. Alternative splicing at the 3' end of the primary transcript generates GRα and GRβ mRNAs, which encode GRα and GRβ proteins differing only at their carboxyl-terminus. Alternative translation initiation from 8 different AUG start codons derived from exon 2 generates additional protein isoforms with progressively shorter NTDs. Numbers shown denote the first and last residues for the human GR isoforms. For simplicity, only the most proximal of 9 alternate exon 1s (1H) is shown.

Moreover, A3669G carriers exhibit an increased risk of myocardial infarction and coronary heart disease, two pathologies with inflammatory underpinnings.[62]

A broader role for GRβ in cell signaling has recently emerged with the demonstration that this isoform can modulate gene expression apart from its effects on GRα. In a genome-wide microarray analysis performed in cells selectively expressing GRβ, the isoform was found to alter the expression of over 5000 genes.[63] Less than 20% of the genes were commonly regulated by ligand-activated GRα, indicating that GRβ possesses its own unique gene-regulatory profile. GRβ was also shown to bind the glucocorticoid antagonist mifepristone (RU486), and binding of this ligand abolished most of the GRβ-mediated changes in gene expression.[63] As a bona fide transcription factor, GRβ may contribute to alterations in glucocorticoid responsiveness in healthy and diseased tissues by genomic effects independent of its dominant negative activity on GRα.

Alternative translation initiation of the GR mRNA produces an additional cohort of receptor subtypes (see Fig. 3-2).[10,64,65] Eight GR isoforms with progressively shorter NTDs are generated from one GRα mRNA transcript via different AUG start codons: GRα-A, GRα-B, GRα-C1, GRα-C2, GRα-C3, GRα-D1, GRα-D2, and GRα-D3. GRα-A is the classic, full-length 777 amino acid protein that is generated from the first initiator AUG codon. The GRβ mRNA also contains the identical start codons and would be expected to give rise to a similar complement of subtypes. The GRα translational isoforms show a widespread tissue distribution; however, the relative levels of the subtypes differ both between and within tissues.[64,66] Functionally, the isoforms bind glucocorticoids with similar affinity and bind GREs with similar capacity.[66] Additionally, all eight isoforms occupy the nucleus of cells following glucocorticoid treatment. In the absence of hormone, however, the subcellular distribution of the subtypes differ, with the GRα-D isoforms residing predominantly in the nucleus and the others predominantly in the cytoplasm.[64]

Marked differences have also been reported in the transcriptional properties of the GRα translational isoforms.[64,66] On GRE-containing reporter and endogenous genes, the GRα-C3 isoform was the most active stimulating gene expression, whereas the GRα-D subtypes were the most deficient. These isoform-selective effects have been attributed to differences among the subtypes in their ability to recruit various transcriptional factors and coregulators, such as CBP and RNA polymerase II, to the promoter. In contrast to these divergent effects on gene induction, no significant differences have been observed so far in the ability of the GRα isoforms to repress NF-κB.[66] In a whole-genome microarray analysis performed on U2OS osteosarcoma cells selectively expressing the individual receptor isoforms, each subtype was found to regulate both a common and a unique set of genes.[66] Of the approximately 6500 genes regulated by at least one GRα isoform, less than 500 were regulated commonly by all the receptor isoforms. Thus the majority of glucocorticoid-responsive genes were selectively regulated by different GRα subtypes. These isoform-unique gene regulatory profiles were further shown to produce functional differences in cellular responsiveness to glucocorticoids; the GRα translational isoforms exhibited distinct capabilities to induce apoptosis.[66] Cells expressing GRα-C3 were the most sensitive to the apoptosis-inducing actions of glucocorticoids, whereas cells expressing GRα-D3 were the most resistant. Isoform-selective differences in the induction of the proapoptotic enzymes granzyme A and caspase-6 may account for the observed phenotype.

GR Control of Inflammation and Immune Response

There are two general mechanisms by which ligand-activated GR controls inflammation and the immune response. First, GR protects cells at sites of injury or inflammation from undergoing inflammation-induced apoptosis. This is accomplished by both positive and negative regulation of gene transcription and protein expression. GR stimulates production of antiinflammatory proteins such as secretory leukocyte protease inhibitor, IL-1 receptor antagonist, IL-10, and neutral endopeptidase.[2] In addition, by regulating the activity of NF-κB, AP-1, and STATs, GR inhibits the expression of a variety genes important to the control of inflammation and the immune response, including proinflammatory cytokines (e.g., IL-2, IL-3, IL-6, and TNF-α), chemokines that attract inflammatory cells to sites of inflammation, nitric oxide synthase (NOS), and cyclooxygenase 2 (COX-2), among others.[2] The second mechanism by which GR controls inflammation and the immune response is by inducing programmed cell death in immune cells that underlie inflammation. Glucocorticoids reduce the survival of eosinophils, T lymphocytes, mast cells, and dendritic cells.[2] Although the mechanisms and target proteins responsible for GR-induced apoptosis are not well understood, GR-dependent control of transcription has been reported to be involved in the initiation of programmed cell death in lymphocytes.[67]

The proper modulation of immune system activity and inflammation is critical to normal human function. A blunted immune response leaves the door open for potentially fatal infections, whereas an overstimulated immune response can result in autoimmune activity that damages organs. Glucocorticoids are potent modulators of the immune response and use a variety of GR-dependent mechanisms to accomplish this regulation on target genes. The traditional view that glucocorticoids exert these effects through one receptor isoform has changed dramatically in recent years with the discovery of a family of receptor isoforms arising from alternative processing of the single GR gene. These receptor isoforms possess unique expression, functional, and gene-regulatory profiles. Moreover, the potential for these isoforms to undergo posttranslational modifications and to function as monomers, homodimers, and/or heterodimers on both common and unique sets of genes provides cells with a wealth of possibilities for controlling the immune response with fine-tuned precision. Important goals of future research will be to determine the contribution each isoform makes to the specificity and sensitivity of glucocorticoid responsiveness and to assess whether changes in the cellular expression of these isoforms contribute to the etiology of various inflammatory and immune diseases.

GLUCOCORTICOID RECEPTOR RESISTANCE*

Generalized glucocorticoid resistance (GGR) is a rare disorder characterized by ACTH-dependent hypercortisolism and the absence of the clinical features of glucocorticoid excess. Adrenocorticotropin (ACTH)-mediated overproduction of adrenal

---

*The section titled "Glucocorticoid Receptor Resistance" was written by Carl D. Malchoff and Diana Malchoff.

androgens and mineralocorticoids produces a clinical syndrome in some individuals. The disorder is often receptor-mediated, and 10 distinct human glucocorticoid receptor alpha (hGR) mutations have been described. Therapy is reserved for those patients with significant clinical abnormalities.

History

Vingerhoeds et al. first described generalized glucocorticoid resistance, also known as *primary cortisol resistance*, in 1976.[68] It is quite rare; fewer than 30 separate probands have been reported.[68-79] It is sometimes caused by functionally abnormal hGRs. The clinical presentation of glucocorticoid resistance varies from asymptomatic hypercortisolism to clinical syndromes of mineralocorticoid or adrenal androgen excess. Since the first description of a pathogenetic hGR mutation in 1990,[80,81] nine other pathogenetic hGR mutations have been identified.[69,77-79,82-85]

Pathogenesis

ENDOCRINE PATHOPHYSIOLOGY

GGR may be caused by abnormal hGR. This was first demonstrated in assays of hGR function.[70-76] More recent studies have validated this expectation by identifying hGR mutations[69,77-85] that decrease hGR-mediated gene transcription.

The clinical findings are a consequence of impaired hGR function. The HPA axis and its negative feedback regulation of cortisol production are described elsewhere. The glucocorticoid sensitivity of all tissues is decreased in GGR. The entire HPA axis is reset (Fig. 3-3). At the pituitary and hypothalamus, serum cortisol concentrations, which otherwise would be considered

normal, are insufficient to suppress corticotropin-releasing hormone (CRH) and adrenocorticotropic hormone (ACTH) secretion. Consequently, ACTH secretion is increased. ACTH stimulates the adrenal glands to produce greater-than-normal amounts of cortisol, adrenal androgens, and mineralocorticoids. In the peripheral tissues, the glucocorticoid resistance is equal to that of the pituitary and hypothalamus; however, sensitivity to androgens and mineralocorticoids is normal. Hence, the clinical findings are not those of glucocorticoid excess but rather those of mineralocorticoid or androgen excess. The glucocorticoid circadian rhythm and response to stress are maintained.

The resistance to cortisol is partial, and plasma ACTH concentrations can be suppressed by high doses of exogenous glucocorticoids. Complete glucocorticoid resistance may be incompatible with life, as suggested by animal models.[86]

GLUCOCORTICOID RECEPTOR ABNORMALITIES

Functionally abnormal hGRs with mutations in the primary hGR alpha structure cause GGR. However, some individuals with glucocorticoid resistance have apparently normal hGR primary structure.[79,87,88] Functional changes include decreased receptor number,[70,73] decreased receptor affinity for glucocorticoids,[70-72,84,85] decreased DNA binding,[74] thermolability,[75] delayed translocation into the nucleus,[89] and impaired coactivator interaction.[78]

No assay is completely sensitive for all hGR functional abnormalities. Binding of [³H] dexamethasone to fresh mononuclear leukocytes is used most commonly, but this is normal in some subjects.[70] Dexamethasone induction of aromatase in cultured skin fibroblasts[90] and dexamethasone suppression of mitogen-stimulated thymidine incorporation into mononuclear leukocytes[70] have been used as assays for glucocorticoid resistance.

Pathogenetic mutations of the hGR gene have been found in some subjects. A splice-site microdeletion, which interferes with hGR messenger RNA (mRNA) processing and reduces the hGR number by 50%, causes glucocorticoid resistance in one kindred.[69] Fig. 3-4 summarizes the nine missense point mutations that are known to cause glucocorticoid resistance. The original subject of Vingerhoeds et al., who presented with hyper-

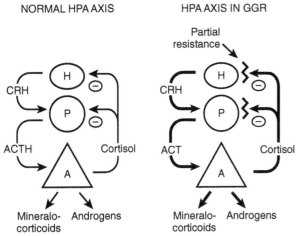

NORMAL HPA AXIS   **HPA AXIS IN GGR**

FIGURE 3-3. Hypothalamic-pituitary-adrenal (HPA) axis in normal and in generalized glucocorticoid resistance subjects. Normally, corticotropin-releasing hormone (CRH) from the hypothalamus (H) stimulates the pituitary (P) to produce adrenocorticotropic hormone (ACTH). ACTH stimulates the adrenal (A) to produce of mineralocorticoids, cortisol, and adrenal androgens. Cortisol inhibits (−) secretion of CRH and ACTH from the hypothalamus and pituitary, respectively. In GGR, there is partial blockade of the negative feedback at the pituitary and hypothalamus. This causes increased secretion of CRH and ACTH. ACTH stimulates the adrenal gland to make excess glucocorticoids, mineralocorticoids, and androgens. The HPA axis is qualitatively normal but quantitatively reset at higher hormone concentrations than normal. (Adapted from Javier EC, Reardon GE, Malchoff CD: Glucocorticoid resistance and its clinical presentations. Endocrinologist 1:141–148, 1991.)

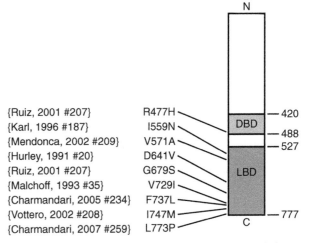

{Ruiz, 2001 #207}   R477H
{Karl, 1996 #187}   I559N
{Mendonca, 2002 #209}   V571A
{Hurley, 1991 #20}   D641V
{Ruiz, 2001 #207}   G679S
{Malchoff, 1993 #35}   V729I
{Charmandari, 2005 #234} F737L
{Vottero, 2002 #208}   I747M
{Charmandari, 2007 #259} L773P

FIGURE 3-4. Diagrammatic representation of the human glucocorticoid receptor (hGR) point mutations in generalized glucocorticoid resistance. The DNA-binding domain (*light gray*) and ligand-binding domain (*dark gray*) are two of the major functional units of the receptor. Point mutations have been identified at the indicated amino acids (aa).[77-79,81-85] Not shown is a splice-site microdeletion that disrupts processing of the hGR messenger RNA.[69]

tension and hypokalemia, is homozygous for an aspartate-to-valine change at amino acid 641.[82] The heterozygous I559N and I747M mutations cause more severe glucocorticoid resistance than would be expected for a single allele defect, suggesting a dominant negative effect.[78,83,89] Most hGR mutations causing glucocorticoid resistance are located in the LBD and interfere with ligand binding.[77,79-85] Only one has been described within the DNA-binding domain.[79] Some hGR mutations are silent polymorphisms.[87] Therefore, identification of an hGR gene mutation is not conclusive evidence of GGR. In some subjects, no hGR mutation is identified, and the cause remains unknown.[79]

At high concentrations, the beta isoform of the glucocorticoid receptor (hGRβ), which does not bind ligand, interferes with the action of the alpha isoform of the hGR.[49] Increased expression of the hGRβ combined with markedly decreased expression of the hGR is suggested to be the cause of GGR in one subject.[91]

In large population studies, the relatively common R23K hGR polymorphism is associated with decreased glucocorticoid sensitivity,[92,93] whereas the N363S polymorphism is associated with increased glucocorticoid sensitivity[94] in peripheral tissues. This suggests that the effects of these polymorphisms are not precisely equal in the pituitary and in different peripheral tissues. In support of this hypothesis, the wild-type and N363S hGR were found to mediate different gene expression profiles, as determined by microarray analysis, even though they demonstrated similar glucocorticoid sensitivity in reporter gene assays.[95]

Clinical Features

PHENOTYPIC CHARACTERISTICS

The clinical characteristics of GGR are based on the rare cases reported in the literature. Therefore, the apparent relative frequencies of the different clinical presentations may change as more affected individuals are completely evaluated.

The most common characteristic is hypercortisolism without features of glucocorticoid excess. It was this finding that led to the first description of the syndrome,[68] and occasionally it is discovered during the investigation of other problems unrelated to glucocorticoid resistance.[73] However, the diagnosis of glucocorticoid resistance may not be straightforward. Hypercortisolism is most frequently characterized by an elevated urinary cortisol excretion. However, this may not be a universal finding; some subjects demonstrate resistance only upon testing with dexamethasone.[70] It may be difficult to differentiate glucocorticoid resistance from Cushing's syndrome based on clinical features, since many clinical features of Cushing's syndrome are nonspecific.

Although hypercortisolism without cushingoid features usually suggests the diagnosis, this constellation of features usually does not bring the patient to clinical attention. The presenting clinical features are secondary to excess androgens or mineralocorticoids. The most common clinical presentation is evidence of increased androgens in women. This was the presentation in four of the six probands described by Lamberts et al.[70] and in two probands with hGR mutations described by Ruiz et al.[79] Characteristics include hirsutism, acne, and menstrual irregularities. This presentation is caused by the increased adrenal androgens. In children, isosexual precocious pseudopuberty was the clinical presentation in a 6½-year-old boy[71] but has not been described in others. Although heterosexual precocious pseudopuberty has not been described in a girl, a female newborn did present with ambiguous genitalia.[77] It is not clear why presentations in childhood are not more common. The clinical features may be overlooked because they are subtle. Infertility in men has been reported and is secondary to the increased adrenal androgen production and subsequent suppression of the hypothalamic-pituitary-testicular axis.[83] Hypertension and hypokalemia were the presenting clinical findings of the first subject described by Vingerhoeds et al.[68] Hypertension with severe thiazide-induced hypokalemia occurred in another patient.[70] Other subjects have been found to be hypertensive without hypokalemia.[70,73,74] In these latter cases, the contribution of GGR to the hypertension is less clear, since essential hypertension is common.

At least one subject with glucocorticoid resistance developed nodular adrenal hyperplasia.[70] The frequency of this event in all affected subjects has not been ascertained.

In general, individuals with the greatest degree of hypercortisolism produce the most androgens and mineralocorticoids and subsequently have the most obvious clinical findings. Variability of clinical characteristics within a kindred may be due in part to a gene dose effect. Homozygotes are affected to a greater degree than heterozygotes. In addition, some mutations have a dominant negative effect, so that heterozygotes are more severely affected than expected for inactivation of a single allele.[89] Women seem to be affected more frequently than men. This may be an ascertainment bias, since women are most likely to present with clinical features of increased adrenal androgens. It is not clear why androgen effects predominate in some patients, whereas the mineralocorticoid effects predominate in others.

One subject with severe GGR and a missense hGR mutation developed Cushing's syndrome due to an ACTH-secreting pituitary adenoma.[83] Presumably, the hGR mutation was the initial tumorigenic abnormality, which combined with other somatic pituitary gene mutations to effect the adenoma phenotype.

The possibility of tissue-specific or localized glucocorticoid resistance is in early stages of investigation. It does occur in some neoplasms. In ACTH-dependent Cushing's syndrome, the pituitary or the ectopic ACTH source is well known to be more resistant to glucocorticoids than are the normal tissues. The molecular basis of this resistance is being probed; hGR mutations, gene deletions, or both, occur in some circumstances.[83,94,96,97] Some neoplasms of hematopoietic origin demonstrate glucocorticoid resistance to apoptosis, and in some cell lines derived from these neoplasms, hGR mutations have been shown to cause glucocorticoid resistance.[98,99] It is attractive to speculate that differences in tissue sensitivity to glucocorticoids could contribute to the development of clinical disorders such as glucocorticoid-resistant asthma,[100] rheumatoid arthritis,[101] obesity,[102] hypertension,[103] insulin resistance, and diabetes.[104] It is also possible that infection with the HIV virus may increase[105,106] or decrease[107] glucocorticoid sensitivity. Studies of these possible relationships and their mechanisms are evolving.

INHERITANCE PATTERN

Initial studies suggested an autosomal-dominant transmission of GGR. The inheritance pattern may vary depending upon the exact hGR mutation. It is clearly autosomal dominant in the kindred, with a splice-site microdeletion of one allele.[69] In the kindred described by Vingerhoeds et al.[68] and investigated further in collaboration with Loriaux and Chrousos,[72,108] the proband, who is most severely affected, is homozygous for a mutation of the hGR ligand-binding domain. The son and nephew, who are mildly affected, are both heterozygous.[68,72,82,108] Therefore, in this kindred, the disorder is recessive, or there is a gene dose effect. The hGR mutation in one family arose as a new mutation, so that both parents were unaffected.[83] However, this individual had more severe glucocorticoid resistance than would be expected from an abnormality of a single allele, and subsequent in vitro studies indicate that the mutant receptor had a dominant negative effect.[89] Extensive family studies noting genotype-phenotype correlations have not been performed. In summary, inheritance patterns vary, and biochemical investigation of familial members may not identify all the subjects carrying the mutant hGR allele.

BIOCHEMICAL CHARACTERISTICS

Hypercortisolism, usually measured as increased urinary cortisol excretion, was found in most affected individuals.[68,70,72-74,76] Occasionally, urinary cortisol excretion is normal, and resistance to dexamethasone suppression is the only abnormality.[70] In contrast, in the most severely affected patients, urinary cortisol excretion may exceed the upper-normal limit by 200-fold.[68,70] This considerable variability suggests heterogeneity in the degree of resistance and in the pathogenetic receptor abnormality.

Hypercortisolism of GGR is distinguished from that of Cushing's syndrome by the presence of a diurnal variation in serum cortisol. As discussed before, the HPA axis is qualitatively normal but quantitatively reset with higher-than-normal hormone concentrations. Serum cortisol concentrations usually decrease by at least 50% from 8 AM to 8 PM in normal subjects[109] and in glucocorticoid-resistant subjects,[70-72] whereas in Cushing's syndrome, there is loss of the diurnal variation.[110] An example of the diurnal variation of serum cortisol reset at higher-than-normal concentrations in a subject with generalized glucocorticoid resistance is shown in Fig. 3-5.

Serum cortisol concentrations can be increased up to eightfold above normal but may be normal if the resistance is mild.[68,70,72] Comparison of cortisol concentrations must be made with controls from the same time of day. The 8 AM serum cortisol is normally not suppressed by 1 mg of dexamethasone given orally at 11 PM the previous evening.[70] Cortisol production is ACTH-dependent, and plasma ACTH concentrations can be suppressed by supraphysiologic glucocorticoid doses.[71,72] Plasma ACTH concentrations are less frequently increased above the normal range than are cortisol concentrations but tend to be the highest in individuals with the greatest resistance.

Adrenal androgens (androstenedione, dehydroepiandrosterone, and dehydroepiandrosterone sulfate) are increased in most children and women.[68,70-74,76] These increases range from mild to fivefold above the upper normal limit, and they can be suppressed by high doses of glucocorticoids.

The mineralocorticoids have been less extensively studied. However, when they have been measured, deoxycorticosterone (DOC) and corticosterone are usually increased by two- to fivefold above the upper-normal limit, aldosterone concentrations are low, and plasma renin activity is suppressed.[71-74] Production of DOC and corticosterone is ACTH-dependent.[111] The high concentrations of DOC and/or cortisol cause hypokalemia and volume-dependent hypertension by activating the aldosterone receptor. Volume expansion suppresses plasma renin activity.

Diagnosis

GGR is suspected in the setting of hypercortisolism without cushingoid features. The differential diagnosis includes Cushing's syndrome, depression, increased cortisol-binding globulin, and drug interference with cortisol assays.

It can be difficult to distinguish cortisol resistance from Cushing's syndrome, since no single test is completely discriminatory. Individuals with glucocorticoid resistance lack clinical features of glucocorticoid excess. However, many features of glucocorticoid excess can be subtle, and others are nonspecific. The usual tests used to distinguish Cushing's syndrome subjects from normal subjects do not distinguish Cushing's syndrome subjects from GGR subjects. In both Cushing's syndrome and GGR, urinary cortisol excretion is elevated, dexamethasone suppression tests are abnormal, and (presumably) late-night salivary cortisol will be elevated. Studies that demonstrate the qualitative integrity of the HPA axis help to distinguish Cushing's syndrome from GGR. The diurnal rhythm is found in glucocorticoid resistance but is absent in Cushing's syndrome (see Fig. 3-5). There is a normal response to hypoglycemic stress in GGR[71] but not in Cushing's syndrome.[112] These tests have been useful in a limited number of patients, but cortisol concentrations in Cushing's syndrome may vary throughout the day[110] and mimic a diurnal variation. Clinical judgment and repeated evaluations over time are essential.

In children, the growth curves may help to distinguish subjects with GGR from those with Cushing's syndrome. In Cushing's syndrome, growth is slowed. Although the growth curves in most GGR subjects have not been carefully examined, it seems unlikely that growth would be slowed. In one GGR child presenting with isosexual precocious pseudopuberty, growth was accelerated compared to the expected normal rate. This accelerated growth was associated with advanced bone age, and both were caused by increased adrenal androgens.[71]

Other diagnostic considerations include increased cortisol-binding globulin (CBG) and pharmaceuticals that interfere with the cortisol assays. Increased CBG may imitate glucocorticoid resistance, since it causes high serum cortisol concentrations with a diurnal variation. Radioimmunoassays for CBG are commercially available, and CBG is normal in glucocorticoid resistance.[71,72] Carbamazepine interferes with testing of the HPA axis in multiple ways. It increases the rate of dexamethasone metabolism, so patients may appear dexamethasone resistant. Patients taking carbamazepine demonstrate increased circulating cortisol

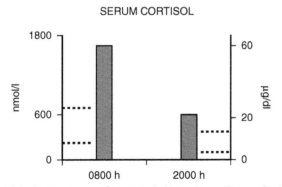

SERUM CORTISOL

FIGURE 3-5. Diurnal variation of serum cortisol in a subject with generalized glucocorticoid resistance. Serum cortisol concentrations are represented in nanomoles per liter on the left ordinate and in micrograms per deciliter on the right ordinate. The 8 AM and 8 PM serum cortisol concentrations from a patient with glucocorticoid resistance are shown. The results are the mean of three separate determinations. The normal range of serum cortisol at 8 AM is shown by the dotted lines on the left ordinate, and the normal range at 8 PM is shown by the dotted lines on the right ordinate. (Adapted from Malchoff CD, Javier EC, Malchoff DM et al: Primary cortisol resistance presenting as isosexual precocity. J Clin Endocrinol Metab 70:503–507, 1990. © The Endocrine Society.)

concentrations and increased urinary cortisol excretion, although usually not out of the normal range, as occurs in glucocorticoid resistance.[113] Finally, both carbamazepine and fenofibrate or their metabolites may interfere with some of the commercial high-performance liquid chromatography (HPLC) assays for cortisol and produce a false elevation.[114,115]

Since the most common clinical presentation of generalized glucocorticoid resistance is hyperandrogenism in women, this disorder should be considered in the differential diagnosis of the polycystic ovary syndrome and idiopathic hirsutism. Subjects with hypertension and hypokalemia but without increased aldosterone should be evaluated for glucocorticoid resistance so they are not mistaken for other rare causes of volume-dependent hypertension.

If the clinical and biochemical studies suggest the diagnosis of glucocorticoid resistance, then direct hGR functional studies may be confirmatory. As discussed, a number of functional receptor abnormalities have been reported.[70-76] Unfortunately, these different studies require fresh or cultured mononuclear leukocytes or fibroblasts and are not commercially available. In addition, there may be other causes of abnormal ligand-binding assays. The apparent receptor number may be slightly decreased in Cushing's syndrome,[116] and in patients with AIDS, the hGR may have a decreased affinity for glucocorticoids.[117] Finally, there are some glucocorticoid-resistant subjects with normal hGR ligand binding. Therefore, even this research tool is not completely sensitive or specific.

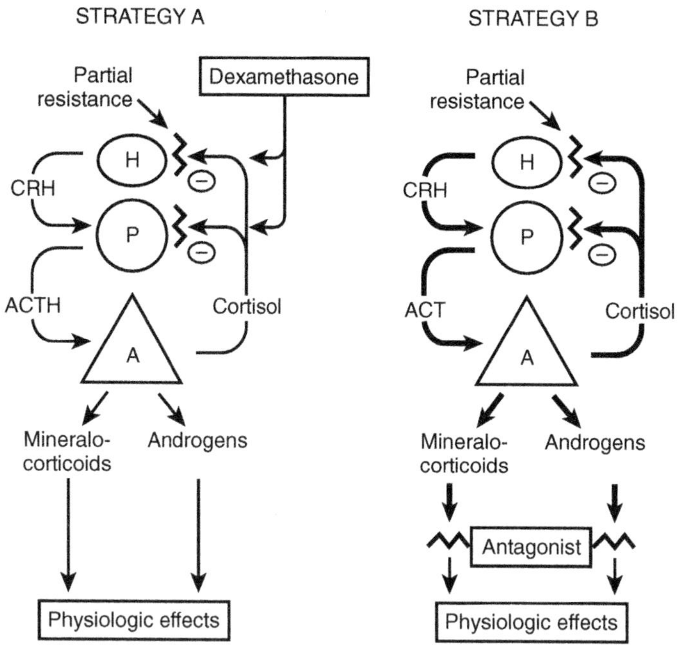

Treatment

There is limited experience with treatment of this rare disorder. Therapy is reserved for those with significant clinical features.

The most common approach to therapy is the use of exogenous glucocorticoids (Fig. 3-6, strategy A). It has been used for patients with hypertension and hypokalemia,[70,118] with sexual precocity,[111] and for women with hirsutism.[70,76] The goal is to suppress adrenal androgen and mineralocorticoid concentrations without using so much dexamethasone as to cause Cushing's syndrome. Dexamethasone, which does not interfere with radioimmunoassays for cortisol, is chosen so that serum cortisol concentrations can be monitored and titrated into the normal range.[70,76,111] With this therapy, androgens and mineralocorticoids fall, and the clinical features improve.[70,76,111,118]

An alternative approach (see Fig. 3-6, strategy B) is to use mineralocorticoid or androgen antagonists. For example, hyper-

FIGURE 3-6. Treatment strategies for generalized glucocorticoid resistance. Two strategies have been proposed. In the first strategy (A), exogenous glucocorticoids (usually dexamethasone) are administered to decrease adrenocorticotropic hormone (ACTH) secretion and subsequently decrease the secretion of adrenal mineralocorticoids and androgens. The dose is adjusted to titrate cortisol into the normal range. In the second (B), mineralocorticoid and androgen antagonists block the peripheral effects of the hormones, producing clinical effects. CRH, Corticotropin-releasing hormone; H, hypothalamus; P, pituitary; A, adrenal gland. (Adapted from Malchoff CD, Malchoff DM, Reardon G: Glucocorticoid resistance. In Bardin CW (ed): Current Therapy in Endocrinology and Metabolism, 5th ed. St. Louis: Mosby-Year Book, 1994, pp 167–171.)

tension and hypokalemia should be treatable with spironolactone, which blocks the mineralocorticoid receptor, or with amiloride, which blocks the sodium-potassium exchange in the distal tubule.

No therapy is indicated for biochemically affected subjects who are otherwise asymptomatic. Adrenal insufficiency is not a common feature of this disease, since the block of glucocorticoid effects is partial, and there is considerable reserve for increased cortisol production by the adrenal gland. However, glucocorticoids should not be withheld from a resistant subject if adrenal insufficiency is suspected during a significant physical stress.

REFERENCES

1. Rhen T, Cidlowski JA: Antiinflammatory action of glucocorticoids—new mechanisms for old drugs, N Engl J Med 353:1711–1723, 2005.
2. Barnes PJ: Anti-inflammatory actions of glucocorticoids: molecular mechanisms, Clin Sci (Lond) 94:557–572, 1998.
3. Sapolsky RM, Romero LM, Munck AU: How do glucocorticoids influence stress responses? Integrating permissive, suppressive, stimulatory, and preparative actions, Endocr Rev 21:55–89, 2000.
4. Miner JN, Hong MH, Negro-Vilar A: New and improved glucocorticoid receptor ligands, Expert Opin Investig Drugs 14:1527–1545, 2005.
5. Chrousos GP, Kino T: Intracellular glucocorticoid signaling: a formerly simple system turns stochastic, Sci STKE 48: 2005.
6. Evans RM: The steroid and thyroid hormone receptor superfamily, Science 240:889–895, 1988.
7. Kumar R, Thompson EB: Gene regulation by the glucocorticoid receptor:structure:function relationship, J Steroid Biochem Mol Biol 94:383–394, 2005.
8. Duma D, Jewell CM, Cidlowski JA: Multiple glucocorticoid receptor isoforms and mechanisms of post-translational modification, J Steroid Biochem Mol Biol 102:11–21, 2006.
9. Pratt WB, Toft DO: Steroid receptor interactions with heat shock protein and immunophilin chaperones, Endocr Rev 18:306–360, 1997.
10. Lu NZ, Cidlowski JA: Glucocorticoid receptor isoforms generate transcription specificity, Trends Cell Biol 16:301–307, 2006.
11. Beato M: Gene regulation by steroid hormones, Cell 56:335–344, 1989.
12. Freedman LP: Anatomy of the steroid receptor zinc finger region, Endocr Rev 13:129–145, 1992.
13. Drouin J, Sun YL, Tremblay S, et al: Homodimer formation is rate-limiting for high affinity DNA binding by glucocorticoid receptor, Mol Endocrinol 6:1299–1309, 1992.
14. McNally JG, Muller WG, Walker D, et al: The glucocorticoid receptor: rapid exchange with regulatory sites in living cells, Science 287:1262–1265, 2000.
15. Lonard DM, O'Malley BW: Expanding functional diversity of the coactivators, Trends Biochem Sci 30:126–132, 2005.
16. Dostert A, Heinzel T: Negative glucocorticoid receptor response elements and their role in glucocorticoid action, Curr Pharm Des 10:2807–2816, 2004.
17. Meyer T, Gustafsson JA, Carlstedt-Duke J: Glucocorticoid-dependent transcriptional repression of the osteocalcin gene by competitive binding at the TATA box, DNA Cell Biol 16:919–927, 1997.

18. Diamond MI, Miner JN, Yoshinaga SK, et al: Transcription factor interactions: selectors of positive or negative regulation from a single DNA element, Science 249:1266–1272, 1990.

19. Malkoski SP, Dorin RI: Composite glucocorticoid regulation at a functionally defined negative glucocorticoid response element of the human corticotropin-releasing hormone gene, Mol Endocrinol 13:1629–1644, 1999.

20. Chandran UR, Warren BS, Baumann CT, et al: The glucocorticoid receptor is tethered to DNA-bound Oct-1 at the mouse gonadotropin-releasing hormone distal negative glucocorticoid response element, J Biol Chem 274:2372–2378, 1999.

21. Martens C, Bilodeau S, Maira M, et al: Protein-protein interactions and transcriptional antagonism between the subfamily of NGFI-B/Nur77 orphan nuclear receptors and glucocorticoid receptor, Mol Endocrinol 19:885–897, 2005.

22. Necela BM, Cidlowski JA: Mechanisms of glucocorticoid receptor action in noninflammatory and inflammatory cells, Proc Am Thorac Soc 1:239–246, 2004.

23. Newton R, Holden NS: Separating transrepression and transactivation: a distressing divorce for the glucocorticoid receptor? Mol Pharmacol 72:799–809, 2007.

24. De Bosscher K, Vanden Berghe W, Haegeman G: The interplay between the glucocorticoid receptor and nuclear factor-kappaB or activator protein-1: molecular mechanisms for gene repression, Endocr Rev 24:488–522, 2003.

25. Caelles C, Gonzalez-Sancho JM, Munoz A: Nuclear hormone receptor antagonism with AP-1 by inhibition of the JNK pathway, Genes Dev 11:3351–3364, 1997.

26. Smoak K, Cidlowski JA: Glucocorticoids regulate tristetraprolin synthesis and posttranscriptionally regulate tumor necrosis factor alpha inflammatory signaling, Mol Cell Biol 26:9126–9135, 2006.

27. Ogawa S, Lozach J, Benner C, et al: Molecular determinants of crosstalk between nuclear receptors and toll-like receptors, Cell 122:707–721, 2005.

28. Nissen RM, Yamamoto KR: The glucocorticoid receptor inhibits NF-kappaB by interfering with serine-2 phosphorylation of the RNA polymerase II carboxy-terminal domain, Genes Dev 14:2314–2329, 2000.

29. Rogatsky I, Luecke HF, Leitman DC, et al: Alternate surfaces of transcriptional coregulator GRIP1 function in different glucocorticoid receptor activation and repression contexts, Proc Natl Acad Sci U S A 99:16701–16706, 2002.

30. Ito K, Barnes PJ, Adcock IM: Glucocorticoid receptor recruitment of histone deacetylase 2 inhibits interleukin-1beta-induced histone H4 acetylation on lysines 8 and 12, Mol Cell Biol 20:6891–6903, 2000.

31. Rogatsky I, Ivashkiv LB: Glucocorticoid modulation of cytokine signaling, Tissue Antigens 68:1–12, 2006.

32. Lerner L, Henriksen MA, Zhang X, et al: STAT3-dependent enhanceosome assembly and disassembly: synergy with GR for full transcriptional increase of the alpha 2-macroglobulin gene, Genes Dev 17:2564–2577, 2003.

33. Takeda T, Kurachi H, Yamamoto T, et al: Crosstalk between the interleukin 6 (IL-6)-JAK-STAT and the glucocorticoid-nuclear receptor pathway: synergistic activation of IL-6 response element by IL-6 and glucocorticoid, J Endocrinol 159:323–330, 1998.

34. Zhang Z, Jones S, Hagood JS, et al: STAT3 acts as a co-activator of glucocorticoid receptor signaling, J Biol Chem 272:30607–30610, 1997.

35. Stocklin E, Wissler M, Gouilleux F, et al: Functional interactions between Stat5 and the glucocorticoid receptor, Nature 383:726–728, 1996.

36. Stoecklin E, Wissler M, Moriggl R, et al: Specific DNA binding of Stat5, but not of glucocorticoid receptor, is required for their functional cooperation in the regulation of gene transcription, Mol Cell Biol 17:6708–6716, 1997.

37. Lechner J, Welte T, Tomasi JK, et al: Promoter-dependent synergy between glucocorticoid receptor and Stat5 in the activation of beta-casein gene transcription, J Biol Chem 272:20954–20960, 1997.

38. Hermoso MA, Matsuguchi T, Smoak K, et al: Glucocorticoids and tumor necrosis factor alpha cooperatively regulate toll-like receptor 2 gene expression, Mol Cell Biol 24:4743–4756, 2004.

39. Cella N, Groner B, Hynes NE: Characterization of Stat5a and Stat5b homodimers and heterodimers and their association with the glucocorticoid receptor in mammary cells, Mol Cell Biol 18:1783–1792, 1998.

40. Wyszomierski SL, Yeh J, Rosen JM: Glucocorticoid receptor/signal transducer and activator of transcription 5 (STAT5) interactions enhance STAT5 activation by prolonging STAT5 DNA binding and tyrosine phosphorylation, Mol Endocrinol 13:330–343, 1999.

41. Biola A, Lefebvre P, Perrin-Wolff M, et al: Interleukin 2 inhibits glucocorticoid receptor transcriptional activity through a mechanism involving STAT5 (signal transducer and activator of transcription 5) but not AP-1, Mol Endocrinol 15:1062–1076, 2001.

42. De Miguel F, Lee SO, Onate SA, et al: Stat3 enhances transactivation of steroid hormone receptors, Nucl Recept 1:3, 2003.

43. Encio IJ, Detera-Wadleigh SD: The genomic structure of the human glucocorticoid receptor, J Biol Chem 266:7182–7188, 1991.

44. Francke U, Foellmer BE: The glucocorticoid receptor gene is in 5q31-q32 [corrected], Genomics 4:610–612, 1989.

45. Oakley RH, Sar M, Cidlowski JA: The human glucocorticoid receptor beta isoform. Expression, biochemical properties, and putative function, J Biol Chem 271:9550–9559, 1996.

46. Theriault A, Boyd E, Harrap SB, et al: Regional chromosomal assignment of the human glucocorticoid receptor gene to 5q31, Hum Genet 83:289–291, 1989.

47. Hollenberg SM, Weinberger C, Ong ES, et al: Primary structure and expression of a functional human glucocorticoid receptor cDNA, Nature 318:635–641, 1985.

48. Oakley RH, Webster JC, Sar M, et al: Expression and subcellular distribution of the beta-isoform of the human glucocorticoid receptor, Endocrinology 138:5028–5038, 1997.

49. Bamberger CM, Bamberger AM, de Castro M, et al: Glucocorticoid receptor beta, a potential endogenous inhibitor of glucocorticoid action in humans, J Clin Invest 95:2435–2441, 1995.

50. Lewis-Tuffin LJ, Cidlowski JA: The physiology of human glucocorticoid receptor beta (hGRbeta) and glucocorticoid resistance, Ann N Y Acad Sci 1069:1–9, 2006.

51. Oakley RH, Jewell CM, Yudt MR, et al: The dominant negative activity of the human glucocorticoid receptor beta isoform. Specificity and mechanisms of action, J Biol Chem 274:27857–27866, 1999.

52. Hauk PJ, Hamid QA, Chrousos GP, et al: Induction of corticosteroid insensitivity in human PBMCs by microbial superantigens, J Allergy Clin Immunol 105:782–787, 2000.

53. Orii F, Ashida T, Nomura M, et al: Quantitative analysis for human glucocorticoid receptor alpha/beta mRNA in IBD, Biochem Biophys Res Commun 296:1286–1294, 2002.

54. Strickland I, Kisich K, Hauk PJ, et al: High constitutive glucocorticoid receptor beta in human neutrophils enables them to reduce their spontaneous rate of cell death in response to corticosteroids, J Exp Med 193:585–593, 2001.

55. Tliba O, Cidlowski JA, Amrani Y: CD38 expression is insensitive to steroid action in cells treated with tumor necrosis factor-alpha and interferon-gamma by a mechanism involving the up-regulation of the glucocorticoid receptor beta isoform, Mol Pharmacol 69:588–596, 2006.

56. Webster JC, Oakley RH, Jewell CM, et al: Proinflammatory cytokines regulate human glucocorticoid receptor gene expression and lead to the accumulation of the dominant negative beta isoform: a mechanism for the generation of glucocorticoid resistance, Proc Natl Acad Sci U S A 98:6865–6870, 2001.

57. Goecke IA, Alvarez C, Henriquez J, et al: Methotrexate regulates the expression of glucocorticoid receptor alpha and beta isoforms in normal human peripheral mononuclear cells and human lymphocyte cell lines in vitro, Mol Immunol 44:2115–2123, 2007.

58. Derijk RH, Schaaf MJ, Turner G, et al: A human glucocorticoid receptor gene variant that increases the stability of the glucocorticoid receptor beta-isoform mRNA is associated with rheumatoid arthritis, J Rheumatol 28:2383–2388, 2001.

59. Schaaf MJ, Cidlowski JA: AUUUA motifs in the 3′ UTR of human glucocorticoid receptor alpha and beta mRNA destabilize mRNA and decrease receptor protein expression, Steroids 67:627–636, 2002.

60. Syed AA, Irving JA, Redfern CP, et al: Association of glucocorticoid receptor polymorphism A3669G in exon 9beta with reduced central adiposity in women, Obesity (Silver Spring) 14:759–764, 2006.

61. van den Akker EL, Nouwen JL, Melles DC, et al: Staphylococcus aureus nasal carriage is associated with glucocorticoid receptor gene polymorphisms, J Infect Dis 194:814–818, 2006.

62. van den Akker EL, Koper JW, van Rossum EF, et al: Glucocorticoid receptor gene and risk of cardiovascular disease, Arch Intern Med 168:33–39, 2008.

63. Lewis-Tuffin LJ, Jewell CM, Bienstock RJ et al: Human glucocorticoid receptor β binds RU-486 and is transcriptionally active, Mol Cell Biol 27:2266–2282, 2007.

64. Lu NZ, Cidlowski JA: Translational regulatory mechanisms generate N-terminal glucocorticoid receptor isoforms with unique transcriptional target genes, Mol Cell 18:331–342, 2005.

65. Yudt MR, Cidlowski JA: Molecular identification and characterization of a and b forms of the glucocorticoid receptor, Mol Endocrinol 15:1093–1103, 2001.

66. Lu NZ, Collins JB, Grissom SF, et al: Selective regulation of bone cell apoptosis by translational isoforms of the glucocorticoid receptor, Mol Cell Biol 27:7143–7160, 2007.

67. Distelhorst CW: Recent insights into the mechanism of glucocorticosteroid-induced apoptosis, Cell Death Differ 9:6–19, 2002.

68. Vingerhoeds A, Thijssen J, Shwarz F: Spontaneous hypercortisolism without Cushing's syndrome, J Clin Endocrinol Metab 43:1128–1133, 1976.

69. Karl M, Lamberts SWJ, Detera-Wadleigh SD, et al: Familial glucocorticoid resistance caused by a splice site deletion in the human glucocorticoid receptor gene, J Clin Endocrinol Metab 76:683–689, 1993.

70. Lamberts SWJ, Koper JW, Biemond P, et al: Cortisol receptor resistance: the variability of its clinical presentation and response to treatment, J Clin Endocrinol Metab 74:313–321, 1992.

71. Malchoff C, Javier E, Malchoff D, et al: Primary cortisol resistance presenting as isosexual precocity, J Clin Endocrinol Metab 70:503–507, 1990.

72. Chrousos GP, Vingerhoeds ACM, Brandon D, et al: Primary cortisol resistance in man: a glucocorticoid receptor-mediated disease, J Clin Invest 69:1261–1269, 1982.

73. Iida S, Gomi M, Moriwaki K, et al: Primary cortisol resistance accompanied by a reduction in glucocorticoid receptors in two members of the same family, J Clin Endocrinol Metab 60:967–971, 1985.

74. Nawata H, Sekiya K, Higuchi K, et al: Decreased deoxyribonucleic acid binding of glucocorticoid-receptor complex in cultured skin fibroblasts from a patient with glucocorticoid resistance syndrome, J Clin Endocrinol Metab 65:219–226, 1987.

75. Bronnegard M, Werner S, Gustafsson J: Primary cortisol resistance associated with a thermolabile glucocorticoid receptor in a patient with fatigue as the only symptom, J Clin Invest 78:1270–1278, 1986.

76. Lamberts SWJ, Poldermans D, Zweens M, et al: Familial cortisol resistance: differential diagnostic and therapeutic aspects, J Clin Endocrinol Metab 63:1328–1333, 1986.

77. Mendonca B, Leite M, de Castro M, et al: Female pseudohermaphroditism caused by a novel homozygous missense mutation of the GR gene, J Clin Endocrinol Metab 87:1805–1809, 2002.

78. Vottero A, Kino T, Combe H, et al: A novel, C-terminal dominant negative mutation of the GR causes familial glucocorticoid resistance through abnormal interactions with p160 steroid receptor coactivators, J Clin Endocrinol Metab 87:2658–2667, 2002.

79. Ruiz M, Lind U, Gafvels M, et al: Characterization of two novel mutations in the glucocorticoid receptor gene in patients with primary cortisol resistance, Clin Endocrinol 55:363–371, 2001.

80. Brufsky A, Malchoff D, Javier E, et al: A glucocorticoid receptor mutation in a subject with primary cortisol resistance, Trans Assoc Am Phys 103:53–63, 1990.

81. Malchoff DM, Brufsky A, Reardon G, et al: A point mutation of the human glucocorticoid receptor in primary cortisol resistance, J Clin Invest 91:1918–1925, 1993.

82. Hurley D, Accili D, Stratakis C, et al: Point mutation causing a single amino acid substitution in the hormone

binding domain of the glucocorticoid receptor in familial glucocorticoid resistance, J Clin Invest 87:680–686, 1991.

83. Karl M, Lamberts SW, Koper JW, et al: Cushing's disease preceded by generalized glucocorticoid resistance: clinical consequences of a novel, dominant-negative glucocorticoid receptor mutation, Proc Assoc Am Phys 108:296–307, 1996.

84. Charmandari E, Raji A, Kino T, et al: A novel point mutation in the ligand-binding domain (LBD) of the human glucocorticoid receptor (hGR) causing generalized glucocorticoid resistance: the importance of the C terminus of HGR LBD in conferring transactivational activity, J Clin Endocrinol Metab 90:3696–3705, 2005.

85. Charmandari E, Kino T, Ichijo T, et al: A novel pint mutation in helix 11 of the ligand-binding domain of the human glucocorticoid receptor gene causing generalized glucocorticoid resistance, J Clin Endocrinol and Metab 92:3986–3990, 2007.

86. Cole TJ, Blendy JA, Monaghan AP, et al: Targeted disruption of the glucocorticoid receptor gene blocks adrenergic chromaffin cell development and severely retards lung maturation, Genes Dev 9:1608–1621, 1995.

87. Koper JW, Stolk RP, de Lange P, et al: Lack of association between five polymorphisms in the human glucocorticoid receptor gene and glucocorticoid resistance, Hum Genet 99:663–668, 1997.

88. Huizenga N, de Lange P, Koper J, et al: Five patients with biochemical and/or clinical generalized glucocorticoid resistance without alterations in the glucocorticoid receptor gene, J Clin Endocrinol Metab 85: 2076–2081, 2000.

89. Kino T, Stauber RH, Resau JH, et al: Pathologic human GR mutant has a transdominant negative effect on the wild-type GR by inhibiting its translocation into the nucleus: importance of the ligand-binding domain for intracellular GR trafficking, J Clin Endocrinol Metab 86:5600–5608, 2001.

90. Berkovitz GD, Carter KM, Levine MA, et al: Abnormal induction of aromatase activity by dexamethasone in fibroblasts from a patient with cortisol resistance, J Clin Endocrinol Metab 70:1608–1611, 1990.

91. Shahadi H, Vottero A, Stratakis C, et al: Imbalanced expression of the glucocorticoid receptor isoforms in cultured lymphocytes from a patient with systemic glucocorticoid resistance and chronic lymphocytic leukemia, Biochem Biophys Res Commun 254:559–565, 1999.

92. van Rossum E, Koper J, Huizenga N, et al: A polymorphism in the glucocorticoid receptor gene, which decreases sensitivity to glucocorticoids in vivo, is associated with low insulin and cholesterol levels, Diabetes 51:3128–3134, 2002.

93. van Rossum E, Voorhoeve P, te Velde S, et al: The ER2/23EK polymorphism in the glucocorticoid receptor gene is associated with a beneficial body composition and muscle strength in young adults, J Clin Endocrinol and Metab 89:4004–4009, 2004.

94. Huizenga NA, de Lange P, Koper JW, et al: Human adrenocorticotropin-secreting pituitary adenomas show frequent loss of heterozygosity at the glucocorticoid receptor gene locus, J Clin Endocrinol Metab 83:917–921, 1998.

95. Jewell CM, Cidlowski JA: Molecular evidence for a link between the N363S glucocorticoid receptor polymorphism and altered gene expression, J Clin Endocrinol Metab 92:3268–3277, 2007.

96. Karl M, Von Wichert G, Kempter E, et al: Nelson's syndrome associated with a somatic frame shift mutation in the glucocorticoid receptor gene, J Clin Endocrinol Metab 81:124–129, 1996.

97. Dahia PL, Honegger J, Reincke M, et al: Expression of glucocorticoid receptor gene isoforms in corticotropin-secreting tumors, J Clin Endocrinol Metab 82:1088–1093, 1997.

98. Strasser-Wozak EM, Hattmannstorfer R, Hala M, et al: Splice site mutation in the glucocorticoid receptor gene causes resistance to glucocorticoid-induced apoptosis in a human acute leukemic cell line, Cancer Res 55:348–353, 1995.

99. Hala M, Hartmann BL, Bock G, et al: Glucocorticoid-receptor gene defects and resistance to glucocorticoid-induced apoptosis in human leukemic cell lines, Int J Cancer 68:663–668, 1996.

100. Sher ER, Leung DY, Surs W, et al: Steroid resistant asthma. Cellular mechanisms contributing to inadequate response to glucocorticoid therapy, J Clin Invest 93:33–39, 1994.

101. Schlaghecke R, Kornely E, Wollenhaupt J, et al: Glucocorticoid receptors in rheumatoid arthritis, Arthritis Rheum 35:740–744, 1992.

102. Huizenga NA, Koper JW, de Lange P, et al: A polymorphism in the glucocorticoid receptor gene may be associated with an increased sensitivity to glucocorticoids in vivo. J Clin Endocrinol Metab 83:144–151, 1998.

103. Panarelli M, Holloway CD, Fraser R, et al: Glucocorticoid receptor polymorphism, skin vasoconstriction, and other metabolic intermediate phenotypes in normal human subjects, J Clin Endocrinol Metab 83:1846–1852, 1998.

104. Nyirenda MJ, Lindsay RS, Kenyon CJ, et al: Glucocorticoid exposure in late gestation permanently programs rat hepatic phosphoenolpyruvate carboxykinase and glucocorticoid receptor expression and causes glucose intolerance in adult offspring, J Clin Invest 101:2174–2181, 1998.

105. Guo WX, Antakly T, Cadotte M, et al: Expression and cytokine regulation of glucocorticoid receptors in Kaposi's sarcoma, Am J Pathol 148:1999–2008, 1996.

106. Refaeli Y, Levy DN, Weiner DB: The glucocorticoid receptor type II complex is a target of the HIV-1 *vpr* gene product, Proc Natl Acad Sci U S A 92:3621–3625, 1995.

107. Norbiato G, Bevilacqua M, Vago T, et al: Glucocorticoids and interferon-alpha in the acquired immunodeficiency syndrome, J Clin Endocrinol Metab 81: 2601–2606, 1996.

108. Chrousos G, Vingerhoeds A, Loriaux D, et al: Primary cortisol resistance: a family study, J Clin Endocrinol Metab 56:1243–1245, 1983.

109. Rivest R, Schulz P, Lustenberger S, et al: Differences between circadian and ultradian organization of cortisol and melatonin rhythms during activity and rest, J Clin Endocrinol Metab 68:721–729, 1989.

110. Van Cauter E, Refetoff S: Evidence for two subtypes of Cushing's disease based on the analysis of episodic cortisol secretion, N Engl J Med 312:1343–1349, 1985.

111. Malchoff CD, Reardon G, Javier EC, et al: Dexamethasone therapy for isosexual precocious pseudopuberty caused by generalized glucocorticoid resistance, J Clin Endocrinol Metab 79:1632–1636, 1994.

112. Besser G, Edwards C: Cushing's syndrome, Clin Endocrinol Metab 1:451–490, 1972.

113. Perini G, Devinsky O, Hauser P, et al: Effects of carbamazepine on pituitary-adrenal function in health volunteers, J Clin Endocrinol Metab 74:406–412, 1992.

114. Findling J, Pinkstaff SM, Shaker J, et al: Pseudohypercortisoluria: spurious elevation of urinary cortisol due to carbamazepine, Endocrinologist 8:51–54, 1998.

115. Meikle A, Findling J, Kushnir M, et al: Pseudo-Cushing's syndrome caused by fenofibrate interference with urinary cortisol assayed by high-performance liquid chromatography, J Clin Endocrinol Metab 88:3521–3524, 2003.

116. Kontula K, Pelkonen R, Andersson L, et al: Glucocorticoid receptors in adrenocorticoid disorders, J Clin Endocrinol Metab 51:654–657, 1980.

117. Norbiato G, Bevilacqua M, Vago T, et al: Cortisol resistance in acquired immunodeficiency syndrome, J Clin Endocrinol Metab 74:608–613, 1992.

118. Lipsett M, Tomita M, Brandon D, et al: Cortisol resistance in man, Adv Exp Med Biol 196:97–110, 1986.

Chapter 4

ALDOSTERONE: Secretion and Action

PETER FULLER

The steroid hormone aldosterone first appeared in evolution with the appearance of terrestrial life and the consequent need to conserve sodium and water.[1] The primary and best characterized actions of aldosterone are those that stimulate sodium retention in transporting epithelia, particularly the distal nephron, distal colon, and salivary glands.[2] At these epithelia, the conservation of sodium is associated with increased secretion of both potassium and hydrogen ions. Aldosterone also has so-called nonclassical actions at the heart, the vasculature, and the central nervous system.

The existence of an adrenal corticoid natriuretic factor, distinct from the other adrenocorticoid steroid hormones, had been suspected for several years before its isolation in 1953.[3] Using the toad urinary bladder as a model system, Crabbè[4] was the first to show that in vitro aldosterone increases sodium transport. Subsequent studies demonstrated the presence of binding sites for aldosterone in the toad bladder and in other target tissues, particularly the principal cell of the cortical collecting duct of the kidney.[5]

Feedback Control of Aldosterone Secretion

Both serum sodium concentration and total body sodium are maintained within a narrow range by a complex set of endocrine feedback loops (Fig. 4-1). The most important of these involves the renin-angiotensin system, which responds to volume status. The feedback loops involved with potassium homeostasis operate in parallel and overlap those for sodium.

Volume status is sensed by the renin-secreting juxtaglomerular cells of the kidney. Where the sodium status (and hence, volume) is low, renin will be secreted. Renin, an aspartyl protease, is synthesised as inactive prorenin that is activated by the action of a protease. Renin release from the juxtaglomerular cells is influenced by a number of factors (Table 4-1), including renal perfusion pressure, the sympathetic nervous system, and prostaglandins (which are stimulatory), dopamine, atrial natriuretic peptide (ANP), and angiotensin II, all of which are inhibitory. Renin acts on angiotensinogen to release the decapeptide angiotensin I, which in turn is subject to further proteolysis by angiotensin-converting enzyme, primarily in the pulmonary vascular bed, to yield the octapeptide angiotensin II. Angiotensin II acts via its specific G protein–coupled receptor in the vasculature as a potent vasoconstrictor (thereby defending plasma volume and blood pressure) and on the adrenocorticoid glomerulosa cells to stimulate aldosterone synthesis.[6] The latter response promotes sodium retention with a consequent increase in plasma volume. Aldosterone biosynthesis in the zona glomerulosa of the adrenal cortex is regulated by transcription of the aldosterone synthase gene (CYP11B2). As with other steroidogenic enzymes, steroidogenic factor-1 (SF-1) is required for aldosterone synthase expression. Members of the NR4A family of nuclear receptors have been shown to be regulators of aldosterone synthase gene expression.[7] Although angiotensin II is important in the regulation of aldosterone, a response to low-salt or high-potassium diet is also seen in mice in which the angiotensinogen gene has been deleted.[8] In these mice, the regulation of aldosterone is directed primarily by serum potassium levels.

The secretion of aldosterone is also stimulated by potassium, so a negative feedback loop exists for potassium and aldosterone. It should be noted that aldosterone also affects acid-base balance by increasing the exchange of hydrogen ions for sodium.

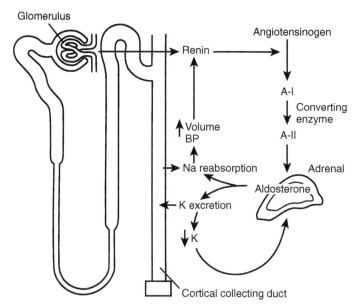

FIGURE 4-1. Interacting feedback loops controlling aldosterone secretion. Volume is regulated through the renin-angiotensin system, and potassium is regulated through direct feedback. *A-I*, Angiotensin I; *A-II*, angiotensin II; *BP*, blood pressure.

Table 4-1. Factor Regulating Renin Release

Stimulatory	Inhibitory
Decreased perfusion pressure	Increased chloride delivery at the macula densa
PGI_2	Angiotensin II
ACTH	Atrial natriuretic factor
	Vasopressin
β-Adrenergic stimulation	α-Adrenergic stimulation
	Dopamine

ACTH, Adrenocorticotropic hormone; *PGI₂,* prostacyclin.

Therefore, the net effect of an increase in aldosterone levels, as may result from an aldosterone-producing tumor (Conn's syndrome) or exogenous mineralocorticoid administration (e.g., 9α-fludrocortisol), is sodium resorption with consequent volume expansion, hypertension and suppression of plasma renin activity, hypokalemia, and a metabolic alkalosis.

Aldosterone secretion is also subject to negative regulation. ANP is a potent inhibitor of aldosterone secretion, consistent with its role to promote natriuresis. Dopamine is a well-characterized inhibitor of aldosterone secretion.[9] Other inhibitors have been described, but their physiologic relevance is not clear (Table 4-2).

Dietary sodium has a major impact on the state of the renin-angiotensin-aldosterone system (RAS). Sodium deficiency increases adrenal sensitivity to angiotensin II over time; the converse is true of the vasopressor response. Aldosterone-induced sodium retention restores volume status by maintaining the balance between volume and capacity.[10]

The response of the individual to aldosterone-mediated sodium retention is self-limiting in that after 3 to 4 days, expansion of the extracellular volume plateaus and of sodium secretion returns to control levels. This process is termed *escape*.[11] It should be noted that the kaliuretic effect persists despite the escape of sodium retention. Intrarenal regulators, particularly prostaglan-

Table 4-2. Factors Regulating Aldosterone Secretion

Factor	Stimulatory	Inhibitory
Peptides	Angiotensin II	Atrial natriuretic peptide
	Angiotensin III	Somatostatin
	ACTH	
	Vasopressin	
	Endothelin	
Ions	Plasma potassium	
Other	Serotonin	Dopamine
		Ouabain

ACTH, Adrenocorticotropic hormone.

dins, are probably the critical mediators of the escape, although other factors (e.g., ANP) may play a role.[12,13]

A local renin-angiotensin system has been reported to operate in a number of tissues, including the submaxillary glands, gonads, smooth muscle cells, adipose tissue, pituitary, brain, and adrenal cortex. The existence of this system is often determined by the presence of mRNA for renin, angiotensinogen, and angiotensin-converting enzyme (ACE); the relative physiologic importance of these local systems has recently been called into question.[14]

Potassium Homeostasis

Aldosterone is primarily involved in the chronic regulation of plasma potassium levels.[15] Acute regulation involves nonrenal mechanisms such as those mediated by insulin and β-adrenergic agonists. Aldosterone regulates potassium homeostasis through direct effects on transport of epithelia, including its effects on sodium homeostasis. Small fluctuations in plasma potassium influence aldosterone secretion. Although the mechanism of these effects has not been determined, it is known to be independent of angiotensin II levels; however, plasma potassium levels do alter the sensitivity of the adrenal to angiotensin II. The local adrenal RAS has been implicated in the adrenal response to potassium; the circulating system is inhibited by potassium, whereas local adrenal production is increased.

Aldosterone secretion is also subject to regulation by adrenocorticotropic hormone (ACTH); however, aldosterone regulation is normal in patients with hypopituitarism.[16]

Mineralocorticoid Receptors

The classic actions of aldosterone involve epithelial cells in the distal nephron and distal colon; these mediate sodium flux. As with other steroid hormones, the principal mode of action, at least in sodium transport, involves an intracellular receptor that when activated by ligand-binding regulates gene transcription, a so-called genomic mechanism of action.

High-affinity cytosol and nuclear binding of ^3H-aldosterone were first described in classic mineralocorticoid target tissues such as kidney[5,17] and parotid[18] more than 30 years ago. Spironolactone was shown to block aldosterone binding and action on urinary electrolytes in parallel,[19] providing evidence that these sites are physiologic mineralocorticoid receptors (MRs). MR were subsequently cloned from human kidney,[20] and the rat homologue was cloned from a hippocampal cDNA library.[21] In contrast to glucocorticoid receptors (GRs), which are expressed ubiqui-

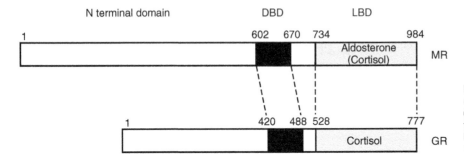

FIGURE 4-2. Domain structure of the mineralocorticoid receptor (MR) and the closely related glucocorticoid receptor (GR) showing the three principal functional domains: the N-terminal domain, the DNA-binding domain (DBD), and the ligand-binding domain (LBD). These domains share less than 15%, 94%, and 57% identity, respectively.

tously, MRs have a tissue-specific pattern of expression, with highest levels observed in the distal nephron,[22] distal colon,[23] and hippocampus.[20] Lower levels of expression are observed elsewhere in the gastrointestinal tract; in cardiovascular tissues; and in a range of other tissues, both epithelial and nonepithelial.[20,22,23]

The human mineralocorticoid receptor is a protein of 984 amino acids and, together with the GR, progesterone receptor (PR), and androgen receptor (AR), forms a distinct subfamily within the steroid/thyroid/retinoid/orphan receptor superfamily.[24] This receptor superfamily is defined by a central cysteine-rich DNA-binding domain. At the C terminus is the ligand-binding domain (LBD), which has a highly conserved tertiary structure. The N-terminal domain has little or no homology between receptors. Within the MR/GR/PR/AR subfamily, MR and GR are closely related, with 94% amino acid identity in the central cysteine-rich DNA-binding domain, and 57% identity in the C-terminal ligand-binding domain (Fig. 4-2). The MR and GR, however, are located on different chromosomes (MR on 4q31.2[25]; GR on 5q31[26]).

The cysteine residues of the DNA-binding domain complex around two zinc atoms to form two α-helices, one of which lies in the major groove and binds with a common consensus sequence in the DNA, the hormone response element.[27] The LBD consists of 11 α-helices, which form a three-layered structure with the ligand-binding pocket buried in the middle.[28-30] The N-terminal domain contains a transcription activation function that is relatively unstructured. The N-terminal domains are not conserved between steroid receptors, although in several (including the MR[31]), a functional interaction has been described between the N-terminal and ligand-binding domains. It is curious that for the MR, this interaction is seen only with aldosterone; cortisol acts as an antagonist.

The unliganded receptor is predominantly cytoplasmic,[32] being complexed with the heat shock proteins 70 and 90 and their co-chaperones.[33] This configuration maintains the receptor in a transcriptionally inactive high-affinity binding state. The interaction of the ligand-binding domain with this complex is an important determinant of ligand-binding affinity and specificity.[34] The mineralocorticoid receptor antagonists, spironolactone and eplerenone, appear to be accommodated into the ligand-binding pocket without distortion,[35] suggesting that the mechanism of their antagonism differs from that of the estrogen receptor antagonists such as tamoxifen and raloxifene. These latter compounds exhibit tissue-specific antagonism, in contrast to spironolactone, which is a pure antagonist. Evidence that cortisol/corticosterone may antagonize the actions of aldosterone at the MR in certain tissues suggests that different ligands may induce differing conformations on binding the receptor.[31] At a cellular level, these differing conformations result in differential interac-

tions with the transcriptional machinery through the mediators of this signaling, the co-regulatory molecules. In contrast to the other steroid receptors, such interactions are only now being characterized for the MR.[36]

Very good evidence suggests that not all MRs are physiologic receptors for aldosterone. In brief, cortisol and corticosterone (the physiologic glucocorticoid in the rat) have an affinity for the MR equivalent to that for aldosterone and substantially higher than their affinity for the GR.[20] MRs are distributed widely in tissues in which a physiologic effect of aldosterone on Na^+ homeostasis is unlikely (e.g., the hippocampus[20,37]). Given the much higher circulating levels of glucocorticoids than of aldosterone, these sites appear to be high-affinity GRs in such tissues. In nonepithelial tissues, the response of MR to cortisol/corticosterone and aldosterone often is not equivalent,[38] leading to speculation about the relationship of epithelial to nonepithelial MR. Most evidence to date would suggest that although the MR gene uses multiple, tissue-specific promoters,[39-41] the coding region is unaltered between tissues, with the possible exception of some minor isoforms.[42] The explanation for such differences between tissues may lie in the nature of the conformation that the MR adopts after ligand binding.[43] Such conformational differences may alter some but not all transactivation functions, such that tissue-specific receptor co-activators or co-repressors[36] may mediate different responses in different tissues.

A second question, given the equivalent affinity of MR for glucocorticoids and aldosterone, is that of the mechanism(s) allowing aldosterone occupancy of MR in physiologic mineralocorticoid target tissues. This matter is discussed later in this chapter. Not only do MRs appear unable to distinguish between physiologic mineralocorticoids and glucocorticoids, but evidence suggests an equivalent lack of selectivity at the level of the response elements, where both MR and GR act as transcription factors.[20,44] Because no MR-selective response elements have been characterized to date, the evidence for this lack of specificity is indirect but clearly established for epithelial tissues.[45] In vitro studies on cultured cortical collecting tubule cells have shown aldosterone, dexamethasone, and the highly specific GR agonist RU28362 to have indistinguishable effects on unidirectional Na^+ and K^+ fluxes and on the transepithelial potential difference as measured by short-circuit current.[46] In vivo studies on adrenalectomized rats given the highly specific GR agonist RU28362 similarly have shown that GR, appropriately activated by ligand, can activate the same genes as the MR[2] and can produce a classic mineralocorticoid effect on urinary electrolytes. On the other hand, differences in the action of MR and GR in the same cells can be demonstrated,[44,45,47,48] suggesting the possibility of greater complexity in certain circumstances (e.g., when GR but not MR can be shown to interact with other transcription factors such as adaptor protein-1 [AP-1]).[47]

In addition to its effects on ion flux in classic mineralocorticoid target tissues, aldosterone has been shown to have effects via MR occupancy in a variety of other tissues. Aldosterone elevates blood pressure in the rat when infused into the cerebral ventricles[49]; this effect clearly results from unprotected MR, because it is blocked by simultaneous infusion of low doses of corticosterone. Thus, corticosterone in the AV3V region acts as an aldosterone antagonist on MR, in contrast with the kidney and other epithelia, where its action is to mimic aldosterone.[46,50] An additional difference between epithelial and nonepithelial tissues is that in the former, activation of GR has been shown to mimic that of MR,[46,50] whereas in nonepithelial tissues, this clearly is not the case. In the heart, a nonepithelial tissue that expresses MR, studies conducted in vivo show that levels of aldosterone inappropriately high for the Na+ status of the rat produce diffuse perivascular and interstitial fibrosis, an effect that can be antagonized by corticosterone or spironolactone.[51] The clinical correlation of these observations is found in two recent large trials, which show a benefit of the addition of a mineralocorticoid antagonist to the conventional regimen in the treatment of individuals with severe cardiac failure, with respect to both morbidity and mortality.[52,53]

Mice homozygous for inactivating mutations in the *MR* gene[54] (MR knockout, or MRKO) show classical features of aldosterone deficiency—salt-wasting, hyperkalemia, and dehydration—but have marked hyperaldosteronism; these features are also seen in the syndrome of pseudohypoaldosteronism (PHA) (see Chapter 13). MRKO mice are born at the expected frequency from heterozygote matings; untreated, they begin to deteriorate from day 5, and they die between day 8 and day 11; treatment by salt supplementation allows survival and normal growth. Mutations of the *MR* have been reported in the autosomal dominant form of PHA,[55-57] which thus appear to be equivalent to mice heterozygous for the MR gene knockout. In the more severe autosomal recessive form and in many sporadic cases of PHA, mutations of the *MR* are not observed.[56,57]

GENOMIC VERSUS NONGENOMIC ALDOSTERONE ACTIONS

Considerable interest has been expressed with respect to steroid hormone action in terms of whether all responses are mediated through the classical nuclear receptor with direct regulation of gene expression, or whether other pathways, perhaps involving novel cell membrane receptors, exist[58]; the evidence for novel receptors is not compelling.[59] Clear evidence has been found both in vitro and in vivo for rapid nongenomic signaling. This can involve activation by src kinase of the epidermal growth factor (EGF) receptor with consequent downstream signaling through the mitogen-activated protein (MAP)-kinase pathway; the signaling appears to require only the LBD of the MR.[60] McEneaney et al.[61] defined rapid effects on protein kinase signaling, Mihailidou et al.[62] reported rapid effects in isolated cell patches from cardiomyocytes, and Alzamora et al.[63] observed rapid effects in vascular cells. Karst et al.[64] found rapid nongenomic effects of corticosterone on glutamate release from the CA1 pyramidal neurons of the hippocampus. This response also involves mitogen-activated protein kinase/extracellular signal–related kinase (MAPK/ERK) signaling.[65] In each case, the receptor involved is the classical MR. The relative contribution to the mineralocorticoid response by this signaling has not yet been evaluated, although it is speculated that this rapid response may prime the transcriptional response[65] or may alter the dynamic range of the response.[65]

Specificity-Conferring Enzymes

11β-HYDROXYSTEROID DEHYDROGENASE TYPE 2

Although the affinity of MR in vitro[20,37] is equal for aldosterone, corticosterone, and cortisol, in vivo cortisol is excluded from such receptors in the kidney, parotid, and colon (but not in the hippocampus).[66] This reflects the activity of the enzyme 11β-hydroxysteroid dehydrogenase (11β-HSD), which is responsible for the interconversion of cortisol and cortisone (in the rat, corticosterone and 11-dehydrocorticosterone). In the kidney, the predominant direction of conversion is cortisol to cortisone, as is shown by the reduced cortisol-to-cortisone ratio in human renal venous blood.[67] Initially, rat liver 11β-HSD was purified, cloned, and sequenced,[68] as was its human homologue[69]; it is expressed at high levels in the liver, testis, lung, and renal proximal tubule,[70] none of which are physiologic mineralocorticoid target tissues. Subsequently, a second isoform (11β-HSD2, with the "liver" isoform termed 11β-HSD1) was isolated by expression cloning[71] and was shown to be the enzyme responsible for the aldosterone selectivity of MR in epithelial aldosterone target tissues.[72,73] Unlike 11β-HSD1, it co-localizes with MR[32] in renal distal tubular elements, colon, sweat, and salivary glands[74]; it is also expressed at high abundance in the placenta[71] and in select areas (subcommissural organ, ventromedial ventrolateral hypothalamus) of the rat brain.[75] It has a low K_m (i.e., high affinity) for both corticosterone ($\approx$5 nM) and cortisol ($\approx$50 nM), unlike the micromolar K_m of 11β-HSD1; in vivo, it appears operationally unidirectional, acting uniquely as a dehydrogenase, whereas 11β-HSD1 appears to act predominantly as a reductase.[72] Deletion of the 11β-HSD2 gene in mice yields a phenotype[76] consistent with the clinical syndrome of human apparent mineralocorticoid excess (AME).[72,73,77]

In AME, 11β-HSD2 activity is congenitally low, indicated by a markedly increased ratio of urinary cortisol to cortisone metabolites; abnormally high intrarenal cortisol levels occupy receptors normally protected by the enzyme, resulting in increased Na+ retention and elevation of blood pressure.[72,73,78] Kindred with AME have been examined for the presence of mutations in the gene coding for 11β-HSD2.[77,79,80] The mutations are autosomal recessive and thus are commonly seen in the context of consanguinity, although compound heterozygosity has also been reported.[77] Although heterozygotes may show subtle departures from normal in terms of their ratio of urinary cortisol to cortisone metabolites, little evidence indicates a substantial deficit in such individuals (see also Chapter 13).

Licorice ingestion has long been known to cause Na+ retention, hypokalemia, and hypertension; the mechanism of its action was elucidated by elegant studies[78] on human volunteers, in whom ingestion of 250 g of licorice a day for 10 days produced a clinical picture equivalent to a mild form of apparent mineralocorticoid excess. When rats were given glycyrrhetinic acid (the active principal of licorice)[81] or carbenoxolone (glycyrrhetinic acid hemisuccinate)[82] to block 11β-HSD, the normal aldosterone selectivity of epithelial MR was abolished.

These studies demonstrate the crucial specificity-conferring role in mineralocorticoid target tissues for 11β-HSD2. Aldosterone is not a substrate for 11β-HSD, because its 11β-OH group is stabilized as an 11,18-hemiketal via cyclization with the highly reactive aldehyde group unique to aldosterone at C18.

Cellular Actions of Aldosterone

As the term *mineralocorticoid* implies, the classical effects of aldosterone reflect its role in the regulation of electrolyte flux across transporting epithelia. The molecular basis of this regulation, particularly the steps downstream of receptor binding, has yet to be fully established.[2,83,84] The more recently defined roles of aldosterone in the central regulation of blood pressure,[47] in salt appetite,[85] and in the pathogenesis of cardiac fibrosis[51,86] are even less well understood in terms of their cellular basis.

SODIUM TRANSPORT

Aldosterone increases transepithelial sodium flux in a number of target tissues, of which the amphibian bladder, the mammalian distal nephron, and the mammalian distal colon are the best characterized.[2,83] The temporal pattern of response comprises a lag period of 30 to 60 minutes, followed by an early phase in which preexisting pumps and channels are activated; this is followed by a so-called late phase.[83] The late phase starts 3 to 6 hours after steroid exposure and is characterized by an increase in the number of pumps and channels; with longer exposure, morphologic and functional changes are observed.[87] The latent phase is consistent with the concept that the effects of aldosterone are primarily genomic, with genes primarily regulated by the MR as it mediates sodium transport per se, or by modulating components of the transport pathway. In the classic model of aldosterone-induced transport, sodium entry at the apical membrane occurs through an amiloride-sensitive electrogenic sodium channel, and efflux via the sodium pump at the basolateral membrane is energy dependent, with ATP generation needed to drive the efflux process (Fig. 4-3).[88]

EPITHELIAL SODIUM CHANNELS

Although a variety of amiloride-sensitive sodium channels have been identified in various epithelia,[89] only one has been shown clearly to be directly involved in aldosterone-dependent sodium transport. The epithelial sodium channel (ENaC) genes cloned from the rat distal colon encode three homologous subunits (α, β, and γ).[90] Each subunit consists of two transmembrane domains

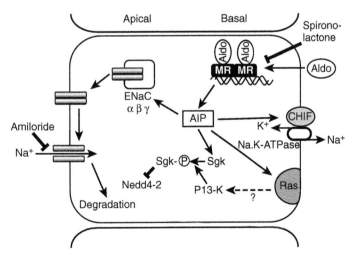

FIGURE 4-3. Aldosterone (Aldo) acts on epithelial cells of the distal nephron and the distal colon via the mineralocorticoid receptor (MR) to induce aldosterone-induced proteins (AIP). *ENaC,* Epithelial sodium channels; *sgk,* serum and glucocorticoid-induced kinase; *CHIF,* channel-inducing factor; *PI 3-K,* phosphoinositide 3-kinase.

with intracellular N and C termini. When the α subunit is expressed in *Xenopus* oocytes, a weak, amiloride-sensitive sodium flux can be demonstrated; expression of the other subunits alone occurs without activity, and co-expression of all three subunits is required for maximal amiloride-sensitive sodium transport.[90] The subunits exhibit a heterotrimeric complex, as is demonstrated by the recent characterization of the tertiary structure of a closely related acid-sensing ion channel.[91]

The genes for the ENaC subunits are members of the DEG/ENaC superfamily of sodium channels; the degenerins (DEGs) mediate mechanosensory transduction in *Caenorhabditis elegans*.[92] Insights into the structural determinants of function of the ENaC subunits have been derived from a combination of both naturally occurring and engineered mutations.[92] Deletion of the αENaC gene in transgenic mice results in early neonatal death caused by defective clearance of lung liquid[93]; partial restoration of αENaC expression in these mice by transgenesis results in a phenotype very similar to that seen in PHA.[94] Mice with the βENaC or the γENaC gene deleted show a less severe pulmonary phenotype but die between 24 and 36 hours with salt wasting and profound hyperkalemia, again reminiscent of PHA[95,96]; low levels of expression of the βENaC subunit gene in mice in which the βENaC gene has been disrupted also result in a milder phenotype analogous to PHA.[97] Autosomal recessive PHA indeed is associated with inactivating mutations of all three of the ENaC subunits[98,99] (see also Chapter 13).

The molecular characterization of Liddle's syndrome[100] has also provided important insights into the function of the C-terminal intracellular domain and emphasizes the central role of the channel in amiloride-sensitive sodium transport[2,94] (see also Chapter 13). Liddle's syndrome, or pseudoaldosteronism, has the reciprocal pathophysiology to PHA,[100] with apparent aldosterone excess (i.e., hypertension, hypokalemia, and suppressed plasma renin activity) but low aldosterone levels, and no response to spironolactone but a response to amiloride. Several studies have identified mutations in the β- or γENaC gene in various kindred.[100,101] The mutations are either nonsense or missense mutations localized to the C terminus; the latter are particularly informative because they identify a key motif, proline-proline-proline-X-tyrosine (PY), which is conserved across the subunits and is disrupted in all cases of Liddle's syndrome.[92,101] ENaC is a relatively short-lived protein that is ubiquinated on residues in the N terminus of the α and γ but not β subunits; the PY motif interacts with Nedd4-2, a ubiquitin protein-ligase, whose role is to target the channels for proteosomal degradation.[102] Nedd4-2 is not itself regulated by aldosterone.[103]

These studies demonstrated the central role of the ENaC in mediating aldosterone-induced epithelial sodium transport. ENaC subunit gene expression is regulated by aldosterone. Both β and γENaC subunit mRNA levels were increased in the colon by sodium depletion[104] and by dexamethasone or aldosterone treatment for 6[105] or 24 hours[106,107]; in the kidney, however, levels remained unaltered, although when separate regions of the kidney were distinguished, an increase in αENaC mRNA levels was seen in the inner medulla.[108] Cultured medullary collecting duct cells show increased α- but not β- or γENaC mRNA levels after 3 hours of aldosterone exposure; in cultured cortical collecting duct cells, a γENaC subunit response to aldosterone required 24 hours of treatment.[109] Although it is clear from the above studies that aldosterone can increase ENaC synthesis (at least in the late phase), an effect in the early phase (i.e., a primary effect) has not been demonstrated. This is in agreement with a number of electrophysiologic[88] and biosynthetic studies.[110]

Studies in amphibian A6 cells[111] and rabbit cortical collecting duct cells[112] provided the first conclusive evidence for an early phase, direct mediator of aldosterone action in the kidney. Aldosterone treatment in vivo rapidly increased levels of the serine, threonine kinase, serum, and glucocorticoid-regulated kinase (sgk[111]), with a time course clearly consistent with an effect of aldosterone on transcription.[113,114] Sgk directly interacts with Nedd4-2 to block its binding of the ENaC and, as a consequence, slows ENaC degradation.[115,116] Regulation of ENaCα subunit gene expression involves sgk-1 through relief of Dotla-Af9–mediated transcriptional repression.[117] Nedd4-2 is also regulated by Usp2-45, a deubiquitinylation enzyme that itself is regulated by aldosterone.[118] Sgk requires phosphorylation by the phosphatidylinositol 3-kinase (PI 3-kinase) pathway for full activity.[119] This may be a point at which the signaling of nuclear receptors and that of membrane-associated receptors such as the insulin receptor are integrated.[119] PI 3-kinase may be activated by small monomeric G proteins, including ras. *K-ras 2A* has been identified as an aldosterone-induced gene in an amphibian-derived renal cell line[84]; this has been confirmed in the rodent distal colon.[120] The glucocorticoid-induced leucine zipper protein (GIL2) is also aldosterone-induced; it acts to repress ERK signaling.[121]

Na+/K+-ATPase

Active extrusion of Na^+ from the cell reflects sodium pump activity in the basolateral cell membrane. Na^+/K^+-ATPase activity is increased in a number of epithelia by aldosterone. Toad bladder and A6 cells provide evidence that Na^+/K^+-ATPase α and β subunit gene expression is significantly increased in the early phase of the response to aldosterone,[83] although this does not appear to be the case in mammalian systems.[122] Na^+/K^+-ATPase activity is very sensitive to intracellular sodium concentrations, and in isolated cortical tubules the early Na^+/K^+-ATPase response to aldosterone is blocked by amiloride, suggesting that the increased activity is secondary to sodium influx at the apical membrane.[123] In the late phase of the aldosterone response, levels of Na^+/K^+-ATPase mRNA, protein, and activity are all increased.[124] Channel-inducing factor (*CHIF*) was first identified as a novel corticosteroid-induced gene in the rat distal colon.[125] CHIF is a member of the FXYD family of small transmembrane proteins that includes the γ subunit of Na^+/K^+-ATPase.[126] Under experimental conditions, CHIF is upregulated in the distal colon in response to aldosterone[127,128]; this appears to be a primary transcriptional response.[129] It has been shown recently[126] that CHIF increases the affinity of Na^+/K^+-ATPase for sodium. It would appear that the early aldosterone-induced increase in Na^+/K^+-ATPase activity is mediated by CHIF.

POTASSIUM TRANSPORT

Potassium flux occurs in transporting epithelia in response to aldosterone as a result of Na^+/K^+-ATPase–mediated exchange at the basolateral membrane, with the resulting electrochemical gradient favoring potassium excretion.[130] Regulation of potassium homeostasis by aldosterone is independent of its effects on sodium transport, and Na^+/K^+-ATPase–mediated basolateral membrane exchange of sodium and potassium[130] has been described; recent evidence[131] suggests that a mediator of potassium transport, the α subunit of a putative K^+-ATPase, is regulated by dietary potassium and corticosteroids. Aldosterone and dexamethasone treatment for 2 days upregulates levels of K^+-ATPase mRNA in the epithelial cells of both the outer medullary collecting duct and the distal colon.[131] Sgk-1 has been reported to increase the channel density of ROMK, a potassium channel, through direct phosphorylation or perhaps through Nedd4-2.[132]

HYDROGEN ION TRANSPORT

As for potassium, aldosterone also has effects on proton excretion over and above a simple cation exchange for sodium across the epithelium to maintain electroneutrality.[133] The targets for this effect are carbonic anhydrase–rich cells, particularly the intercalated cells within the outer medullary collecting ducts. Transport across the apical membrane occurs through an H^+-ATPase activity[134] (which is upregulated by aldosterone), coupled with increased activity of the basolateral Cl^-/HCO_3^- exchanger.[135] These effects are largely sodium independent, as demonstrated by the lack of an effect of amiloride. Aldosterone also has an effect on the Na^+-H^+ antiporter in a range of tissues; in some tissues, the response is very rapid and represents a nongenomic action.

OTHER TISSUES

Although the last decade has seen significant advances in our understanding of the molecular responses to aldosterone in epithelial cells, the nature of the response in other tissues is much less well characterized. In the heart, for instance, the acute inflammatory response to mineralocorticoid treatment in the presence of salt loading is likely to involve a distinctively different set of genes.[51,86] Responses in the central nervous system also appear to differ.[136] The role of aldosterone in other tissues, particularly those of the cerebrovascular and cardiovascular systems, has been a major focus of recent research. In the heart, mineralocorticoid treatment in the presence of salt loading results in an inflammatory response that leads to cardiac fibrosis.[34] Several studies have identified aldosterone-induced genes in the heart,[137,138] although their full physiologic significance remains to be determined. The same is true in the central nervous system.[139,65] It is important to note that in several, but not all of these tissues, the biology may be that of cortisol activation of the MR rather than of aldosterone.

REFERENCES

1. Vinson GP, Whitehouse BJ, Goddard C, et al: Comparative and evolutionary aspects of aldosterone secretion and zona glomerulosa function, J Endocrinol 81:5P–24P, 1979.
2. Rogerson FM, Fuller PJ: Mineralocorticoid action, Steroids 65:61–73, 2000.
3. Simpson SA, Tait JF, Wettstein A, et al: Isolierung eines neuen kristallisierten Hormons aus Nebennieren mit besonders hoher Wirksamkeit auf den Mineralstoffwechsel, Experientia 9:333–335, 1953.
4. Crabbé J: Stimulation of active sodium transport across toad bladder with aldosterone *in vitro*, J Clin Invest 76:2103–2110, 1961.
5. Feldman D, Funder JW, Edelman IS: Subcellular mechanisms in the action of adrenal steroids, Am J Med 53:545–560, 1972.
6. Weir MR, Dzau VJ: The renin-angiotensin-aldosterone system: a specific target: hypertension management, Am J Hypertens 12:205S–213S, 1999.
7. Nogueira EF, Vargas CA, Otis M, et al: Angiotensin-II acute regulation of rapid response genes in human, bovine, and rat adrenocortical cells, J Mol Endocrinol 39:365-374, 2007.

8. Okubo S, Niimura F, Nishimura H, et al: Angiotensin-independent mechanism for aldosterone synthesis during chronic extracellular fluid volume depletion, J Clin Invest 99:855–860, 1997.

9. Carey RM: Physiologic and possible pathophysiologic relevance of dopaminergic mechanisms in the control of aldosterone secretion. In Mantero F, Biglieri EG, Funder JW, Scoggins BA, editors: The Adrenal and Hypertension, New York, 1995, Raven, pp 55–69.

10. Hollenberg NK, Chenitz WR, Adams DF, et al: Reciprocal influence of salt intake on adrenal glomerulosa and renal vascular responses to angiotensin II in normal man, J Clin Invest 54:34–42, 1974.

11. Knox F, Burnett JJ, Kohan D, et al: Escape from the sodium-retaining effects of mineralocorticoids, Kidney Int 17:263–276, 1980.

12. Zimmerman RS, Edwards BS, Schwab TR, et al: Atrial natriuretic peptide during mineralocorticoid escape in the human, J Clin Endocrinol Metab 64:624–627, 1987.

13. Gaillard CA, Koomans HA, Rabelink TJ, et al: Enhanced natriuretic effect of atrial natriuretic factor during mineralocorticoid escape in humans, Hypertension 12:450–456, 1988.

14. Ye P, Kenyon CJ, MacKenzie SM, et al: The aldosterone synthase (CYP11B2) and 11β-hydroxylase (CYP11B1) genes are not expressed in the rat heart, Endocrinology 146:5287-5293, 2005.

15. Young DB: Quantitative analysis of aldosterone's role in potassium regulation, Am J Physiol 55:F811–F822, 1988.

16. Williams GH, Rose LI, Dluhy RG, et al: Aldosterone response to sodium restriction and ACTH stimulation in panhypopituitarism, J Clin Endocrinol Metab 32:27–35, 1971.

17. Rousseau G, Baxter JD, Funder JW, et al: Glucocorticoid and mineralocorticoid receptors for aldosterone, J Steroid Biochem 3:219–227, 1972.

18. Funder JW, Feldman D, Edelman IS: Specific aldosterone binding in rat kidney and parotid, J Steroid Biochem 3:209–218, 1972.

19. Marver D, Stewart J, Funder JW, et al: Renal aldosterone receptors: studies with (^{3}H)aldosterone and the anti-mineralocorticoid (^{3}H)spirolactone (SC-26304), Proc Natl Acad Sci U S A 71:1431–1435, 1974.

20. Arriza JL, Weinberger C, Cerelli G, et al: Cloning of human mineralocorticoid receptor complementary DNA: structural and functional kinship with the glucocorticoid receptor, Science 237:268–275, 1987.

21. Patel PD, Sherman TG, Goldman DJ: Molecular cloning of a mineralocorticoid (type I) receptor complementary DNA for rat hippocampus, Mol Endocrinol 3:1877–1885, 1989.

22. Todd-Turla MD, Schnermann J, Fejes-Toth G, et al: Distribution of mineralocorticoid glucocorticoid receptor mRNA along the nephron, Am J Physiol 264:F781–F791, 1993.

23. Fuller PJ, Verity K: Mineralocorticoid receptor gene expression in the gastrointestinal tract: distribution and ontogeny, J Steroid Biochem 36:263–267, 1990.

24. Mangelsdorf DJ, Thummel C, Beato M, et al: The nuclear receptor superfamily: the second decade, Cell 83:835–839, 1995.

25. Fan Y-S, Eddy RL, Byers LL, et al: The human mineralocorticoid receptor gene (MLR) is located on chromosome 4 at q31.2, Cytogenet Cell Genet 52:83–84, 1989.

26. Theriault A, Boyd E, Harrap SB, et al: Regional chromosomal assignment of the human glucocorticoid receptor gene to 5q31, Hum Genet 83:289–291, 1989.

27. Luisi BF, Xu WX, Itwubiwsju Z, et al: Crystallographic analysis of the interaction of the glucocorticoid receptor with DNA, Nature 352:497–505, 1991.

28. Fagart J, Huyet J, Pinon GM, et al: Crystal structure of a mutant mineralocorticoid receptor responsible for hypertension, Nature Struct Mol Biol 12, 554-555, 2005.

29. Bledsoe, R.K., Madauss KP, Holt JA, et al: A ligand-mediated hydrogen bond network required for the activation of the mineralocorticoid receptor, J Biol Chem 280:31283-31293, 2005.

30. Li Y, Suino K, Daugherty J, et al: Structural and biochemical mechanisms for the specificity of hormone binding and coactivator assembly by mineralocorticoid receptor, Mol Cell 19:367-380, 2005.

31. Rogerson FM, Fuller PJ: Interdomain interactions in the mineralocorticoid receptor, Mol Cell Endocrinol 200:45–55, 2003.

32. Odermatt A, Arnold P, Frey FJ: The intracellular localization of the mineralocorticoid receptor is regulated by 11beta-hydroxysteroid dehydrogenase type 2, J Biol Chem 276:28484–28492, 2001.

33. Bruner KL, Derfoul A, Robertson NM, et al: The unliganded mineralocorticoid receptor is associated with heat shock proteins 70 and 90 and the immunophilin FKBP-52, Recept Signal Transduct 7:85–98, 1997.

34. Fuller PJ, Young MJ: Mechanisms of mineralocorticoid action, Hypertension 46:1227-1235, 2005.

35. Rogerson FM, Yao YZ, Smith BJ, et al: Determinants of spironolactone binding specificity in the mineralocorticoid receptor, J Mol Endocrinol 31:573–582, 2003.

36. Viengchareun S, Le Menuet D, Martinerie L, et al: The mineralocorticoid receptor: insights into its molecular and (patho)physiological biology, Nucl Recept Signal 5:1-16, 2007.

37. Krozowski ZS, Funder JW: Renal mineralocorticoid receptors and hippocampal corticosterone binding species have identical intrinsic steroid specificity, Proc Natl Acad Sci U S A 80:6056–6060, 1983.

38. de Kloet ER, Vreugdenhil E, Oitzl MS, et al: Brain corticosteroid receptor balance in health and disease, Endocr Rev 19:269–301, 1998.

39. Kwak SP, Patel PD, Thompson RC, et al: 5'-heterogeneity of the mineralocorticoid receptors messenger ribonucleic acid: differential expression and regulation of splice variants within the rat hippocampus, Endocrinology 133:2344–2350, 1993.

40. Zennaro M-C, Keightley MC, Kotelevtsev Y, et al: Human mineralocorticoid receptor genomic structure and identification of expressed isoforms, J Biol Chem 270:21016–21020, 1995.

41. Zennaro M-C, Le Menuet D, Lombes M: Characterization of the human mineralocorticoid receptor gene 5'-regulatory region: evidence for differential hormonal regulation of two alternative promoters via non-classical mechanisms, Mol Endocrinol 10:1549–1560, 1996.

42. Zennaro MC, Souque A, Viengchareun S, et al: A new human MR splice variant is a ligand-independent transactivator modulating corticosteroid action, Mol Endocrinol 15:1586–1598, 2001.

43. Couette B, Fagart J, Jalaguier S, et al: Ligand-induced conformational change in the human mineralocorticoid receptor occurs within its hetero-oligomeric structure, Biochem J 315:421–427, 1996.

44. Farman N, Rafestin-Oblin ME: Multiple aspects of mineralocorticoid selectivity, Am J Physiol Renal Physiol 280:F181–F192, 2001.

45. Lim-Tio SS, Keightley M-C, Fuller PJ: Determination of specificity of transactivation by the mineralocorticoid or glucocorticoid receptors, Endocrinology 138:2537–3543, 1997.

46. Naray-Fejes-Toth A, Fejes-Toth G: Glucocorticoid receptors mediate mineralocorticoid-like effects in cultured collecting duct cells, Am J Physiol 259:F672–F678, 1990.

47. Pearce D, Yamamoto KR: Mineralocorticoid and glucocorticoid receptor activities are distinguished by nonreceptor factors at a composite response element, Science 259:1661–1665, 1993.

48. Lim-Tio SS, Fuller PJ: Intracellular signaling pathways confer specificity of transactivation by mineralocorticoid and glucocorticoid receptors, Endocrinology 139:1653–1661, 1998.

49. Gomez-Sanchez EP, Venkataraman MT, Thwaites D, et al: Intracerebroventricular infusion of corticosterone antagonizes ICV-aldosterone hypertension, Am J Physiol 258:E649–E653, 1990.

50. Funder JW, Pearce P, Myles K, et al: Apparent mineralocorticoid excess, pseudohypoaldosteronism and urinary electrolyte excretion: towards a redefinition of "mineralocorticoid" action, FASEB J 4:3234–3238, 1990.

51. Young MJ, Funder JW: Mineralocorticoid receptors and pathophysiological roles for aldosterone in the cardiovascular system, J Hypertens 20:1465–1468, 2002.

52. Pitt B, Zannad F, Remme WJ, et al: The effect of spironolactone on morbidity and mortality in patients with severe heart failure. Randomized Aldactone Evaluation Study Investigators, N Engl J Med 341:709–717, 1999.

53. Pitt B, Remme W, Zannad F, et al: Eplerenone post-acute myocardial infarction heart failure efficacy and survival study investigators, N Engl J Med 348:1309–1321, 2003.

54. Berger S, Bleich M, Schmid W, et al: Mineralocorticoid receptor knockout mice: pathophysiology of Na$^+$ metabolism, Proc Natl Acad Sci U S A 95:9424–9429, 1998.

55. Geller DS, Rodriguez-Soriano J, Boado AV, et al: Mutations in the mineralocorticoid receptor gene cause autosomal dominant pseudohypoaldosteronism type 1, Nat Genet 19:279–281, 1998.

56. Pujo L, Fagart J, Gary F, et al: Mineralocorticoid receptor mutations are the principal cause of renal type 1 pseudohypoaldosteronism, Hum Mutat 28:33-40, 2007.

57. Geller DS, Zhang J, Zennaro MC, et al: Autosomal dominant pseudohypoaldosteronism type 1: mechanisms, evidence for neonatal lethality, and phenotypic expression in adults, J Am Soc Nephrol 16:1429–1436, 2006.

58. Losel RM, Feuring M, Falkenstein E, et al: Nongenomic effects of aldosterone: cellular aspects and clinical implications, Steroids 67:493–498, 2002.

59. Funder JW: The nongenomic actions of aldosterone, Endocr Rev 26:313–321,2005.

60. Grossmann C, Freudinger R, Mildenbergr S, et al: EF-domains are sufficient for nongenomic mineralocorticoid receptor actions, J Biol Chem 283:7109–7116, 2008.

61. McEneaney V, Harvey BJ, Thomas W: Aldosterone regulates rapid trafficking of ENaC subunits in renal cortical collecting duct cells via protein kinase D activation, Mol Endocrinol 22:881–882, 2008.

62. Mihailidou AS, Mardini M, Funder JW: Rapid, nongenomic effects of aldosterone in the heart mediated by epsilon protein kinase C, Endocrinology 145:773–780, 2003.

63. Alzamora R, Marusic ET, Gonzalez M, et al: Nongenomic effect of aldosterone on Na+,K+-adenosine triphosphatase in arterial vessels, Endocrinology 144:1266–1272, 2003.

64. Karst H, Berger S, Turiault M, et al: Mineralocorticoid receptors are indispensable for nongenomic modulation of hippocampal glucamate transmission by corticosterone, Proc Natl Acad Sci U S A 102:19204–19207, 2005.

65. Joels M, Karst H, DeRijk R, et al: The coming out of the brain mineralocorticoid receptor, Trends Neurosci 31:1–7, 2008.

66. Sheppard K, Funder JW: Type I receptors in parotid, colon and pituitary are aldosterone-selective in vivo, Am J Physiol 253:E467–E471, 1987.

67. Walker BR, Campbell JC, Fraser R, et al: Mineralocorticoid excess and inhibition of 11β-hydroxysteroid dehydrogenase in patients with ectopic ACTH syndrome, Clin Endocrinol 37:483–489, 1992.

68. Agarwal AK, Monder C, Eckstein B, et al: Cloning and expression of rat cDNA encoding corticosteroid 11β-dehydrogenase, J Biol Chem 264:18939–18943, 1989.

69. Tannin GM, Agarwal AK, Monder C, et al: The human gene for 11β-hydroxysteroid dehydrogenase: Structure, tissue distribution, and chromosomal localization, J Biol Chem 266:16653–16658, 1991.

70. Monder C, Lakshmi V: Corticosteroid 11β-dehydrogenase of rat tissues: immunological studies, Endocrinology 126:2435–2443, 1990.

71. Albiston AL, Obeyesekere VR, Smith RE, et al: Cloning and tissue distribution of the human 11 beta-hydroxysteroid dehydrogenase type 2 enzyme, Mol Cell Endocrinol 105:R11–R17, 1994.

72. Quinkler M, Stewart PM: Hypertension and the cortisol-cortisone shuttle, J Clin Endocrinol Metab 88:2384–2392, 2003.

73. White PC, Mune T, Agarwal AK: 11β-Hydroxysteroid dehydrogenase and the syndrome of apparent mineralocorticoid excess, Endocr Rev 18:135–156, 1997.

74. Smith RE, Li KXZ, Andrews RK, et al: Immunohistochemical and molecular characterization of the rat 11 beta-hydroxysteroid dehydrogenase type II enzyme, Endocrinology 138:540–547, 1997.

75. Roland BL, Li KX, Funder JW: Hybridization histochemical localization of 11 beta-hydroxysteroid dehydrogenase type 2 in rat brain, Endocrinology 136:4697–4700, 1995.

76. Kotelevtsev Y, Brown RW, Fleming S, et al: Hypertension in mice lacking 11β-hydroxysteroid dehydrogenase type 2, J Clin Invest 103:683–689, 1999.

77. Wilson RC, Nimkarn S, New MI: Apparent mineralocorticoid excess, Trends Endocrinol Metab 12:104–111, 2001.

78. Stewart PM, Valentino R, Wallace AM, et al: Mineralocorticoid activity of licorice: 11β-hydroxysteroid dehydrogenase activity comes of age, Lancet 2:821–824, 1987.

79. Wilson RC, Krozowski ZS, Obeyesekere VR, et al: A mutation in the HSD11B2 gene in a family with apparent mineralocorticoid excess, J Clin Endocrinol Metab 80:2263–2266, 1995.

80. Mune T, Rogerson FM, Nikkila H, et al: Human hypertension caused by mutations in the kidney isozyme of 11 beta-hydroxysteroid dehydrogenase, Nat Genet 10:394–399, 1995.

81. Edwards CRW, Stewart PM, Burt D, et al: Localization of 11β-hydroxysteroid dehydrogenase: tissue-specific protector of the mineralocorticoid receptor, Lancet 2:986–989, 1988.

82. Funder JW, Pearce PT, Smith R, et al: Mineralocorticoid action: target-tissue specificity is enzyme, not receptor-mediated, Science 242:583–585, 1988.

83. Verrey F: Early aldosterone action: toward filling the gap between transcription and transport, Am J Physiol 277:F319–F327, 1999.

84. Stockand JD: New ideas about aldosterone signalling in epithelia, Am J Physiol 282:F559–F576, 2002.

85. McEwen BS, Lambdin LT, Rainbow TC, et al: Aldosterone effects on salt appetite in adrenalectomized rats, Neuroendocrinology 43:38–43, 1986.

86. Rocha R, Funder JW: The pathophysiology of aldosterone in the cardiovascular system, Ann N Y Acad Sci 970:89–100, 2002.

87. Wade JB, Stanton BA, Field MJ, et al: Morphological and physiological responses to aldosterone: time course and sodium dependence, Am J Physiol 259:F88–F94, 1990.

88. Garty H, Palmer LG: Epithelial sodium channels: function, structure and regulation, Physiol Rev 77:359–396, 1997.

89. Benos DJ, Awayda MS, Ismailov II, et al: Structure and function of amiloride-sensitive Na+ channels, J Membr Biol 143:1–18, 1995.

90. Canessa CM, Schild L, Buell G, et al: Amiloride-sensitive epithelial Na+ channel is made of three homologous subunits, Nature 367:463–467, 1994.

91. Jasti J, Furukawa H, Gonzales EB, et al: Structure of acid-sensing ion channel 1 at 1.9A resolution and low pH, Nature 449:316–323, 2007.

92. Barbry P, Hofman P: Molecular biology of Na+ absorption, Am J Physiol 273:G571–G585, 1997.

93. Hummler E, Barker P, Gatzy J, et al: Early death due to defective neonatal lung liquid clearance in αENaC-deficient mice, Nat Genet 12:325–328, 1996.

94. Gründer S, Rossier BC: A reappraisal of aldosterone effects on the kidney: new insights provided by epithelial sodium channel cloning, Curr Opin Nephrol Hypertens 6:35–39, 1997.

95. Barker PM, Nguyen MS, Gatzy JT, et al: Role of gamma ENaC subunit in lung liquid clearance and electrolyte balance in newborn mice. Insights into perinatal adaptation and pseudohypoaldosteronism, J Clin Invest 102:1634–1640, 1998.

96. McDonald FJ, Yang B, Hrstka RF, et al: Disruption of the beta subunit of the epithelial Na+ channel in mice: hyperkalemia and neonatal death associated with a pseudohypoaldosteronism phenotype, Proc Natl Acad Sci U S A 96:1727–1731, 1999.

97. Pradervand S, Barker PM, Wang Q, et al: Salt restriction induces pseudohypoaldosteronism type 1 in mice expressing low levels of the beta-subunit of the amiloride-sensitive epithelial sodium channel, Proc Natl Acad Sci U S A 96:1732–1737, 1999.

98. Chang SS, Grunder S, Hanukoglu A, et al: Mutations in subunits of the epithelial sodium channel cause salt wasting with hyperkalaemic acidosis, pseudohypoaldosteronism type 1, Nat Genet 12:248–253, 1996.

99. Strautnieks SS, Thompson RJ, Gardiner RM, et al: A novel splice-site mutation in the γ-subunit of the epithelial sodium channel gene in three pseudohypoaldosteronism type 1 families, Nat Genet 13:248–250, 1996.

100. Shimkets RA, Warnock DG, Bositis CM, et al: Liddle's syndrome: Heritable human hypertension caused by mutations in the β subunit of the epithelial sodium channel, Cell 79:407–414, 1994.

101. Lifton RP, Gharavi AG, Geller DS: Molecular mechanisms of human hypertension, Cell 104:545–556, 2001.

102. Staub O, Gautschi I, Ishikawa T, et al: Regulation of stability and function of the epithelial Na+ channel ENaC by ubiquitination, EMBO J 16:6325–6336, 1997.

103. Rogerson FM, Brennan FE, Fuller PJ: Dissecting mineralocorticoid receptor structure and function, J Steroid Biochem Mol Biol 85:389–396, 2003.

104. Lingueglia E, Renard S, Waldmann R, et al: Different homologous subunits of the amiloride-sensitive Na+ channel are differently regulated by aldosterone, J Biol Chem 269:13736–13739, 1994.

105. Stokes JB, Sigmund RD: Regulation of rENaC mRNA by dietary NaCl and steroids: organ, tissue, and steroid heterogeneity, Am J Physiol 274:C1699–C1707, 1998.

106. Renard S, Voilley N, Bassilana F, et al: Localization and regulation by steroids of the α, β and γ subunits of the amiloride-sensitive Na+ channel in colon, lung and kidney, Pflugers Arch 430:299–307, 1995.

107. Asher C, Wald H, Rossier BC, et al: Aldosterone-induced increase in the abundance of Na+ channel subunits, Am J Physiol 271:C605–C611, 1996.

108. Volk KA, Sigmund RD, Snyder PM, et al: rENaC is the predominant Na+ channel in the apical membrane of the rat renal inner medullary collecting duct, J Clin Invest 96:2748–2757, 1995.

109. Denault DL, Fejes-Tóth G, Naray-Fejes-Tóth A: Aldosterone regulation of sodium channel γ-subunit mRNA in cortical collecting duct cells, Am J Physiol 271:C423–C428, 1996.

110. May A, Puoti A, Gaeggeler H-P, et al: Early effect of aldosterone on the rate of synthesis of the epithelial sodium channel α subunit in A6 renal cells, J Am Soc Nephrol 8:1813–1822, 1997.

111. Chen SY, Bhargava A, Mastroberardino L, et al: Epithelial sodium channel regulated by aldosterone-induced protein sgk, Proc Natl Acad Sci U S A 96:2514–2519, 1999.

112. Naray-Fejes-Toth A, Canessa C, Cleaveland ES, et al: sgk is an aldosterone-induced kinase in the renal collecting duct, J Biol Chem 274:16973–16978, 1999.

113. Brennan FE, Fuller PJ: Rapid up-regulation of serum and glucocorticoid-regulated kinase (sgk) gene expression by corticosteroids in vivo, Mol Cell Endocrinol 30:129–136, 2000.

114. Bhargava A, Fullerton MJ, Myles K, et al: The serum- and glucocorticoid-induced kinase is a physiological mediator of aldosterone action, Endocrinology 142:1587–1594, 2001.

115. Debonneville C, Flores SY, Kamynina E, et al: Phosphorylation of Nedd4-2 by Sgk1 regulates epithelial Na+ channel cell surface expression, EMBO J 20:7052–7059, 2001.

116. Snyder PM, Olson DR, Thomas BC: Serum and glucocorticoid-regulated kinase modulates Nedd4-2-mediated inhibition of the epithelial Na+ channel, J Biol Chem 277:5–8, 2002.

117. Zhang W, Xia X, Reisenauer MR, et al: Aldosterone-induced Sgk1 relieves Dot1a-Af9-mediated transcriptional repression of epithelial Na+ channel α, J Clin Invest 117:773–783, 2007.

118. Fakitsas P, Adam G, Daidié D, et al: Early aldosterone-induced gene product regulates the epithelial sodium channel by deubiquitylation, J Am Soc Nephrol 18:1084–1092, 2007.

119. Wang J, Barbry P, Maiyar AC, et al: SGK integrates insulin and mineralocorticoid regulation of epithelial sodium transport, Am J Physiol 280:F303–F313, 2001.

120. Brennan FE, Fuller PJ: Mammalian K-ras2 is a corticosteroid-induced gene in vivo, Endocrinology 147:2809–2816, 2006.

121. Soundarajan R, Wang J, Melters D, et al: Differential activities of glucocorticoid-induced leucine zipper protein isoforms, J Biol Chem 282:36303–36313, 2007.

122. Fuller PJ, Verity K: Colonic sodium-potassium adenosine triphosphate subunit gene expression: ontogeny and regulation by adrenocortical steroids, Endocrinology 127:32–38, 1990.

123. Petty KJ, Kokko JP, Marver D: Secondary effect of aldosterone on Na-K,ATPase activity in the rabbit cortical collecting tubule, J Clin Invest 68:1514–1521, 1981.

124. Sansom SC, O'Neil RG: Mineralocorticoid regulation of apical cell membrane Na+ and K+ transport of the cortical collecting duct, Am J Physiol 248:F858–F868, 1985.

125. Attali B, Latter H, Rachamim N, et al: A corticosteroid-induced gene expressing an "IsK-like" K+ channel activity in Xenopus oocytes, Proc Natl Acad Sci U S A 92:6092–6096, 1995.

126. Beguin P, Crambert G, Guennoun S, et al: CHIF, a member of the FXYD protein family, is a regulator of Na,K-ATPase distinct from the gamma-subunit, EMBO J 20:3993–4002, 2001.

127. Wald H, Goldstein O, Asher C, et al: Aldosterone induction and epithelial distribution of CHIF, Am J Physiol 271:F322–F329, 1996.

128. Brennan FE, Fuller PJ: Acute regulation by corticosteroids of CHIF mRNA in the distal colon, Endocrinology 140:1213–1218, 1999.

129. Brennan FE, Fuller PJ: Transcriptional control by corticosteroids of CHIF gene expression in the rat distal colon, Clin Exp Physiol Pharmacol 26:489–491, 1999.

130. Young DB: Quantitative analysis of aldosterone's role in potassium regulation, Am J Physiol 255:F811–F822, 1988.

131. Jaisser F, Escoubet B, Coutry N, et al: Differential regulation of putative K+-ATPase by low-K+ diet and corticosteroids in rat distal colon and kidney, Am J Physiol 270:C679–C687, 1996.

132. Yoo D, Kim BY, Campo C, et al: Cell surface expression of the ROMK (Kir 1.1) channel is regulated by the aldosterone-induced kinase, sgk-1, and protein kinase A, J Biol Chem 278:23066–23075.

133. Stone DK, Seldin DW, Kokko JP, et al: Mineralocorticoid modulation of rabbit medullary collecting duct acidification, J Clin Invest 72:77–83, 1983.

134. Kuwahara M, Sasaki S, Marumo F: Mineralocorticoids and acidosis regulate H+/HCO3 transport of intercalated cells, J Clin Invest 89:1388–1394, 1992.

135. Hays TR: Mineralocorticoid modulation of apical and basolateral membrane H+/OH-/HCO3 transport processes in the rabbit inner stripe of outer medullary collecting duct, J Clin Invest 90:1–8, 1992.

136. Obradovic D, Tirard M, Nemethy ZS, et al: DAXX, FLASH, and FAF-1 modulate mineralocorticoid and glucocorticoid receptor-mediated transcription in hippocampal cells: toward a basis for the opposite actions elicited by two nuclear receptors? Mol Pharmacol 65:761–769, 2004.

137. Turchin A, Guo CZ, Adler GK, et al: Effect of acute aldosterone administration on gene expression profile in the heart, Endocrinology 147:3183–3189, 2006.

138. Fejes Tóth G, Náray-Fejes-Tóth A: Early aldosterone-regulated genes in cardiomyocytes: clues to cardiac remodeling? Endocrinology 148:1502–1510, 2007.

139. Rigsby CS, Cannady WE, Dorrance AM: Aldosterone: good guy or bad guy in cerebrovascular disease? Trends Endocrinol Metab 16:401–406, 2005.

Chapter 5

GLUCOCORTICOID THERAPY

LLOYD AXELROD

This chapter examines the risks associated with the use of glucocorticoids as antiinflammatory or immunosuppressive agents and provides guidelines for the administration of these commonly prescribed substances.

Structure of Commonly Used Glucocorticoids

Fig. 5-1 presents the structures of several commonly used glucocorticoids.[1,2] Cortisol (hydrocortisone) is the principal circulat-

ing glucocorticoid in humans. The presence of a hydroxyl group at carbon 11 of the steroid molecule is an absolute requirement for glucocorticoid activity. Cortisone and prednisone, which are 11-keto compounds, lack glucocorticoid activity until they are converted in vivo to cortisol and prednisolone, the corresponding 11β-hydroxyl compounds.[3,4] This conversion occurs predominantly in the liver. Thus, topical application of cortisone is ineffective in the treatment of dermatologic diseases that respond to topical application of cortisol.[4] Similarly, the antiinflammatory action of cortisone injected into joints is minimal compared with the effect of cortisol administered in the same manner.[3] Cortisone and prednisone are used only for systemic therapy. All glucocor-

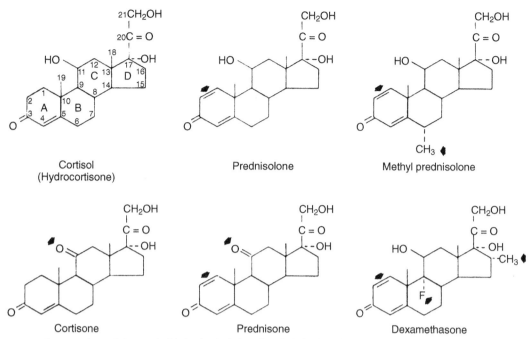

FIGURE 5-1. The structures of commonly used glucocorticoids. In the depiction of cortisol, the 21 carbon atoms of the glucocorticoid skeleton are indicated by *numbers*, and the four rings are designated by *letters*. The *arrowheads* indicate the structural differences between cortisol and each of the other molecules. (Data from Axelrod L: Glucocorticoid therapy. Medicine [Baltimore] 55:39–65, 1976.)

Table 5-1. Commonly Used Glucocorticoids

Duration of Action*	Glucocorticoid Potency[†]	Equivalent Glucocorticoid Dose (mg)	Mineralocorticoid Activity
Short-Acting			
Cortisol (hydrocortisone)	1.0	20	Yes[‡]
Cortisone	0.8	25	Yes[‡]
Prednisone	4.0	5.0	No
Prednisolone	4.0	5.0	No
Methylprednisolone	5.0	4.0	No
Intermediate-Acting			
Triamcinolone	5.0	4.0	No
Long-Acting			
Betamethasone	25	0.60	No
Dexamethasone	30	0.75	No

Data from Axelrod L: Glucocorticoid therapy. Medicine (Baltimore); 55:39–65, 1976.
*The classification by duration of action is based on Harter JG: Corticosteroids. NY State J Med 66:827–840, 1966.
[†]The values given for glucocorticoid potency are relative. Cortisol is arbitrarily assigned a value of 1.
[‡]Mineralocorticoid effects are dose related. At doses close to or within the basal physiologic range for glucocorticoid activity, no such effect may be detectable.

ticoid preparations marketed for topical or local use are 11β-hydroxyl compounds, obviating the need for biotransformation.

Pharmacodynamics

HALF-LIFE, POTENCY, AND DURATION OF ACTION

The important differences among the systemically used glucocorticoid compounds are duration of action, relative glucocorticoid potency, and relative mineralocorticoid potency[1,2] (Table 5-1). The commonly used glucocorticoids are classified as *short-acting*, *intermediate-acting*, and *long-acting* on the basis of the duration of adrenocorticotropic hormone (ACTH) suppression after a single dose, equivalent in antiinflammatory activity to 50 mg of prednisone[5] (see Table 5-1). The relative potencies of the glucocorticoids correlate with their affinities for the glucocorticoid receptor.[6] The observed potency of a glucocorticoid, however, is determined not only by the intrinsic biological potency but also by the duration of action.[6,7] The relative potency of two glucocorticoids varies as a function of the time interval between the administration of the two steroids and the determination of the potency. In particular, failure to consider the duration of action may lead to a marked underestimation of the potency of dexamethasone.[7]

Little correlation exists between the circulating half-life (T$_{1/2}$) of a glucocorticoid and its potency. The T$_{1/2}$ of cortisol in the circulation is 80 to 115 minutes.[1] The T$_{1/2}$ values of other commonly used agents are as follows: cortisone, 0.5 hour; prednisone, 3.4 to 3.8 hours; prednisolone, 2.1 to 3.5 hours;

methylprednisolone, 1.3 to 3.1 hours; and dexamethasone, 1.8 to 4.7 hours.[1,7,8] Although prednisolone and dexamethasone have comparable $T_{1/2}$ values, dexamethasone is clearly more potent. Similarly, little correlation is found between the $T_{1/2}$ of a glucocorticoid and its duration of action. The many actions of glucocorticoids do not have an equal duration.

The duration of action is a function of the dose. For example, the duration of ACTH suppression produced by an individual glucocorticoid is dose related.[5] The duration of ACTH suppression is not simply a function of the level of antiinflammatory activity, because variations in the duration of ACTH suppression are achieved by doses of glucocorticoids with comparable antiinflammatory activity.

In short, the slight differences in the $T_{1/2}$ values of the glucocorticoids contrast with their marked differences in potency and duration of ACTH suppression. Thus the potency and the duration of action of a glucocorticoid are not determined solely by its presence in the circulation; this is consistent with the mechanism of action of steroid hormones. Steroid molecules bind to a specific intracellular receptor protein, the glucocorticoid receptor. The steroid-receptor complex modifies the process of transcription by which RNA is transcribed from the DNA template, among other mechanisms of action (see later discussion). This process alters the rate of synthesis of specific proteins. The steroid thereby modifies the phenotypic expression of the genetic information. Thus a glucocorticoid continues to act inside the cell after it has disappeared from the circulation. Moreover, the events initiated by a glucocorticoid may continue to occur, or a product of these events (such as a specific protein) may be present, after the disappearance of the glucocorticoid from the circulation.

BIOAVAILABILITY, ABSORPTION, AND BIOTRANSFORMATION

Normally the plasma cortisol level is much lower after oral administration of cortisone than after an equal dose of cortisol.[9] Although oral cortisone may be adequate replacement therapy in chronic adrenal insufficiency, the oral form of this agent should not be used when pharmacologic effects are sought. Comparable plasma prednisolone levels are achieved in normal persons after equivalent oral doses of prednisone and prednisolone.[8,10] After the administration of either of these substances, a wide variation is found in individual prednisolone concentrations, which may reflect variability in absorption.[8]

In contrast to the marked increase in the plasma cortisol level that follows the intramuscular injection of hydrocortisone, the plasma cortisol level increases little or not at all after an intramuscular injection of cortisone acetate. When given intramuscularly, cortisone acetate does not provide an adequate plasma cortisol level and offers no advantage over hydrocortisone delivered by the same route. The explanation for the failure of intramuscular cortisone acetate to provide adequate plasma cortisol levels is not known. It may reflect poor absorption from the site of injection. Intramuscular cortisone acetate, which reaches the liver through the systemic circulation, also may be metabolically inactivated before it can be converted to cortisol in the liver, in contrast to oral cortisone acetate, which reaches the liver through the portal circulation.

PLASMA TRANSPORT PROTEINS

In normal people, circadian fluctuations occur in the capacity of corticosteroid-binding globulin (transcortin) to bind cortisol and prednisolone. Patients who have received prednisone for a prolonged period have no diurnal variation in the binding capacity of corticosteroid-binding globulin for cortisol or prednisolone, and both capacities are reduced in comparison with normal persons. Thus, long-term glucocorticoid therapy not only changes the endogenous secretion of steroids but also affects the transport of some glucocorticoids in the circulation. This may explain why the disappearance of prednisolone from the circulation is more rapid in those persons who have previously received glucocorticoids.

Glucocorticoid Therapy in the Presence of Liver Disease

Plasma cortisol levels are normal in patients with liver disease. Although the clearance of cortisol is reduced in patients with cirrhosis, the hypothalamopituitary-adrenal (HPA) homeostatic mechanism remains intact. Consequently, the decreased clearance rate is accompanied by decreased synthesis of cortisol.

The conversion of prednisone to prednisolone is impaired in patients with active liver disease.[11] This is offset in large part by a decreased rate of elimination of prednisolone from the plasma.[11] In patients with liver disease, the plasma availability of prednisolone is quite variable after oral doses of either prednisone or prednisolone.[11] The percentage of plasma prednisolone that is bound to protein is reduced in patients with active liver disease; the unbound fraction is inversely related to the serum albumin concentration. The frequency of prednisone side effects is increased at low serum albumin levels.[12] Both findings may reflect impaired hepatic function. Because the impairment of conversion of prednisone to prednisolone is quantitatively small in patients with liver disease and is offset by the decreased clearance rate of prednisolone, and because of the marked variability in plasma prednisolone levels after the administration of either corticosteroid, no clear mandate exists to use prednisolone rather than prednisone in patients with active liver disease or cirrhosis.[8] If prednisone or prednisolone is used, however, a dose somewhat lower than usual should be given if the serum albumin level is low.[8]

Glucocorticoid Therapy and the Nephrotic Syndrome

When hypoalbuminemia is caused by the nephrotic syndrome, the fraction of prednisolone that is protein bound is decreased. The unbound fraction is inversely related to the serum albumin concentration. The unbound prednisolone concentration remains normal, however.[13,14] Because the pharmacologic effect is determined by the unbound concentration, altered prednisolone kinetics do not explain the increased frequency of prednisolone-related side effects in patients with the nephrotic syndrome.

Glucocorticoid Therapy and Hyperthyroidism

The bioavailability of prednisolone after an oral dose of prednisone is reduced in patients with hyperthyroidism because of decreased absorption of prednisone and increased hepatic clearance of prednisolone.[15]

Glucocorticoids During Pregnancy and in the Early Postnatal Period

Glucocorticoid therapy is well tolerated by the mother in pregnancy.[16] Glucocorticoids cross the placenta, but no compelling evidence indicates that this produces clinically significant adrenal insufficiency or Cushing's syndrome in the neonate, although subnormal responsiveness to exogenous ACTH may occur.[16] Maternal glucocorticoid exposure during the first 8 weeks after conception is associated with an increased risk of cleft lip and palate but not cleft palate alone.[17] Otherwise, no evidence exists that glucocorticoids during pregnancy increase the incidence of congenital defects in humans.[16] Studies in animals indicate that maternal treatment with glucocorticoids programs the offspring, causing increases in blood pressure, glucose levels, HPA activity, and anxiety-related behaviors.[18] In humans, antenatal glucocorticoid therapy may be associated with hypertension in adolescence, hyperinsulinemia, and subtle effects on neurologic function in offspring.[18] Glucocorticoids during pregnancy decrease the birth weight of term infants; the long-term consequences of this are unknown. Glucocorticoid therapy initiated within the first 12 hours after birth is followed by reduced stature and head circumference and impaired neuromotor and cognitive function at school age.[19,20] Because the concentrations of prednisone and prednisolone in breast milk are low, the administration of these drugs to the mother of a nursing infant is unlikely to produce deleterious effects in the infant.

Glucocorticoid Therapy and Aging

The clearance of prednisolone and methylprednisolone decreases with age.[21,22] Although prednisolone levels are higher in elderly subjects than in young subjects after comparable doses, endogenous plasma cortisol levels are suppressed to a lesser extent in the elderly.[21] These findings may be associated with an increased incidence of side effects and suggest the need to use smaller doses in the elderly than in young patients.

Drug Interactions

The concomitant use of other medications can alter the effectiveness of glucocorticoids; the reverse also is true.[23]

EFFECTS OF OTHER MEDICATIONS ON GLUCOCORTICOIDS

The metabolism of glucocorticoids is accelerated by substances that induce hepatic microsomal enzyme activity, such as phenytoin, barbiturates, and rifampicin. The administration of these medications can increase the corticosteroid requirements of patients with adrenal insufficiency or lead to deterioration in the condition of patients whose underlying disorders are well controlled by glucocorticoid therapy. These substances should be avoided if possible in patients receiving corticosteroids. Diazepam does not alter the metabolism of glucocorticoids and is preferable to barbiturates in this setting. If drugs that induce hepatic microsomal enzyme activity must be used in patients taking corticosteroids, an increase in the required dose of corticosteroids should be anticipated.

Conversely, ketoconazole increases the bioavailability of large doses of prednisolone (0.8 mg/kg) because of inhibition of hepatic microsomal enzyme activity.[24] Oral contraceptive use decreases the clearance of prednisone and increases its bioavailability.[25]

The bioavailability of prednisone is decreased by antacids in doses comparable to those used clinically.[26] The bioavailability of prednisolone is not impaired by sucralfate, H_2-receptor blockade, or cholestyramine.

EFFECTS OF GLUCOCORTICOIDS ON OTHER MEDICATIONS

The concurrent administration of a glucocorticoid and a salicylate may reduce the serum salicylate level. Conversely, reduction of the glucocorticoid dose during the administration of a fixed dose of salicylate may produce a higher and possibly toxic serum salicylate level. This interaction may reflect the induction of salicylate metabolism by glucocorticoids.[27]

Glucocorticoids may increase the required dose of insulin or other agents used to treat hyperglycemia, blood-pressure medications, or glaucoma medications. They also may alter the required dose of sedative-hypnotic or antidepressant therapy. Digitalis toxicity can result from hypokalemia caused by glucocorticoids, as from hypokalemia of any cause. Glucocorticoids can reverse the neuromuscular blockade induced by pancuronium.

Considerations Before Initiating Use of Glucocorticoids as Pharmacologic Agents

Cushing's syndrome is a life-threatening disorder. The 5-year mortality rate was more than 50% at the beginning of the era of glucocorticoid and ACTH therapy.[28] Infections and cardiovascular complications were frequent causes of death. High-dose exogenous glucocorticoid therapy is similarly hazardous.

Table 5-2 presents the important questions to consider before initiating glucocorticoid therapy.[29] These questions enable the physician to assess the potential risks of treatment that must be weighed against the possible benefits. The more severe the underlying disorder, the more readily systemic glucocorticoid therapy can be justified. Thus, corticosteroids are commonly

Table 5-2. Considerations Before the Use of Glucocorticoids as Pharmacologic Agents

1. How serious is the underlying disorder?
2. How long will therapy be required?
3. What is the anticipated effective corticosteroid dose?
4. Is the patient predisposed to any of the potential hazards of glucocorticoid therapy?
   Diabetes mellitus
   Osteoporosis
   Peptic ulcer, gastritis, or esophagitis
   Tuberculosis or other chronic infections
   Hypertension and cardiovascular disease
   Psychological difficulties
5. Which glucocorticoid preparation should be used?
6. Have other modes of therapy been used to minimize the glucocorticoid dose and to minimize the side effects of glucocorticoid therapy?
7. Is an alternate-day regimen indicated?

Data from Thorn GW: Clinical considerations in the use of corticosteroids. N Engl J Med 274:775–781, 1966.

used in patients with severe forms of systemic lupus erythematosus, sarcoidosis, active vasculitis, asthma, transplantation rejection, pemphigus, or diseases of comparable severity. Systemic corticosteroids should not be administered to patients with mild bronchial asthma, who should receive more conservative therapy first, including inhaled glucocorticoids.[30] Inhaled glucocorticoids are the most effective long-term control medication for asthma across all age groups.[30]

DURATION OF THERAPY

The anticipated duration of glucocorticoid therapy is a critical consideration. The use of glucocorticoids for 1 to 3 weeks for a condition such as poison ivy or allergic rhinitis is unlikely to be associated with serious side effects in the absence of a contraindication. An exception to this rule is a corticosteroid-induced psychosis, which may occur after only a few days of high-dose glucocorticoid therapy, even in patients with no previous history of psychiatric disease.[31,32] The risk of most complications is related to the dose and duration of therapy.[33-36] Consequently, one should prescribe the smallest possible dose for the shortest possible period. If hypoalbuminemia is present, the dose should be reduced. If long-term treatment is indicated, the use of alternate-day glucocorticoid therapy should be considered (see later).

LOCAL USE

Local corticosteroid preparations should be used whenever possible because they produce fewer side effects than do systemically administered agents. Examples include topical therapy in dermatologic disorders such as bullous pemphigoid, corticosteroid aerosols in bronchial asthma and allergic rhinitis, and corticosteroid enemas in ulcerative proctitis.[30,37,38] Inhaled glucocorticoids have a markedly better safety profile than do orally administered agents.[39] Nevertheless, adrenal suppression and other complications may develop from topical, inhaled, and regional administration of glucocorticoids. The risk factors for the development of these side effects from topical steroids for dermatologic indications include application to a large surface area of skin, application for a prolonged period, use of occlusive dressings, and use of a highly potent (class I) glucocorticoid. In sufficient doses, inhaled glucocorticoids produce an acute but apparently temporary decrease in growth velocity in children, cause osteoporosis, and may increase the risk of cataracts, glaucoma, skin atrophy, and ecchymoses.[39] The development of adrenal suppression from inhaled steroids is related to dose, duration of therapy, and use of a potent agent (e.g., fluticasone).[40] The intraarticular injection of corticosteroids may be of value in carefully selected patients if strict aseptic techniques are used and if frequent injections are avoided.

SELECTING A SYSTEMIC PREPARATION

Agents with no mineralocorticoid activity should be used when a glucocorticoid is prescribed for pharmacologic purposes. If the dosage is to be tapered over a few days, a long-acting agent should be avoided. For alternate-day therapy, one should use a short-acting agent that generally does not cause sodium retention (e.g., prednisone, prednisolone, or methylprednisolone). The use of supplemental medications to minimize the systemic corticosteroid dose and to reduce the side effects of systemic glucocorticoids should always be considered. In asthma, for example, treatment should include inhaled glucocorticoids and bronchodilators such as β-adrenergic agonists and theophylline.

Effects of Exogenous Glucocorticoids

ANTIINFLAMMATORY AND IMMUNOSUPPRESSIVE EFFECTS

Among their many actions, endogenous glucocorticoids protect the organism from damage caused by its own defense reactions and the products of these reactions during stress. They do this by confining inflammatory responses to the area of injury. Consequently, the use of glucocorticoids as antiinflammatory and immunosuppressive agents represents an application of the physiologic effects of glucocorticoids to the treatment of disease (see Chapter 3).

Chronic inflammation is characterized by the increased expression of multiple inflammatory genes that are regulated by transcription factors such as nuclear factor (NF)-κB and activator protein-1 (AP-1).[41-45] These transcription factors bind to and activate coactivator molecules, which acetylate core histone proteins, causing the DNA to unwind, thereby switching on gene transcription, a process called *chromatin remodeling*.[44,45] Glucocorticoids switch off multiple inflammatory genes (including those related to synthesis of cytokines, chemokines, adhesion molecules, inflammatory enzymes, receptors, and other proteins) that are activated during the chronic inflammatory process.[41-45] They do so principally by reversing histone acetylation of activated inflammatory genes through binding of glucocorticoid receptors to coactivators (which have been activated by transcription factors such as NF-κB and AP-1) and recruitment of histone deacetylase-2 to the activated transcription site.[44,45] In high concentrations, glucocorticoids increase the synthesis of antiinflammatory proteins, notably annexin-1 (also called lipocortin-1), an inhibitor of phospholipase A2 (see following); inhibit transcription of genes linked to proteins related to the pathogenesis of glucocorticoid side effects; and have postgenomic effects.[44,45]

Influence on Blood Cells and on Microvasculature

Glucocorticoid effects on inflammatory and immune phenomena include effects on leukocyte movement, leukocyte function, and humoral factors. In general, glucocorticoids have a greater effect on leukocyte traffic than on function and more effect on cellular than on humoral processes.[46,47] Glucocorticoids alter the traffic of all the major leukocyte populations in the circulation.

Perhaps the most important antiinflammatory effect of glucocorticoids is the ability to inhibit the recruitment of neutrophils and monocyte-macrophages to an inflammatory site.[47] Glucocorticoids modify the increased capillary and membrane permeability that occurs in an area of inflammation. By decreasing the microvasculature dilatation and increased capillary permeability that occur during an inflammatory response, the exudation of fluid and the formation of edema may be reduced, and the migration of leukocytes may be impaired.[2,47,48] The decrease in the accumulation of inflammatory cells also is related to decreased adherence of inflammatory cells to the vascular endothelium. This may reflect decreased expression of adhesion molecules E-selectin and intercellular adhesion molecule 1 (ICAM-1) by stimulated endothelial cells.[49]

Glucocorticoids have many effects on leukocyte function.[47] Glucocorticoids suppress cutaneous delayed hypersensitivity responses. Monocyte-macrophage traffic and function are sensitive to glucocorticoids. Glucocorticoids, in divided daily doses, depress the bactericidal activity of monocytes. The sensitivity of monocytes to glucocorticoids may explain the effectiveness of these agents in many granulomatous diseases, because the monocyte is the principal cell involved in granuloma formation.[47] Although neutrophil traffic is sensitive to glucocorticoids, neutrophil function appears to be relatively resistant to these agents.[47] Whereas most in vivo studies of neutrophil phagocytosis have found no evidence for impairment of phagocytosis or bacterial killing,[47] other studies suggest that glucocorticoids induce a generalized phagocytic defect, affecting both granulocytes and monocytes.

Glucocorticoid therapy retards the disappearance of sensitized erythrocytes, platelets, and artificial particles from the circulation.[47] This may account for the efficacy of glucocorticoids in the treatment of idiopathic thrombocytopenic purpura and autoimmune hemolytic anemia.

Influence on Arachidonic Acid Derivatives

Glucocorticoids inhibit prostaglandin (PG) and leukotriene synthesis by inhibiting the release of arachidonic acid from phospholipids.[50] The inhibition of arachidonic acid release appears to be mediated by the induction of annexin-1 (lipocortin-1) and other lipocortins, a family of related proteins that inhibit phospholipase A_2, an enzyme that liberates arachidonic acid from phospholipids.[51,52] This mechanism is distinct from the mechanism of action of the nonsteroidal antiinflammatory agents, such as salicylates and indomethacin, which inhibit the cyclooxygenase that converts arachidonic acid to the cyclic endoperoxide intermediates in the PG synthetic pathway; in some tissues, glucocorticoids inhibit cyclooxygenase activity. Thus the glucocorticoids and the nonsteroidal antiinflammatory agents exert their antiinflammatory effects at two distinct but adjacent loci in the pathway of arachidonic acid metabolism. Glucocorticoids and nonsteroidal antiinflammatory agents have different therapeutic effects. Some of the therapeutic effects of glucocorticoids that are not produced by the nonsteroidal antiinflammatory agents may be related to the inhibition of leukotriene formation.[50]

SIDE EFFECTS

The side effects of glucocorticoids include the diverse manifestations of Cushing's syndrome and HPA suppression[36,53] (Table 5-3) Exogenous Cushing's syndrome differs from endogenous Cushing's syndrome in several respects. Hypertension, acne, menstrual disturbances, male erectile dysfunction, hirsutism or virilism, striae, purpura, and plethora are more common in endogenous Cushing's syndrome. Benign intracranial hypertension, glaucoma, posterior subcapsular cataract, pancreatitis, and avascular necrosis of bone are virtually unique to exogenous Cushing's syndrome. Obesity, psychiatric symptoms, and poor wound healing have nearly equal frequency in endogenous and exogenous Cushing's syndrome.[53,54] These differences may be explained as follows. When Cushing's syndrome is caused by exogenous glucocorticoids, ACTH secretion is suppressed; in spontaneous, ACTH-dependent Cushing's syndrome, the elevated ACTH output causes bilateral adrenal hyperplasia. In the former circumstance, the secretion of adrenocortical androgens and mineralocorticoids is not increased. Conversely, when ACTH output is elevated, the secretion of adrenal androgens and mineralocorticoids may be increased.[1] The augmented secretion of adrenal androgens may account for the higher prevalence of virilism, acne, and menstrual irregularity in the endogenous form of Cushing's syndrome, and the enhanced production of mineralocorticoids may explain the higher prevalence of hypertension.[1] Some of the complications that are virtually unique to exogenous Cushing's syndrome arise after the prolonged use of large doses of glucocorticoids. Examples are benign intracranial

Table 5-3. Adverse Reactions to Glucocorticoids

Ophthalmic

Posterior subcapsular cataracts, increased intraocular pressure and glaucoma, exophthalmos

Cardiovascular

Hypertension
Congestive heart failure in predisposed patients

Gastrointestinal

Peptic ulcer disease, pancreatitis

Endocrine-Metabolic

Truncal obesity, moon facies, supraclavicular fat deposition, posterior cervical fat deposition (buffalo hump), mediastinal widening (lipomatosis), hepatomegaly caused by fatty liver
Acne, hirsutism or virilism, erectile dysfunction, menstrual irregularities
Suppression of growth in children
Hyperglycemia; diabetic ketoacidosis; hyperglycemic, hyperosmolar state; hyperlipoproteinemia
Negative balance of nitrogen, potassium, and calcium
Sodium retention, hypokalemia, metabolic alkalosis
Secondary adrenal insufficiency

Musculoskeletal

Myopathy
Osteoporosis, vertebral compression fractures, other fractures
Avascular necrosis of femoral and humeral heads and other bones

Neuropsychiatric

Convulsions
Benign intracranial hypertension (pseudotumor cerebri)
Alterations in mood or personality
Psychosis

Dermatologic

Facial erythema, thin fragile skin, petechiae and ecchymoses, violaceous striae, impaired wound healing

Immune, Infectious

Suppression of delayed hypersensitivity
Neutrophilia, monocytopenia, lymphocytopenia, decreased inflammatory responses
Susceptibility to infections

hypertension, posterior subcapsular cataract, and avascular necrosis of bone.[1]

Glucocorticoids appear to increase the risk of peptic ulcer disease and also gastrointestinal hemorrhage.[55] The magnitude of the association between glucocorticoid therapy and these complications is small and is related to the total dose and duration of therapy.[55,56] The risk of peptic ulcer disease and related gastrointestinal problems is increased by the concurrent use of glucocorticoids and nonsteroidal antiinflammatory drugs.[57,58]

Glucocorticoid therapy, especially daily therapy, may suppress the immune response to skin tests for tuberculosis. When possible, a tuberculin skin test should be performed before the initiation of glucocorticoid therapy, with the intention to treat with isoniazid if the skin test meets the criteria of the American Thoracic Society.[59]

Some patients respond to (and experience side effects of) glucocorticoids more readily than others at comparable doses. Increased responsiveness to glucocorticoids may be a consequence of hypoalbuminemia, the nephrotic syndrome, impaired renal function, age, drug interactions, and variations in the severity of the underlying disease (see earlier). Impaired renal function may contribute to a decrease in the clearance of prednisolone and an increase in the prevalence of cushingoid features.[60] In patients who experience side effects, the metabolic clearance rate of prednisolone and the volume of distribution are lower[10,61] and the $T_{1/2}$ is longer than in those who do not.[61] Patients who have a cushingoid habitus while taking prednisolone have higher endogenous plasma cortisol levels than do those without this complication, perhaps because of resistance of the HPA axis to suppression by exogenous glucocorticoids.[62] Alterations in bioavailability probably do not account for variations in the therapeutic response to glucocorticoids.

Variations in the effectiveness of corticosteroids may be the result of altered cellular responsiveness to the drugs.[63-66] In patients with primary open-angle glaucoma, exogenous glucocorticoids produce a more pronounced increase of intraocular pressure[63]; a greater suppression of the 8:00 AM plasma cortisol level when dexamethasone, 0.25 mg, is administered the previous evening at 11:00 PM;[65] and greater suppression of phytohemagglutinin-induced lymphocyte transformation[64,66] than in normal persons. Primary open-angle glaucoma is relatively common. These findings suggest that a distinct subpopulation of patients is hyperresponsive to glucocorticoids and that this sensitivity is genetically determined.

PREVENTION OF SIDE EFFECTS

The issues of concern to physicians and patients with respect to glucocorticoid therapy are not only HPA suppression but also long-term complications such as glucocorticoid-induced osteoporosis and *Pneumocystis carinii* pneumonia. The risk of most complications can be reduced by the use of the lowest possible dose of a glucocorticoid for the shortest possible period, by the use of regional or topical rather than systemic steroids, and by the use of alternate-day steroid therapy. In addition, pharmacologic interventions to prevent specific complications such as bone disease and *P. carinii* pneumonia are now widely used.

OSTEOPOROSIS

Patients who receive long-term glucocorticoid therapy develop low bone-mineral density. Fractures occur in as many as 30% to 50% of patients chronically receiving systemic glucocorticoid therapy.[67] The prevalence of vertebral fractures in asthmatic patients on glucocorticoid therapy for at least a year is 11%.[68] Patients with rheumatoid arthritis who are treated with glucocorticoids have an increased incidence of fractures of the hip, ribs, spine, leg, ankle, and foot.[68] Skeletal wasting occurs most rapidly during the first 6 to 12 months of therapy, presumably due to excessive bone resorption. This is followed by a slower progressive phase related to impaired bone formation.[67] Trabecular bone is affected more than cortical bone. Fractures occur at higher levels of bone-mineral density than in postmenopausal osteoporosis.[67] The effects on the skeleton are related to the cumulative dose and duration of treatment.[68] Alternate-day glucocorticoid therapy does not reduce the risk of osteopenia. Inhaled steroids are associated with bone loss.[39]

Glucocorticoids have both direct and indirect effects on the skeleton.[67] They impair the replication, differentiation, and function of osteoblasts and also induce the apoptosis of mature osteoblasts and osteocytes. These effects result in suppression of bone formation. Glucocorticoids promote the formation of osteoclasts with a prolonged life span, which results in enhanced and prolonged bone resorption. Glucocorticoids also affect bone cells by their effects on growth factors present in the bone microenvironment.[67] In particular, glucocorticoids suppress transcription of the insulin-like growth factor 1 (IGF-1) gene.[67] The indirect effects of glucocorticoids on bone metabolism include inhibition of intestinal calcium absorption (by antagonizing the

actions of vitamin D and decreasing the expression of specific calcium channels in the duodenum) and inhibition of renal tubular calcium absorption.[67] These changes may lead to secondary hyperparathyroidism in at least some patients. Glucocorticoids reduce sex steroid–hormone production, probably by inhibition of gonadotropin release as the most important mechanism. Reduced sex steroid–hormone production also may result from reduced ACTH secretion from the pituitary, with consequent diminution of adrenal androgen production. Importantly, some of the disorders for which glucocorticoids are given may themselves cause osteoporosis.[67]

The evaluation of the patient should emphasize risk factors for osteoporosis, including inadequate dietary calcium and vitamin D intake, alcohol consumption, smoking, menopause, and hypogonadism in males. Attention also should be devoted to the possibility of thyrotoxicosis, overtreatment with thyroid hormone medication, renal osteodystrophy, multiple myeloma, osteomalacia, or primary hyperparathyroidism. In selected patients, laboratory studies should be ordered for evaluation of these disorders. Serial assessment of bone-mineral density by using dual energy x-ray absorptiometry, especially in the lateral projection of the spine, is the best way to assess the effects of glucocorticoids on bone.

All patients treated with glucocorticoids systemically should receive calcium and vitamin D supplementation to correct any nutritional deficiency. Calcium therapy alone is associated with rapid rates of spinal bone loss and offers only partial protection from this loss. No evidence suggests that the combination of calcium and vitamin D prevents bone loss due to glucocorticoids.[69] Bisphosphonates (such as etidronate, alendronate, and risedronate) are effective as antiresorptive agents in the prevention of bone loss and fractures resulting from glucocorticoid therapy.[67,70] These agents are the treatment of choice for the prevention and treatment of glucocorticoid-induced osteoporosis.

Daily subcutaneous injections of teriparatide (human parathyroid hormone 1-34) stimulate bone formation and dramatically increase bone mass in the spines of women with glucocorticoid-induced osteoporosis.[71] In glucocorticoid-treated patients with osteoporosis at high risk for fracture, bone-mineral density increases more in patients treated with teriparatide than in those treated with alendronate.[72] Also, fewer new vertebral fractures occur in those on teriparatide than in those on alendronate.[72] Teriparatide, an expensive agent that requires daily subcutaneous injections, should be considered for selected patients who are at high risk for fracture by virtue of low bone-mineral density and long-term glucocorticoid therapy.[70,72]

Women with a premature menopause should receive hormone-replacement therapy unless contraindicated. In postmenopausal women, alternatives to hormone-replacement therapy such as those just indicated should be used. Hypogonadotropic men should receive testosterone therapy unless contraindicated. Patients should be educated about the risks and the consequences of osteoporosis and the factors in their own lives that may contribute thereto. Because steroids also affect muscle mass and function, the patient should be advised about exercises to maintain muscle strength and about the need for adequate protein intake.

PNEUMOCYSTIS CARINII PNEUMONIA

Glucocorticoids predispose patients to many different infections. In the past, prophylaxis against infections for patients treated with glucocorticoids was limited to patients receiving transplantation of organs, who also receive other forms of immunosuppression. Currently, prophylaxis is often used for patients with other disorders who are treated with glucocorticoids, particularly for *P. carinii* pneumonia.[73,74]

In a series of 116 patients without acquired immunodeficiency syndrome (AIDS) who experienced a first episode of *P. carinii* pneumonia between 1985 and 1991, 105 (90.5%) had received glucocorticoids within 1 month before the diagnosis of *P. carinii* pneumonia was established.[73] The median daily dose was equivalent to 30 mg of prednisone; 25% of the patients had received as little as 16 mg/day. The median duration of glucocorticoid therapy was 12 weeks before the development of the pneumonia. In 25% of the patients, *P. carinii* pneumonia developed after 8 weeks or less of glucocorticoid therapy. However, the attack rate in patients with primary or metastatic central nervous system tumors who receive glucocorticoid therapy is about 1.3% and may be lower in other conditions.[74] Prophylactic therapy also may produce side effects.

Many physicians recommend prophylaxis (e.g., trimethoprimsulfamethoxazole, one double-strength tablet per day) for patients with impaired immunocompetence conferred by chemotherapy, transplantation, or an inflammatory disease who have received prednisone, 20 mg or more per day, for more than 1 month. Controlled studies with such prophylaxis in steroid-treated patients are not available. Physicians at the Mayo Clinic detected no cases of *P. carinii* pneumonia in patients who received adequate chemoprophylaxis, when not contraindicated, in recipients of bone marrow or organ transplantation from 1989 to 1995.[73]

WITHDRAWAL FROM GLUCOCORTICOIDS

The symptoms associated with glucocorticoid withdrawal include anorexia, myalgia, nausea, emesis, lethargy, headache, fever, desquamation, arthralgia, weight loss, and postural hypotension. Many of these symptoms can occur with normal plasma glucocorticoid levels and in patients with normal responsiveness to conventional tests of HPA function.[75,76] These patients may have abnormal responses to a low-dose ACTH test with 1 μg of α1-24 ACTH rather than the conventional 250-μg dose.[77,78] Because glucocorticoids inhibit PG production and because many of the features of the glucocorticoid withdrawal syndrome can be produced by PGs such as PGE_2 and PGI_2, this syndrome may be caused by a sudden increase in PG production after the withdrawal of exogenous corticosteroids. In addition, increased circulating interleukin 6 (IL-6) levels may mediate the signs and symptoms of glucocorticoid deficiency.[79] The glucocorticoid withdrawal syndrome may contribute to psychological dependence on glucocorticoid treatment and to difficulties in discontinuing such therapy.

Suppression of the Hypothalamo-Pituitary-Adrenal System

DEVELOPMENT OF HYPOTHALAMO-PITUITARY-ADRENAL SUPPRESSION

Adrenal suppression (i.e., abnormal adrenocortical function as a consequence of glucocorticoid therapy) occurs without hypotension. Secondary adrenal insufficiency caused by glucocorticoid therapy is a clinical entity in which hypotension is always present.[35] Adrenal suppression is much more common than adrenal insufficiency and may indicate susceptibility to overt

adrenal insufficiency, especially under stressful circumstances such as general anesthesia and surgery.

Few well-documented cases of acute adrenocortical insufficiency after prolonged glucocorticoid therapy have been reported, and none after ACTH therapy.[1] After ACTH and glucocorticoids were introduced into clinical practice in the late 1940s, patients were reported in whom shock was attributed to adrenocortical insufficiency caused by these agents, but biochemical evidence of adrenocortical insufficiency was not available to substantiate the diagnosis.[1] Prolonged hypotension or an apparent response of hypotension to intravenous hydrocortisone is not a reliable means of assessing adrenocortical function; one must demonstrate simultaneously that the plasma cortisol level is lower than the values found in normal persons experiencing a comparable degree of stress. When measurement of plasma cortisol levels became available in the early 1960s, three cases were described that met these criteria. The paucity of reports may relate to acute adrenocortical insufficiency after glucocorticoid therapy being uncommon in properly treated patients and physicians being reluctant to report such events.

The minimal duration of glucocorticoid therapy that can produce HPA suppression must be determined from studies of adrenocortical weight and adrenocortical responsiveness to provocative tests.[1,2] Any patient who has received a glucocorticoid in a dose equivalent to 20 to 30 mg/day of prednisone for more than 5 days should be suspected of having HPA suppression.[1,2] If the dose is closer to, but still above, the physiologic range, 1 month is probably the minimal interval.[1,2]

The stress of general anesthesia and surgery is not hazardous to patients who have received only replacement doses ($\leq$25 mg of hydrocortisone, 5 mg of prednisone, 4 mg of triamcinolone, or 0.75 mg of dexamethasone), as long as the corticosteroid is given early in the day. If doses of this size are given late in the day, suppression may occur because of inhibition of the diurnal surge of ACTH release.

ASSESSMENT OF HYPOTHALAMO-PITUITARY-ADRENAL FUNCTION

When HPA suppression is suspected, it may be helpful to assess the integrity of the HPA system. A test of HPA reserve is required only when the result will modify therapy. In practice, this applies to patients who may need an increase in the glucocorticoid dosage to cover a stressful event (such as general anesthesia and surgery) and to patients in whom discontinuation of glucocorticoid therapy is contemplated. In the latter group, a test of the HPA axis is indicated only when the glucocorticoid dosage has been reduced to replacement levels (for example, prednisone, 5 mg/day, or an equivalent dose of another glucocorticoid). In stable patients receiving prolonged glucocorticoid therapy, frequent tests of HPA reserve function are not indicated. For example, it is not necessary to test before each reduction in dose during tapering of the steroid regimen. The responsiveness of the HPA system may change as glucocorticoid therapy continues, and repeated testing is costly.

The short ACTH test is a valuable guide to the presence or absence of HPA suppression in glucocorticoid-treated patients (Table 5-4). Although this test assesses directly only the adrenocortical response to ACTH, it is usually an effective measure of the integrity of the entire HPA axis. Because hypothalamo-pituitary function returns before adrenocortical function during recovery from HPA suppression, a normal adrenocortical response to ACTH in this setting implies that hypothalamo-pituitary function also is normal. This rationale is supported by

Table 5-4. Assessment of Hypothalamo-Pituitary-Adrenal Function in Patients Treated With Glucocorticoids

Method

Withhold exogenous glucocorticoids for 24 h.

Give cosyntropin (synthetic α1-24 ACTH) 250 μg as intravenous bolus or intramuscular injection.

Obtain plasma cortisol level 30 or 60 min after administration of ACTH.

Performance of test in the morning is customary but not essential.

Interpretation

Normal response: plasma cortisol level >18 μg/dL at 30 or 60 min after ACTH administration

Note: Traditional recommendations also specify an increment above baseline of 7 μg/dL at 30 min or 11 μg/dL at 60 min and a doubling of the baseline value at 60 min. These values are valid in normal, unstressed subjects but are frequently misleading in ill patients with a normal HPA axis, in whom stress may raise the baseline plasma cortisol level by an increase in endogenous ACTH levels.

clinical studies. Thus the maximal response of the plasma cortisol level to ACTH corresponds to the maximal plasma cortisol level observed during the induction of general anesthesia and surgery in patients who have received glucocorticoid therapy.[1,2] A normal response to ACTH before surgery is not likely to be followed by impaired secretion of cortisol during anesthesia and surgery in glucocorticoid-treated patients. An abnormal response to ACTH is a necessary but not a sufficient condition for the occurrence of adrenal insufficiency in a steroid-treated patient who undergoes surgery, because some patients with an abnormal response to ACTH tolerate surgery without steroid treatment.[80] Furthermore, hypotension in the operative or postoperative period in a patient who has been treated previously with glucocorticoid therapy is often due to another cause, such as volume depletion or a reaction to anesthetic medication, and may respond to treatment of the other factor. The serum total cortisol response to ACTH may be abnormal in critically ill patients with hypoalbuminemia and reduced levels of corticosteroid-binding globulin, in whom the serum free (bioactive) cortisol levels are normal.[81,82] Thus the abnormal circulating cortisol response to ACTH may reflect decreased circulating binding proteins rather than adrenocortical insufficiency.

Other tests of HPA function generally are not indicated. The low-dose (1-μg) short ACTH test is more sensitive than the conventional ACTH test in patients treated with glucocorticoids.[77,83] The conventional dose of ACTH used in the short ACTH test (and other ACTH tests) produces circulating ACTH levels that are well above the physiologic range. These supraphysiologic levels may result in a normal plasma cortisol level in patients with partial adrenocortical insufficiency. Nevertheless, the low-dose short ACTH test has not yet replaced the conventional-dose short ACTH test in clinical practice. The lower limit of the normal range for the low-dose ACTH test has not been defined.[78] No commercial preparations of ACTH are available for use in the low-dose short ACTH test. The injection for the low-dose short ACTH test must be prepared by dilution, a source of inconvenience and potential error. Insulin-induced hypoglycemia may be dangerous (especially in patients with cardiac or neurologic disease), and the symptoms may be uncomfortable, but it is the only test of the entire HPA axis and is preferred by some. This procedure is more time-consuming and expensive than the ACTH test, because more cortisol values must be obtained. The measurement of plasma cortisol levels before and after the administration of corticotropin-releasing hormone also has been proposed.[84] This test also is longer and more expensive than the ACTH test and has not been compared with

a physiologic stress such as anesthesia and surgery; it offers no advantage over the short ACTH test.[35]

ADRENOCORTICOTROPIC HORMONE AND THE HYPOTHALAMO-PITUITARY-ADRENAL SYSTEM

Pharmacologic doses of ACTH produce elevated cortisol secretory rates and increased plasma cortisol levels. The elevated plasma cortisol levels might be expected to suppress ACTH secretion, but no evidence indicates that ACTH therapy causes significant hypothalamo-pituitary suppression in patients.[1] The failure of ACTH therapy to suppress hypothalamo-pituitary function is not explained by the dose of ACTH used, the frequency of injection, the time of administration, or the plasma cortisol pattern after ACTH administration. Alternatively, the hyperplastic and overactive adrenal cortex that results from ACTH therapy may compensate for hypothalamo-pituitary suppression. Although the threshold adrenocortical sensitivity to ACTH is not changed in patients who have received daily ACTH therapy, adrenocortical responsiveness to ACTH in the physiologic range may be enhanced. The normal response of the plasma cortisol level in patients treated with ACTH also may be preserved, at least in part, because ACTH treatment reduces the rate of endogenous ACTH secretion but not the total amount secreted, whereas glucocorticoids reduce both the rate of secretion and the total amount secreted.[85]

RECOVERY FROM HYPOTHALAMO-PITUITARY-ADRENAL SUPPRESSION

During recovery from HPA suppression, hypothalamo-pituitary function returns before adrenocortical function.[1,2,86] Twelve months must elapse after the discontinuation of large glucocorticoid doses given for a prolonged period before HPA function, including responsiveness to stress, returns to normal.[1,2,86] In contrast, recovery from HPA suppression induced by a brief course of glucocorticoids (i.e., prednisone, 25 mg, twice daily for 5 days) occurs within 5 days.[87] Patients with mild suppression of the HPA axis (i.e., normal basal plasma and urine corticosteroid levels but impaired responses to ACTH and insulin-induced hypoglycemia) resume normal HPA function more rapidly than do those with severe depression of the HPA axis (i.e., low basal plasma and urine corticosteroid levels and impaired responses to ACTH and insulin-induced hypoglycemia).[88] The time course of recovery correlates with the total duration of previous glucocorticoid therapy and the total previous glucocorticoid dose.[88-90] However, in an individual patient, one cannot predict the duration of recovery from a course of glucocorticoid therapy at supraphysiologic doses lasting more than a few weeks. Therefore, the physician should suspect persistence of HPA suppression for 12 months after such treatment. The recovery interval after suppression of the contralateral adrenal cortex by the products of an adrenocortical tumor may exceed 12 months. The recovery from HPA suppression induced by glucocorticoid therapy may be more rapid in children than in adults.

Withdrawal of Patients from Glucocorticoid Therapy

RISKS OF WITHDRAWAL

The decision to discontinue glucocorticoid therapy provokes apprehension among physicians. The potentially harmful consequences of such an action include precipitation of adrenocortical insufficiency, development of the glucocorticoid withdrawal syndrome, and exacerbation of the underlying disease. Adrenocortical insufficiency after the withdrawal of glucocorticoids is an appropriate concern. The probability of precipitating an exacerbation of the underlying disease depends on the activity and natural history of the condition under treatment. When any possibility exists of an exacerbation of the underlying illness, the glucocorticoid should be withdrawn gradually, over an interval of weeks to months, with frequent reassessment of the patient. Changes in dose should be about 10 mg of prednisone (or equivalent) at total daily doses of more than 30 mg, 5 mg at total doses of more than 20 mg, and 2.5 mg at lower doses. Sometimes smaller changes are necessary. The interval between changes in dosage may be as short as 1 day or as long as many weeks.

TREATMENT OF PATIENTS WITH HYPOTHALAMO-PITUITARY-ADRENAL SUPPRESSION

No proven method is known for hastening a return to normal HPA function once inhibition has resulted from glucocorticoid therapy. The administration of ACTH does not prevent or reverse the development of glucocorticoid-induced adrenal insufficiency. Conversion to an alternate-day schedule permits recovery to occur but does not accelerate it. In children, alternate-day glucocorticoid therapy may delay recovery.

The recovery from glucocorticoid-induced adrenal insufficiency is time dependent and spontaneous. The rate of recovery is determined not only by the doses given when the glucocorticoid is being tapered but also by the doses administered during the initial phase of treatment, before tapering is commenced. During the course of recovery, a small dose of hydrocortisone (10 to 20 mg) or prednisone (2.5 to 5.0 mg) given in the morning may alleviate withdrawal symptoms. Recovery of HPA function continues to occur when a small dose of a glucocorticoid is administered in the morning. The possibility cannot be excluded, however, that a small dose of a glucocorticoid given in the morning retards the rate of recovery from HPA suppression.

Alternate-Day Glucocorticoid Therapy

Alternate-day glucocorticoid therapy is defined as the administration of a short-acting glucocorticoid with no appreciable mineralocorticoid effect (i.e., prednisone, prednisolone, or methylprednisolone) once every 48 hours in the morning at about 8:00 AM. The purpose of this approach is to minimize the adverse effects of glucocorticoids while retaining the therapeutic benefits. The original basis for this schedule was the hypothesis that the antiinflammatory effects of glucocorticoids persist longer than the undesirable metabolic effects.[91-93] This hypothesis is not supported by observations of the duration of glucocorticoid effects. A second hypothesis emphasizes that intermittent rather than continuous administration produces a cyclic, although not diurnal, pattern of glucocorticoid levels in the circulation and within the target cells that simulates the normal diurnal cycle.[46] This may prevent the development of Cushing's syndrome and HPA suppression and provide therapeutic benefit. The full expression of a disease frequently occurs only when the level of inflammatory activity is elevated over a prolonged period. The intermittent administration of a glucocorticoid may be sufficient to shorten the interval during which the disorder develops without interruption and thereby prevent the level of disease

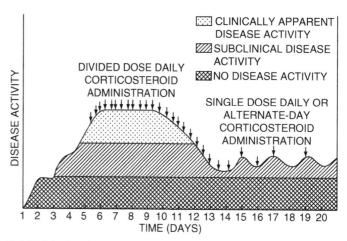

FIGURE 5-2. The effect of glucocorticoid administration on the activity of the underlying disease. A divided daily dose schedule may be necessary initially in some disorders. When the disease is controlled, or from the start of therapy in certain diseases, alternate-day therapy may be effective. (Data from Fauci AS, Dale DC, Balow JE: Glucocorticosteroid therapy: mechanisms of action and clinical considerations. Ann Intern Med 84:304–315, 1976.)

activity from becoming apparent clinically[46] (Fig. 5-2). The duration of action of the glucocorticoid is an important consideration. The selection of prednisone, prednisolone, and methylprednisolone as the agents of choice for alternate-day therapy and of 48 hours as the appropriate interval between doses has an empirical basis. Intervals of 36, 24, and 12 hours are accompanied by adrenal suppression, and an interval of 72 hours is therapeutically ineffective when prednisone is used.[93] An interval of 48 hours is optimal.

ALTERNATE-DAY GLUCOCORTICOID THERAPY AND MANIFESTATIONS OF CUSHING'S SYNDROME

An alternate-day regimen can prevent or ameliorate the manifestations of Cushing's syndrome.[1,2] The susceptibility to infections that characterizes Cushing's syndrome may be diminished. Patients have been described in whom refractory infections cleared after conversion from daily to alternate-day regimens. In addition, the frequency of infections is low in patients receiving alternate-day therapy. Children treated with alternate-day steroid therapy regain or retain tonsillar and peripheral lymphoid tissue. The available information strongly suggests that alternate-day regimens are associated with a lower incidence of infections than are daily regimens but does not firmly establish this point.

Host defense mechanisms have been studied in patients receiving alternate-day therapy. Patients maintained on such schedules have normal blood neutrophil and monocyte counts, normal cutaneous inflammatory responses, and normal neutrophil $T_{1/2}$ values on the days they do not take the glucocorticoid. Patients receiving daily therapy, however, demonstrate neutrophilia, monocytopenia, decreased cutaneous neutrophil and monocyte inflammatory responses, and prolongation of the neutrophil $T_{1/2}$. Patients studied on the days they do not receive treatment do not have the lymphocytopenia observed in patients who receive daily therapy. Monocyte cellular function is normal at 4 hours and at 24 hours after a dose in patients receiving alternate-day therapy. Intermittently normal leukocyte kinetics, preservation of delayed hypersensitivity, and preservation of monocyte cellular function may explain the apparently reduced susceptibility to infection in patients receiving alternate-day therapy.[94-96]

EFFECTS OF ALTERNATE-DAY GLUCOCORTICOID THERAPY ON HYPOTHALAMO-PITUITARY-ADRENAL RESPONSIVENESS

Patients receiving alternate-day glucocorticoid therapy may have some suppression of basal corticosteroid levels, but they have normal or nearly normal responsiveness to provocative tests such as the corticotropin-releasing hormone stimulation test, the ACTH stimulation test, insulin-induced hypoglycemia, and the metyrapone test.[1,2,97] They have less suppression of HPA function than do patients receiving daily therapy.

EFFECTS OF ALTERNATE-DAY THERAPY ON UNDERLYING DISEASE

Alternate-day glucocorticoid therapy is as effective, or nearly as effective, in controlling diverse disorders as is daily therapy in divided doses.[1,2] This approach has provided apparent benefit in patients with the following disorders: childhood nephrotic syndrome, adult nephrotic syndrome, membranous nephropathy, renal transplantation, mesangiocapillary glomerulonephritis, lupus nephritis, ulcerative colitis, rheumatoid arthritis, acute rheumatic fever, myasthenia gravis, Duchenne's muscular dystrophy, dermatomyositis, idiopathic polyneuropathy, asthma, Sjögren's syndrome, sarcoidosis, alopecia areata and other chronic dermatoses, and pemphigus vulgaris. Prospective, controlled studies demonstrate the efficacy of alternate-day therapy in membranous nephropathy and renal transplantation. The role of alternate-day therapy in giant cell arteritis is controversial.[98-100]

USE OF ALTERNATE-DAY THERAPY

Because alternate-day therapy can prevent or ameliorate the manifestations of Cushing's syndrome, can avert or permit recovery from HPA suppression, and is as effective (or nearly as effective) as continuous therapy, patients for whom long-term glucocorticoid administration is indicated should receive such therapy whenever possible. Many efforts fail because of lack of familiarity with the indications for, and use of, such therapy.

The benefits of alternate-day glucocorticoid therapy are demonstrable only when corticosteroids are used for a prolonged period. No need exists to use an alternate-day schedule when the anticipated duration of therapy is a few weeks or less.

Alternate-day glucocorticoid therapy may not be necessary or appropriate during the initial stages of therapy or during exacerbation of the underlying disease. Conversely, patients with many chronic disorders have been treated with an alternate-day regimen as initial therapy with apparent benefit.[1,2] In patients with rheumatoid arthritis, it may be easier to establish treatment with alternate-day corticosteroids than to convert from daily therapy. Physicians treating recipients of renal transplants initially use daily therapy and then convert to an alternate-day schedule.

Alternate-day therapy may be hazardous in the presence of adrenocortical insufficiency of any cause because patients are not protected against glucocorticoid insufficiency during the last 12 hours of the 48-hour cycle. In patients who have been taking glucocorticoids for more than a brief period, or in those who may have adrenal insufficiency on another basis, the adequacy of HPA function should be determined before the initiation of an alternate-day program. It may be possible to address this issue by giving a small dose of a short-acting glucocorticoid (i.e.,

10 mg of hydrocortisone) during the afternoon of the second day; this approach has not been studied systematically.

Alternate-day glucocorticoid therapy may fail to prevent or ameliorate the manifestations of Cushing's syndrome or HPA suppression if a short-acting glucocorticoid is not used, or if it is used incorrectly. For example, the use of prednisone four times a day on alternate days may be less successful than the use of the same total dose once every 48 hours.

An abrupt alteration from daily to alternate-day therapy should be avoided. First, the prolonged use of glucocorticoids in divided daily doses may have caused HPA suppression. In addition, patients with normal HPA function may experience withdrawal symptoms and have an exacerbation of the underlying disease.

No schedule of conversion from daily therapy in divided doses to alternate-day therapy has been shown to be optimal. One approach is to reduce the frequency of drug administration until the total dose for each day is given in the morning, and then to increase the dose gradually on the first day of each 2-day period and to decrease the dose on the second day. Another approach is to double the dose on the first day of each 2-day cycle, to give this as a single morning dose if possible, and then to taper the dose gradually on the second day.[101] It is not clear how often changes in dosage should be made with any approach. This depends on many variables, including the disease under treatment, the duration of previous glucocorticoid therapy, the personality of the patient, and the physician's ability to use adjunctive therapy. Nonetheless, the conversion should be made as quickly as the patient can tolerate it. If adrenal insufficiency, the glucocorticoid withdrawal syndrome, or an exacerbation of the underlying disease develops, the previously effective regimen should be reinstituted and then tapered more gradually. Occasionally it is necessary to resume full daily doses temporarily.

Optimal results from alternate-day glucocorticoid therapy may not be achieved because of failure to use supplemental (steroid-sparing) therapy for the underlying disorder. Conservative (non-glucocorticoid) therapy often is used until a glucocorticoid is initiated, at which time these less toxic therapeutic measures are ignored. Adjunctive therapeutic measures may facilitate the use of the lowest possible glucocorticoid dose. With alternate-day therapy, these measures should be used especially during the end of the second day when symptoms may be prominent. Supplemental therapy may be especially helpful in disorders in which patients are likely to experience symptoms of the disease on the day off therapy, such as asthma and rheumatoid arthritis. In illnesses in which disabling symptoms are less likely to appear on the alternate day, such as the childhood nephrotic syndrome, less difficulty may be encountered.

Alternate-day therapy may be unsuccessful because of failure to inform patients about the purposes of this regimen. Because glucocorticoids may induce euphoria, patients may be reluctant to accept modification of a schedule of frequent doses. A careful explanation about the risks of glucocorticoid excess, attuned to each patient's intellectual and emotional ability to comprehend, enhances the prospects of success.

Daily Single-Dose Glucocorticoid Therapy

Sometimes, alternate-day therapy fails because the patient experiences symptoms of the underlying disease during the last few hours of the second day. In these situations, daily single-dose glucocorticoid therapy may be of value.[1,2] This regimen appears to be as effective as divided daily doses in controlling such underlying diseases as rheumatoid arthritis, systemic lupus erythematosus, polyarteritis, and proctocolitis. In giant cell arteritis, a daily dose in the morning is nearly as effective as daily therapy in divided doses.[98] Daily single-dose therapy reduces the likelihood that HPA suppression will develop. The manifestations of Cushing's syndrome probably are not prevented or ameliorated by a daily single-dose schedule.

Glucocorticoids or Adrenocorticotropic Hormone?

Disorders that respond to glucocorticoid therapy also respond to ACTH therapy if the adrenal cortex is normal. No evidence exists, however, that ACTH is superior to glucocorticoids for the treatment of any disorder when comparable doses are used.[1,2,102] Hydrocortisone and ACTH given intravenously in pharmacologically equivalent doses (determined by plasma cortisol levels and urinary corticosteroid excretion rates) are equally effective in the treatment of inflammatory bowel disease.[103] Similarly, no difference is found in the effectiveness of prednisone and ACTH in the treatment of infantile spasms.[104] Because ACTH does not appear to offer any therapeutic advantage, glucocorticoids are preferable for therapeutic purposes. They can be administered orally, the dose can be regulated precisely, their effectiveness does not depend on adrenocortical responsiveness (an important consideration in patients who have been treated with glucocorticoids), and they produce a lower frequency of certain side effects such as acne, hypertension, and increased skin pigmentation.[1,2] If alternate-day therapy cannot be used, ACTH might appear to be preferable because it does not suppress the HPA axis. This benefit usually is outweighed by the advantages of glucocorticoids and by the fact that daily injections of ACTH are not superior to single daily doses of short-acting glucocorticoids; in both cases, HPA suppression is unlikely to result, but Cushing's syndrome is not prevented. In life-threatening situations, glucocorticoids are indicated because maximal blood levels are obtained immediately after intravenous administration, whereas with ACTH infusion, the plasma cortisol level increases to a plateau over a several-hour period. The principal indication for ACTH continues to be the assessment of adrenocortical function.

Dosage

ANTIINFLAMMATORY OR IMMUNOSUPPRESSIVE THERAPY

The glucocorticoid dose required for antiinflammatory or immunosuppressive therapy is variable and depends on the disease under treatment. In general, the dose ranges from just above that needed for long-term replacement therapy up to 60 to 80 mg of prednisone or its equivalent daily. Although much larger dosages sometimes are recommended for diseases such as asthma, systemic lupus erythematosus, and cerebral edema, controlled studies have not shown the need for such large quantities. The role of massive doses of corticosteroids in asthma is controversial.[105,106] Most studies report no advantage of high-dose therapy (e.g., >60 to 80 mg of prednisone per day). Many physicians use intravenous pulse therapy (e.g., 1 g/day of methylprednisolone intravenously for 3 consecutive days) for severe manifestations of systemic lupus erythematosus, rapidly progressive glomerulonephritis, or other entities. No controlled studies compared

pulse therapy with a dose of 60 to 80 mg/day of prednisone, so the superiority of pulse therapy has not been demonstrated.[107,108]

When alternate-day therapy is used, the dose is variable and depends on the disease under treatment. It may range from just above that needed for long-term replacement therapy to 150 mg of prednisone every other day.

PERIOPERATIVE MANAGEMENT

Traditional doses of glucocorticoids recommended for perioperative coverage in glucocorticoid-treated patients (for example, hydrocortisone, 100 mg intravenously every 8 hours, or methylprednisolone, 20 mg intravenously every 8 hours on the day of surgery, with a gradual taper over the ensuing days) are arbitrary and have no empirical basis.[80] A study in cynomolgus monkeys explored the doses required to prevent postoperative hypotension.[109] Bilateral adrenalectomies were performed, and replacement glucocorticoid (hydrocortisone) and mineralocorticoid doses were given for 4 months. The animals were then divided into three groups, given normal, one-tenth normal, or 10 times the normal replacement doses of glucocorticoid (hydrocortisone) for 4 days before surgery (a cholecystectomy) while the mineralocorticoid replacement continued. The animals that received the one-tenth normal replacement dose had an increased mortality rate, decreased peripheral vascular resistance, and hypotension. The group that received a normal replacement dose of steroids had no more hypotension or postoperative complications than did the group receiving 10 times the replacement dose. A double-blind study in patients yielded similar results.[110] The investigators studied patients who had taken at least 7.5 mg of prednisone per day for several months and had an abnormal response to an ACTH test. All patients received their usual daily dose of prednisone on the day of surgery. One group of 12 patients received perioperative injections of saline. The other group of six patients received hydrocortisone in saline. No significant difference in outcome appeared between the groups in this small study. It appears that patients with adrenal suppression due to glucocorticoid therapy do not experience hypotension or tachycardia when given only their usual daily dose of steroids for surgical procedures such as joint replacements and abdominal operations.

Based on an analysis of the literature, an interdisciplinary group suggests the use of variable doses, depending on the magnitude of the surgical stress.[80] For minor surgical stress (e.g., an inguinal herniorrhaphy), the glucocorticoid target dose is 25 mg of hydrocortisone or equivalent. For moderate surgical stress (e.g., a lower-extremity revascularization or total joint replacement), the target is 50 to 75 mg of hydrocortisone or equivalent. This might constitute continuation of the patient's usual dose of prednisone, such as 10 mg/day, and 50 mg of hydrocortisone intravenously intraoperatively. For major surgical stress (e.g., esophagogastrectomy or cardiopulmonary bypass), the patient might receive his or her usual steroid dose (for example, prednisone, 40 mg) and 50 mg of hydrocortisone intravenously every 8 hours after the initial dose for the first 48 to 72 hours.

Glucocorticoid therapy should not be tapered inadvertently to a dosage below that known to control the underlying disease.

OTHER CONSIDERATIONS

The glucocorticoid dose may have to be modified in patients with certain diseases, in the setting of hypoalbuminemia, in elderly patients, and in patients receiving certain other medications. These considerations are addressed elsewhere in this chapter.

REFERENCES

1. Axelrod L: Glucocorticoid therapy, Medicine (Baltimore) 55:39–65, 1976.
2. Axelrod L: Glucocorticoids. In Kelley WN, Harris ED Jr, Ruddy S, et al, editors: Textbook of Rheumatology, ed 4, Philadelphia, 1993, WB Saunders, pp 779–796.
3. Hollander JL, Brown EM Jr, Jessar RA, et al: Hydrocortisone and cortisone injected into arthritic joints, JAMA 147:1629–1635, 1951.
4. Robinson RCV, Robinson HM Jr: Topical treatment of dermatoses with steroids, South Med J 49:260–266, 1956.
5. Harter JG: Corticosteroids: their physiologic use in allergic disease, NY State J Med 66:827–840, 1966.
6. Ballard PL, Carter JP, Graham BS, et al: A radioreceptor assay for evaluation of the plasma glucocorticoid activity of natural and synthetic steroids in man, J Clin Endocrinol Metab 41:290–304, 1975.
7. Meikle AW, Tyler FH: Potency and duration of action of glucocorticoids: effects of hydrocortisone, prednisone and dexamethasone on human pituitary-adrenal function, Am J Med 63:200–207, 1977.
8. Pickup ME: Clinical pharmacokinetics of prednisone and prednisolone, Clin Pharmacokinet 4:111–128, 1979.
9. Jenkins JS, Sampson PA: Conversion of cortisone to cortisol and prednisone to prednisolone, BMJ 2:205–207, 1967.
10. Gambertoglio JG, Amend WJC Jr, Benet LZ: Pharmacokinetics and bioavailability of prednisone and prednisolone in healthy volunteers and patients: a review, J Pharmacokinet Biopharm 8:1–52, 1980.
11. Davis M, Williams R, Chakraborty J, et al: Prednisone or prednisolone for the treatment of chronic active hepatitis? A comparison of plasma availability, Br J Clin Pharmacol 5:501–505, 1978.
12. Lewis GP, Jusko WJ, Burke CW, et al: Prednisone side-effects and serum-protein levels: a collaborative study, Lancet 2:778–781, 1971.
13. Frey FJ, Frey BM: Altered prednisolone kinetics in patients with the nephrotic syndrome, Nephron 32:45–48, 1982.
14. Gatti G, Perucca E, Frigo GM, et al: Pharmacokinetics of prednisone and its metabolite prednisolone in children with nephrotic syndrome during the active phase and in remission, Br J Clin Pharmacol 17:423–431, 1984.
15. Frey FJ, Horber FF, Frey BM: Altered metabolism and decreased efficacy of prednisolone and prednisone in patients with hyperthyroidism, Clin Pharmacol Ther 44:510–521, 1988.
16. Schatz M, Patterson R, Zeitz S, et al: Corticosteroid therapy for the pregnant asthmatic patient, JAMA 233:804–807, 1975.
17. Carmichael SL, Shaw GM, Ma C, et al: Maternal corticosteroid use and orofacial clefts, Am J Obstet Gynecol 197:585–586, 2007.
18. Seckl JR, Holmes MC: Mechanisms of disease: glucocorticoids, their placental metabolism and fetal "programming" of adult pathophysiology, Nature Clinical Practice Endocrinology & Metabolism 3:479–488, 2007.
19. Yeh TF, Lin YJ, Lin HC, et al: Outcomes at school age after postnatal dexamethasone therapy for lung disease of prematurity, N Engl J Med 350:1304–1313, 2004.
20. Jobe AH: Postnatal corticosteroids for preterm infants: do what we say, not what we do, N Engl J Med 350:1349–1351, 2004.
21. Stuck AE, Frey BM, Frey FJ: Kinetics of prednisolone and endogenous cortisol suppression in the elderly, Clin Pharmacol Ther 43:354–362, 1988.
22. Tornatore KM, Logue G, Venuto RC, et al: Pharmacokinetics of methylprednisolone in elderly and young healthy males, J Am Geriatr Soc 42:1118–1122, 1994.
23. Jubiz W, Meikle AW: Alterations of glucocorticoid actions by other drugs and disease states, Drugs 18:113–121, 1979.
24. Zürcher RM, Frey BM, Frey FJ: Impact of ketoconazole on the metabolism of prednisolone, Clin Pharmacol Ther 45:366–372, 1989.
25. Legler UF, Benet LZ: Marked alterations in dose-dependent prednisolone kinetics in women taking oral contraceptives, Clin Pharmacol Ther 39:425–429, 1986.

26. Uribe M, Casian C, Rojas S, et al: Decreased bioavailability of prednisone due to antacids in patients with chronic active liver disease and in healthy volunteers, Gastroenterology 80:661–665, 1981.
27. Graham GG, Champion GD, Day RO, et al: Patterns of plasma concentrations and urinary excretion of salicylate in rheumatoid arthritis, Clin Pharmacol Ther 22:410–420, 1977.
28. Plotz CM, Knowlton AI, Ragan C: The natural history of Cushing's syndrome, Am J Med 13:597–614, 1952.
29. Thorn GW: Clinical considerations in the use of corticosteroids, N Engl J Med 274:775–781, 1966.
30. Expert Panel Report 3 (EPR-3): Guidelines for the diagnosis and management of asthma-summary report 2007, J Allergy Clin Immunol 120:S94–S138, 2007.
31. Boston Collaborative Drug Surveillance Program: Acute adverse reactions to prednisone in relation to dosage, Clin Pharmacol Ther 13:694–698, 1972.
32. Perry PJ, Tsuang MT, Hwang MH: Prednisolone psychosis: clinical observations, Drug Intell Clin Pharm 18:603–609, 1984.
33. Stuck AE, Minder CE, Frey FJ: Risk of infectious complications in patients taking glucocorticoids, Rev Infect Dis 11:954–963, 1989.
34. Lionakis MS, Kontoyiannis DP: Glucocorticoids and invasive fungal infections, Lancet 362:1828–1838, 2003.
35. Axelrod L: Perioperative management of patients treated with glucocorticoids, Endocrinol Metab Clin North Am 32:367–383, 2003.
36. McDonough AK, Curtis JR, Saag KG: The epidemiology of glucocorticoid-associated adverse events, Curr Opin Rheumatol 20:131–137, 2008.
37. Joly P, Roujeau J-C, Benichou J, et al: A comparison of oral and topical corticosteroids in patients with bullous pemphigoid, N Engl J Med 346:321–327, 2002.
38. Stern RS: Bullous pemphigoid therapy-think globally, act locally, N Engl J Med 346:364–367, 2002.
39. Allen DB, Bielory L, Derendorf H, et al: Inhaled corticosteroids: past lessons and future issues, J Allergy Clin Immunol 112: S1–S40, 2003.
40. Lipworth BJ: Systemic adverse effects of inhaled glucocorticoid therapy: a systematic review and meta-analysis, Arch Intern Med 159:941–955, 1999.
41. Scheinman RI, Cogswell PC, Lofquist AK, et al: Role of transcriptional activation of IκBα in mediation of immunosuppression by glucocorticoids, Science 270:283–286, 1995.
42. Auphan N, DiDonato JA, Rosette C, et al: Immunosuppression by glucocorticoids: inhibition of NF-κB activity through induction of IκB synthesis, Science 270:286–290, 1995.
43. Marx J: How the glucocorticoids suppress immunity, Science 270:232–233, 1995.
44. Barnes PJ: How corticosteroids control inflammation: Quintiles Prize Lecture 2005, Br J Pharmacol 148:245–254, 2006.
45. Buckingham JC: Glucocorticoids: exemplars of multitasking, Br J Pharmacol 147: S258–S268, 2006.
46. Fauci AS, Dale DC, Balow JE: Glucocorticosteroid therapy: mechanisms of action and clinical considerations, Ann Intern Med 84:304–315, 1976.
47. Parrillo JE, Fauci AS: Mechanisms of glucocorticoid action on immune processes, Annu Rev Pharmacol Toxicol 19:179–201, 1979.
48. Cupps TR, Fauci AS: Corticosteroid-mediated immunoregulation in man, Immunol Rev 65:133–155, 1982.
49. Cronstein BN, Kimmel SC, Levin RI, et al: A mechanism for the antiinflammatory effects of corticosteroids: the glucocorticoid receptor regulates leukocyte adhesion to endothelial cells and expression of endothelial-leukocyte adhesion molecule 1 and intercellular adhesion molecule 1, Proc Natl Acad Sci U S A 89:9991–9995, 1992.
50. Samuelsson B: Leukotrienes: mediators of immediate hypersensitivity reactions and inflammation, Science 220:568–575, 1983.
51. DiRosa M, Flower RJ, Hirata F, et al: Anti-phospholipase proteins, Prostaglandins 28:441–442, 1984.
52. Parente L, DiRosa M, Flower RJ, et al: Relationship between the anti-phospholipase and anti-inflammatory effects of glucocorticoid-induced proteins, Eur J Pharmacol 99:233–239, 1984.

53. Axelrod L: Side effects of glucocorticoid therapy. In Schleimer RP, Claman HN, Oronsky AL, editors: Anti-inflammatory Steroid Action: Basic and Clinical Aspects, San Diego, 1989, Academic Press, pp 377–408.
54. Ragan C: Corticotropin, cortisone and related steroids in clinical medicine: practical considerations, Bull N Y Acad Med 29:355–376, 1953.
55. Messer J, Reitman D, Sacks HS, et al: Association of adrenocorticosteroid therapy and peptic ulcer disease, N Engl J Med 309:21–24, 1983.
56. Conn HO, Blitzer BL: Nonassociation of adrenocorticosteroid therapy and peptic ulcer, N Engl J Med 294:473–479, 1976.
57. Piper JM, Ray WA, Daugherty JR, et al: Corticosteroid use and peptic ulcer disease: role of nonsteroidal anti-inflammatory drugs, Ann Intern Med 114:735–740, 1991.
58. Gabriel SE, Jaakkimainen L, Bombardier C: Risk for serious gastrointestinal complications related to use of nonsteroidal anti-inflammatory drugs: a meta-analysis, Ann Intern Med 115:787–796, 1991.
59. American Thoracic Society: Targeted tuberculin testing and treatment of latent tuberculosis infection, Am J Respir Crit Care Med 161:S221–S247, 2000.
60. Bergrem H, Jervell J, Flatmark A: Prednisolone pharmacokinetics in cushingoid and non-cushingoid kidney transplant patients, Kidney Int 27:459–464, 1985.
61. Kozower M, Veatch L, Kaplan MM: Decreased clearance of prednisolone, a factor in the development of corticosteroid side effects, J Clin Endocrinol Metab 38:407–412, 1974.
62. Frey FJ, Amend WJC Jr, Lozada F, et al: Endogenous hydrocortisone, a possible factor contributing to the genesis of cushingoid habitus in patients on prednisone, J Clin Endocrinol Metab 53:1076–1080, 1981.
63. Becker B: Intraocular pressure response to topical corticosteroids, Invest Ophthalmol 4:198–205, 1965.
64. Bigger JF, Palmberg PF, Becker B: Increased cellular sensitivity to glucocorticoids in primary open angle glaucoma, Invest Ophthalmol 11:832–837, 1972.
65. Becker B, Podos SM, Asseff CF, et al: Plasma cortisol suppression in glaucoma, Am J Ophthalmol 75:73–76, 1973.
66. Becker B, Shin DH, Palmberg PF, et al: HLA antigens and corticosteroid response, Science 194:1427–1428, 1976.
67. Canalis E, Mazziotti G, Giustina A, et al: Glucocorticoid-induced osteoporosis: pathophysiology and therapy, Osteoporos Int 18:1319–1328, 2007.
68. American College of Rheumatology Task Force on Osteoporosis Guidelines: Recommendations for the prevention and treatment of glucocorticoid-induced osteoporosis, Arthritis Rheum 39:1791–1801, 1996.
69. Sambrook PN: Calcium and vitamin D therapy in corticosteroid bone loss: what is the evidence? J Rheumatol 23:963–964, 1996.
70. Sambrook PH: Anabolic therapy in glucocorticoid-induced osteoporosis, N Engl J Med 357:2084–2086, 2007.
71. Lane NE, Sanchez S, Modin GW, et al: Parathyroid hormone treatment can reverse corticosteroid-induced osteoporosis: results of a randomized controlled clinical trial, J Clin Invest 102:1627–1633, 1998.
72. Saag KG, Shane E, Boonen S, et al: Teriparatide or alendronate in glucocorticoid-induced osteoporosis, N Engl J Med 357:2028–2039, 2007.
73. Yale SH, Limper AH: *Pneumocystis carinii* pneumonia in patients without acquired immunodeficiency syndrome: associated illnesses and prior corticosteroid therapy, Mayo Clin Proc 71:5–13, 1996.
74. Sepkowitz KA: *Pneumocystis carinii* pneumonia without acquired immunodeficiency syndrome: who should receive prophylaxis? Mayo Clin Proc 71:102–103, 1996.
75. Amatruda TT Jr, Hollingsworth DR, D'Esopo ND, et al: A study of the mechanism of the steroid withdrawal syndrome: evidence for integrity of the hypothalamic-pituitary-adrenal system, J Clin Endocrinol Metab 20:339–354, 1960.
76. Amatruda TT Jr, Hurst MM, D'Esopo ND: Certain endocrine and metabolic facets of the steroid with-

drawal syndrome, J Clin Endocrinol Metab 25:1207–1217, 1965.

77. Dickstein G, Shechner C, Nicholson WE, et al: Adrenocorticotropin stimulation test: effects of basal cortisol level, time of day, and suggested new sensitive low-dose test, J Clin Endocrinol Metab 72:773–778, 1991.

78. Streeten DHP: Shortcomings in the low-dose (1 μg) ACTH test for the diagnosis of ACTH deficiency states, J Clin Endocrinol Metab 84:835–837, 1999.

79. Papanicolaou DA, Tsigos C, Oldfield EH, et al: Acute glucocorticoid deficiency is associated with plasma elevations of interleukin-6: does the latter participate in the symptomatology of the steroid withdrawal syndrome and adrenal insufficiency? J Clin Endocrinol Metab 81:2303–2306, 1996.

80. Salem M, Tainsh RE Jr, Bromberg J, et al: Perioperative glucocorticoid coverage: a reassessment 42 years after emergence of a problem, Ann Surg 219:416–425, 1994.

81. Hanrahian AH, Oseni TS, Arafah BM: Measurements of serum free cortisol in critically ill patients, N Engl J Med 350:1629–1638, 2004.

82. Loriaux L: Glucocorticoid therapy in the intensive care unit, N Engl J Med 350:1601–1602, 2004.

83. Henzen C, Suter A, Lerch E, et al: Suppression and recovery of adrenal response after short-term, high-dose glucocorticoid treatment, Lancet 355:542–545, 2000.

84. Schlaghecke R, Kornely E, Santen RT, et al: The effect of long-term glucocorticoid therapy on pituitary-adrenal responses to exogenous corticotropin-releasing hormone, N Engl J Med 326:226–230, 1992.

85. Daly JR, Fletcher MR, Glass D, et al: Comparison of effects of long-term corticotropin and corticosteroid treatment on responses of plasma growth hormone, ACTH, and corticosteroid to hypoglycaemia, BMJ 2:521–524, 1974.

86. Graber AL, Ney RL, Nicholson WE, et al: Natural history of pituitary-adrenal recovery following long-term suppression with corticosteroids, J Clin Endocrinol Metab 25:11–16, 1965.

87. Streck WF, Lockwood DH: Pituitary adrenal recovery following short-term suppression with corticosteroids, Am J Med 66:910–914, 1979.

88. Spitzer SA, Kaufman H, Koplovitz A, et al: Beclomethasone dipropionate and chronic asthma: the effect of long-term aerosol administration on the hypothalamic-pituitary-adrenal axis after substitution for oral therapy with corticosteroids, Chest 70:38–42, 1976.

89. Westerhof L, Van Ditmars MJ, Der Kinderen PJ, et al: Recovery of adrenocortical function during long-term treatment with corticosteroids, BMJ 4:534–537, 1970.

90. Westerhof L, Van Ditmars MJ, Der Kinderen PJ, et al: Recovery of adrenocortical function during long-term treatment with corticosteroids, BMJ 2:195–197, 1972.

91. Haugen HN, Reddy WJ, Harter JG: Intermittent steroid therapy in bronchial asthma, Nord Med 63:15–18, 1960.

92. Reichling GH, Kligman AM: Alternate-day corticosteroid therapy, Arch Dermatol 83:980–983, 1961.

93. Harter JG, Reddy WJ, Thorn GW: Studies on an intermittent corticosteroid dosage regimen, N Engl J Med 269:591–596, 1963.

94. MacGregor RR, Sheagren JN, Lipsett MB, et al: Alternate-day prednisone therapy: evaluation of delayed hypersensitivity responses, control of disease and steroid side effects, N Engl J Med 280:1427–1431, 1969.

95. Dale DC, Fauci AS, Wolff SM: Alternate-day prednisone: Leukocyte kinetics and susceptibility to infections, N Engl J Med 291:1154–1158, 1974.

96. Fauci AS, Dale DC: Alternate-day therapy and human lymphocyte sub-populations, J Clin Invest 55:22–32, 1975.

97. Schürmeyer TH, Tsokos GC, Avgerinos PC, et al: Pituitary-adrenal responsiveness to corticotropin-releasing hormone in patients receiving chronic, alternate-day glucocorticoid therapy, J Clin Endocrinol Metab 61:22–27, 1985.

98. Hunder GG, Sheps SG, Allen GL, et al: Daily and alternate-day corticosteroid regimens in treatment of giant cell arteritis: comparison in a prospective study, Ann Intern Med 82:613–618, 1975.

99. Abruzzo JL: Alternate-day prednisone therapy, Ann Intern Med 82:714, 1975.

100. Bengtsson B-A, Malmvall B-E: An alternate-day corticosteroid regimen in maintenance therapy of giant cell arteritis, Acta Med Scand 209:347–350, 1981.

101. Fauci AS: Alternate-day corticosteroid therapy, Am J Med 64:729–731, 1978.

102. Allander E: ACTH or corticosteroids? A critical review of results and possibilities in the treatment of severe chronic disease, Acta Rheum Scand 15:277–296, 1969.

103. Kaplan HP, Portnoy B, Binder HJ, et al: A controlled evaluation of intravenous adrenocorticotropic hormone and hydrocortisone in the treatment of acute colitis, Gastroenterology 69:91–95, 1975.

104. Hrachovy RA, Frost JD Jr, Kellaway P, et al: Double-blind study of ACTH vs prednisone therapy in infantile spasms, J Pediatr 103:641–645, 1983.

105. Steroids in acute severe asthma (editorial), Lancet 340:1384–1386, 1992.

106. McFadden ER Jr: Dosages of corticosteroids in asthma, Am Rev Respir Dis 147:1306–1310, 1993.

107. Elenbaas J: Steroid pulse therapy in systemic lupus erythematosus, Drug Intell Clin Pharm 17:342–344, 1983.

108. Kurki P, editor: High-dose intravenous corticosteroid therapy of systemic lupus erythematosus and primary crescenteric rapidly progressive glomerulonephritis: proceedings of a symposium, Scand J Rheumatol Suppl 54:1–34, 1984.

109. Udelsman R, Ramp J, Gallucci WT, et al: Adaptation during surgical stress: a reevaluation of the role of glucocorticoids, J Clin Invest 77:1377–1381, 1986.

110. Glowniak JV, Loriaux DL: A double-blind study of perioperative steroid requirements in secondary adrenal insufficiency, Surgery 121:123–129, 1997.

Chapter 6

ADRENAL INSUFFICIENCY

TENG-TENG CHUNG, ASHLEY GROSSMAN, and ADRIAN J.L. CLARK

Adrenal insufficiency was the first clinical disorder linked unequivocally to pathologic changes in an endocrine organ. It is characterized by impaired adrenocortical function, which causes decreased production of glucocorticoids, mineralocorticoids, and/or adrenal androgens. Primary adrenal insufficiency is caused by diseases that affect the adrenal cortex; it is uncommon, with a recorded incidence of 6 per million population per year.[1,2] Although rare, if overlooked this disorder can be life threatening. Secondary adrenal insufficiency occurs as the consequence of pituitary or hypothalamic pathology and also can be due to abrupt withdrawal of long-term glucocorticoid replacement, resulting in decreased production of adrenocorticotropic hormone (ACTH) from the anterior pituitary or decreased production of cortictropin-releasing hormone (CRH) from the hypothalamus.

History

The recognition of this disease by Addison is generally accepted as the beginning of clinical endocrinology as a specialty. The adrenal glands were first recognized as organs distinct from the kidneys by Bartolomeo Eustachi in 1563.[3] The clinical importance of the adrenal glands was recognized by Addison, a British surgeon, and was described in one of the classic papers in medicine.[4] He showed that destruction of the adrenal glands in humans was associated with a fatal outcome. Of the 11 patients who were described, 5 had bilateral adrenal tuberculosis, 1 had unilateral adrenal tuberculosis, 3 had carcinomatous adrenal involvement, 1 had adrenal hemorrhage, and 1 showed atrophy and fibrosis. Addison's findings were quickly confirmed by Brown-Sequard (1856),[5] who verified Addison's hypothesis in several laboratory animals and showed that bilateral adrenalectomy was a uniformly fatal intervention. The clinical syndrome was named after Addison by Trousseau in 1856.[6] Osler[7] attempted unsuccessfully to treat a young patient with Addison's disease, employing a glycerine extract of fresh pig adrenals given orally. The effects were inconclusive. Wintersteiner and Pfiffner,[8] Kendall,[9] de Fremery and coworkers,[10] and Grollman[11] isolated and characterized cortisone and cortisol in the 1930s, and Sarett[12] devised a partial synthesis for cortisone from deoxycholic acid in 1945. The clinical effects of cortisone soon were made apparent by the work of Hench and coworkers[13] in the treatment of rheumatoid arthritis, and by Thorn and Forsham[14] in the treatment of adrenal insufficiency. The role of the pituitary gland in regulating adrenal function was clarified largely by Cushing,[15] and the role of the hypothalamus in regulating pituitary function was clarified by Harris[16] in the 1950s. ACTH was isolated and characterized by Li and coworkers[17] in 1958, and CRH, in turn, was characterized by Vale and coworkers[18] in 1983. Finally, the syndrome of acute adrenal insufficiency was first recognized in a surgical patient who had atrophic adrenal glands secondary to long-standing glucocorticoid treatment in 1961 by Sampson.[19]

Pathogenesis

Adrenal insufficiency can be categorized into two types, depending on the locus of the pathologic lesion causing the disorder. Primary adrenal insufficiency (Addison's disease) is caused by disordered adrenal function. It is characterized by a low cortisol production rate and a high plasma ACTH concentration. Secondary adrenal insufficiency is caused by disordered function of the hypothalamus and pituitary gland and is characterized by a low cortisol production rate and a normal or low plasma ACTH concentration. The two major adrenal steroids that play an important role in the syndromes of adrenal insufficiency are cortisol and aldosterone; both are usually deficient in primary adrenal insufficiency. In secondary adrenal insufficiency, however, only cortisol is deficient, because the adrenal gland is normal in this condition, and aldosterone is regulated primarily by the renin-angiotensin system, which is independent of the hypothalamus and the pituitary. This difference underlies the relatively different clinical presentations of primary and secondary adrenal insufficiency. The actions and mechanisms of action of glucocorticoids and mineralocorticoids are treated extensively elsewhere in this text. The actions of each class of steroid that have a role in the clinical syndromes of adrenal insufficiency, however, are limited in number. Glucocorticoid modulates ACTH secretion,[20,21] maintains cardiac contractility,[22-24] modulates vascular response to the β-adrenoceptor agonists,[25] and is required for hepatic glycogen deposition.[21,26] Mineralocorticoid modulates the renal handling of sodium, potassium, and hydrogen ions, in effect promoting sodium retention at the expense of potassium and hydrogen excretion.[27] Thus, glucocorticoid deficiency is clinically manifested as ACTH-mediated hyperpigmentation (if the hypothalamo-pituitary unit is normal), hypotension characterized by tachycardia, reduced stroke volume, decreased peripheral vascular resistance, and (in some cases) hypoglyce-mia. Mineralocorticoid deficiency is clinically manifested through isosmotic dehydration, leading to hyponatremia, hyperkalemia, and metabolic acidosis. Thus, in primary adrenal insufficiency, the combined effects of glucocorticoid and mineralocorticoid deficiency lead to orthostatic hypotension, hyponatremia, hyperkalemia, and a mild metabolic acidosis. This is associated with hyperpigmentation due to the high circulating levels of ACTH, which stimulates melanocortin-1 receptors on cutaneous melanocytes. Hyperpigmentation is evident, especially in areas of skin most exposed to increased friction, such as palmar creases, scars, knuckles, and oral mucosa. In secondary adrenal insufficiency, the isolated effects of glucocorticoid insufficiency lead to hypotension and hyponatremia. Hyponatremia occurs secondary (at least in part) to antidiuretic hormone (ADH)-mediated water retention, with normal potassium and hydrogen ion concentrations. ACTH hyperpigmentation is absent in secondary adrenal insufficiency.

Etiology

PRIMARY ADRENAL INSUFFICIENCY

Primary adrenal insufficiency has many causes; these are listed in Table 6-1.[28-32]

Autoimmune Adrenal Insufficiency

When Thomas Addison first described this clinical syndrome, tuberculous adrenalitis was by far the most prevalent cause

Table 6-1. Causes of Primary Adrenal Insufficiency

Diagnosis	Pathogenesis
Autoimmune Adrenal Insufficiency	
Autoimmune Addison's disease	Antibodies against 21-hydroxylase most common, other steroidogenic enzymes such as 17α-hydroxylase, side-chain cleavage enzyme and *CTLA-4*
APS type I or APCED	Autosomal recessive defect in *AIRE-1* gene (autoimmune-regulator-1)
APS type II	HLA DR3/4 locus, including DRB1, DQA1, DQB1, and *CTLA-4*
X-linked polyendocrinopathy	*FOXP3*
Infectious	
Tuberculosis	Tuberculous adrenalitis
Systemic fungal infections	Histoplasmosis, cryptococcosis, blastomycosis
AIDS	Opportunistic infection with CMV, bacteria, protozoa, Kaposi's sarcoma
Adrenal infiltration	Metastases, lymphoma, sarcoidosis, amyloidosis, hemochromatosis
Bilateral adrenalectomy	Result of unresolved Cushing's, treatment with mitotane, ketoconazole, and etomidate, bilateral pheochromocytoma, bilateral nephrectomy
Bilateral adrenal hemorrhage	Meningococcal meningitis, antiphospholipid syndrome, anticoagulation therapy, coagulation disorder, septic shock
Genetic Disorders	
Congenital adrenal hyperplasia	Mutations in the genes encoding 21-hydroxylase (*CYP21A2*), 11β-hydroxylase (*CYB11B1*), 17-hydroxylase (*CYP17A1*), or 3β-hydroxysteroid dehydrogense type 2 (*HSD3B2*)
Adrenoleukodystrophy	Excessive accumulation of the very long chain fatty acid in brain and adrenal cortex. Due to mutations in the *ABCD-1*
Adrenomyeloneuropathy	gene, which encodes the peroxisomal transporter protein ALP
Familial Glucocorticoid Deficiency	
Type 1	Melanocortin 2 receptor (*MC2R*) mutation
Type 2	Melanocortin 2 accessory protein (*MRAP*) gene mutation
Type 3	Genetic origin unknown
Congenital lipoid adrenal hyperplasia	Mutations in the gene encode the steroidogenic acute regulatory protein (*StAR*)
Triple A syndrome	Mutations in *AAAS* encoding ALADIN, a component of the nuclear pore of unknown function
Congenital adrenal hypoplasia	Mutation in the orphan nuclear receptor DAX-1, SF-1, or other unidentified genes

AIDS, Acquired immunodeficiency syndrome; *APCED,* autoimmune polyendocrinopathy, mucocutaneous candidiasis, and ectodermal dystrophy; *APS,* autoimmune polyendocrine syndrome; *CMV,* cytomegalovirus.

of adrenal insufficiency, and this remains a major cause in the developing world. In developed countries, 80% to 90% of patients with primary adrenal insufficiency have autoimmune adrenalitis, which can be isolated or seen as part of an autoimmune polyendocrine syndrome.

Autoimmune Addison's disease involves the autoimmune destruction of the adrenal cortex and is the most common cause of idiopathic adrenal insufficiency in the developed world. The 21-hydroxylase enzyme is the major autoantigen targeted by antiadrenal autoantibodies, and 21-hydroxylase antibodies are present in more than 90% of recent-onset patients.[33] It has been reported that the cumulative risk of developing autoimmune Addison's disease in the presence of 21-hydoxylase antibodies was 48.5%.[34] This cumulative risk was higher in children than in adults (100% vs. 31.9%), and a male preponderance was noted. The presence of autoantibodies against other steroidogenic enzymes, such as the cholesterol side-chain cleavage enzyme (P-450cc) and 17α-hydroxylase, does not correlate with the degree of adrenal dysfunction or the risk of progression. The cytotoxic T cell antigen (*CTLA-4*) gene has been suggested to play an important role in the predisposition to autoimmune Addison's disease,[35] and this locus is linked to type 1 diabetes and autoimmune thyroid disease. However, when found in isolation or in the context of autoimmune polyendocrine syndrome type II (APS II), no significant correlation with the development of Addison's disease is apparent.

About 50% of all Addison's patients have isolated autoimmune adrenal failure; the remainder exhibit an autoimmune polyendocrinopathy, including adrenal failure in association with other gland-specific failure. This latter syndrome has two forms, designated types I and II.[36] The clinical features are summarized in Table 6-2.

Autoimmune polyendocrine syndrome type I (APS I) is also known as autoimmune polyendocrinopathy, mucocutaneous candidiasis, and ectodermal dystrophy (APCED). This is a rare monogenic autosomal recessive disease[37] that is most prevalent in certain stable populations, including Finns and Iranian Jews. The gene that causes this syndrome is located on human chromosome 21q22 and encodes a novel protein known as autoimmune regulator (AIRE).[38,39] AIRE is a nuclear protein that is expressed in cells of the immune system and has structural features that suggest a role as a transcription factor. To date, more than 40 mutations have been discovered in the AIRE gene in patients with APCED. The typical presentation is persistent candidal infection of the skin and mucous membranes, without features of severe systemic infection and with an average onset at 5 years of age, followed by hypoparathyroidism (8 years) and adrenal failure (12 years).[40,41] Affected individuals may suffer from various other autoimmune manifestations such as type 1 diabetes, primary hypogonadism, pernicious anemia, malabsorption, hepatitis, hypothyroidism, alopecia, and vitiligo.

After diagnosis, patients with autoimmune polyendocrine syndrome type I should be closely monitored to prevent delay in diagnosis of additional autoimmune diseases, such as Addison's disease and hypoparathyroidism (which may present during adulthood) and oral cancer, due to inadequate treatment for candidiasis.[42]

Recent attempts have been made to predict occurrences of the disease. In a large European cohort, APS I subjects were screened for 10 different autoantibodies, which revealed several interesting findings. First, redundancy in testing was noted for antibodies to multiple steroidogenic enzymes, and 21-hydroxylase and side-chain cleavage enzymes were deemed sufficient for the prediction of adrenocortical and gonadal failure, respectively.[43] Furthermore, antibodies against tryptophan hydroxylase, which was recognized as an antigen associated with intestinal dysfunction in APS I, have now been identified as a strong predictor of autoimmune hepatitis. These advances should allow early screening for the disease and should improve early intervention rates.

Hypoparathyroidism, a hallmark of APS I, affects more than 80% of patients with this syndrome. A parathyroid-specific antigen called NACHT leucine-rich-repeat protein 5 (NALP5) has recently been identified and is highly specific to hypoparathyroidism. NALP5-specific antibodies were detected in 49% of patients with APS I with hypoparathyroidism and were absent in patients without hypoparathyroidism.[44]

Autoimmune polyendocrine syndrome type II presents more commonly in adulthood, mainly in the third or fourth decade, with a female-to-male ratio of 1.8 to 1.0. It is the most common of the immunoendocrinopathies, estimated at about 5 cases per 100,000 in the United States[45] and 11 to 14 per 100,000 in Europe.[46] It has a complex pattern of inheritance.

Table 6-2. Features of APS I, II and X-Linked Polyendocrinopathy

Features	Type I	Type II	X-Linked Polyendocrinopathy Immune Dysfunction and Diarrhea
Prevalence	Rare	Common	Very rare
Time of onset	Infancy	Adulthood	Neonatal period
Genetic and inheritance	Monogenic, *AIRE*	Polygenic	*FOXP2*, X-linked
Immunodeficiency	Asplenism, susceptibility to candidiasis	None	Overwhelming autoimmunity Loss of regulatory T cells
Adrenal insufficiency	60%-70%	40%-50%	+
Diabetes mellitus	<20%	50%-60%	80%
Autoimmune thyroid disease	10%	70%-75%	+
Hypoparathyroidism	80%-85%	0%-5%	−
Mucocutaneous candidiasis	70%-80%	Nil	−
Hypogonadism	12%	Rare	−
Hypopituitarism	0%-2%	<0.1%	−
Chronic active hepatitis	+	−	+
Pernicious anemia	+	0.5%	−
Skin manifestation	Vitiligo, alopecia	Vitiligo	Eczema, psoriasis or atopic dermatitis
Gastrointestinal	Diarrhea, constipation	Celiac	Enteropathy, malabsorption

This disorder often occurs in multiple generations of the same family, with autosomal dominant inheritance and incomplete penetrance,[47] and it shows a strong association with HLA-DR3 and *CTLA-4*. The HLA locus plays a key role in determining T cell responses to antigens. Various alleles within the HLA-DR3/4 locus, including the DRB1*0301, DQA1*0501, DQB1*0201, and DBP1*0101 or DRB1*0404 haplotypes, have been associated with APS type II patients.[48,49]

The presence of autoimmune adrenal insufficiency with autoimmune thyroid disease (Schmidt's syndrome) and/or type 1 diabetes mellitus defines APS II. Adrenal failure may precede other endocrinopathies.[50] Other features (see Table 6-2) that can be part of this syndrome include hypergonadotrophic hypogonadism, vitiligo, alopecia, myasthenia gravis, pernicious anemia, celiac disease, central diabetes insipidus, and lymphocytic hypophysitis. The major distinction between APS types I and II is the absence of mucocutaneous candidiasis and hypoparathyroidism in APS type II.

X-linked polyendocrinopathy immune dysfunction and diarrhea (XPID) is a rare inborn error of immune regulation that presents as neonatal diabetes and is often fatal. The disorder is also known as X-linked autoimmunity and allergic dysregulation (XLAAD) and immune dysfunction, polyendocrinopathy, and enteropathy, X-linked (IPEX). XPID is caused by mutations in *FOXP3,* which is a critical determinant of CD4+ and CD25+ T regulatory cell development and function.[51] It is characterized by fulminant, widespread autoimmunity, type 1 diabetes, and enteropathy, which leads to diarrhea. Immunosuppressants and bone marrow transplantation can prolong life but are rarely curative.

Infectious Adrenalitis

Infectious diseases represent the most common cause of primary adrenal failure worldwide, with generalized tuberculosis the most frequent single cause. On abdominal computed tomography (CT), an enlarged adrenal with necrotic areas can be seen in the early stages of the disease, and adrenal calcification is seen at a later stage. All the clinically important fungi except *Candida* can also cause adrenal insufficiency. The most common is histoplasmosis, which is particularly prominent in the Ohio and Tennessee River Valleys and along the Piedmont Plateau of the Middle Atlantic States[52,53] and in South India; South American blastomycosis is the next most common fungal cause of adrenal insufficiency,[54] followed by North American blastomycosis,[55] coccidioidomycosis, and cryptococcosis, although all are rare causes of adrenal destruction. The pathophysiology of this process is much like that of tuberculosis, with early adrenal enlargement due to caseating granuloma formation. If healing occurs, the adrenal glands can shrink and sometimes resume a relatively normal volume. This healing process may be accompanied by calcification.

Acquired immunodeficiency syndrome (AIDS) can be associated with adrenal insufficiency in its late stages. The adrenals are involved with infection or tumor in well over half the autopsy cases, although less than 50% of the adrenal gland is destroyed in 97% of cases.[56] This explains the rarity of overt symptoms. Cytomegalovirus infection of the adrenal glands is common in this condition, as is infection with *Mycobacterium avium-intracellulare* and the various fungi that can colonize and destroy the adrenal glands. The plasma cortisol response to ACTH administration, however, is abnormal in only 10% to 15% of these patients.[57] A further occasional cause of adrenal failure is amyloidosis,[58] which often is underdiagnosed and masked by other clinical manifestations of the disease. Although medications may precipitate adrenal insufficiency, they are rarely the cause (fluconazole, ketoconazole, phenytoin sodium, rifampicin, barbiturates). However, one should be aware that the anesthetic agent etomidate can cause significant adrenal insufficiency. Finally, high circulating levels of cytokines in patients with AIDS may suppress the hypothalamic-pituitary-adrenal axis without overt adrenal destruction.

Adrenal Infiltration

The adrenal glands are common sites of metastasis from several different primary tumors. Metastases to the adrenal gland can be as high as 60% in patients with disseminated breast or lung cancer. However, adrenal insufficiency as a result of metastases is uncommon,[59] because clinical manifestations do not occur until more than 90% of the cortex is destroyed. Tumors that are commonly associated with adrenal insufficiency are cancers of the breast, lung, stomach, and colon; melanoma; and some lymphomas. Lymphomas in particular may be bilateral.

Bilateral Adrenalectomy

Bilateral adrenalectomy may be used in failed control of ACTH-dependent Cushing's disease, or for bilateral pheochromocytoma.

Adrenal Hemorrhage

With the advent of the abdominal CT, adrenal hemorrhage is recognized much more frequently as a cause of adrenal insufficiency than it was in years past. The usual setting is a stressed individual anticoagulated for the prevention of pulmonary emboli or other thrombotic phenomena. Other scenarios include trauma, sepsis, or extensive burns. A more frequently recognized relationship is that of adrenal hemorrhage and the antiphospholipid syndrome.[60] It also is well recognized in children or infants with severe infection, particularly those with meningococcemia or *Pseudomonas* sepsis. Typically, the patient will complain of back pain, which is followed in a few days by the acute onset of the first signs and symptoms of adrenal insufficiency. Rarely, these patients may recover adrenal function.[61]

Genetic Disorders

Congenital adrenal hyperplasia (CAH) is a family of inborn errors of steroidogenesis, each characterized by a specific enzyme deficiency that leads to impairment of cortisol synthesis from the adrenal, and can lead to sexual ambiguity, particularly in genetic females. This autosomal recessive disease involves impaired enzymatic function at any of the various steps of synthesis of cortisol from cholesterol. Most often affected are 21-hydroxylase, 11β-hydroxylase, and 3β-hydroxylase dehydrogenase, and less often, 17α-hydroxylase/17,20-lyase and cholesterol desmolase.[62] Blocks in cortisol synthesis impair the negative feedback control of ACTH secretion, and chronic stimulation of the adrenal cortex by ACTH leads to excessive secretion of androgens, resulting in altered development of primary and secondary sexual characteristics. The clinical features of the different forms of CAH are detailed extensively elsewhere in this text.

Congenital lipoid adrenal hyperplasia is a rare form of adrenal steroidogenic defect and is inherited in an autosomal recessive pattern. The disease results from mutations in the gene that encodes the steroidogenic acute regulatory protein (StAR) on chromosome 8p11, which regulates cholesterol uptake into the mitochondria in readiness for conversion to pregnenolone, the first step of steroidogenesis.[63] The pathogenic mechanism has been described as a two-step process. Initially, the biallelic StAR defect leads to impaired steroid biosynthesis in both the adrenal cortex and gonads. Steroidogenesis is reduced to about 15% of normal, the residue resulting presumably because of alternative cholesterol import processes. Consequently, ACTH is stimulated, resulting in increased expression of the adrenocortical low-density lipoprotein receptor and thus increased cholesterol uptake into the adrenals. On histologic examination, the steroidogenic cells of the adrenal cortex and gonads exhibit a characteristic vacuolated appearance due to the florid lipid deposit, ultimately destroying the gland. It is the most severe form of adrenal hyperplasia; affected infants, who experience salt loss from impaired mineralocorticoid and glucocorticoid synthesis, are at risk of death, but hormonal replacement permits long-term survival. In addition, 46XY genetic males have complete lack of androgenization and appear phenotypically female owing to impaired testicular androgen secretion in utero.

Adrenoleukodystrophy (ALD) and adrenomyeloneuropathy (AMN) are two clinical presentations of the same disorder that may exhibit a very broad phenotype. ALD, also known as *Brown Schilder's disease* (brown being an adjective describing the hyperpigmentation of the skin) or *sudanophilic leukodystrophy,* is typically a disease of children characterized by rapidly progressive central demyelination that eventuates in seizures, dementia, cortical blindness, coma, and death. Death usually occurs before puberty is complete.[64,65] However, clinical manifestations can be highly variable, and long survival may occur. Adrenomyeloneuropathy is a disease of young adults that is characterized by a slowly progressive mixed motor and sensory peripheral neuropathy associated with an upper motor neuropathy, leading to an ascending spastic paraparesis. Both forms of the disease are associated with progressive failure of the steroid-secreting cells leading to adrenal and gonadal failure,[66,67] but adrenal failure may occur in isolation. Usually an X-linked disorder, ALD might be underrecognized as a cause of adrenal failure. In one large series, it accounted for a significant proportion of young adult males believed to have autoimmune Addison's disease.[68] The metabolic marker for these diseases is an elevated circulating level of very long chain fatty acids (VLCFAs), C_{26} and greater in length, which rises in response to the primary abnormality, which is a peroxisomal defect in VLCFA metabolism. Peroxisomes are small, intracytoplasmic, membrane-enclosed bodies that contain the enzyme pathways for a number of metabolic and detoxification processes. The gene underlying ALD, identified in 1993 by positional cloning from its location on chromosome Xq28, was found to be a half-transporter of the adenosine triphosphate (ATP)-binding cassette membrane transporter class.[69] It includes six transmembrane domains and an ATP-binding site. This gene probably functions as a heterodimer with another half-transporter to regulate the import of VLCFA into the peroxisome. Many missense, nonsense, and splicing defects in the ALD gene have been described in patients with this disorder. Accumulation of VLCFA in the adrenals seems to be the pathogenic mechanism, although the neuronal pathogenic process may differ. Several treatments have been tried, but only autologous bone marrow transplantation appears to be effective.[70]

Familial glucocorticoid deficiency (FGD) is an autosomal recessive syndrome characterized by cortisol deficiency despite high plasma ACTH and a preserved renin-aldosterone axis. Considerable phenotypic variation has been noted within this disorder. Patients with this syndrome usually present in early childhood with features of glucocorticoid deficiency with undetectable circulating cortisol, although some pass unrecognized

until later childhood, and the diagnosis is then made after a short ACTH stimulation test. It is interesting to note that these children tend to be tall, for reasons that are obscure, and also tend to be highly resistant to suppression of their pigmentation in terms of hydrocortisone replacement. This latter phenomenon, which can be clinically problematic, may indicate the presence of ACTH-mediated auto-feedback at the level of the pituitary.[71] The first molecular abnormality demonstrated was a mutation of the ACTH receptor, located on chromosome 18p11,[72] although it is now known that these cases, known as FGD type 1, represent only some 25% of cases of FGD.[72a] FGD type 2 appears to relate to an entirely novel gene on chromosome 21 that encodes a single transmembrane protein called melanocortin-2 receptor accessory protein (MRAP).[73] This accounts for approximately 20% of all FGD cases,[74] implying that about half of all FGD cases result from other genes yet to be identified.

Triple A syndrome (Allgrove's syndrome) is the association of alacrima, achalasia, and Addison's disease. It is associated with a variety of progressive motor, sensory and autonomic neurologic defects plus mineralocorticoid insufficiency, and it occurs in approximately 15% of cases. This recessive condition results from abnormalities in *AAAS* on chromosome 12q13, which encodes a putative nuclear pore complex protein, ALADIN.[75,76] Furthermore, the expression of clinical features can be highly variable, even within families with the same mutation.[77]

Congenital adrenal hypoplasia (also known as adrenal hypoplasia congenital [AHC]) most often occurs as an X-linked disorder caused by mutation in the nuclear receptor DAX1 (*NR0B1*),[78] which is expressed in the adrenal cortex, gonads, and gonadotrophs, and the ventromedial nucleus of the hypothalamus.[79] Boys with this condition tend to present with salt-losing primary adrenal insufficiency in early infancy (60%) or throughout childhood (40%), followed by hypogonadotrophic hypogonadism secondary to abnormal development of both the hypothalamus and the pituitary. In addition, these boys also show disordered tubular structures and Leydig cell hyperplasia. Recent evidence points to the existence of a milder form with onset in adult life presenting with mild adrenal insufficiency and partial hypogonadotropic hypogonadism.[80] The genetic basis for the recessive form of congenital adrenal hypoplasia remains unknown, but homozygous and heterozygous mutations have been described in the *SF-1* gene that produce primary adrenal failure and a female phenotype complete with uterus in an XY male.[80]

SECONDARY ADRENAL INSUFFICIENCY

The causes of secondary adrenal insufficiency are listed in Table 6-3. The most common cause of secondary adrenal insufficiency is the suppression of CRH and ACTH synthesis with secretion that occurs as a result of exogenous steroid administration. If the exogenous steroids are discontinued for any reason, a period of absolute or relative adrenal insufficiency will ensue. Symptoms usually begin in the first 48 hours after discontinuation of the steroid medication. The likelihood of adrenal suppression in this situation, its magnitude, and its duration all depend on the dose of steroid given, its administration schedule, and the duration of administration (see Chapter 5). The least suppressive regimen is a dose of glucocorticoid that is less than the replacement dose given once a day in the morning for 2 weeks or less. In this case, meaningful adrenal suppression is unlikely.[20] At the other extreme is the administration of supraphysiologic doses of glucocorticoid given in divided doses around the clock for a period long enough to allow early signs of Cushing's syndrome to develop. In this

Table 6-3. Causes of Secondary Adrenal Insufficiency

1. Hypothalamic-pituitary-adrenal suppression
   A. Exogenous
      i. Glucocorticoids
      ii. ACTH
   B. Endogenous: Cushing's syndrome, ACTH dependent or ACTH independent
2. Lesions of the hypothalamus or pituitary gland
   A. Neoplasm
      i. Pituitary tumor
      ii. Metastatic tumor
   B. Craniopharyngioma
   C. Infection
      i. Tuberculosis
      ii. Actinomycosis
      iii. *Nocardia*
3. Sarcoid
4. Head trauma
5. Isolated deficiency of ACTH

ACTH, Adrenocorticotropic hormone.

case, the chance for meaningful adrenal suppression is almost a certainty, and its duration can be as long as 1 year or even longer.[81] Although rare, topical steroid cream can cause adrenal suppression, as can high-dose progesterone therapy such as that employed for treatment of breast carcinoma.[82,83] Secondary adrenal insufficiency is also increasingly a risk in patients with inhaled high-dose potent glucocorticoids used in the treatment of asthma.

Suppression of hypothalamic and pituitary function also can result from endogenous glucocorticoid overproduction, as is seen in Cushing's syndrome caused by an ACTH-secreting pituitary microadenoma, or a cortisol-secreting adrenal adenoma or carcinoma. Therapeutic interventions that eliminate the glucocorticoid excess unmask the secondary adrenal insufficiency.

Tumors and other destructive processes in the region of the sella turcica can lead to secondary adrenal insufficiency. Examples include pituitary tumors,[84] metastatic tumors to the region, sarcoids,[85] amyloids,[86] craniopharyngiomas, and Rathke's pouch cysts. Infections such as actinomycosis and nocardiosis and vascular accidents such as Sheehan's syndrome also can lead to adrenal insufficiency. Finally, isolated ACTH deficiency can occur. When this arises in adulthood, the probable cause is an autoimmune lymphocytic hypophysitis.[87,88] This disorder is more common in females and may be associated with pituitary enlargement, headache, and visual field disturbances, often around the time of pregnancy.[89] Inherited forms of isolated ACTH deficiency present in childhood. Some of these patients demonstrate mutations in the *T-Pit* gene, which encodes an essential transcription factor for the pro-opiomelanocortin gene expression in the corticotroph.[90]

Clinical Features

The symptoms of adrenal insufficiency are the same for primary and secondary disease. Addison's description of the clinical presentation remains as accurate today as it was in 1855: "anaemia, general languor and debility, remarkable weakness of the heart's action, irritability of the stomach, and a peculiar change of colour in the skin."[91] Certain characteristic symptoms distinguish whether it had a primary adrenal cause or a pituitary/hypothalamic cause, and whether onset of disease was gradual or acute.

CHRONIC ADRENAL INSUFFICIENCY

In chronic primary adrenal insufficiency, the presentations are of glucocorticoid and mineralocortioid deficiency. This is different from secondary adrenal insufficiency, where the mineralcorticoid function is often preserved. Onset of disease is usually insidious as the symptoms are nonspecific. Unfortunately, about 50% of patients have signs and symptoms of Addison's disease for longer than 1 year before the diagnosis is made.[92]

Usual complaints center on weakness, fatigue, loss of appetite, and weight loss. Frequent gastrointestinal complaints may include nausea, vomiting, diarrhea, constipation, and abdominal pain, possibly related to loss of gut motility, but the pathophysiology is poorly understood. Some patients complain of dizziness on standing, and some report darkening of the skin, hair, and nails with primary adrenal failure: this is due to ACTH-mediated hyperpigmentation. In many cases, the symptoms are so vague and ill defined that the patient may survive for many years with chronic ill health until a relatively minor infection leads to cardiovascular collapse. The differential diagnosis in such patients will usually include cancer cachexia, but in younger patients some form of functional disorder such as depression or anorexia nervosa can be misdiagnosed. The signs of primary adrenal insufficiency include weight loss and electrolyte abnormalities (hyponatremia, hyperkalemia, mild metabolic acidosis, and hypoglycemia).

Symptoms of salt craving and postural dizziness are characteristic of primary adrenal failure and are attributable to aldosterone deficiency and hypovolemia. In secondary adrenal insufficiency, hyponatraemia is also seen; this is due to cortisol deficiency, increased vasopressin secretion, and water retention.[93] The most specific sign of primary adrenal insufficiency is hyperpigmentation of the skin and mucosa (Fig. 6-1), caused by enhanced stimulation of the skin MC1 receptor by ACTH and possibly other pro-opiomelanocortin–related peptides. In secondary adrenal insufficiency, hyperpigmentation is not present. Other features specific to primary disease are vitiligo in autoimmune adrenal insufficiency and adrenal calcification (Figs. 6-2 and 6-3). In females, decreased axillary and pubic hair, loss of libido, and amenorrhea may be associated.[93,94]

Adrenal insufficiency inevitably leads to dehydroepiandrosterone (DHEA) deficiency, which is a substrate for peripheral sex hormone biosynthesis. Loss of production could result in pronouned androgen deficiency in women. Clinical manifestations in women frequently include loss of axillary and pubic hair, dry skin, and reduced libido. It has also been suggested that DHEA exerts direct effects on neurotransitter receptors in the brain and may have potential antidepressant properties,[95] although the clinical benefits of replacement remain controversial (see Chapter 9).

ACUTE ADRENAL INSUFFICIENCY

Acute adrenal insufficiency or adrenal crisis could be the initial presentation of undiagnosed chronic adrenal insufficiency, precipitated by acute stress or a serious infection. This is of vital importance in critically ill patients and should be suspected in the presence of hypotension that is refractory to therapy with volume expansion and inotropes.

Supraventricular tachycardia, reduced stroke volume, and decreased peripheral resistance are usual.[96] Furthermore, the possiblity of bilateral adrenal hemorrhage or adrenal vein thrombosis will have to be considered in patients with unexplained abdominal or loin pain, vomiting, fever, and altered mental state.

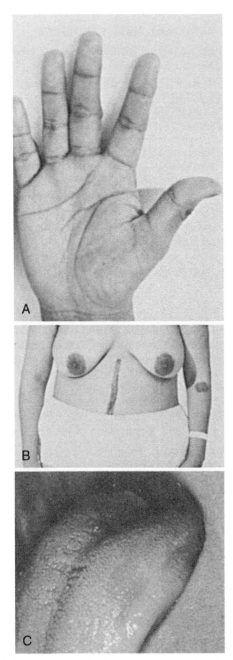

FIGURE 6-1. Hyperpigmented hand, scar, areolae, and buccal mucosa. (From Loriaux L, Cutler G Jr: Disease of the adrenal gland. In Kohler P [ed]: Clinical Endocrinology. New York, Churchill-Livingstone, 1986, p 211.)

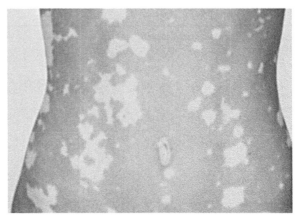

FIGURE 6-2. Vitiligo. (From Loriaux L, Cutler G Jr: Disease of the adrenal gland. In Kohler P [ed]: Clinical Endocrinology. New York, Churchill-Livingstone, 1986, p 211.)

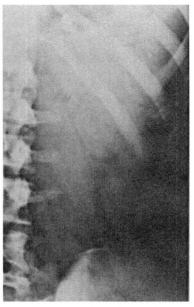

FIGURE 6-3. Adrenal calcification on "flat plate" of the abdomen. (From Loriaux L, Cutler G Jr: Disease of the adrenal gland. In Kohler P [ed]: Clinical Endocrinology. New York, Churchill-Livingstone, 1986, p 211.)

Biochemical Pathology

The traditional laboratory abnormalities that are associated with adrenal insufficiency include normochromic, normocytic anemia, relative lymphocytosis with an increased eosinophil count, a mild metabolic acidosis, and some degree of prerenal azotemia. Electrolyte abnormalities include hyponatremia and hyperkalemia in primary disease and hyponatremia alone in secondary disease.[97] In the former case, electrolyte abnormalities are attributable primarily to mineralocorticoid deficiency with its attendant salt wasting,[98] whereas in the second case, abnormalities can be attributed primarily to free water retention mediated by vasopressin secreted to defend the "relative" volume deficiency caused by glucocorticoid deficiency.[99] This is not "inappropriate ADH," as the excess vasopressin is appropriate to the hypovolemic state.

Diagnosis of Adrenal Insufficiency

Diurnal variation related to the pulsatile release of plasma concentrations of ACTH and cortisol throughout the day makes random sampling unreliable; therefore cortisol measurements (and tests) should be taken between 8 AM and 9 AM. In addition, total cortisol measured can be increased by increased hepatic cortisol-binding globulin production when concomitant medication such as estrogen is prescribed, therefore giving a falsely high reading. A morning plasma cortisol ≤3 μg/dL (83 nmol/L) is indicative of adrenal insufficiency, whereas ≥19 μg/dL (525 nmol/L) rules out the disorder.[93] Plasma ACTH separates patients with primary adrenal insufficiency from those with secondary disease. In primary disease, plasma ACTH usually is greatly increased with values greater than 100 pg/mL (22.0 pmol/L).

CORTICOSYN/SYNACTHEN TEST

This test has become the standard screening test for the diagnosis of primary adrenal insufficiency. The test depends on the fact that the normal adrenal gland, under maximal and acute ACTH stimulation, produces a plasma cortisol concentration of 20 μg/dL (550 nmol/L) at the lower boundary of the normal range.[100] The test is simply done and simply interpreted. Synthetic ACTH, 250 μg, is administered as an intravenous bolus at any time of day, and a blood sample for the measurement of cortisol is drawn at 0, 30, and 60 minutes. Values greater than 20 μg/dL (550 nmol/L) are normal; values less than 20 μg/dL (550 nmol/L; 18 μg/dL [500 nmol/L] in some laboratories) imply dysfunction of the adrenal "axis." The test is quick, stable, insensitive to interference from diet or medication, simple to interpret, and reliable and can be applied to people of all ages without fear of untoward effect, although anaphylaxis has been reported rarely. Similar times and criteria have been demonstrated after intramuscular administration. A completely normal response in this test renders adrenal insufficiency extremely unlikely.

However, some cautions need to be considered. First, this is a test of *adrenal* function; therefore, if it is used as an assessment of *pituitary*-adrenal function, the indirect nature of the test must be appreciated. For example, although hypothalamo-pituitary failure eventually will lead to adrenal hypofunction, and in general a reasonably close correlation has been noted between tests of hypothalamo-pituitary-adrenal function (such as the insulin tolerance test; see below) and the ACTH stimulation test, there are exceptions. In particular, a patient who recently has been rendered hypopituitary, as after pituitary surgery, might show a maintained response to ACTH stimulation while being profoundly ACTH and cortisol deficient.[101] In addition, some patients with chronic fatigue syndrome or fibromyalgia might show marginally low cortisol responses to ACTH,[102] and in general, such patients show little or no clinical response to glucocorticoid replacement therapy. Finally, patients who are severely stressed or ill may show cortisol levels basally or in response to ACTH that are "normal," but these are still insufficient for the degree of systemic upset. Nevertheless, the standard ACTH stimulation test remains the bedrock for the diagnosis of adrenal insufficiency. There has been some support for the use of a "low-dose" test using just 1 μg of ACTH,[103] but although this might be useful in a research setting for diagnosing subtle abnormalities of the pituitary-adrenal axis, in clinical practice the test is difficult to organize and has not found widespread applicability.

In general, with suspected primary adrenal failure, a low 9 AM serum cortisol and a greatly elevated plasma ACTH are sufficient to make the diagnosis. However, if the results of the ACTH assay are delayed, then it is reasonable to perform an ACTH stimulation test as a more rapid surrogate in order to make the diagnosis quickly.

INSULIN TOLERANCE TEST

Insulin-induced hypoglycemia is a powerful stimulus for the secretion of cortisol. This stimulus depends on an intact hypothalamic stimulation of pituitary ACTH secretion and on the ability of the adrenal gland to respond to ACTH with the secretion of cortisol. Thus, a normal test indicates a normally functioning complete adrenal axis. An abnormal test implies a lesion in this system that can be anywhere between the hypothalamus and the adrenal gland. The usual test is done by administering 0.15 unit/kg of regular insulin intravenously as a bolus and measuring blood glucose and cortisol at 15 minute intervals over the subsequent 2 hours. The blood glucose level must fall below 45 mg/mL (<2.2 mmol/L) to ensure adequate stimulation for interpretation of the test. The normal response is a plasma cortisol of greater than 20 μg/dL (550 nmol/L) at any time during the test. With careful observation and adherence to strict guidelines, the test is safe[104] and provides the only complete assessment of the whole hypothalamic-pituitary-adrenal axis.

ADRENAL AUTOANTIBODY TESTS

Antibodies against 21-hydroxylase are present in more than 80% of patients with recent-onset autoimmune adrenalitis.[105] Antibodies against the adrenal side-chain cleavage enzyme and 17-hydroxylase are present less frequently in some patients.

Males with isolated adrenal insufficiency, without evidence of autoimmunity, should be tested for very long chain fatty acids to exclude adrenoleukodystrophy or adrenomyeloneuropathy.

Adrenal Imaging

Imaging is not usually useful for the diagnosis of autoimmune adrenal insufficiency, as the gland would be atrophic. In patients with suspected hemorrhage, infection, infiltration, or neoplastic disease, abdominal CT should be performed.

Treatment

CHRONIC ADRENAL INSUFFICIENCY

Treatment for adrenal insufficiency consists of replacement of the missing steroid hormones: cortisol in secondary adrenal insufficiency and cortisol and aldosterone in primary adrenal insufficiency. Many glucocorticoid preparations are available for this use, but only one, hydrocortisone itself, is entirely appropriate for this purpose. Most of the synthetic steroids such as prednisone and dexamethasone are longer-acting and have no mineralocorticoid activity. Hence, these steroids are ideally suited for pharmacologic intervention in diseases of inflammation and as probes for differential diagnosis, but not for physiologic replacement. Cortisone acetate has a reputation for reduced efficacy and is no longer used frequently.[106,107] The usual dose of hydrocortisone (cortisol) ranges between 12 and 15 mg/m² of body surface area. Hydrocortisone can be given as a once-a-day oral dose, and compliance is enhanced with this regimen. However, most patients feel best when the total daily dose of approximately 20 mg is given in divided doses, usually 10 mg on rising, 5 mg at lunchtime, and 5 mg in the early evening. We usually would advise that the first dose of the day be taken before arising from bed and note that maximal blood levels occur 30 to 60 minutes after the dose taken on an empty stomach. Some actually would advise that the initial morning dose be taken an hour before rising. The dosage can be tapered according to clinical response, and many clinicians also perform measurements of serum cortisol at critical points in the day, just before each dose, or as a day curve to measure levels at several time points after each dose throughout the day. The final dose regimen then is modulated according to clinical response, blood levels, and patient lifestyle, in an attempt to mirror as far as possible the normal circadian rhythm of cortisol. It is particularly important not to overtreat children, in whom growth can be compromised. It should be remembered that exogenous estrogens will dramatically increase cortisol-binding globulin and will vitiate biochemical blood levels. Finally, delayed-release preparations are under clinical trial as a more convenient once-daily form of replacement.

The only preparation that is available to replace mineralocorticoid activity is fludrocortisone, which we normally give as a single daily dose of 50 to 200 µg/day by mouth. Response is best monitored in terms of plasma renin levels, which we measure basally on recumbence and then after 2 to 4 hours of ambulation. No parenteral preparation of fludrocortisone is available, but deoxycorticosterone is available in some countries for parenteral mineralocorticoid substitution.

Replacement of Dehydroepiandrosterone (DHEA)

Approximately 90% of DHEA and DHEA sulfate originates from the adrenal; in women with adrenal insufficiency, this will result in profound androgen deficiency, but the clinical significance remains controversial. Patients with adrenal insufficiency on optimal glucocorticoid and mineralocorticoid replacement have been reported to have a reduced quality of life when compared with normal individuals.[108,109] Several short-term trials in primary and secondary adrenal insufficiency have shown that DHEA replacement potentially improves mood and well-being,[110,111] but beneficial effects have not been reported by all.[112,113] For more detailed discussion, please see Chapter 9. DHEA should be reserved for patients whose well-being is severely impaired, despite optimal glucocorticoid and mineralocorticoid replacement. A daily dose of 25 to 50 mg DHEA taken in the morning with monitoring of therapy with serum DHEA to target the middle of the normal range is recommended.

CHRONIC ADRENAL SUPPRESSION

The goal in treating chronic adrenal suppression is to replace glucocorticoid in a fashion that will permit a reasonable quality of life and at the same time encourage recovery of normal hypothalamo-pituitary-adrenal function. This usually is accomplished by prescribing a dose of hydrocortisone in the range of 12 mg/m² as a once-every-morning dose. Recovery can be gauged by the response of plasma cortisol to an intravenous injection of cosyntropin (Cortrosyn), recovery being indicated by a plasma cortisol level greater than 20 µg/dL (550 nmol/L). This test can be done reasonably at 6 months and every 3 months thereafter until recovery is documented. When recovery is documented, hydrocortisone replacement therapy can be discontinued safely.

ACUTE ADRENAL INSUFFICIENCY

Acute adrenal insufficiency should be considered in any ill patient who has been taking glucocorticoids or has a systemic disease associated with adrenal insufficiency, such as metastatic cancer, AIDS, or tuberculosis. At one extreme are unexplained fever, abdominal pain, and orthostatic hypotension, and at the other extreme is shock that is unresponsive to vasopressors and volume replacement. In this case, a blood sample should be drawn for the measurement of cortisol after administration of ACTH, if time permits. Depending on the severity of the illness and the availability of rapid cortisol measurements, the physician may elect to treat on the assumption that the illness is acute adrenal insufficiency or to hold treatment pending results of the diagnostic evaluation. Obviously, in cases of shock or "pending" shock, waiting is imprudent. Treatment consists of replacing intravascular volume, sodium chloride, and glucocorticoid. Volume and sodium chloride can be replaced together in the form of normal saline infused as quickly as cardiovascular status will permit. Infusions of 2 to 3 L/hr are not unusual. As hypotension improves, the rate of infusion should be metered back to 3 to 4 L/day of normal saline. Glucocorticoid should be given intravenously or intramuscularly, 50 to 100 mg hydrocortisone every 6 hours. If adrenal insufficiency is the sole cause of the clinical picture, clear improvement can be expected within hours. This regimen should be maintained until the results of the blood tests are returned. In critically ill patients, particularly if treatment needs to be prolonged in a critical care unit, hydrocortisone 1 mg/hr by continuous intravenous infusion normally will keep the blood level in the range of 20 to 40 µg/dL (550 to 1100 nmol/L), but occasional blood levels are helpful in modulating the infusion rate. If the diagnosis is confirmed, the hydrocortisone dose can be tapered gradually into the normal range. If the diagnosis is not confirmed, the regimen should be discontinued.

STRESS

The adjustment of glucocorticoid dose with stress remains a problematic issue. The standard of practice is to double the dose with minor stresses such as febrile illness, minor surgical procedures such as dental work, and minor trauma such as small lacerations and contusions. The general practice is to increase the daily dose of hydrocortisone to about 200 to 400 mg/day for major stresses such as intracavitary surgical procedures. Few data are available to support this practice other than the early observations that cortisol excretory products rise with stress, and recent laboratory evidence suggests that cortisol supplementation may not be necessary in all cases. Nonetheless, until it is convincingly demonstrated that the practice has no value, the prudent course is to conform.[114] It is also important that patients understand how to manage their condition, including the need to double their oral dose of hydrocortisone during stress; we also advise that patients always carry a "steroid card" on them and, ideally, that they wear a bracelet or necklace that carries their diagnosis or a contact number to supply details (Medi-Alert/Medi-Tag). The provision of a hydrocortisone emergency pack, consisting of an ampule of 100 mg hydrocortisone, a syringe, and a needle, is also useful for urgent administration during an incipient adrenal crisis, especially in the presence of vomiting and/or diarrhea. This is particularly useful for patients to have available if they travel frequently to places where there might be less familiarity with their diagnosis, and we believe it is important that the patient, wherever possible, be taught to self-inject in an emergency situation. Finally, membership in one of the self-help patient groups can be helpful in allowing these patients to associate with others with the same condition and can encourage a more active and independent role in their self-management.

Adrenal Insufficiency in Critical Illness

Patients with critical illnesses have elevated glucocorticoid secretion, marked by an increase in the serum total cortisol concentration.[115] Evaluation of adrenal function in critical illness is difficult, as there are many confounding factors.[116] These are related to drugs used such as etomidate and ketoconazole, which could decrease cortisol production, or estrogen, which would increase cortisol-binding globulin (CBG) and increase total cortisol. The severity of the illness which often causes profound hypoalbuminemia, will lead to lowering of CBG and therefore decreased total cortisol measurement, although the biologically active free cortisol is normal.[117] Therefore, in interpreting serum total cortisol levels, one should consider the limitations of these measurements when the CBG is increased or decreased. It is clear from previous studies[117-119] that measurement of serum free cortisol represents the most ideal approach in assessing glucocorticoid production in critically ill patients, especially in patients with hypoalbuminemia, yet this assay is not available for routine clinical use. It is possible that salivary cortisol may be a useful surrogate.

The use of hydrocortisone in sepsis as an adjuvant therapy has been controversial for decades.[120] Multiple negative studies have been conducted on the effect of hydrocortisone on septic shock[121,122]; this controversial entity was once again challenged when a study with 229 of 299 patients tested positive for "relative adrenal insufficiency."[123] It was shown that significant mortality improvement occurred when the "nonresponders" were treated with both hydrocortisone and fludrocortisone. However, the most limiting factor of this study is that 24% of the patients had

received etomidate within 8 hours of testing. Etomidate is a short-acting intravenous anesthetic agent that selectively inhibits adrenal corticosteroid synthesis. In the face of this finding, Sprung et al.[124] conducted the Corticosteroid Therapy of Septic Shock (CORTICUS) study, with 499 patients in a randomized double-blinded design. In all, 251 patients given 6-hourly intravenous hydrocortisone versus placebo demonstrated no improvement in survival or reversal of septic shock. A short Synacthen test did not appear to be useful for determining patient therapy, thus questioning the concept of relative adrenal insufficiency.

No consensus has been reached as to which patients in intensive care should be tested with the short Synacthen test, or who would benefit from treatment. The latest guideline from the "Surviving Sepsis Campaign 2008" recognizes that hydrocortisone therapy is not to be used as a routine adjuvant therapy; however, it is suggested for patients who are poorly responsive to fluid resuscitation and concomitant inotropes.[125]

REFERENCES

1. Lovas K, Husebye ES: High prevalence and increasing incidence of Addison's disease in western Norway, Clin Endocrinol 56:787–791, 2002.
2. Kong MF, Jeffcoate W: Eighty-six cases of Addison's disease, Clin Endocrinol 41:757–761, 1994.
3. Eustachi B, Fallopio G: Opuscula Anatomica, Venice, 1563, M.A. Ulmus.
4. Addison T: On the Constitutional and Local Effects of Disease of the Suprarenal Capsules, London, 1855, Highly.
5. Brown-Sequard CE: Recherches experimentales sur la physiologie et la pathologie des capsules surrenales, Acad Sci Paris 43:422–425, 1856.
6. Trousseau A: Bronze Addison's disease, Arch Gen Med 8:478, 1856.
7. Osler W: Case of Addison's disease: death during treatment with the supravital extra, Bull Johns Hopkins Hosp 7:208–209, 1896.
8. Wintersteiner OP, Pfiffner J: Chemical studies on the adrenal cortex: II, J Biol Chem 111:599–612, 1935.
9. Kendall EC: A chemical and physiological investigation of the suprarenal cortex, Symp Quant Biol 5:299, 1937.
10. de Fremery P, Laquer E, Reichstein T, et al: Corticosterone: a crystalloid compound with biological activity of the adrenal-cortical hormone, Nature 139:26–27, 1937.
11. Grollman A: Physiological and chemical studies on the adrenal cortical hormone, Symp Quant Biol 5:313, 1937.
12. Sarett L: The synthesis of hydrocortisone from desoxycholic acid, J Biol Chem 162:601, 1946.
13. Hench PS, Slocumb CH, Barnes AR, et al: The effects of the adrenal cortical hormone, compound E, on the acute phase of rheumatic fever: a preliminary report, Proc Mayo Clin 24:277–297, 1949.
14. Thorn GW, Forsham PH: The treatment of adrenal insufficiency, Rec Prog Horm Res 4:229, 1949.
15. Cushing HW: The Pituitary Body and Its Disorders, Philadelphia, 1912, JB Lippincott.
16. Harris GW: Neural control of the pituitary gland, Physiol Rev 28:139, 1948.
17. Li CH, Dixon JS, Chung D: The structure of bovine corticotropin, J Am Chem Soc 80:2587–2596, 1958.
18. Vale W, Spiers J, Rivier C, et al: Characterization of a 41 residue ovine hypothalamic peptide that stimulates secretion of corticotropin and beta-endorphin, Science 213:585–587, 1981.
19. Sampson PA, Brooke BN, Winstone NE: Biochemical confirmation of collapse due to adrenal failure, Lancet 1:1377, 1961.
20. Speigel RJ, Vigersky RA, Oliff AI: Adrenal suppression after short term corticosteroid therapy, Lancet 1:630–632, 1979.
21. Olefsky JM: The effect of dexamethasone on insulin binding, glucose transport, and glucose oxidation of isolated rat adipocytes, J Clin Invest 56:1499–1508, 1975.

22. Reidenberg MM, Ohler EA, Seuy RW, et al: Hemodynamic changes in adrenalectomized dogs, Endocrinology 72:918–923, 1963.
23. Clarke APW, Cleghorn RA, Ferguson JKW, et al: Factors concerned in the circulatory failure of adrenal insufficiency, J Clin Invest 26:359–363, 1947.
24. Lefer AM, Verrier RL, Carson WW: Cardiac performance in experimental adrenal insufficiency, Circ Res 22:817–827, 1968.
25. Rodan SB, Rodan GA: Dexamethasone effects on beta-adrenergic receptors and adenylate cyclase regulatory proteins Gs and Gi in ROS 17/2.8 cells, Endocrinology 118:2510–2518, 1986.
26. Livingstone JN, Lockwood DH: Effect of glucocorticoids on the glucose transport system of isolated fat cells, J Biol Chem 250:8353–8360, 1975.
27. Marver D, Kokko JP: Renal target sites and the mechanism of action of aldosterone, Miner Electrolyte Metab 9:1–32, 1983.
28. Neufeld M, MacLaren N, Blizzard R: Autoimmune polyglandular syndromes, Pediatr Ann 9:154–162, 1980.
29. Betterle C, Greggio NA, Valpato M: Clinical review 93: autoimmune polyglandular syndrome type 1, J Clin Endocrinol Metab 83:1049–1055, 1998.
30. Betterle C, Valpato M, Greggio NA, et al: Type 2 polyglandular autoimmune disease (Schmidt's syndrome), J Pediatr Endocrinol Metab 9:113–123, 1996.
31. Dittmar M, Kahaly GJ: Extensive personal experience. Polyglandular autoimmune syndromes: immunogenetics and Long-Term follow up, J Clin Endocrinol Metab 88:2983–2992, 2003.
32. Eisenbarth GS, Wilson PN, Ward F, et al: The polyglandular failure syndrome: disease inheritance, HLA-type, and immune function studies in patients and families, Ann Intern Med 91:528–533, 1979.
33. Devendra D, Eisenbarth GS: Immunologic endocrine disorders, J Allergy Clin Immunol 111:S624-S636, 2003.
34. Coco G, Dal Pra C, Presotto F, et al: Estimated Risk for Developing Autoimmune Addison's Disease in Patients with Adrenal Cortex Autoantibodies, J Clin Endocrinol Metab 91:1637–1645, 2006.
35. Betterle C, Dal Pra C, Mantero F, et al: Autoimmune adrenal insufficiency and autoimmune polyendocrine syndromes: autoantibodies, autoantigens, and their applicability in diagnosis and disease prediction, Endocr Rev 23:327–364, 2002.
36. Neufeld M, Maclaren NK, Blizzard RM: Two types of autoimmune Addison's disease associated with different polyglandular autoimmune syndromes, Medicine 60:355–362, 1981.
37. Ahonen P, Myllärniemi S, Sipila I, et al: Clinical variation of autoimmune polyendocrinopathy-candidiasis-ectodermal dystrophy (APECED) in a series of 68 patients, N Engl J Med 322:1829–1836, 1990.

38. An autoimmune disease, APECED, caused by mutations in a novel gene featuring two PHD-type zinc-finger domains: Finnish-German APEED Consortium. Autoimmune Polyendocrinopathy-Candidiasis-Ectodermal Dystrophy, Nat Genet 17:399–403, 1997.
39. Nagamine K, Peterson P, Scott HS, et al: Positional cloning of the APECED gene, Nat Genet 17:393–398, 1997.
40. Perheentupa J: APS1/APECED: the clinical disease and therapy, Endocrinol Metab Clinic North Am 31:295–320, 2002.
41. Pearce SH, Cheetham TD: Autoimmune polyendocrinopathy syndrome type 1: treat with kid gloves, Clin Endocrinol (Oxf) 54:433–435, 2001.
42. Barker JM, Eisenbarth GS: Autoimmune polyendocrine syndromes. In Eisenbarth GS, editor: Type 1 diabetes: molecular, cellular, and clinical immunology, Denver, 2003, Barbara Davis Center for Childhood Diabetes, (Web only).
43. Söderbergh A, Myhre AG, Ekwall O, et al: Prevalence and clinical associations of 10 defined autoantibodies in autoimmune polyendocrine syndrome type I, J Clin Endocrinol Metab 89:557–562, 2004.
44. Alimohammadi M, Björklund P, Hallgren A, et al: Autoimmune polyendocrine syndrome type 1 and NALP5, a parathyroid autoantigen, N Engl J Med 358:1018–1028, 2008.
45. Falorni A, Laurenti S, Santeusanio F: Autoantibodies in autoimmune polyendocrine syndrome type II, Endocrinol Metab Clin North Am 31:369–389, 2002.
46. Laureti S, Vecchi L, Santeusanio F, et al: Is the prevalence of Addison's disease underestimated? J Clin Endocrinol Metab 84:1762, 1999.
47. Eisenbarth GS, Wilson PN, Ward F, et al: The polyglandular failure syndrome: disease inheritance, HLA-type, and immune function studies in patients and families, Ann Intern Med 91:528–533, 1979.
48. Peterson P, Uibo R, Krohn KJ: Adrenal autoimmunity: results and developments, Trends Endocrinol Metab 11:285–290, 2000.
49. Partanen J, Peterson P, Westman P, et al: Major histocompatibility complex class II and III in Addison's disease: MHC alleles do not predict autoantibody specificity and 21-hydroxylase gene polymorphism has no independent role in disease susceptibility, Hum Immunol 41:135–140, 1994.
50. Ten S, New M, MacLaren N: Clinical review 130: Addison's disease, J Clin Endocrinol Metab 86:2909–2922, 2001.
51. Wildin RS, Freitas A: IPEX and FOXP3: clinical and research perspectives, J Autoimmun 25:56–62, 2005.
52. Sarosi GA, Voth DW, Dahl BA, et al: Disseminated histoplasmosis: results of long term follow-up, Ann Intern Med 75:511–516, 1971.
53. Levine E: CT evaluation of active adrenal histoplasmosis, Urol Radiol 13:103–106, 1991.

54. Osa SR, Peterson RE, Roberts RB: Recovery of adrenal reserve following treatment of South American blastomycosis, Am J Med 71:298–301, 1981.
55. Abernathy RS, Melby JC: Addison's disease in North American blastomycosis, N Engl J Med 266:552–554, 1962.
56. Glasgow BJ, Steinsapir BS, Anders K, et al: Adrenal pathology in the acquired immunodeficiency syndrome, Am J Clin Pathol 84:594–597, 1985.
57. Guerra I, Kimmel PL: Hypokalemic adrenal crisis in a patient with AIDS, South Med J 84:1265–1267, 1991.
58. Arik N, Tasdemir I, Karaaslan Y, et al: Subclinical adrenocortical insufficiency in renal amyloidosis, Nephron 56:246–248, 1990.
59. Hasan RI, Yonan NA, Lawson RA: Adrenal insufficiency due to bilateral metastases from oat cell carcinoma of the esophagus, Eur J Cardiothorac Surg 5:336–337, 1991.
60. Satta MA, Corsello SM, Della Casa S, et al: Adrenal insufficiency as the first clinical manifestation of the primary antiphospholipid antibody syndrome, Clin Endocrinol (Oxf) 52:123–126, 2000.
61. Feurstein B, Streeten DHF: Recovery of adrenal function after failure resulting from traumatic bilateral adrenal hemorrhages, Ann Intern Med 115:785–786, 1991.
62. New MI: Diagnosis and management of congenital adrenal hyperplasia, Annu Rev Med 49:311–328, 1998.
63. Lin D, Sugawara T, Strauss JF, et al: Role of steroidogenic acute regulatory protein in adrenal and gonadal steroidogenesis, Science 267:1828–1831, 1995.
64. Schaumberg H, Powers JM, Raine CS, et al: Adrenoleukodystrophy: a clinical and pathological study of 17 cases, Arch Neurol 32:577–585, 1975.
65. Johnson AB, Ascauberg HH, Powers TM: Histochemical characteristics of the striated inclusions of adrenoleukodystrophy, J Histochem Cytochem 24:725–730, 1976.
66. Griffen JW, Goren E, Schaumberg H: Adrenomyelopathy: a probable variant of adrenoleukodystrophy, Neurology 27:1107–1111, 1977.
67. Schaumberg H, Powers JM, Raine CS: Adrenomyeloneuropathy: general, pathologic, neuropathologic, and biochemical aspects, Neurology 27:1114–1120, 1977.
68. Laureti S, Casucci G, Santeusanio F, et al: X-linked adrenoleukodystrophy is a frequent cause of idiopathic Addison disease in young adult male patients, J Clin Endocrinol Metab 81:470–474, 1996.
69. Mosser J, Douar AM, Sarde CO, et al: Putative X-linked adrenoleukodystrophy gene shares unexpected homology with ABC transporters, Nature 361:726–730, 1993.
70. Aubourg P, Blanche S, Jambaqué I, et al: Reversal of early neurologic and neuroradiologic manifestations of X-linked adrenoleukodystrophy by bone marrow transplantation, N Engl J Med 322:1860–1866, 1990.
71. Morris DG, Kola B, Borboli N, et al: Identification of ACTH receptor mRNA in the human pituitary and its loss of expression in pituitary adenomas, J Clin Endocrinol Metab 88:6080–6087, 2003.
72. Clark AJ, McLoughlin L, Grossman A: Familial glucocorticoid deficiency associated with point mutation in the adrenocorticotropin receptor, Lancet 341:461–462, 1993.
72a.Clark AJ, Weber A: Adrenocorticotropin insensitivity syndromes, Endocr Rev 19:828–843, 1998.
73. Metherell LA, Chapple JP, Cooray S, et al: Mutations in MRAP, encoding a novel interacting partner of the ACTH receptor, cause Familial Glucocorticoid Deficiency Type 2, Nat Genet 37:166–170, 2005.
74. Clark AJL, Metherell LA, Cheetham ME, et al: Inherited ACTH insensitivity illuminates the mechanisms of ACTH action, Trends Endocrinol Metab 16:451–457, 2005.
75. Tullio-Pelet A, Salomon R, Hadj-Rabia S, et al. Mutant WD-repeat protein in triple-A Syndrome, Nat Genet 26:332–335, 2000.
76. Handschug K, Sperling S, Yoon S-JK, et al: Triple A syndrome is caused by mutations in AAAs, a new WD-repeat protein gene, Hum Mol Genet 10:283–290, 2001.
77. Houlden H, Smith S, de Carvalho M, et al: Clinical and genetic characterisation of families with triple A (Allgrove) syndrome, Brain 25:2681–2690, 2002.

78. Phelan JK, McCabe ER: Mutations in NR0B1 (DAX1) and NR5A1 (SF1) responsible for adrenal hypoplasia congenital, Hum Mutat 18:472–487, 2001.
79. Reutens AT, Achermann JC, Ito M, et al: Clinical and functional effects of mutations in DAX-1 gene in patients with adrenal hypoplasia congenital, J Clin Endocrinol Metab 84:504–511, 1999.
80. Lin L, Achermann JC: Inherited adrenal hypoplasia: Not just for kids! Clin Endocrinol (Oxf) 60:529–537, 2004.
81. Graber AL, Ney RL, Nicholson WE, et al: Natural history of pituitary-adrenal recovery following long-term suppression with corticosteroids, J Clin Endocrinol Metab 25:11–17, 1965.
82. Staughten RCD, August PJ: Cushing's syndrome and pituitary-adrenal suppression due to clobetasol propionate, Br Med J 2:419–421, 1975.
83. Hug V, Kau S, Hertobagi GN, et al: Adrenal failure in patients with breast carcinoma after long-term treatment of cyclic alternating oestrogen progesterone, Br J Cancer 63:454–456, 1991.
84. Comtois R, Beauregard H, Somma M, et al: The clinical and endocrine outcome to transsphenoidal microsurgery of non-secreting pituitary adenomas, Cancer 68:860–866, 1991.
85. Verhage TL, Godfried MH, Alberts C: Hypothalamic-pituitary dysfunction with adrenal insufficiency and hyperprolactinemia in sarcoidosis, Sarcoidosis 7:139–141, 1990.
86. Erdkamp FL, Gams RO, Hoorntje SJ: Endocrine organ failure due to systemic AA-amyloidosis, Neth J Med 38:24–28, 1991.
87. Asa SL, Bilbao JM, Kovacs K, et al: Lymphocytic hypophysitis of pregnancy resulting in hypopituitarism: a distinct clinicopathologic entity, Ann Intern Med 95:166–171, 1981.
88. Mirakian R, Cudworth AG, Bottazzo GF, et al: Autoimmunity to anterior pituitary cells and the pathogenesis of insulin-dependent diabetes mellitus, Lancet 1:755–759, 1982.
89. Bellastella A, Bizzarro A, Coronella C, et al: Lymphocytic hypophysitis: a rare or underestimated disease? Eur J Endocrinol 149:363–376, 2003.
90. Pulichino AM, Vallette-Kasic S, Couture C, et al: Human and mouse TPIT gene mutations cause early onset pituitary ACTH deficiency, Genes Dev 15:711–716, 2003.
91. Oelker W: Hyponatremia in inappropriate secretion of vasopressin (antidiuretic hormone) in patients with hypopituitarism, N Engl J Med 321:492–496, 1989.
92. Zelissen PM: Addison patients in the Netherlands: medical report of the survey, The Hague, 1994, Dutch Addison Society.
93. Oelkers W: Adrenal Insufficiency, N Engl J Med 335:1206–1212, 1996.
94. Stewart PM: The adrenal cortex. In Larsen PR, Kronenberg HM, Melmed S, et al, editors: Williams Textbook of Endocrinology, Philadelphia, PA, 2003, Saunders, pp 525–532.
95. Allolio B, Arlt W: DHEA treatment: myth or reality? Trends Endocrinol Metab 13:288–294, 2002.
96. Claussen MS, Landercasper J, Cogbill TH: Acute adrenal insufficiency presenting as shock after trauma and surgery: three cases and a review of the literature, J Trauma 32:94–100, 1992.
97. Pearson OH, Whitmore WF, West CD: Clinical and metabolic studies of bilateral adrenalectomy for advanced cancer in man, Surgery 34:543–552, 1953.
98. Lipsett MB, Pearson OH: Pathophysiology and treatment of adrenal crisis, N Engl J Med 254:511–515, 1956.
99. Boykin T, DeTorrente A, Erikson A: The role of plasma vasopressin in impaired water excretion of glucocorticoid deficiency, J Clin Invest 62:738–746, 1978.
100. Kehlet H, Binder C: Value of an ACTH test in assessing hypothalamic-pituitary-adrenocortical function in glucocorticoid-treated patients, Br Med J 2:147–152, 1973.
101. Mukherjee JJ, Jacome de Castro J, Kaltsas G, et al: A comparison of insulin tolerance/glucagon tests with the short ACTH stimulation test for assessment of hypothalamo-pituitary-adrenal axis in the early post-operative period after hypophysectomy, Clin Endocrinol (Oxf) 47:51–60, 1997.

102. Calis M, Gokce C, Ates F, et al: Investigation of the hypothalamo-pituitary-adrenal axis (HPA) by 1 microg ACTH test and metyrapone test in patients with primary fibromyalgia syndrome, J Endocrinol Invest 27:42–46, 2004.
103. Rasmuson S, Olsson T, Hagg E: A low dose ACTH test to assess the function of the hypothalamic-pituitary-adrenal axis, Clin Endocrinol (Oxf) 44:151–156, 1996.
104. Jones SL, Trainer PJ, Perry L, et al: An audit of the insulin tolerance test in adult subjects in an acute invesigation unit over one year, Clin Endocrinol 41:123–128, 1994.
105. Betterle C, Volpato M, Pedini B, et al: Adrenal-cortex autoantibodies and steroid-producing cells autoantibodies in patients with Addison's disease: comparison of immunofluorescence and immunoprecipitation assays, J Clin Endocrinol Metab 84:618–622, 1999.
106. Kehlet H, Madsen SN, Binder C: Cortisol and cortisone acetate in parenteral glucocorticoid therapy, Acta Med Scand 195:421–425, 1974.
107. Fariss BL, Hane S, Shinsako H: Comparison of absorption of cortisone acetate and hydrocortisone hemisuccinate, J Clin Endocrinol Metab 47:1137–1140, 1978.
108. Baker SJK, Hunt PJ, Wass JAH: Assessing the potential for fine tuning the management of Addison's disease/steroid replacement therapy. 188th Society for Endocrinology (UK) meeting, London, J Endocrinol Abstract Suppl 155:P2, 1997.
109. Lovas K, Loge JH, Husebye ES: Subjective health status in Norwegian patients with Addison's disease, Clin Endocrinol (Oxf) 56:581–588, 2002.
110. Arlt W, Callies F, van Vlijmen JC, et al: Dehydroepiandrosterone replacement in women with adrenal insufficiency, N Engl J Med 341:1013–1020, 1999.
111. Hunt PJ, Gurnell EM, Huppert FA, et al: Improvement in mood and fatigue after dehydroepiandrosterone replacement in Addison's disease in a randomized, double blind trial, J Clin Endocrinol Metab 85:4650–4656, 2000.
112. Lovas K, Gebre-Medhin G, Trovik TS, et al: Replacement of dehydroepiandrosterone in adrenal failure: no benefit for subjective health status and sexuality in a 9-month, randomized, parallel group clinical trial, J Clin Endocrinol Metab 88:1112–1118, 2003.
113. Gurnell EM, Hunt PJ, Curran SE, et al: Long term DHEA replacement in primary adrenal insufficiency: a randomized, controlled trial, J Clin Endcrinol Metab 93:400–409, 2008.
114. Udelsman R, Chrousos GP, Loriaux DL: Adaptation during surgical stress, J Clin Invest 77:1377–1381, 1986.
115. Cooper MS, Stewart PM: Corticosteroid insufficiency in acutely ill patients, N Engl J Med 348:727–734, 2003.
116. Arafah BM: Review: hypothalamic pituitary adrenal function during critical illness: limitations of current assessment methods, J Clin Endocrinol Metab 91:3725–3745, 2004.
117. Hamrahian AH, Oseni TS, Arafah BM: Measurements of serum free cortisol in critically ill patients, N Engl J Med 350:1629–1638, 2004.
118. Ho JT, Al-Musalhi H, Chapman MJ, et al: Septic shock and sepsis: a comparison of total and free plasma cortisol levels, J Clin Endocrinol Metab 91:105–114, 2006.
119. Loriaux L: Glucocorticoid therapy in the intensive care unit, N Engl J Med 350:1601–1602, 2004.
120. Russell JA: Management of sepsis, N Engl J Med 355:1699–1713, 2006.
121. The Veterans Administration Systemic Sepsis Cooperative Study Group: Effect of high-dose glucocorticoid therapy on mortality in patients with clinical signs of systemic sepsis, N Engl J Med 317:659–665, 1987.
122. Bone RC, Fisher CJ Jr, Clemmer TP, et al: A controlled clinical trial of high-dose methylprednisolone in the treatment of severe sepsis and septic shock, N Engl J Med 317:653–658, 1987.
123. Annane D, Sebille V, Charpentier C, et al: Effect of treatment with low doses of hydrocortisone and fludrocortisone on mortality in patients with septic shock, JAMA 288:862–871, 2002.
124. Sprung CL, Annane D, Keh D, et al: for the CORTICUS Study Group: hydrocortisone therapy for patients with septic shock, N Engl J Med 358:111–124, 2008.
125. Surviving Sepsis Campaign. http://www.survivingsepsis.org, accessed December, 2008.

Chapter 7

ADRENAL CAUSES OF HYPERCORTISOLISM

FRANCESCO CAVAGNINI and FRANCESCA PECORI GIRALDI

Cushing's syndrome defines sustained hypercortisolism irrespective of its etiology. This disorder recognizes two main etiologies: adrenocorticotropic hormone (ACTH)-dependent, that is, pituitary or ectopic ACTH secretion; and ACTH-independent, that is, adrenal disorders. At variance with other endocrine diseases, excess cortisol exposure is not classified into primary or secondary but defined as *Cushing's disease*, which identifies only pituitary ACTH-secreting adenomas, and *Cushing's syndrome*, which encompasses all causes of hypercortisolism including Cushing's disease.

Adrenal causes of Cushing's syndrome are diverse, including both tumoral and genetic disorders. Tumors arising from the zona fasciculata of the adrenal cortex may be benign or malignant and are thus classified as adenomas and carcinomas, respectively, a distinction that is by no means always straightforward (see also Chapter 11). ACTH-independent adrenal hyperplasia, both macro- and micronodular, is characterized by nodular hyperplasia of the zona fasciculata, possibly a consequence of inappropriate or excessive stimulation by factors other than ACTH. Lastly, familial causes of adrenal Cushing's syndrome include primary pigmented nodular adrenal dysplasia (PPNAD), usually in the context of Carney's complex, and the McCune-Albright syndrome (MAS).

HISTORICAL NOTES

The first description of Cushing's syndrome dates back to 1899 when William Osler presented a patient with "an acute mixoedematous condition," which he ascribed to thyroid gland dysfunction, but in hindsight was actually due to excess glucocorticoid secretion.[1] Some 10 years later, Harvey Cushing summarized the symptoms featured in his namesake syndrome and established the causative link with "pituitary basophilism." The second case in his landmark monograph, however, was ascribed to an adrenal disorder, and he himself recognized that the syndrome of "diabetes in bearded women" was often associated with hyperplasia or tumors of the suprarenal glands.[2] In 1934, Walters et al. demonstrated that removal of the adrenals was curative in these patients,[3] thus validating the importance of the adrenal gland as a target of pituitary hyperproduction or primary cause of glucocorticoid excess. This distinction was by no means straightforward; pituitary Cushing's disease was also being called "ACTH-dependent adrenal hyperplasia," necessitating bilateral adrenalectomy, and "nodular adrenal hyperplasia" was considered partially ACTH dependent.

Over time, primary adrenal Cushing's syndrome finessed its etiologic status, thanks in part to the widespread availability of radioimmunoassay measurements, and adrenal autonomy became associated with suppressed ACTH levels rather than nodular adrenal morphology. The importance of aberrant or

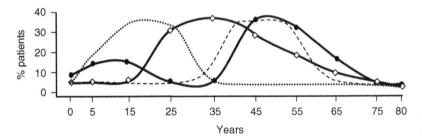

FIGURE 7-1. Age distribution in adrenal Cushing's syndrome according to etiology, depicted as percentage of patients at different ages: adenoma (-◇-), carcinoma (-●-), PPNAD (.......), and AIMAH (- - -).

inappropriate receptors as causative factors for bilateral adrenal hyperplasia, the isolation of genes linked with PPNAD, and the identification of molecular markers for the distinction between malignant and benign adrenal tumors are all recent developments in the field of adrenal Cushing's syndrome.

EPIDEMIOLOGY

Cushing's syndrome is a rare disease. Its incidence has been estimated at around 2 to 10 patients per million population per year, with less than half due to adrenal causes.[4,5] Of interest, adrenal adenomas appear to affect the Japanese population with greater frequency, reportedly presenting over 20 new patients per million per year.[6] The ratio between benign and malignant adrenal tumors varies from roughly equal in some series[5,7] to 10:1 in Japanese studies.[6] Oncologic surveys report an annual incidence of adrenal neoplasms of around 2 per million[8,9] and 0.6 to 1 per million for adrenocortical cancer.[8] Approximately one third of these patients will present with Cushing's syndrome,[10,11] resulting in 0.2 to 0.3 cortisol-secreting adrenal cancers per million per year, which tallies nicely with estimates garnered from endocrinologic studies.[5]

Age and gender distribution vary somewhat between the different adrenal etiologies of Cushing's syndrome, with adrenal cancer presenting a bimodal distribution (peak in childhood/adolescence then again after 45 years of age), and adrenal adenoma occurring mostly in young adults (25 to 45 years of age) (Fig. 7-1). PPNAD gives rise to hypercortisolism during infancy and adolescence in over half of cases,[12] whereas ACTH-independent macronodular adrenocortical hyperplasia (AIMAH) has been reported mostly in adults older than 50.[13,14] Adrenal Cushing's syndrome in the majority of adult patients is due to benign adenomas (50% to 80%, according to different series). Adrenal-cortex carcinoma accounts for another 20%, and a scattering of cases are due to ACTH-independent adrenal hyperplasia and PPNAD.[15,16] Conversely, in childhood, malignant forms make up the major share, the remainder due to adenomas or even genetic causes such as PPNAD or MAS.[12,17]

Adrenal adenoma occurs mostly in females, as does—to a lesser extent—cortisol-secreting adrenal cancer.[5,18,19] No clear-cut sex-related pattern has been observed for Cushing's associated with AIMAH and PPNAD.

Mortality from untreated Cushing's syndrome is high, with 50% survival 5 years after the diagnosis,[20] mostly due to cerebrovascular events and infections. Upon removal of a benign adenoma, taking perisurgical mortality into consideration, 5-year survival averaged 77%[21] in the 1980s, but is nowadays comparable to mortality in the general population.[5,22] As regards mortality from malignant adrenocortical cancer, outcome is dismal, with high mortality for stage III and IV disease and slightly better survival for patients diagnosed with localized disease.[23-25] In Cushing's syndrome due to PPNAD within Carney's complex, a familial multiple endocrine neoplasia syndrome, extraendocrine

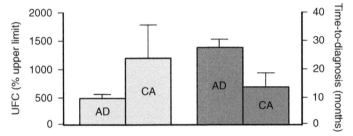

FIGURE 7-2. Urinary free cortisol (UFC) and time to diagnosis in patients with Cushing's syndrome due to adrenal adenoma (AD) or adrenal carcinoma (CA). UFC is expressed as percent of the upper limit of the normal range.

manifestations such as cardiac myxomas or malignant Schwannomas contribute to excess mortality.[26]

Clinical Features of Hypercortisolism

Cushing's syndrome features all the consequences of tissue exposure to excessive cortisol concentrations, including aspecific alterations such as obesity, hypertension, and mood changes, and more unique signs such as proximal muscle wasting, purple striae, and easy bruising. The severity of clinical manifestations varies according to the extent and duration of cortisol hypersecretion, with adrenal cancer characterized by rapid attainment of very high cortisol levels and severe clinical signs; adenomas present milder glucocorticoid hypersecretion and a more indolent course. In fact, the clinical presentation of adrenal adenomas closely resembles that of pituitary-driven Cushing's disease, whereas adrenal cancer mimics ectopic ACTH secretion due to poorly differentiated neuroendocrine tumors. On average, over 2 years are necessary for a cortisol-secreting adrenal adenoma to be diagnosed after the appearance of the first symptoms, but the remarkable clinical presentation of adrenal carcinoma leads to the diagnosis in half that time.[7,27] Indeed, the time to diagnosis is inversely related to mean cortisol levels (Fig. 7-2).

Specifically, patients with hypercortisolism usually present with central obesity, a round and erythematous face, supraclavicular fat pads, cervical fat accumulation (the so-called "buffalo hump"), thinning of the skin, purple striae, and proximal muscle weakness. Hirsutism, a common feature of ACTH-dependent Cushing's syndrome, is usually absent in benign tumors that secrete only cortisol but, conversely, accompanies malignant transformation.[7] Hypertension as well as osteopenia and pathologic fractures (ribs, feet, and vertebrae are frequently affected sites) are common, and osteopenia in young patients with Cushing's syndrome should raise the suspicion for PPNAD (see later). Derangements in blood chemistry include increased white blood cell count with granulocytosis, lymphopenia, and eosinopenia; a

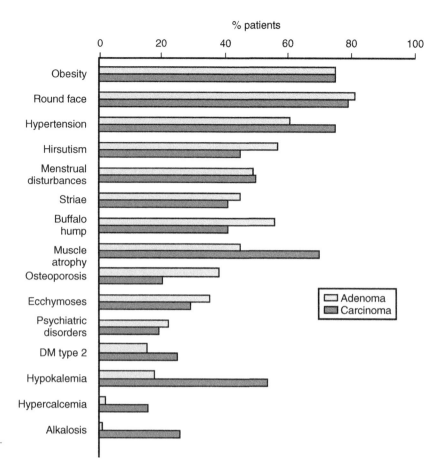

FIGURE 7-3. Clinical presentation in patients with Cushing's syndrome due to adrenal adenoma or adrenal carcinoma.

slightly elevated red blood cell count; increased VLDL, LDL, and HDL cholesterol and triglycerides; and frequently, impaired glucose tolerance or overt type 2 diabetes mellitus. Electrolyte imbalances such as hypokalemia are more common in severe hypercortisolism. Case history will reveal menstrual irregularities or even amenorrhea, reduced libido or impotence, fatigue, easy bruising, insomnia, and psychiatric alterations. These latter range from changes in mood, irritability with rage fits, anxiety, impaired memory, and concentration to psychosis with frank depression and manic episodes. Curiously, in children and adolescents, hypercortisolism has been associated with overachievement both in school and in extracurricular activities. Less frequent signs are cutaneous fungal infections, wound dehiscence, exophthalmos, nephrolithiasis, glaucoma, and headache. As mentioned before, severity of the clinical presentation often reflects the underlying etiology and features such as extreme muscle atrophy, hypokalemia, hypercalcemia, and the abrupt appearance of diabetes should increase the suspicion of adrenocortical cancer (Fig. 7-3). Except for signs of virilization, however, no single sign or symptom is significantly overrepresented in either etiology.[7,16] The hormonal secretory pattern of adrenal carcinoma may change over time. Curiously, Cushing's syndrome developed in two previously asymptomatic patients after recurrence of adrenocortical carcinoma, but conversely, no sign of hypercortisolism accompanied relapse of a previously symptomatic adrenocortical carcinoma.[18]

In addition to cortisol hypersecretion, adrenal androgens may also be produced in excess, most notably in adrenocortical cancer and more rarely in adenomas. Androgen secretion reflects inefficient steroidogenesis, since enzymes involved in the later steps of cortisol synthesis (e.g., 11β-hydroxylase or 21β-hydroxylase) are unable to transform their substrate overload. Precursors, therefore, accumulate and are shunted to alternative biosynthetic pathways, leading to accumulation of DHEA, DHEAS, androstenedione, and estrogen (see Chapter 1). This alteration is the biochemical correlate of progressive dedifferentiation of adrenal tumors, with steroidogenesis proceeding to its final product, cortisol, in benign and hyperplastic lesions, whereas poorly differentiated carcinomas are unable to efficiently carry steroidogenesis to term.[28] From a clinical viewpoint, androgen hypersecretion gives rise to significant hirsutism, acne, and temporal balding in adult patients and contributes to menstrual alterations in women. In children, hyperandrogenism may arrest linear growth in boys or lead to sexual precocity and virilization in girls.[29] Excess estrogen secretion may lead to gynecomastia in men.[30] Mixed cortisol- and aldosterone-producing adenomas have also been reported,[31] as have mixed cortisol-, androgen-, and estrogen-producing adenomas.[32]

Adrenal cortex carcinomas may present with mass-related signs, symptoms of metastatic disease, or nonspecific features of malignancy such as weight loss, fever, and anorexia. Palpable and painful abdominal masses, an acute abdomen, and vascular obstruction by tumor thrombi of hepatic veins (Budd-Chiari syndrome) or the inferior vena cava may first raise suspicion of adrenal cancer. Metastases occur most frequently to liver, lungs, retroperitoneal lymph nodes, and bone and may give rise to back pain and osteoporotic fractures, or hypoglycemia if the liver is extensively infiltrated[18,24] (see Chapter 11).

The clinical picture of the other etiologies of adrenal Cushing's syndrome, AIMAH and PPNAD, presents certain unique features such as overt hypercortisolism only during particular phases of life—for example, pregnancy and menopause in luteinizing hormone (LH)-dependent AIMAH or signs of Carney's complex in familial PPNAD. These issues will be discussed in more detail in specific sections (see later).

Diagnosis

DIAGNOSIS OF CUSHING'S SYNDROME

The diagnosis of Cushing's syndrome due to adrenal tumors is first raised by the clinical presentation then confirmed by both biochemical and radiologic investigations. Hormonal measurements reflect the functional derangement of the hypothalamo-pituitary-adrenal (HPA) axis consequent to sustained autonomous cortisol production by the adrenal gland. Two features of the HPA axis are relevant to pathophysiology of primary adrenal hypercortisolism: (1) homeostasis of the HPA axis is assured through long and short feedback loops acting at hypothalamic (i.e., corticotropin-releasing hormone [CRH]), pituitary (i.e., ACTH), and adrenal (i.e., cortisol) levels, with cortisol levels as the effector of feedback; (2) cortisol and ACTH are secreted in pulsatile fashion, inscribed within a circadian rhythm with high secretory output in the early morning, progressive decrease during the day, and nadir around midnight. If adrenal cortisol production is autonomous, as occurs in adrenal-derived Cushing's syndrome, high steroid secretion will activate negative-feedback loops leading to suppression of hypothalamic and pituitary secretion and thus disruption of physiologic pulsatility and circadian rhythmicity of ACTH and cortisol secretion. The HPA axis will also be resistant to further inhibition by exogenous steroids. The diagnosis of Cushing's syndrome is performed by looking for these alterations: evaluation of integrated daily cortisol secretion and its circadian rhythmicity and suppressibility with dexamethasone. Details of these investigations are given elsewhere, but specific changes expected in adrenal-driven disease are given in following discussions.

Urinary free cortisol (UFC) levels are usually very high in patients with adrenocortical cancer (up to 100 times greater than normal), whereas such striking elevations are less frequent in patients with cortisol-secreting adenoma (Fig. 7-4). Indeed, UFC concentrations may occasionally fall within the normal range in these latter patients,[27] and this underlines the need for multiple UFC measurements.[33,34] In patients with AIMAH, UFC concentrations are rarely very high and may fluctuate according to stimulation by the causative aberrant receptor. For example, patients in whom hypercortisolism was dependent upon adrenal cortex stimulation by LH, who exhibit markedly elevated UFC concentrations and develop Cushingoid features only during pregnancy and menopause.[35,36] In young patients with PPNAD, again, UFC rarely reaches very high levels and may present slow, periodic progression.[12,37,38] Other tests usually involve assessment of cortisol daily variations or its suppressibility by dexamethasone. In patients with full blown hypercortisolism, two clearly pathologic results or even one are sufficient to establish the diagnosis of Cushing's syndrome and proceed with the diagnostic workup. However, in patients with mildly elevated or fluctuating cortisol values (as often occurs with AIMAH or even PPNAD), repeat evaluations over time are necessary. A secure diagnosis of Cushing's syndrome is essential before performing tests for the etiologic diagnosis of hypercortisolism, because the results obtained with these procedures may overlap with normal physiology.

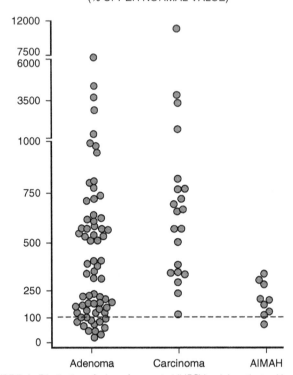

FIGURE 7-4. Distribution of urinary free cortisol (UFC) levels in patients with adrenal Cushing's syndrome. Values are expressed as percentage of the upper limit of normal range (dashed line = 100%). (Adapted from Invitti C, Pecori Giraldi F, De Martin M, Cavagnini F: Diagnosis and management of Cushing's syndrome: results of an Italian multicentre study, J Clin Endocrinol Metab 84:442, 1999. © Endocrine Society.)

DIAGNOSIS OF ADRENAL CUSHING'S SYNDROME

Once the existence of Cushing's syndrome is firmly established, the etiology of the disease has to be defined. In adrenal Cushing's syndrome of any given etiology, autonomous cortisol secretion by the adrenals feeds back at hypothalamo-pituitary level to inhibit CRH and ACTH secretion. Plasma ACTH levels will therefore be suppressed in adrenal Cushing's syndrome, whereas inappropriately high ACTH concentrations characterize ACTH-dependent Cushing's syndrome (i.e., pituitary or ectopic ACTH secreting tumor. Measurement of plasma ACTH levels is therefore pivotal to the differentiation of ACTH-dependent from ACTH-independent Cushing's syndrome. As mentioned above, ACTH is secreted in pulsatile fashion, dictating the same circadian rhythm to cortisol. Further, ACTH is extremely sensitive to stress, has a short plasma half life, and is easily degraded by plasma peptidases. For these reasons, blood samples for ACTH measurement have to be collected in unstressed conditions, preferably two or three samples over 30 minutes, into tubes containing enzyme inhibitors and conserved at low temperatures prior to separation into aliquots. Repeated freeze/thaw cycles should be avoided.

In the vast majority of patients with adrenal Cushing's syndrome, plasma ACTH concentrations are suppressed, thus providing clear distinction from ACTH-dependent Cushing's syndrome. Initially formulated guidelines indicated that morning ACTH concentrations lower than 10 pg/mL (2 pmol/L) or evening ACTH levels lower than 5 pg/mL (1 pmol/L) were indic-

ACTH (% LOWER NORMAL VALUE)

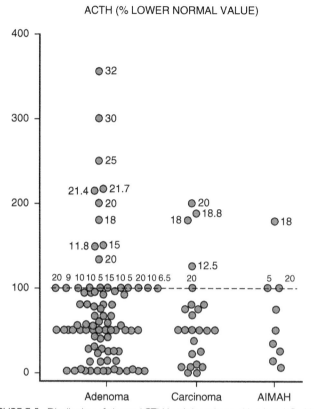

FIGURE 7-5. Distribution of plasma ACTH levels in patients with adrenal Cushing's syndrome. Values are expressed as percentage of the lower limit of the normal range. For values within the normal range, numbers close to individual points indicate absolute ACTH concentrations in pg/mL measured using different assays. (Adapted from Invitti C, Pecori Giraldi F, De Martin M, Cavagnini F: Diagnosis and management of Cushing's syndrome: results of an Italian multicentre study, J Clin Endocrinol Metab 84:442, 1999. © Endocrine Society.)

ACTH (% BASELINE)

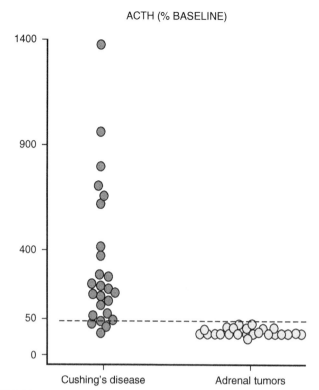

FIGURE 7-6. ACTH response (% baseline) to stimulation with CRH in patients with Cushing's syndrome presenting with adrenal nodules.

ative of ACTH-independent Cushing's syndrome.[39] In RIA assays with 5 to 10 pg/mL sensitivity, this corresponds to values below the detection limit. With the newly developed IRMA or chemiluminescent assays capable of measuring plasma ACTH concentrations as low as 1 pg/mL (0.2 pmol/L), ACTH values may be detectable in patients with adrenal Cushing's syndrome but usually are below the lower limit of the normal range.[16,27,40,41] However, in an Italian study on over 50 patients with adrenal Cushing's syndrome, up to one fourth presented ACTH concentrations within the normal range[27] (Fig. 7-5), but whether this is because of issues in assay methodology, as seems more likely, or to incomplete suppression of pituitary ACTH secretion remains to be established. Occasionally, ACTH concentrations are frankly non-suppressed[40,42,43]; in one patient bearing an adrenal carcinoma, ACTH concentrations were persistently high because the tumor itself produced ACTH.[44] In addition to patients with adrenal Cushing's syndrome presenting measurable or normal ACTH concentrations, some 10% of patients with Cushing's disease display ACTH values below 10 pg/mL (2 pmol/L),[27] thus blurring the boundaries between the two etiologies. To correctly diagnose patients falling into this grey area, stimulation with CRH proves of use; patients with pituitary-dependent hypercortisolism will mount an ACTH response to the stimulus, whereas patients with ACTH-independent hypercortisolism will not[27,45,46] (Fig. 7-6).

In the past, tests such as stimulation with metyrapone or suppression with high-dose dexamethasone have been employed to distinguish between adrenal and pituitary Cushing's syndrome,[47] but their suboptimal specificity has superseded their routine use for this purpose. However, the high-dose dexamethasone suppression test has been re-proposed for the etiologic diagnosis of adrenal Cushing's syndrome (see later).

DIFFERENTIAL DIAGNOSIS OF ADRENAL CAUSES OF CUSHING'S SYNDROME

The etiology of adrenal Cushing's syndrome is usually established by imaging of the adrenals (see also Chapter 10), since biochemical and clinical features overlap considerably between adenoma, carcinoma, and adrenal hyperplasia.[7,14,16] Hormonal measurements provide useful adjunctive information but rarely establish the diagnosis with certainty. Genetic causes, such as PPNAD or MAS, may be recognized by features typical to the syndrome (e.g., lentigines or myxomas and fibrous osseous dysplasia, respectively; see later).

Steroid Markers

Dehydroepiandrosterone Sulfate

Measurement of serum dehydroepiandrosterone sulfate (DHEAS) may aid in the distinction between benign and malignant adrenal tumors. Indeed, although no cutoff value ensures absolute diagnostic accuracy, low age-and-gender-adjusted DHEAS levels are usually found in Cushing's syndrome due to adrenal adenoma, whereas DHEAS levels are markedly increased in adrenal carcinoma (Fig. 7-7), especially in children.[16,29,48,49] Two mechanisms underlie this diversity: on the one hand, DHEAS is an ACTH-dependent androgen, so inhibition of the normal adrenal gland in patients with cortisol-secreting adrenal adenoma will lead to reduced DHEAS secretion. On the other hand, inefficient steroidogenesis in malignant neoplasms leads to the release of

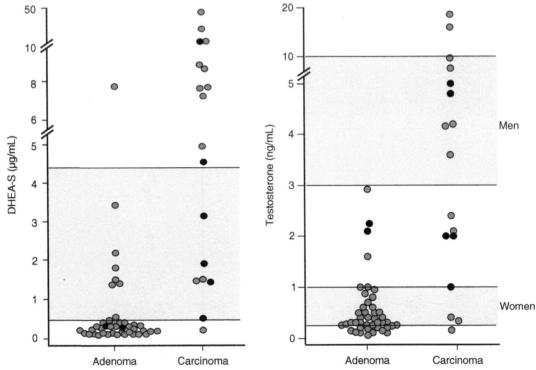

FIGURE 7-7. DHEAS and total testosterone levels in patients with Cushing's syndrome due to adrenal adenoma or adrenal carcinoma. *Black circles,* women; *gray circles,* men; *shaded area* represents the normal range.

several steroid precursors, including delta-5 steroids such as DHEAS. Of interest, DHEAS levels often remain suppressed long after removal of the hypersecreting adrenal gland, occasionally up to 8 years after surgery.[48,50] This is in contrast with the recovery of ACTH and cortisol secretion, which usually occurs 12 to 18 months after surgery and indicates a dissociation of adrenal DHEAS and cortisol regulation.[48,50] Enhanced sensitivity of the reticular zone to ACTH deficiency and preferential inhibition of 17,20-lyase in the atrophic adrenal gland have been hypothesized as causal factors.

Testosterone and Androstenedione

Plasma testosterone levels are within the lower centiles of the normal range in men with cortisol-secreting adrenal adenoma,[51] reflecting testosterone suppression (see Fig. 7-7). This is in line with the 30% to 50% fall in testosterone levels reported after administration of high doses of cortisol or dexamethasone[52] and its rebound increase following removal of the adenoma.[51] Normal testosterone levels have been reported in women with cortisol-secreting adrenal adenomas[7] (see Fig. 7-7). Androstenedione levels are mostly low-normal in patients of both sexes with cortisol-secreting adrenal adenomas.[29,53] Conversely, in adrenal carcinoma, androstenedione and testosterone levels may be high in both men and women (see Fig. 7-7) when impairment of downstream steroidogenic enzymes in the tumor, in particular 21-hydroxylase and 11β-hydroxylase, leads to accumulation of progesterone or pregnenolone and shunting of these precursors towards 17,20-lyase[53] (see Figure 1-4 in Chapter 1). Accumulated DHEA can be transformed into androstenedione and subsequently into testosterone. Indeed, the detection of elevated testosterone or androstenedione in a patient with an adrenal tumor is virtually diagnostic for adrenal carcinoma.[29,53] In children with adrenal carcinoma, Cushing's syndrome is often

accompanied by virilization, and testosterone, androstenedione, and DHEAS levels may reach extremely high levels.[24,29]

17-Hydroxyprogesterone and 11-Deoxycortisol

These two cortisol precursors are usually normal in patients with benign cortisol-secreting adrenal lesions and elevated in malignant adrenocortical tumors.[24,29,53] Normal plasma hormone levels, however, do not allow adrenocortical cancer to be ruled out.

Urinary Steroid Profile

The hallmark of hypercortisolism is excess urinary excretion of cortisol and its main metabolites, such as tetrahydrocortisol, tetrahydro-11-deoxycortisol, tetrahydrocortisone and derivate cortols and cortolones (see Chapter 1). In addition, minor cortisol metabolic pathways, such as 6β-hydroxylation, are recruited to metabolize excess cortisol. In cortisol-producing adenomas, steroid synthesis is efficient, and only minor amounts of early products of the steroid cascade are excreted in urine.[54,55] Conversely, in adrenocortical carcinoma, steroid precursors accumulate, and 3β-hydroxysteroids, desoxycorticosterone, and pregnanetriol—a 17-hydroxyprogesterone metabolite—become abundant in urine.[54,56] Urinary 3β-hydroxy DHEA metabolites, such as 16alpha DHEA, androstenediol, and androstenetriol, as well as androstenedione-derived products such as etiocholanolone, androsterone, and androstanediols (Fig. 7-8), are usually high in adrenocortical carcinomas.[55,57] In addition to these metabolites of early steroid synthesis products, tetrahydro-11-deoxycortisol, the metabolite of the cortisol substrate, is also typically increased in adrenocortical carcinoma, a consequence of relative 11β-hydroxylase deficiency.[55,56] Investigation of the urinary steroid profile by gas chromatography mass spectrometry may reveal unique steroid excretory patterns, but the wide vari-

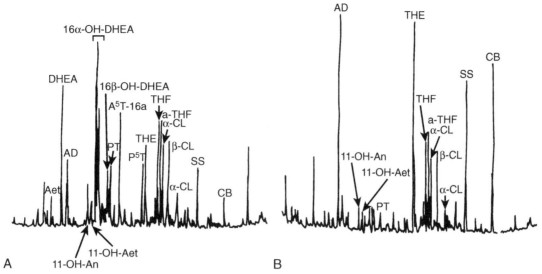

FIGURE 7-8. Chromatographic profile of urinary steroids in **(A)** a 6-year-old girl bearing an adrenal carcinoma and **(B)** an age- and sex-matched normal subject. Androsterone (An), etiocholanolone (Aet), androsten-3β, 16α, 17β-triol (A^5T), pregnanetriol (PT), pregnentriol-5-ene-3βhydroxy (P^5T), tetrahydrocortisone (THE), tetrahydrocortisol (THF), allo-tetrahydrocortisol (a-THF), cortols (C), cortolones (CL); internal standards (AD, SS, CB). (From Homoki J, Holl R, Teller WM: Urinary steroid profiles in Cushing's syndrome and tumors of the adrenal cortex, Klin Wochensch 65:721, Fig. I, 1987; © Springer).

ability of excreted steroids and its changes over time hamper its routine use in clinical setting.

High-Dose Dexamethasone Testing

Adrenal tumors, both benign and malignant, fail to suppress UFC secretion after 2 days of 2 mg of oral dexamethasone every 6 hours; cutoffs for suppression are a 50% decrease from baseline of UFC levels. Patients with PPNAD often exhibit a marked paradoxical rise in UFC levels during high-dose dexamethasone testing.[15,37,41] This test falls short of providing diagnostic certainty in the differential diagnosis of adrenal Cushing's syndrome, since some patients with adrenal adenoma also exhibit an increase in UFC levels after 8 mg dexamethasone for 2 days,[15,27,37] but a doubling of UFC levels is highly suggestive of PPNAD. Parallel evaluation of creatinine clearance should be performed to exclude gross changes in glomerular filtration rate.[58] However, patients with malignancy may also exhibit a paradoxical increase in cortisol levels after high-dose dexamethasone testing,[43,59] so this procedure should be performed only after imaging has narrowed down the choice to benign adrenal lesions.

Stimulation of Aberrant Adrenal Receptors

These procedures are useful if the history suggests hypercortisolism associated with given conditions (e.g., pregnancy, meals) or in the presence of patients with AIMAH. For a detailed discussion, the reader is referred to the heading ACTH-Independent Adrenal Hyperplasia.

Subclinical Cushing's Syndrome

This condition, characterized by subtle alterations of HPA-axis parameters in patients who do not present stigmata of Cushing's syndrome, is being increasingly recognized in subjects with an adrenal incidentaloma. Indeed, a variable percentage of adrenal incidentalomas will reveal themselves as cortisol-secreting adenomas, 5% to 20% according to various series,[60,61] possibly higher (up to 47%) in the Japanese population.[62] This variability can be ascribed in part to the different criteria adopted for the biochemical diagnosis of subclinical Cushing's and in part to the variable degree of cortisol excess; this condition is by no

means homogeneous. Usually, two or more of the following are considered indicative of subclinical Cushing's syndrome: (1) incomplete cortisol suppression after low-dose dexamethasone; (2) low baseline ACTH levels; (3) absent cortisol circadian rhythm; (4) blunted ACTH response to CRH; (5) elevated UFC; (6) decreased DHEAS.[63] Iodocholesterol scintigraphy may also be useful because exclusive uptake by the adrenal mass is indicative of excessive autonomous cortisol secretion with functional inhibition of the contralateral gland.[64] On the other hand, the degree of uptake does not differentiate between overt and subclinical Cushing's syndrome. Patients diagnosed with subclinical Cushing's are somewhat older (mostly older than 50) than those with Cushing's syndrome due to benign cortisol-secreting tumors, and the risk of developing overt Cushing's syndrome in the short term appears low.[46,65] However, even the mild excess in cortisol secretion observed in these patients is deleterious for metabolic, cardiovascular, and bone physiology, and removal of the "pretoxic" adrenal gland is followed in a number of cases by amelioration of diabetes, hypertension, insulin resistance, obesity, and parameters of bone turnover.[66] A note of caution is necessary upon removal of the lesion: Suppression of the contralateral gland may lead to postsurgical adrenal insufficiency.[65]

Subclinical Cushing's syndrome may also be the initial manifestation of AIMAH, and in this case, *preclinical Cushing's syndrome* is the more correct term. In these patients, biochemical derangements and signs and symptoms of hypercortisolism may be subtle and wax and wane over prolonged periods of time. The involvement of both adrenal glands results in bilateral iodocholesterol uptake, although the timing of hyperplasia may be asynchronous (see AIMAH).

Imaging

Radiologic procedures for visualization of adrenal lesions comprise abdominal x-ray, sonography, computed tomography (CT), and magnetic resonance imaging (MRI), while iodocholesterol scintigraphy and the recently developed adrenal-specific positron emission tomography (PET) provide functional assessment of adrenal masses. Additional procedures such as arteriography and CT-guided biopsy are only rarely used in patients with adrenal Cushing's syndrome (for detailed discussion see Chapter 10).

The aim of adrenal radiology in patients with adrenal Cushing's syndrome is to visualize the lesion, define its morphologic features and eventual extension into neighboring structures and provide insights into the nature and function of the tissue. In addition, unrelated adrenal lesions such as silent pheochromocytoma, metastases, collision tumors, and even accessory spleens must be recognized.[67,68] As with adrenal pathology, the results of individual imaging studies may be unequivocal and allow a straightforward diagnosis, whereas in other cases, CT, MRI, and scintigraphy may all be necessary. Unenhanced CT is usually the first-line procedure and may provide sufficient information to diagnose a benign lesion. Should malignancy be suspected, chemical-shift MRI may be performed to confirm the diagnosis and allow the staging of the lesion.

Computed Tomography

This technique provided a breakthrough in adrenal radiology, enabling easy visualization of the glands, given their location, morphology, and composition. Indeed, retroperitoneal fat provides an ideal background for recognition of the Y-shaped hyperlucent adrenal gland. The adrenal rim is usually straight or slightly concave, and any convexity should increase suspicion for underlying lesions. Adrenal size measurements are of little use because they largely depend on gland orientation.[69]

Adrenocortical adenomas, carcinomas, and macronodular hyperplasia are easily identified at unenhanced, thin-section (3 to 5 mm) CT scanning. As to their differentiation, adenomas usually present as a small (<3 cm), homogeneous, round mass with smooth margins and thin peripheral capsule (Fig. 7-9, *left panel*). Given the high steroid content of clear and compact cells, density of the mass is typically low, near that of water, and unenhanced attenuation values below 10 HU are commonly considered indicative of adenoma.[19,70] Black adenomas present somewhat higher density than clear-cell yellow adenomas.[71] Injection of a contrast medium, when performed, leads to homogeneous enhancement of the entire lesion, followed by rapid washout; attenuation values after enhancement do not allow clear distinction from nonadenomatous masses, whereas washout of contrast medium provides useful information for the differentiation from malignant lesions such as metastases.[70] The unaffected gland is usually normal sized or occasionally smaller.[15]

Adrenocortical carcinomas commonly appear as large (>6 cm), irregularly shaped, inhomogeneous lesions with soft tissue density (>20 HU) and patchy enhancement. The borders of the lesion are often "smudged" and only rarely sharp. The heterogeneity of the mass is due to intratumoral necrosis, cystic degeneration, or calcification.[19,69] These latter features, while extremely frequent in adrenal cancer, may be encountered also in degenerated adenomas[72] and are not absolute criteria. Conversely, findings diagnostic for carcinoma are local spread (e.g., extension into the inferior vena cava, lymph node enlargement) or metastases. The size of the lesion, initially considered a useful criterion for the distinction of benign from malignant lesions, has increasingly been questioned; both large adenomas (>6 cm) and small carcinomas (<3 cm) are not infrequent.[24] In addition, both CT and MRI may underestimate the size of the lesion by as much as 20%.[73]

In patients with AIMAH, CT scan most commonly reveals prominent glands with or without multiple large nodules. Massive macronodular hyperplasia is usually easily recognized because the glands appear markedly hypertrophic and multiple macronodules (>1 cm) can be seen in both adrenals[14] (see Fig. 7-9, *right panel*). In other cases, only one gland appears to be affected.[74] Conversely, in micronodular adrenal hyperplasia, the glands appear only slightly enlarged or even indistinguishable from normal. Indeed, a normal adrenal scan in a patient with ACTH-independent Cushing's syndrome may provide indirect evidence of AIMAH.[75]

Adrenal radiology in patients with PPNAD varies from a normal appearance, slight enlargement of one or both adrenal glands, to unilateral or bilateral micronodules.[12,76,77] Macronodules are more rarely encountered and mostly in patients older than 25 years of age.[77] One feature typical to PPNAD is the "knobbly" and irregular outline of the glands, most likely due to internodular atrophy, resulting in a "beads-on-string" appearance.[19,77]

Magnetic Resonance Imaging

MRI easily visualizes both normal adrenal glands and adrenal masses by virtue of the abundant hydrogen ions in lipid tissues. In addition to two-dimensional imaging, which may reveal features typical of benign or malignant adrenocortical tumors (see previous paragraph), MRI allows the assessment of its lipid content and soft-tissue characterization via study of T2 signal intensity and relaxation times, dynamic perfusion studies, or chemical-shift opposed-phase images. Adrenocortical adenomas are isointense and slightly hyperintense relative to the liver on T1- and T2-weighted sequences, respectively,[78,79] whereas carcinomas may display very high signal intensity on T2-weighted images.[77,79] After gadolinium, carcinomas show marked enhancement and slow washout, in contrast with the rapid washout of benign lesions.[79] Chemical-shift imaging reveals loss of signal in out-of-phase images in lipid-rich tissues and is used to differentiate adenomas from metastases[80] but does not reliably distinguish

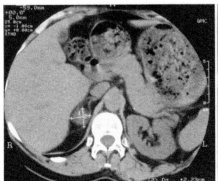 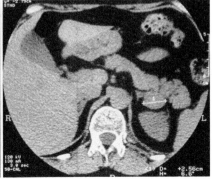

FIGURE 7-9. CT scan of cortisol-secreting adrenal adenoma *(left panel)* and adrenal nodular hyperplasia *(right panel)*. This latter patient presented with a left-sided macronodule and bilateral enlarged glands.

between adenoma and carcinoma, since both usually display a loss of signal intensity.[78] On balance, although some features may be highly indicative, the accuracy of MRI in differentiating adenoma from carcinoma is not absolute,[16,67] and routine MRI is not recommended for patients with adrenal Cushing's syndrome.[19,79] In patients with adrenal carcinoma, however, MRI enables visualization of the mass along sagittal and coronal planes, which allows the definition of anatomic boundaries, compression of surrounding organs, and extent of caval invasion.[24] MRI is the procedure of choice for Cushing's syndrome during pregnancy[81] and in childhood, because of safety concerns and because it allows visualization of the glands even in absence of retroperitoneal fat. The drawback of MRI in pediatric patients is the requirement for absolute standstill, which may be difficult to achieve.

Adrenal Scintigraphy

The advent of CT has shifted adrenal scintigraphy from the center stage of adrenal imaging to an adjunctive, complementary procedure. In the past, evaluation of adrenal uptake was an integral part of the diagnostic workup, providing information also for the differential diagnosis between ACTH-dependent and ACTH-independent Cushing's syndrome. Nowadays it is mostly reserved for differentiation of adenoma from hyperplasia and for those rare cases of ectopic adrenal tissue or adrenal remnants after adrenalectomy. Adrenal scintigraphy relies on the ability of the adrenal cortex to capture and accumulate radiolabeled cholesterol. Tracers are ^{131}I-19 iodocholesterol or its derivative ^{131}I-6β-iodomethyl-19 norcholesterol (NP59), the latter offering sharper adrenal images owing to a fivefold greater adrenal concentration,[82] and ^{75}Se-6β-selenomethyl-19 norcholesterol—used mostly in Europe. For scintigraphy with ^{131}I, adequate preparation with Lugol iodine drops or potassium iodide and laxatives reduces thyroid uptake and intestinal background. Scans can be obtained as early as 48 hours after tracer injection, but usable images are registered up to 7 to 10 days after administration.

Adrenal scintigraphy provides quantitative and qualitative data on adrenal function. In patients with benign adrenal hypercortisolism, radiolabeled cholesterol uptake may be increased compared to normal subjects, usually 0.7% of the administered dose compared to 0.3% in normal subjects[83,84] (Fig. 7-10). This percentage, although indicative of adrenal hyperfunction, does not provide absolute certainty of excessive corticosteroid production and, indeed, does not appear to be directly correlated with indices of adrenal function in these patients.[83] Conversely, qualitative data is of great help for localizing steroid-secreting lesions. Scintigraphy may yield several uptake patterns, as proposed by Gross[83] (Table 7-1).

Exclusive or prevalent uptake on the side of the mass are considered concordant with the mass and confirm its functional activity as a steroid hormone–producing tissue and are taken to indicate a benign adrenocortical adenoma[74,85] (Fig. 7-11A). Inhibition of ACTH secretion by autonomous cortisol production prevents the imaging of the contralateral gland. False-negative results have occasionally been reported with black adenomas, possibly a consequence of the prevalence of lipid-poor compact cells.[86] In adrenocortical carcinoma, bilateral nonvisualization is the rule because the carcinoma itself does not accumulate tracer sufficiently, possibly a consequence of deranged steroidogenesis, and the contralateral gland is inhibited.[85,87] However, some well-differentiated adrenocortical carcinomas and, rarely, also high-grade malignant carcinomas may accumulate the tracer, yielding exclusive or prevalent images.[87]

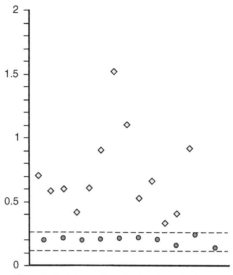

TOTAL ^{131}I-19-IODOCHOLESTEROL UPTAKE (%)

FIGURE 7-10. ^{131}I-19-iodocholesterol total adrenal uptake in normal subjects (●) and patients with Cushing's syndrome (◇). Dotted lines depict mean ±2 SD. (Adapted from Ortega D, Foz M, Doménech-Torné FM, Tresánchez JM: The diagnosis of Cushing's syndrome using ^{131}I-19-iodocholesterol uptake and adrenal imaging, Clin Endocrinol 13:148, 1980.)

Table 7-1. Uptake Patterns at Adrenal Scintigraphy

Exclusive	Uptake on the side of the lesion, with nonvisualization of the contralateral gland
Prevalent	Asymmetric uptake by the tumor, with visualization of the contralateral gland
Symmetric	Comparable uptake by both glands
Discordant	Reduced or absent uptake on the side of the mass
Bilateral nonvisualization	No uptake on either side

Malignant collision tumors may also display concordant uptake because of residual compressed cortical parenchyma within the nonadrenal neoplasm.[59,88] It follows, therefore, that while bilateral nonvisualization is highly indicative of a malignant mass, concordant uptake does not uniformly represent benign disease. On the other hand, in patients with carcinoma concentrating the tracer, scintigraphy may enable the visualization of unsuspected metastases, thus providing invaluable preoperative information.[89]

In patients with ACTH-independent Cushing's syndrome and apparently normal adrenal radiology, scintigraphy becomes paramount in order to localize the lesion and establish the etiologic diagnosis.[85,90] In those rare cases of adrenal adenoma not identified by CT or MRI, exclusive uptake will reveal the side of the lesion and direct the surgeon.[90] In addition, scintigraphy may identify ectopic adenomas or lesions not recognized as adrenals at standard imaging.[91] Bilateral symmetric or slightly asymmetric uptake characterizes adrenal hyperplasia (see Fig. 7-11B) and PPNAD,[12,74,85,92] and adrenal scintigraphy may be the sole procedure to correctly diagnose these clinical entities. Both AIMAH and PPNAD may in fact present with normal or slightly enlarged glands or unilateral or bilateral nodules and need to be differentiated from adrenal adenoma.[74,90,93] However, scintigraphy itself is not foolproof. Bilateral nonvisualization has been reported in patients with hyperplasia or dysplasia,[15,93] as has unilateral uptake in a patient with PPNAD.[12,94]

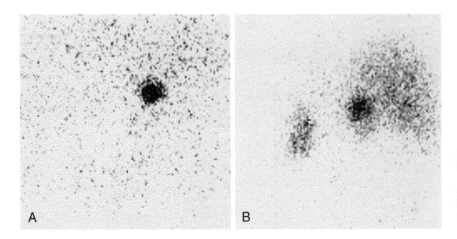

FIGURE 7-11. Scintigraphy in two patients with ACTH-independent Cushing's syndrome due to primary adrenal disease. Images are posterior views obtained 1 week after [131]I-19-norcholesterol injection. **A,** Exclusive uptake by a right-sided adrenocortical adenoma. **B,** Asymmetric uptake in a patient with macronodular adrenocortical hyperplasia. (Courtesy Dr. Eugenio Reschini, Ospedale Maggiore, Milan, Italy.)

Lastly, scintigraphy may be employed in recurrence of adrenal Cushing's syndrome or Cushing's disease after adrenalectomy to localize hyperfunctioning adrenal remnants.[82,93]

Adrenal Venous Sampling

Adrenal venous sampling, performed only in experienced centers, is profitably used to lateralize the source of aldosterone hypersecretion but has been little used in adrenal Cushing's syndrome. It might prove an interesting alternative to adrenal scintigraphy for those patients with bilateral adrenal masses in whom unilateral involvement is suspected[95]; large-scale studies are needed to validate its usefulness in adrenal Cushing's syndrome.

Positron Emission Tomography

Whole-body positron emission tomography (PET) has been used in patients with adrenocortical carcinoma as an adjunctive procedure to detect and monitor metastases. Tracers employed so far are [18]fluorine-fluorodeoxyglucose (FDG), the classical marker of enhanced glycolysis in malignant tumors, and [11]carbon etomidate or metomidate, two inhibitors of 11β-hydroxylase. FDG-PET proved useful for the identification of neoplastic spread both prior to surgery and during follow-up, with markedly increased uptake detected in the site of the neoplasm and in metastases.[96,97] Its use for the distinction between carcinoma and adenoma has been confirmed in larger series,[98] although adrenocortical adenomas and hyperplasias may occasionally yield positive scans.[98] PET using adrenal-specific tracers such as carbon-labeled etomidate or metomidate has yielded promising results for the detection of adrenocortical tumors and their metastases because uptake is clearly increased in adrenal cancer and derived lesions. The aim of this procedure, in contrast to ^{18}F-FDG PET, is to establish the adrenocortical origin of the adrenal lesion; pheochromocytomas, metastases, and nonadrenal masses yield negative scans.[99] Currently, only [11]carbon-labeled metomidate is available, but [18]fluorine tracers are being developed, and these may allow a more widespread use of adrenal-specific tracers in the future.

Interpretation of Adrenal Radiology

Adrenal radiology in patients with adrenal Cushing's syndrome may reveal the presence of normal glands, unilateral or bilateral masses, or uniformly enlarged adrenals. A normal CT scan virtually excludes the presence of adenomatous or malignant lesions and can be taken to indicate micronodular hyperplasia or nodular dysplasia, the latter being more probable in young patients.

Unilateral masses need to be categorized as malignant or benign, and this distinction remains most fraught in cases with intermediate radiologic features, since no procedure is decisive. Benign unilateral masses are most likely adrenocortical adenomas, although dominant nodules in AIMAH and even nodular dysplasia cannot be entirely excluded, and adrenal scintigraphy may be needed to discriminate between unilateral or bilateral disease. On the other hand, hypersecreting and nonhypersecreting adrenocortical adenomas present roughly the same CT/MRI features and cannot be distinguished by radiology.[19,74] Bilateral masses with benign appearance are in all likelihood due to adrenal macronodular hyperplasia and, to a lesser extent, PPNAD. However, the possibility of bilateral carcinoma or adenoma, although exceptional, should not be forgotten. Lastly, bilaterally enlarged glands can be encountered both in adrenal hyperplasia and adrenal dysplasia.

Pathology of Cortisol-Secreting Adrenal Lesions

Adrenal lesions responsible for Cushing's syndrome arise from the zona fasciculata, the middle layer of the adrenal cortex. The adrenal glands are located in the retroperitoneum, immediately above and in front of the kidneys. The mean weight of the adrenal gland is 5 to 6 g, length is approximately 4 cm, width 2.5 cm, and thickness 4 to 6 mm. The left adrenal is usually larger than the right gland and is generally placed more caudally. Men present slightly larger adrenal glands than women. On visual examination, the adrenal gland appears yellowish and triangular or semilunar in shape. The gland is surrounded by abundant retroperitoneal fat and closely wrapped in a thin fibrous capsule transversed by numerous vessels and fibrous branches. In addition to left and right adrenal glands, accessory adrenals may be hidden within the retroperitoneal connective tissue or inside distant organs such as the gonads. The adrenal cortex represents the external portion of the gland between the capsule and the internal adrenal medulla. The glandular epithelium of the cortex is organized into three different zones, each characterized by a different arrangement of polyhedral epithelial cells. The zona fasciculata, the most prominent layer, is composed of large lipid-rich cells, the so-called clear cells, arranged in radial columns. Clear cells present abundant agranular endoplasmic reticulum and well-developed mitochondria, two organelles necessary to steroid hormone production. The outer layer,

Table 7-2. Histologic Features of Adrenal Lesions

	Dysplasia	**Nodule**	**Adenoma**	**Carcinoma**
Size	<1 cm	<1 cm to >3 cm	>1 cm	>3 cm
Shape	Round	Round, oval	Round, oval	Irregular
Number per gland	More than 1	More than 1	Single lesion	Single lesion
Architecture	Fasciculata	Fasciculata or reticularis-like	Cord or alveolar pattern	Sheets, diffuse
Cell population	Homogeneous	Homogeneous	Heterogeneous	Markedly heterogeneous
Pigmentation	Present	Rare	Rare	Exceptional
Nuclear atypia	Absent	Absent	Occasional	Frequent
Regressive changes	Absent	Absent	Rare	Frequent
Necrosis	Absent	Absent	Rare	Frequent
Margins	Clearly demarcated	Circumscribed	Capsulated	Mostly absent
Connective tissue	Lymphoid infiltrates, myelolipomatosis	Fibrovascular trabeculae	Irregular	Large fibrous bands
Extralesional cortex	Atrophied	Normal or hyperplastic	Compressed, atrophied	Normal or compressed
Invasion	Absent	Absent	Rare	Sinusoids, vessels, adrenal capsule

the zona glomerulosa, is composed of highly granular cells arranged in alveolar structures, whereas the inner layer, the zona reticularis, is characterized by irregular nests of compact cells, poor in lipids and rich in lipofuscin granules. The adrenal cortex is extensively innervated by the autonomous nervous system, and nerve terminals abut directly on cortical cells, thereby influencing cortical cell function.

Four main adrenal lesions may be detected in patients with adrenal Cushing's syndrome: a nodule (either isolated or within hyperplastic adrenals), adenoma, carcinoma, and nodular dysplasia. Distinction of hyperplastic nodules from adenoma, as well as adenoma from carcinoma, requires careful pathologic examination not only of the nodule itself but also of the surrounding adrenal tissue (Table 7-2). Indeed, different pathologic systems are used for the diagnosis of these lesions; each offers different advantages and is burdened by different drawbacks (see Chapter 11).

Hyperplastic nodules are usually distinguished from adenomas by the following features: less than 1 cm in diameter, oval or round shape, homogeneous clear-cell population organized in zona fasciculata– or zona reticularis–like architecture, rare smooth cell nests or cordlike structures, with well developed fibrovascular trabeculae.[100-102] Nodules are usually more than one per gland, circumscribed but not encapsulated, and adjacent tissue is normal or hyperplastic. Conversely, adenomas are round or oval lesions of more than 1 cm in diameter, with heterogeneous cell population comprising both clear and compact cells in irregular cord or alveolar patterns. The adenoma is usually a single, encapsulated lesion surrounded by atrophic and compressed cortex. Both hyperplastic nodules and adenomatous lesions are surrounded by a rich network of sinusoidal vessels and dilated intercellular spaces and present well-developed, variably sized and shaped mitochondria and prominent smooth endoplasmic reticulum.[103] Hyperplastic nodules and adenomas present as yellow, lipid-rich lesions, but occasionally lesions are composed of lipofuscin-containing compact cells with abundant eosinophilic cytoplasm, resembling zona reticularis cells and giving rise to black nodules or the so-called black adenoma.[71,102] In patients with AIMAH, adrenal pathology depends on the progression and the extent of the lesions. Most patients present with huge adrenals (up to 500 g) in which the normal architecture is subverted by the presence of big, multiple, yellow or black nodules, some as large as 7 cm, surrounded by internodular hyperplasia (macronodular hyperplasia). Occasionally, the adrenals may be only slightly enlarged, with multiple small nodules (micronodular hyperplasia) or only one gland might be affected,

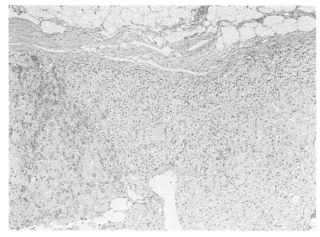

FIGURE 7-12. Pathologic findings in PPNAD. The two nodules are separated by internodular atrophic cortex. Note absence of capsule around nodules and foci of myelolipomatosis. (Courtesy Dr. Aidan Carney, Mayo Clinic, Rochester, MN.)

presenting one or multiple nodules (unilateral hyperplasia). Intriguingly, hyperplastic nodules and adenomas have been reported in the same adrenal gland of patients with Cushing's syndrome,[102] as have bilateral adenomas or multiple adenomas in the same gland.[104,105] In these cases, nodules or adenomas may present different cell composition (e.g., clear or compact cells) and secretory status (hypersecreting or nonhypersecreting) and affect the two glands at different time points. Indeed, bilateral adenomas as well as hyperplastic nodules have been removed several years apart.[106,107]

A unique variant of bilateral nodular involvement is PPNAD, a condition in which adrenals are small to normal-sized and occupied by multiple small, dark nodules (from 1 to 2 mm to 3 cm in diameter) containing large, heavily pigmented, granular eosinophilic cells (rarely clear cells). Pigmented granules contain lipofuscin and neuromelanin.[26,108] Nodules are sharply demarcated, although not encapsulated, and surrounded by atrophic cortical tissue—this provides the major distinction from bilateral hyperplasia. The lesions are usually positioned deep within the adrenal cortex, nearly straddling the corticomedullary junction, whereas the remaining cortex may lose the normal zonation pattern[12] (Fig. 7-12). Some nodules may show lymphocytic infiltration (mostly T-helper cells) within and without the nodule, as well as myelolipomatosis.[109,110] As occurs for cortical tumors, positive immunostaining for neuroendocrine markers, such as synaptophysin and neuron-specific enolase, may be detected.[111] Occasionally, nodularity may be asymmetric and present as a unilateral mass, or more rarely, nodules are markedly prominent, and adrenals appear enlarged,[77] mimicking adrenal macronodular hyperplasia.

The diagnosis of adrenal carcinoma is straightforward if the neoplasm presents typical malignant features ("anaplastic carcinoma") such as necrosis, hemorrhage, abundant mitoses, and nuclear atypia, together with local or hematogenous spread. In most cases, however, Cushing's syndrome is associated with "well-differentiated carcinoma," because steroidogenesis proceeds inefficiently in anaplastic tumors, and these precursors are devoid of significant biological activity.[112] The distinction of well-differentiated carcinoma from adrenocortical adenoma relies on tallies from different pathologic scoring systems, the most used being those of Weiss,[113] Hough,[114] and van Slooten.[115] These diagnostic algorithms are based upon histologic features such as necrosis, architectural changes, nuclear atypia, hyperchromasia, mitotic activity and atypical mitosis, nucleolar appearance, cytoplasmic vacuolization, cellular pleomorphism, fibrosis, and capsular and vascular invasion. The Hough scoring system also takes tumor weight and clinical/endocrine features into account (e.g., 17-ketosteroid excretion and response to ACTH, Cushing's syndrome with or without virilization, body weight loss).[114] While widely accepted, none of these systems offers complete diagnostic certainty,[116] and the definite diagnosis of malignancy remains local invasion or metastasis. Borderline pathologic grading for benign lesions should lead to close follow-up because development of malignant tumors on the same site of a previously removed adenoma[117,118] questions the initial diagnosis of "benign adrenocortical adenoma." Ultrastructural analysis usually reveals lipid-depleted cells with altered mitochondrial and smooth endoplasmic reticulum architecture.[103] Immunohistochemical studies evaluating p53 expression, MiB-1 or Ki-67 labeling, AgNOR counting, MHC class II antigen expression, and c-myc intracellular distribution revealed a differential pattern in benign and malignant lesions, but heterogeneity of neoplastic phenotypes and the resulting overlap between the two neoplasms precludes the identification of a secure profile of malignancy.[119] Likewise, DNA ploidy analysis, comparative genomic hybridization, candidate gene mutations, or differential expression (most notably IGF-II; see Pathogenesis of Adrenal Tumors heading) revealed distinct differences between adenoma and carcinoma but, again, none appeared to ensure absolute diagnostic accuracy.[119] Thus the current state of the art calls for prolonged follow-up also for apparently benign lesions for timely detection of signs of malignancy.

Several variants of adrenocortical tumors have been associated with Cushing's syndrome, such as myxoid adrenocortical carcinoma, composed of polygonal basophilic cells arranged in arborizing cords surrounding myxoma-like large acellular spaces,[120] or oncocytic adrenal tumors, usually benign nonfunctioning lesions composed of mitochondria-rich eosinophilic cells.[121] Combined adrenal adenoma-myelolipoma characterized by intermingled cortical, bone marrow, and lipid cells has also been reported in conjunction with adrenal Cushing's syndrome.[122] Even more complex are mixed corticomedullary tumors, in which tumoral cortical cells are intimately admixed with pheochromocytes,[123] or cortical tumors with neuroendocrine differentiation.[124,125] In the latter case, malignant or benign adrenocortical cells present neuroendocrine features, such as dense core granules and positivity for synaptophysin and neuro-specific enolase, and the tumor may give rise to excess secretion of various peptides, even ACTH itself.[44] Pigmented adrenal lesions are usually benign (i.e., "black adenoma" or PPNAD), although a malignant pigmented lesion has also been reported.[126] Finally, cortisol-secreting adenoma and carcinoma have been reported in the two adrenals of the same subject,[127] as have bilateral carcinomas.[128] On balance, tumors of the adrenal cortex usually display obvious benign or malignant features but occasionally may present with mixed forms or bizarre combinations that challenge the pathologist.

Pathogenesis of Adrenal Tumors

Mechanisms leading to adrenocortical tumorigenesis will be discussed in detail in Chapter 11; this issue will be reviewed briefly here, focusing on features of cortisol-secreting tumors.

Studies performed in the past decade suggest a common multistep process leading from polyclonal hyperplasia, to polyclonal or monoclonal adenomatous lesions, then to single-clone malignant cell expansion. This process, which is in keeping with Knudson's two-hit hypothesis, is apparent in adrenal lesions at different stages,[129,130] possibly even within the same adrenal.[131] Further, genetic heterogeneity in terms of clonality, chromosomal alterations, and proliferation kinetics characterizes all three adrenal lesions, and no single feature allows the distinction between these forms. The common origin of adenoma and carcinoma is also supported by the fact that the same chromosomal regions appear to be affected in benign and malignant lesions.[132] Loci of putative oncogenes (sites of chromosomal gain) and tumor-suppressor genes (sites of chromosomal loss) have been identified on chromosomes 17, 4, 5, and 9 and chromosomes 1, 2, and 11, respectively.[133] Loss of heterozygosity is frequently detected on 11p15.5 (site of IGF2/H19/CDKN1C), 17p13 (site of TP53), 11q13 (site of MEN1), 13q (site of the retinoblastoma gene RB1), 9p (site of CDKN2A), and less frequently on 1p (site of neuroblastoma candidate gene NBL1) and 3p (site of the von Hippel-Lindau gene VHL).[133,134] These changes, most notably the first two, are common in malignant adrenal tumors and are believed to represent pivotal events for adrenocortical tumorigenesis (see Chapter 11). Further, alterations in IGF-2 and p53 can be encountered in Beckwith-Wiedemann and Li-Fraumeni syndromes, respectively, two hereditary conditions presenting, among others, adrenocortical tumors. Germinal TP53 mutations are also linked to adrenal cancer predisposition in southern Brazil, a region with inexplicably high incidence of pediatric adrenal carcinoma.[135] Mutation analysis of factors involved in tumorigenesis in other endocrine tissues (e.g., G proteins, ras) failed to identify significant alterations,[119] nor did the analysis of cortex-specific genes, such as the 21-hydroxylase gene CYP21A2.[136] The ACTH receptor appears unchanged in patients with adrenal disease,[137] although a mutation in MC2R has been reported in one patient with adrenal hyperplasia[138] (see heading ACTH-Independent Adrenal Hyperplasia). Of interest, somatic mutations of PRKAR1A, the gene involved in Carney's complex, and loss of heterozygosity at its locus, 17q22-24, have been detected in adrenal tumors and adrenal hyperplasia,[139,140] as well as alterations in protein kinase A subunits,[141] suggesting an extensive involvement of the cAMP pathway in adrenocortical disease. Lastly, recent microarray studies opened several new avenues of research for adrenocortical lesions, most notably into the Wnt/β-catenin signaling pathway[142] and the inhibin/activin complex.[143]

INHERITED FAMILIAL SYNDROMES

Adrenocortical tumors can be encountered in a number of genetic syndromes, such as multiple endocrine neoplasia (MEN) type 1, MAS, familial adenomatous polyposis and Carney's complex.

Multiple Endocrine Neoplasia Type I

A link between MEN1 (Wermer's syndrome) and adrenal tumors is suggested by the frequent loss of heterozygosity at 11q13, site of the menin gene, in adrenal cancers.[133] However, no mutation in the *MEN1* gene itself has been reported in cortisol-secreting sporadic adrenocortical tumors.[144] Conversely, up to 70% of patients with MEN1 present adrenal lesions, mostly nodular and diffuse hyperplasia, adenomas, or rarely, carcinomas.[145] Cushing's syndrome in the context of MEN1, however, is mostly associated with pituitary ACTH-secreting adenoma, since adrenal lesions are only rarely accompanied by hypercortisolism.[146]

McCune-Albright Syndrome

Since the first description of bony lesions, skin pigmentation, and precocious puberty by Albright in 1937, the spectrum of endocrine abnormalities associated with this syndrome has progressively increased to include thyroid, parathyroid, pituitary, and adrenal disorders. Adrenal Cushing's syndrome develops in less than 10% of patients with MAS, usually in the first year after birth, possibly even before sexual precocity and fibrous dysplasia.[17] Adrenal histology usually reveals bilateral nodular hyperplasia or, rarely, adenoma; interestingly, these lesions have also been detected at autopsy in patients who did not present Cushingoid signs during their lifetime. MAS is known to be due to early postzygotic mutations of the stimulatory guanine nucleotide-binding protein ($G_{s\alpha}$; *GNAS1*), which can be detected in multiple tissues, including the adrenal gland,[147] and also in patients with MAS and adrenal Cushing's syndrome described so far.[17,148] Conversely, *GNAS1* mutations are exceptional in patients with sporadic cortisol-secreting adrenal adenomas.[149] *GNAS1* mutations have been reported in adult patients with Cushing's syndrome due to bilateral adrenal hyperplasia without other features of MAS,[150,151] suggesting that mutational $G_{s\alpha}$ activation could be involved in adrenal hyperplasia.

Familial Adenomatous Polyposis

Patients affected by this autosomal dominant inherited disorder develop extensive adenomatous polyps of the colon and a variety of extracolonic manifestations comprising desmoid tumors, osteomas, pigmented retinal lesions, and adrenocortical neoplasms. Adrenocortical lesions consist in adenomas, bilateral nodular hyperplasia, or rarely, carcinomas and are mostly nonhypersecreting.[152] Cushing's syndrome is a rare occurrence both in classic familial adenomatous polyposis[152] and its variant, Gardner's syndrome.[153] Familial adenomatous polyposis has been causally linked to germline mutations of the adenomatous polyposis coli (*APC*) gene located on chromosome 5, usually inactivating mutations accompanied by loss of the normal allele. It is worth recalling that inactivation of the *APC* gene leads to degradation of β-catenin, a recent putative player in adrenal tumorigenesis.[142] Somatic mutations of *APC* have been detected in a wide variety of other human carcinomas but none so far in sporadic adrenocortical tumors.

Carney's Complex

Carney's complex represents the only etiology of Cushing's syndrome in which a genetic defect has been identified. Indeed, intensive work by two groups of researchers led to the short-listing of two probable loci, on the short arm of chromosome 2 and on 17q24, followed by the identification of inactivating mutations in the protein kinase A regulatory subunit type 1α.[154,155] Carney's complex is discussed in greater detail later (see heading Primary Pigmented Nodular Adrenal Dysplasia).

STEROIDOGENIC ENZYMES IN ADRENAL LESIONS

Several studies have evaluated steroidogenesis in adrenal Cushing's syndrome. Cortisol concentration in tumoral specimens is 2- to 50-fold greater in adenomas than in normal glands,[156] attesting to the greater secretory output. Steroidogenesis usually proceeds without hindrance to its principal end product, cortisol, but individual steroidogenic enzymes may become rate-limiting in hypersecreting adrenals,[157] the extent and involvement of individual enzymes being quite variable. Analysis of steroidogenic enzymes yielded somewhat conflicting results, with increased 21-hydroxylase and 17α-hydroxylase synthesis and activity in cortisol-secreting adenomas as the most constant finding.[112,156,158] Increased 17,20-lyase activity reportedly occurs in adenomas producing androgens in addition to cortisol, possibly a consequence of increased cytochrome b₅ expression.[159] A relative deficiency of 11β-hydroxylase has been suggested by some authors,[160] although not confirmed by others.[158] Conversely, 3β-hydroxysteroid dehydrogenase and cholesterol desmolase appear substantially unchanged in cortisol-secreting adenomas.[112,158] In adrenal carcinoma, cortisol secretion per gram of tumoral tissue is mostly reduced,[160] as are individual steroidogenic enzymes.[28,112,161] Of interest, malignant cells may fail to synthesize the full complement of steroidogenic enzymes,[28,161] thus possibly explaining ineffective steroidogenesis. Shift from excess aldosterone to excess cortisol production has also been reported in malignant tumors, associated with changes in steroidogenic enzyme synthesis and attesting to the plasticity of tumoral tissues.[162] The low efficiency of cortisol secretion is also a feature of macronodular hyperplasia,[100] and variable expression of steroidogenic enzymes in individual cortical cells has been observed.[163] In contrast, nodules from patients with PPNAD all present intense immunostaining for steroidogenic enzymes.[163] Lastly, low levels of expression and activity of 11β-hydroxysteroid dehydrogenase type 2, the enzyme which inactivates cortisol, have been detected in adenomatous cortisol-secreting adrenals and may represent an additional modulator of total cortisol levels.[164,165]

REGULATION OF STEROID SYNTHESIS IN ADRENAL LESIONS

In adrenal Cushing's syndrome, cortisol secretion is by definition ACTH-independent. However, a considerable proportion of adenomas, and to a lesser extent carcinomas, maintain ACTH-responsiveness in vivo and in vitro,[7,166] and the relevance of this preserved ACTH sensitivity in tumors which secrete cortisol autonomously remains unclear. The ACTH receptor (also known as the melanocortin 2 receptor, MC2-R) is expressed in the vast majority of cortisol-secreting adenomas, even overexpressed compared with the normal adrenal cortex, according to some authors,[166,167] whereas cortisol-secreting carcinomas present low levels of *MC2R* mRNA, possibly a consequence of dedifferentiation and loss of heterozygosity at this locus.[167] ACTH is known to up-regulate its own receptor at low concentrations and exert the opposite effect at higher doses,[168] but no direct association between ACTH receptor mRNA and ACTH plasma levels has been detected in various forms of Cushing's syndrome.[169] Stimulation of steroid secretion in adrenocortical tumor cells occurs through activation of protein kinase C, together with the main protein kinase A–cAMP pathway.[170] Of interest, factors other than ACTH may also increase cAMP levels in malignant but not in normal adrenal cells, as has been demonstrated for catecholamines and thyrotropin,[171] indicating a loss of specificity of the transductional machinery in tumoral tissues (see heading ACTH-Independent Adrenal Hyperplasia). Moreover, ACTH is also an indirect adrenocortical mitogen acting through factors such as basic fibroblast growth factor (bFGF), insulin-like growth factor 2 (IGF-2), epidermal growth factor (EGF), and transforming growth factor (TGF) α or β.[172,173] These mediators are responsible for the growth-promoting effect of ACTH in vivo, whereas in vitro, ACTH exerts a direct antimitogenic activity.[172] Similarly divergent are the effects of N-terminal pro-opiomelanocortin (POMC), which appears to stimulate mitogenic activity via the secretory serine protease (AsP) pathway in vitro[174] but is devoid of mitogenic effects in *Pomc*-null mice in vivo.[175]

One brief mention is warranted for the regulation of cortisol synthesis by corticosteroids themselves. Evidence for this ultra-short negative feedback has been garnered by in vivo and in vitro studies, although paradoxically, a stimulatory, permissive effect of cortisol or dexamethasone on ACTH-stimulated cortisol secretion has been reported by some authors.[176] The direct action of corticosteroids on steroidogenesis is presumably mediated by glucocorticoid receptors themselves, since both binding and induction of gene synthesis have been demonstrated in the adrenal cortex.[167,177] Expression of the glucocorticoid receptor is apparently reduced in cortisol-secreting tumors.[167,178]

ACTH-Independent Adrenal Hyperplasia

ACTH-independent adrenal hyperplasia was recognized as a cause of Cushing's syndrome following the description of several case reports which defied classification.[179,180] Considerable confusion arose initially from the fact that some features of ACTH-dependent adrenal hyperplasia (i.e., Cushing's disease) overlapped with ACTH-independent adrenal hyperplasia; indeed, "macronodular Cushing's syndrome" once comprised both entities. Advances in pathology,[100] as well as the identification of factors other than ACTH capable of modulating cortisol hypersecretion, enabled a more precise definition and classification.[14,181,182] In view of its most common presentation, we will refer to this entity with the currently used acronym, *AIMAH*: ACTH-independent macronodular adrenal hyperplasia.

Currently accepted criteria for the diagnosis of AIMAH are the presence of bilaterally enlarged adrenals containing one or more nonpigmented nodules and the presence of suppressed and/or unresponsive ACTH levels.[14,100] Internodular tissue was initially described as atrophic[100] but may also be normal or even hyperplastic, thus does not represent a distinctive element.[14,182] On average, glands weigh five times normal (e.g., 20 to 120 g) and present large, well-circumscribed nodules grossly distorting adrenal cortex architecture (see heading Pathology of Cortisol-Secreting Adrenal Lesions). The size of nodules usually ranges from 0.5 cm to 2 to 3 cm, although exceptionally large lesions, up to 10 cm in diameter, have been described.[183] Nodules are composed of lipid-laden clear cells in cord or nest-like structures interspersed by small islands of lipid-poor compact cells,[100,184] foci of angiomyelolipomatosis and lymphocytic infiltrates. Cellular and nuclear pleomorphism are usually absent.

Unilateral macronodular hyperplasia, as well as diffuse bilateral hyperplasia, have also been described in patients with ACTH-independent hypercortisolism,[14,185] possibly representing different points in the continuum of AIMAH.

The large size of adrenals is in marked contrast with the often mild clinical picture, corroborating in vitro evidence of inefficient steroidogenesis by cortical cells.[100,163,184] Indeed, cytochrome P450 expression and activity are reduced compared to that of cells derived from adrenal adenoma[100,184]; thus the adrenal mass may have to attain a considerable volume for hypercortisolism to become manifest. Subclinical Cushing's syndrome is increasingly reported in patients with ACTH-independent adrenal hyperplasia,[186] occasionally evolving with progressive adrenal enlargement and development of frank hypercortisolism.[187,188]

Salient features of hypercortisolism due to AIMAH are later age at diagnosis (usually around 50 years of age), the even gender distribution, and an unusually long time to diagnosis, on average 4 years from the appearance of the first symptoms, compared to 2 years for cortisol-secreting adenomas.[14,182] One patient developed full-blown hypercortisolism 7 years after the incidental detection of bilateral adrenal masses.[188] The youngest and oldest reported patients with ACTH-independent adrenal hyperplasia were 17 and 74 years old, respectively. In patients with aberrant receptor-induced hyperplasia (see later), hypercortisolism may follow the course of ligand levels, as exemplified by the course of LH-dependent Cushing's syndrome or by low morning serum cortisol levels in the fasted patient with food-dependent Cushing's syndrome.

By definition, ACTH levels are suppressed in patients with ACTH-independent adrenal hyperplasia, but the detection of low-normal ACTH concentrations does not exclude the diagnosis.[14,182] As in other causes of adrenal Cushing's syndrome, CRH testing provides proof of ACTH independency. Inferior petrosal sinus sampling should not be performed, because significant post-CRH center-periphery ACTH gradients have been reported in several patients, presumably reflecting incomplete suppression of pituitary corticotrophs by mild or episodic hypercortisolism.[189] Prior to the availability of ACTH assays, adrenal autonomy from ACTH was established by means of absent dexamethasone suppression or metyrapone stimulation of adrenal steroids. These tests, however, do not guarantee complete diagnostic accuracy; indeed, the number of patients with Cushing's disease and adrenal nodules who fail to suppress after dexamethasone is not negligible,[190] and specificity of metyrapone stimulation is known to be suboptimal.[47] The distinction between ACTH-independent adrenal hyperplasia and unilateral adrenal lesions or PPNAD relies on imaging, both morphologic and functional, and pathology (see earlier discussion).

Major diagnostic difficulties may be encountered in the distinction from longstanding Cushing's disease with ACTH levels in the lower third of the normal range and from adrenal adenoma or even carcinoma, if only one large dominant nodule is visible at adrenal imaging. The distinction is obviously essential to a correct surgical approach.

PATHOGENESIS

ACTH-independent adrenal hyperplasia presents a heterogeneous etiology, comprising legitimate and illegitimate adrenal growth factors and gene mutations. In one of the first descriptions of ACTH-independent adrenal hyperplasia, proliferation of small cortical cells with maturational arrest or incomplete maturation was hypothesized to cause hyperplasia.[100] Causes identi-

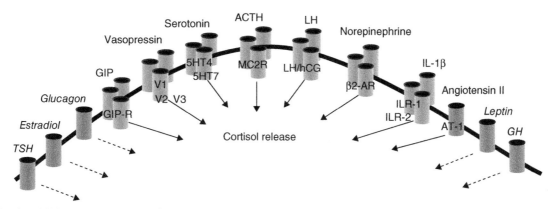

FIGURE 7-13. Ligands and illicit receptors involved in Cushing's syndrome associated with AIMAH. *Single barrelled receptors* and *dashed arrows* indicated putative adrenal-stimulating agents.

fied so far, however, account for only part of reported patients, and other mechanisms are likely to be involved. Indeed, microarray studies in AIMAH tissues identified a host of potential candidate genes,[191,192] in part overlapping with genes involved in adrenal tumorigenesis, such as the Wnt signaling pathway, and cytogenetic analysis revealed frequent allelic losses in 2p16 and 17q22, two sites linked to PPNAD,[140] in adrenal hyperplastic tissues.

Legitimate Adrenal Growth Factor

Adrenal hyperplasia was initially believed to result from prolonged stimulation by ACTH followed by autonomization of adrenal secretion. Several case reports describing transition from ACTH-dependent to ACTH-independent hypercortisolism supported this hypothesis.[193,194] In fact, ACTH induces exaggerated cortisol increases in patients with adrenal hyperplasia, both in vivo and in vitro, attesting to an exquisite adrenal sensitivity to ACTH, in contrast with the barely preserved responsiveness of adrenal adenomas and carcinomas. Indeed, the cortisol response to cosyntropin represents the standard against which responses to other agents are compared (see later). This pathogenetic hypothesis, while theoretically still tenable, has been superseded by subsequent developments.

A role for ACTH cannot be excluded, since locally produced ACTH participates in the intraadrenal CRH/ACTH modulation of corticosteroid release and adrenal proliferation.[195] In two patients with adrenal hyperplasia, cortisol secretion was driven by intraadrenal ACTH production. In one patient, ACTH was produced by an adrenocortical adenoma presenting neuroendocrine features,[196] whereas in the other patient, steroidogenic cells with positivity for Leydig-cell markers were the site of ACTH synthesis.[197] Interestingly, plasma ACTH levels were high in the former but not in the latter patient, and the diagnostic workup comprising adrenal vein sampling was indicative of ectopic ACTH secretion.[196] Altered sensitivity to the adrenal ACTH receptor might be an alternative mechanism. Indeed, a homozygous *MC2R* germline mutation was identified in a patient with Cushing's syndrome and ACTH-independent adrenal hyperplasia; functional studies revealed constitutive activation of the *F278C* mutated receptor.[138] This case is unique; no mutations in *MC2R* were detected in other patients with ACTH-independent adrenal hyperplasia.[151,198] Quantitation of *MC2R* expression in adrenals from patients responsive to illicit receptor stimulants yielded contrasting results, with some studies indicative of increased expression,[199] others observing reduced expression,[192,200] and others again observing expression comparable

to normal adrenocortical tissues.[201] Variability in clinical and molecular phenotypes might explain these differences.

Illicit Adrenal Receptors

The capacity of ligands other than ACTH to stimulate the adrenal cortex had been demonstrated in both animal and human tumoral adrenal specimens,[171,202] but this was initially considered an epiphenomenon to tumoral dedifferentiation. The causative role of aberrant adrenal receptors was later demonstrated by two groups who simultaneously reported that food-induced hypercortisolism was due to stimulation of steroidogenesis by the gastrointestinal-inhibitory peptide (GIP).[203,204] Since then, a variety of adrenal cortisol-stimulating receptors have been described (Fig. 7-13), not only in adrenal hyperplasia but also in patients with adenomas[149] and unilateral or bilateral incidental adrenal lesions associated with subclinical hypercortisolism.[186,205,206] Responses to illicit receptor stimulants appear to occur less frequently in unilateral compared to bilateral lesions.[207,208] Different developmental derangements have been postulated to explain the common etiologic pathway of adenoma and hyperplasia. Sensitivity to illicit adrenal stimulants would be acquired through mutations occurring during early embryogenesis in patients with bilateral hyperplasia, whereas somatic mutations in single adrenal cells would result in unilateral adenoma. The importance of aberrant receptor expression in ACTH-independent adrenal hyperplasia has recently been validated by two elegant xenograft studies.[209,210] These studies have shown that implantation of bovine adrenal tissue transfected with either the GIP or the LH/human chorionic gonadotropin (hCG) receptor into nude mice was accompanied by adrenal growth, elevated cortisol levels, and development of Cushingoid features.[209,210] It appears, therefore, that aberrant expression of the receptor in the adrenal is a primary event, sufficient to initiate adrenal growth and hypersecretion.

The receptors involved in adrenal Cushing's syndrome have been initially called *eutopic* or *ectopic* (or illicit, aberrant), according to their presence or absence in the normal adrenal cortex. Obviously, eutopic receptors would have to function in an altered manner to stimulate cortical cell growth and secretion. Subsequent molecular studies have shown, however, that most ectopic receptors are expressed at low levels in the normal adrenal gland, without significant steroid secretion stimulation. Activation of receptors may occur by hormones secreted elsewhere, in a classical endocrine manner or in paracrine/autocrine fashion if the ligand is produced by the adrenal gland itself. The activation of adrenal growth by ligands extraneous to the HPA axis, thus not

Table 7-3. Testing for Adrenal Responsiveness

1° Test	2° Test	Receptors Involved	In Vitro Stimulation
Upright posture (2 hours supine followed by 2 hours of ambulation)	5% hypertonic saline infusion (0.05 mL/kg × min for 2 hour)	Any AVP receptor	
	0.5 mg terlipressin IV *or* 10 mg terlipressin IM *or* 5 U AVP SC	V1	10 nM vasopressin ±V1 receptor antagonist
	10 μg desmopressin	V2	10-100 nM desmopressin
	5 U AVP SC	V3	10 nM vasopressin ±V3 receptor antagonist
	Angiotensin II: 1 ng/kg × min over 15 min followed by 3 ng/kg × min over 30 min *or* 8 mg candesartan prior to upright posture test	AT-1	10 nM angiotensin
	1 μg isoproterenol IV	Any β-adrenergic receptor	10 μM isoproterenol
		β1 receptor	10 μM dobutamine
		β2 receptor	1 μM salbutamol
		β3 receptor	β3 receptor agonist
Standard mixed meal	75 g oral glucose test	GIP	10–100 nM GIP
	±100 μg octeotide SC 1 hour before the test	GLP-1	1 nM-1 μM GLP-1
100 μg GnRH IV	5000 IU hCG IM	LH/hCG	1 nM-1 μM hCG
	150 IU FSH IM	FSH	1 nM-1 μM FSH
		GnRH	1 nM-1 μM GnRH
200 μg TRH IV		TRH	1 nM-1 μM TRH
		Prolactin	1 nM-1 μM prolactin
		TSH	1 nM-1 μM TSH
10 mg cisapride PO *or* 10 mg metoclopramide IV		5HT4	100 nM-10 μM 5HT ±5HT4 antagonist
		5HT7	100 nM-10 μM 5HT ±5HT7 antagonist
250 μg ACTH IV *Optional:* 1 mg glucagon IM	—	MC2-R	10 nM ACTH
Insulin-induced hypoglycemia	1 μg isoproterenol IV	β-adrenergic	
	100 μg CRH	MC2-R or CRH	
	Any GH stimulatory test	GH or IGF-1	

ACTH, Adrenocorticotropic hormone; *AVP,* arginine vasopressin; *CRH,* corticotropin-releasing hormone; *FSH,* follicle-stimulating hormone; *GnRH,* gonadotropin-releasing hormone; *hCG,* human chorionic gonadotropin; *IGF-1,* insulin-like growth factor 1; *IM,* intramuscularly; *IV,* intravenously; *LH,* luteinizing hormone; *PO,* orally; *SC,* subcutaneously; *TSH,* thyroid-stimulating hormone.

Samples for ACTH, cortisol and other steroid hormones are collected at half-hourly intervals before and for up to 3 hours. Two or three tests can be performed sequentially on the same day. Absent response: cortisol increase <25% baseline levels. Potentially significant response: cortisol increase by 25% to 50% baseline levels. Positive response: cortisol increase over 50% baseline levels.

sensitive to glucocorticoid feedback, will confer selective proliferative advantage to cells presenting the receptor and favor clonal expansion. At the same time, the sensitivity to illicit stimulants may characterize the clinical presentation and hypercortisolism wax and wane according to ligand levels; this is particularly conspicuous for LH/hCG or food-dependent Cushing's syndrome. On the whole, aberrant adrenal sensitivity to endogenous ligands links legitimate events, such as the increase in hCG during pregnancy, with an illegitimate cortisol response.

The demonstration of ectopic receptors or overexpression of eutopic receptors is essential but not sufficient to diagnose illicit receptor-dependent adrenal Cushing's syndrome, because ligand-induced cortisol secretion and adrenal growth or, better, remission of hypercortisolism with specific receptor antagonists are necessary to prove its causative role. Expression of the receptor in the adrenal lesion, in fact, is not invariably associated with responsiveness to the ligand,[211,212] and further, simultaneous expression of multiple aberrant receptors in the same patient is not unusual.[213] Cortisol responsiveness to multiple ligands can often be observed in vivo, and in vitro incubation with potential stimulants may result in significant cortisol increases even if no significant change in cortisol serum levels occurred in vivo.

Protocol for adrenal responsiveness testing is illustrated in Table 7-3 and should be applied to all patients with bilateral adrenal lesions and full-blown or subclinical hypercortisolism. Currently, screening of patients with unilateral, incidental adrenal lesions is not recommended until its usefulness is validated in large-scale studies. Testing usually begins with first-tier tests (see Table 7-3), followed by more specific stimulants if a positive cortisol response is observed.

Gastrointestinal Inhibitory Polypeptide

Food-dependent Cushing's syndrome was the first variant of hypercortisolism due to stimulants other than ACTH to be described. Over 25 cases have been reported since the first description in 1987—mostly in women—so this appears to be the most frequent etiology of ectopic receptor-associated hypercortisolism. A causative role of gastrointestinal hormones was suggested by the increase in cortisol levels after various mixed meals and after oral but not intravenous glucose and by blunting of these responses through octreotide. Candidate hormones were GIP (gastrointestinal or gastric-inhibitory polypeptide or glucose-dependent insulinotropic peptide) and GLP-1 (glucagon-like peptide 1). Evidence in favor of the former accrued with the observation of a close correlation between plasma cortisol and GIP levels in these patients,[203] and the demonstration of a direct stimulatory effect of GIP on cortisol release in vivo[203,204,208] and on adrenal tissue in vitro.[204,213] Conversely, GLP-1 did not stimulate cortisol secretion in either experimental paradigm.[107,213] GIP is a 42-amino-acid gastric peptide which increases after orally ingested meals and stimulates insulin secretion. The GIP receptor (GIP-R) is a member of the secretin-vasoactive intestinal polypeptide family of G protein–coupled receptors normally expressed in pancreatic β cells and in the brain. GIP-R is expressed at very low levels in the normal adrenal, where it appears to be nonfunctional, since no changes in cortisol secretion have been observed in normal adrenals incubated with GIP.[214,215] In contrast, the GIP-R appears to be abundantly expressed in adenomas, nodules, and internodular hyperplastic tissue of patients with food-dependent Cushing's syndrome.[107,208] GIP-R is observed more frequently in tissues from AIMAH than in adenomas, even in patients without signs of food-dependent hypercortisolism[208]; indeed, GIP-R mRNA has also been detected in some patients with Cushing's disease.[216] No mutation in the promoter region and coding sequence of GIP-R has been identified so far,[214,217] and no specific changes in local transcription factors have been detected in patients with food-dependent Cushing's syndrome,[218] thus the mechanisms responsible for GIP responsiveness remain to be established. In GIP-sensitive adrenal cortex nodules, GIP induces cAMP synthesis, coupled to PKA kinase activity as well as ionic currents,[212] thereby activating steroidogenesis. In lesions arising from the zona fasciculata cortisol and to a lesser extent 17OHP will be the main secretory products,[107] whereas in the single adenoma of the zona reticularis described so far, DHEA and androstenedione secretion prevailed.[219]

From a clinical viewpoint, food-dependent Cushing's syndrome is characterized by typically low morning serum cortisol levels, because cortisol will not be stimulated in the fasted patient, and endogenous ACTH will be suppressed by postprandial cortisol bursts.[203,204] Occasionally, ACTH concentrations may fall within the normal range and even respond to CRH stimulation, possibly a consequence of the intermittent nature of food-dependent hypercortisolism.[220] Treatment with octreotide (e.g., 100 to 200 μg t.i.d.) or octreotide LAR achieved clinical and biochemical improvement in several patients.[203,220]

Vasopressin

Arginine vasopressin (AVP) is the second most common "illicit" stimulant in adrenal Cushing's syndrome. The main action of AVP on the HPA axis is stimulation of ACTH with attendant cortisol release,[221] although direct stimulation of adrenocortical cells by AVP has been demonstrated in vitro.[222] However, the importance of this action is unclear, since no cortisol response to AVP is observed in vivo in absence of ACTH.[223] Direct stimulation of AVP on adrenocortical secretion and cell growth most likely subserves the paracrine action of locally produced AVP.[222]

Several patients with AIMAH have been reported in whom AVP, LVP, or the prodrug terlipressin increased serum cortisol in the face of suppressed ACTH levels.[206,224,225] Endogenous AVP plasma levels are usually suppressed in these patients but may increase after stimuli such as upright posture, hypertonic saline, or insulin-induced hypoglycemia in parallel with cortisol.[207,211,226] Aberrant responses to AVP have also been reported in several patients with adrenal hyperplasia and subclinical Cushing's syndrome,[227,228] as well as in a few patients with cortisol-secreting adenoma or carcinoma.[206]

In vitro studies on human adrenal tissue showed that AVP stimulates cortisol secretion via its phospholipase C–coupled V1 receptor,[224,225,229] and that this receptor is abundantly expressed in AVP-responsive patients.[225,227,229] The V1 receptor is also expressed in normal cortical cells[222] and in patients with adrenal hyperplasia and subclinical Cushing's syndrome,[227] but the mechanisms leading to adrenal hypersensitivity in these patients remain to be established. Administration of an oral V1 receptor antagonist did not significantly affect the acute cortisol response to AVP but slightly reduced UFC concentrations.[226] Involvement of other AVP receptor subtypes, namely V2 and V3, has been suspected after the demonstration of these receptors by IHC and RT-PCR in adrenal nodules[229,230] but has yet to be convincingly demonstrated. Desmopressin failed to stimulate cortisol release in patients tested so far, both in vitro and in vivo, and no coincubation experiment using AVP together with selective V3 receptor antagonists has been performed to substantiate V2 or V3 receptor functionality. AVP-dependent adrenal Cushing's syndrome could therefore be due to an aberrant response to the eutopic V1 receptor or ectopic expression of V2 or V3 receptors.

Angiotensin II

Angiotensin induces cortisol secretion by normal and hyperplastic adrenal in vitro, albeit to a consistently greater extent in the latter, especially in patients in whom cortisol increases during the posture test.[213] Involvement of the AT-1 receptor can be demonstrated by blockade of the posture-induced cortisol increase by candesartan, and the drug could be used as medical therapy to contain hypercortisolism.[231] A full description of angiotensin-mediated hypercortisolism has, however, yet to be provided.

Luteinizing Hormone/Human Chorionic Gonadotropin

The observation that some young women develop clinical and biochemical features of hypercortisolism during pregnancy which resolve spontaneously after delivery has long intrigued endocrinologists (Fig. 7-14). Further, the prevalence of adrenal Cushing's syndrome is considerably higher in pregnancy.[81] This suggested an enhanced adrenal sensitivity to some factor produced by the fetoplacental unit and, indeed, aberrant LH/hCG receptors have been shown to mediate the increased adrenal secretion in these patients.[35] The causative role of LH was first demonstrated in a 63-year-old woman who developed Cushingoid features during pregnancy and again after menopause. Cortisol levels increased markedly upon administration of GnRH and chorionic gonadotropin in this patient, whereas FSH was without effect. Treatment with a GnRH agonist over 24 months normalized UFC levels and ameliorated signs of hypercortisolism without, however, affecting adrenal size.[35] Subsequent studies demonstrated that LH can stimulate cortisol secretion in vitro, albeit not in all patients responsive to LH in vivo, and that adenomatous lesions express the LH receptor.[198,213] Low-level synthesis of LH/hCGR can be detected in the zona fasciculata and reticularis of the normal adrenal cortex,[232] but no stimulatory effect of LH/hCG on cortisol secretion by normal adrenals has been observed.[198,213] Support for the role of LH as an adrenal stimulant is supported by animal models. LH-transgenic mice, gonadectomized ferrets, and adrenal xenotransplant studies develop bilateral adrenal hyperplasia.[210,233,234]

Of interest, in the few patients with LH-dependent Cushing's syndrome studied so far, an aberrant response to other stimulants (e.g., 5HT, GIP, AVP) accompanied LH hypersensitivity.[35,186,198,213] In contrast to food-dependent Cushing's syndrome, sustained increases in LH/hCG levels are necessary to induce clinically relevant adrenal hypersecretion; signs of hypercortisolism appeared only during pregnancies and/or menopause. It

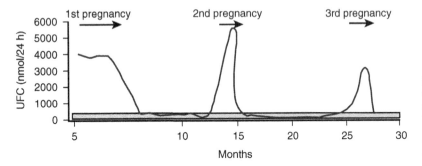

FIGURE 7-14. UFC levels during successive pregnancies in a woman with LH-dependent Cushing's syndrome. The first pregnancy was carried through to the 34th week, the second and third terminated within the first 2 months. *Shaded area* represents normal range. (Data from Hána V, Dokoupilová M, Marek J, et al: Recurrent ACTH-independent Cushing's syndrome in multiple pregnancies and its treatment with metyrapone, Clin Endocrinol 54:277–281, 2001.)

appears that the normal pulsatory gonadotropin pattern is insufficient to activate adrenal steroidogenesis. However, not all patients aberrantly expressing the LH receptor in the adrenal cortex will develop hypercortisolism during periods of increased LH secretion, so factors other than LH must contribute to pregnancy-induced Cushing's syndrome.

Catecholamines

β-Adrenergic receptors were the first aberrant receptors to be demonstrated in cortisol-secreting tumors,[235] but recent studies suggest that the β2-adrenergic type 2 receptor (β2-AR) is expressed also in the normal adrenal cortex, albeit without cortisol-secreting ability.[201] β-Adrenergic agonists have proven capable of stimulating cortisol secretion in a few patients,[207,211,236] and proof of β2-AR involvement was obtained through in vitro experiments with different β-adrenergic receptor agonists.[201] These findings have been translated into medical therapy with long-term beneficial effects in patients,[201,236] thus proving the existence of β-adrenergic-dependent hypercortisolism.

Serotonin

Serotonin is secreted by intraadrenal mast cells and stimulates cortisol secretion in a paracrine fashion, most likely via its type 4 receptor ($5HT_4$). This action can be replicated by incubation of adrenocortical cells with serotonin but not in vivo, because serotonin agonists do not stimulate cortisol secretion in normal subjects.[237] Conversely, significant increases in cortisol levels have been observed in several patients with Cushing's syndrome due to adrenal hyperplasia or adrenocortical adenomas,[149,238] often in patients harboring other types of "aberrant" receptors, attesting to receptor promiscuity in hyperplastic adrenals.[13] Initial studies focused on the $5HT4$ isoform, but no consistent differences in $5HTR4$ expression between normal and hyperplastic adrenal tissues[238,239] or mutations in its coding sequence were detected.[238] Further, some in vivo cisapride-responsive patients failed to release cortisol with cisapride in vitro, and $5HTR_4$ antagonists did not block the cortisol increase evoked by serotonin in vitro.[212] Evaluation of additional serotonin receptor isoforms identified $5HT_{7a}$ as a possible illicit mediator of serotonin responsiveness in AIMAH, given that this receptor does not appear to be expressed by the normal adrenal.[212] No 5HT receptor antagonist has yet been tested in patients with cortisol-hypersecreting adrenal hyperplasia.

Interleukin 1

A single case of Cushing's syndrome due to aberrant expression of interleukin-1 type 1 receptor (*IL1R1*) has been described so far.[240] A role of cytokines in adrenal tumorigenesis was suspected in this patient when pathologic examination of the adrenal adenoma disclosed heavy leukocyte and macrophage infiltration.

Immunohistochemistry, as well as in situ hybridization, revealed the presence of IL1R1, and adenomatous cells released substantial amounts of cortisol in vitro upon incubation with interleukin-1β. In normal adrenal glands, the IL1R1 was not detected by immunohistochemistry, and further, interleukin-1β failed to stimulate cortisol secretion from normal and adenomatous adrenals collected from other patients. The proliferative effect of interleukin-1β is well known,[241] thus it was hypothesized that high concentrations of interleukin-1β released by local immune cells may have favored clonal expansion of adrenocortical cells aberrantly expressing IL1R1.

Estradiol

Mimicking LH-dependent Cushing's syndrome, a young woman presented with features of hypercortisolism during two pregnancies, but in contrast to LH-dependent Cushing's, these features also recurred during contraceptive therapy.[242] Pathology of the adrenals revealed enlarged glands with multiple nonpigmented nodules, and in vitro studies showed marked cortisol release in the presence of estradiol. The authors deduced a causative role of estradiol in cortisol hypersecretion.

Other Putative Stimulants

Additional adrenal receptor ligands include FSH, TSH, GH, glucagon, and leptin. Evidence in favor of these substances is currently only circumstantial, since no patient with hormone-driven hypercortisolism has been fully studied. Finally, a proportion of patients with AIMAH does not present identifiable stimulatory ligands, so a careful clinical history together with specific testing would be necessary to define other, at present unknown, aberrant receptors.

Genetic Causes

As discussed above, no mutation in illicit or licit receptor gene sequences in patients with AIMAH has been reported so far. Conversely, somatic mutations of $G_{s\alpha}$, the so-called *gsp* mutations, have been detected in three out of five patients with adrenal nodular hyperplasia,[151] which is in keeping with adrenal hyperplasia as the most common cause of hypercortisolism in patients with MAS (see earlier). Other genetic causes of ACTH-independent adrenal hyperplasia cannot be excluded, given the increasing number of familial cases, both with and without overt hypercortisolism.[228,230,243]

TREATMENT

Removal of both adrenal glands is obviously the rational approach to curing hypercortisolism in this condition. Laparoscopic adrenalectomy of glands measuring up to 13 cm has been reported, indicating that size need not be a concern in this benign lesion.[244] Likewise, development of Nelson's syndrome has not been reported in patients with ACTH-independent adrenal hyperplasia. Alternative approaches, such as subtotal or unilateral adrenalectomy, may be considered in selected patients. To avoid risks associated with adrenal insufficiency,[245] subtotal adrenalectomy has been performed in a patient with multiple malignancies, whereas removal of the largest adrenal achieved long-term remission in several patients with asymmetric involvement.[189,246] Transitory hypoadrenalism requiring steroid replacement therapy may occur. Should abnormalities in HPA function persist, as appears to occur in patients with comparable enlargement of both adrenal glands, removal of the contralateral gland may be performed,[246] or medical therapy with antagonists to illicit receptors may be used to restrain hypercortisolism.[13] Surgery may not be advisable in all patients with AIMAH, given the often advanced age at diagnosis and the attendant, age-related comorbidities. Thus, administration of steroid synthesis inhibitors may be the treatment of choice, and relatively low doses of steroid blocking agents are usually capable of containing hypercortisolism in these patients. In addition to ketoconazole, metyrapone and mitotane have also been administered with success.[247,248]

Primary Pigmented Nodular Adrenal Dysplasia

Cushing's syndrome due to PPNAD was recognized for the first time at the Mayo Clinic in 1939, but owing to the different terms adopted to identify the adrenal lesion (e.g., *multiple androgenic adenomata, polymicroadenomatosis, primary adrenocortical microadenomatosis*) PPNAD assumed its current nomenclature only in 1982. Some 2000 cases have been described so far, but in all likelihood, this is an under-representation.

PPNAD occurs in a sporadic fashion, without additional clinical conditions, in approximately half of the cases. In the remaining patients, PPNAD is part of Carney's complex, an inherited association of myxomas, spotty pigmentation, and endocrine overactivity.[26] Sporadic and familial PPNAD present similar clinical and pathophysiologic features and, indeed, the same genetic alterations.[155,249]

PPNAD is associated with overt Cushing's syndrome in approximately 70% of cases, the remainder presenting subclinical Cushing's syndrome (i.e., biochemical parameters of adrenal autonomy/hyperfunction without clinical features of hypercortisolism) or latent Cushing's syndrome (no clinical or laboratory alteration but genetic trait present). Salient features of Cushing's syndrome due to PPNAD include its occurrence at a young age (i.e., pre- and postpubertal children in the second decade of life, the youngest patient being a 3-month-old infant), slow progression of features of hypercortisolism, and severe osteoporosis. The mildness, sluggishness, and possibly even cyclical development of Cushingoid features might contribute to the delay in diagnosis (approximately 4 years from the appearance of the first symptoms, against less than 2 years in other forms of Cushing's syndrome). As regards clinical features, osteopenia and stunted growth was the outstanding feature in several young children, whereas hirsutism and menstrual irregularity may be the only sign in young adolescent girls.[12,41] Patients with PPNAD are rarely obese, but skin and muscular atrophy are common. In one young woman, Cushing's syndrome due to PPNAD was diagnosed during pregnancy after vertebral collapse and detection of extensive osteoporosis.[250] In patients in whom PPNAD is part of Carney's complex, other signs of the disease are usually present

Table 7-4. Features of Carney's Complex

Primary Lesions	Affected Patients (%)
Myxomas	
Cardiac	60
Cutaneous	40
Breast	20
Mucocutaneous spotty pigmentation	70
Endocrine overactivity	
PPNAD (ACTH-independent Cushing's syndrome)	50
Testicular tumors (sexual precocity)	35
Pituitary mammosomatotroph tumors (acromegaly, gigantism)	10-15

Additional Lesions
Schwannoma (peripheral nerve root, gastrointestinal tract, skin)
Other multicentric myxomas (uterus, vagina, oral cavity, pharynx)
Thyroid lesions
Osteochondromyxoma
Breast ductal adenoma
Ovarian lesions
Café-au-lait spots
Junctional, compound, and atypical blue nevi

by the time hypercortisolism develops (Table 7-4), most notably pigmented spots and cardiac myxomas, and thus may aid in the diagnosis. However, given the clinical heterogeneity of the complex, all cases of PPNAD should be assumed familial until accurate examination of first-degree relatives excludes Carney's complex.

Diagnosis of Cushing's syndrome due to PPNAD may follow different strategies, depending on the sporadic or familial nature of the disease. In the former, adrenal Cushing's syndrome is suspected in a patient without prior knowledge of Carney's complex and thus requires the differential diagnosis from other forms of adrenal hypercortisolism. Conversely, if the patient or his/her relatives are known to be affected by Carney's complex, then the diagnosis will be aimed at establishing the existence of overt hypercortisolism. In this context, it should be recalled that subclinical or latent hypercortisolism are most probably present in the vast majority of patients with Carney's complex, as attested by typical adrenal lesions, as well as Crooke's hyaline change revealed at autopsy in asymptomatic patients.[12] Further, subtle alterations of cortisol circadian rhythmicity and/or suppressibility by dexamethasone may be encountered in older patients with Carney's complex who did not develop Cushing's syndrome or in first-degree relatives.[12,251]

Patients with Cushing's disease due to PPNAD do not always present suppressed plasma ACTH levels; indeed, low-normal ACTH levels have been reported in several series,[37,41,76] possibly a consequence of the mildness of hypercortisolism (see heading Diagnosis). However, no hormonal response to CRH stimulation was observed.[12] Administration of 8 mg dexamethasone for 2 days is followed by a paradoxical doubling of UFC levels in approximately half of patients with PPNAD,[37] and this may provide useful adjunctive information (see heading Differential Diagnosis of Adrenal Causes of Cushing's Syndrome). CT scan (and possibly adrenal scintigraphy) should be performed in these patients.

PATHOGENESIS

The initial pathogenic hypothesis for PPNAD was based upon the finding of adrenal-stimulating antibodies in sera of patients

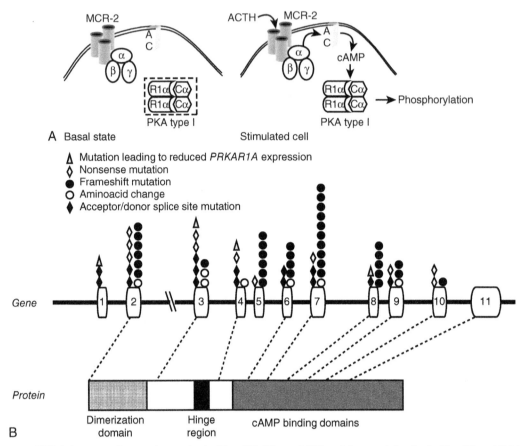

FIGURE 7-15. **A,** Structure of PKA holoenzyme. Four regulatory subunits (RIα, RIβ, R2α, and R2β) and three catalytic subunits (Cα, Cβ, and Cγ) have been identified so far. In the resting state, the PKA holoenzyme tetramer consists of four subunits: two homodimers of regulatory and catalytic subunits. Upon interaction of the receptor with its ligand, the Gα subunit dissociates and activates adenylate cyclase (AC). In turn, cAMP binds to regulatory subunits of PKA enabling dissociation of catalytic subunits which can phosphorylate cytoplasmic and nuclear proteins. Interaction with other intracellular pathways and gene transcription ensues. **B,** Structure of the *PRKAR1A* gene and protein. Mutations identified so far are shown. Of note, gene structure has been revised and exons renumbered starting with exon 4B. See Table 7-5 for list of mutations.

with PPNAD.[92,252] These studies revealed that DNA synthesis, adrenal growth, and cortisol release can be stimulated by circulating immunoglobulins present in patients with PPNAD.[92,110,252] Stimulating immunoglobulins were present independent of the presence of hypercortisolism, suggesting that these antibodies contribute but are not the sole mediator of increased adrenal activity.[252] No additional autoantibodies were detected in sera of affected patients, underlining the specificity of the phenomenon. However, adrenal-stimulating antibodies are not an invariable finding in patients with PPNAD.[253] Studies on resected adrenals showed that nodules present intense immunostaining for steroidogenic enzymes and secrete cortisol in normal amounts.[163,254] Steroidogenesis appears to be extremely sensitive to inhibition by ketoconazole in vitro[254] and increases paradoxically during incubation with dexamethasone.[255] This increase, which may occur also in adrenal adenomas (see earlier) and most likely accounts for the paradoxical responsiveness to high-dose dexamethasone in vivo, has been attributed to the intense expression of the glucocorticoid receptor.[255]

The advent of molecular biology shifted the focus to chromosomal and genetic alterations, leading to the identification of specific chromosomal loci and the first causative genetic alteration. Linkage studies revealed strong LOD scores (≥5.9) for a 6.4 cM region on the short arm of chromosome 2[253] and a 17 cM locus on the long arm of chromosome 17.[256] In keeping with the genetic heterogeneity of Carney's complex, some kindreds map to both loci and others do not segregate to either, thus further sites remain to be identified. The region on chromosome 2 is known to harbor genes involved in tumor suppression and cell-cycle progression, and both genetic losses and gains at 2p16 (Carney complex 2 locus, CNC2) have been reported, suggesting the presence of oncogenes which await definition.[257] Conversely, loss of heterozygosity at 17q22-24 hinted at a possible tumor-suppressor gene, narrowing the field of candidate genes and leading to the detection of mutations in the protein kinase A regulatory subunit 1 alpha (*PRKAR1A*) gene, a mediator involved in inhibition of cAMP signaling.[154,155] *PRKAR1A* spans 11 exons and gives rise to a 2890-bp mRNA species, which in turn is translated into a 381-amino-acid protein (Fig. 7-15B). Heterozygous germline mutations in *PRKAR1A* (Carney complex 1 locus, CNC1) have been detected so far in nearly half of known kindreds with Carney's complex as well as in patients with "sporadic" PPNAD.[155,249] Gene alterations are mostly nonsense point mutations or frameshift mutations with premature stop codons, more rarely large deletions, leading to null alleles due to nonsense-mediated degradation of mutant mRNA or to truncated proteins[154,155,258] (see Fig. 7-15B; Table 7-5). Indeed, the amount of PRKAR1A protein is nearly halved in lymphocytes from patients with Carney's complex compared to normal subjects, reflecting expression of the wild-type allele only.[154] More rarely, *PRKAR1A*

Table 7-5. *PRKAR1A* Mutations Associated With Carney's Complex*

	Current (Former) Nomenclature	Genomic Location	Effect of Mutation
Exon 1	3,876 bp deletion	g.3400-7877del3876	Decreased PKA expression
	12G>A	g.5512G>A	Additional ATG, could abolish translation
	102G>A	g.5580G>A	Activation cryptic splice site
Exon 2	IVS-2A>G	g.8424A>G	Splice acceptor mutation
	c.1A>G (88A>G)	g.8432A>G	Abolishes initiator ATG
	c.26G>A	g.8457G>A	S9N
	139delTG	g.8483delTG	Frameshift
	165insTAAC	g.8505insTAAC	Frameshift
	169C>T	g.8513C>T	Nonsense
	c.85del11 (172del11)	g.8516del11	Frameshift
	c.101_105delCTATT (188delCTATT)	g.8532delCTATT	Frameshift
	c.109C>T (196C>T)	g.8540C>T	Stop codon
	c.124C>T (211C>T)	g.8555C>T	Nonsense
	c.140delT	g.8571delT	Frameshift
	c.177+1G>A	g.8609G>A	Frameshift
Exon 3	4,165 bp deletion	g.12282-16447 del 4165	Exon 3 skipping
	c.178-2A>G	g.15786A>G	Reduced R1a expression
	c.178-348del171	g.15788del171	Exon 3 skipping
	c.187A>T (274A>T)	g.15797A>T	Nonsense
	c.220_21delCG	g.15830delCG	Frameshift
	307C>T	g.15830C>T	R74C
	c.286C>T	g.15896C>T	R96X
	376C>T	g.15899C>T	Nonsense
	IVS3+1G>C	g.15959G>C	Splice donor mutation
Exon 4	IVS3+1G>T	g.16756G>T	Splice acceptor mutation
	c.353_365del13	g.16761del13	Reduced R1a expression
	494delTG	g.16815delTG	Nonsense
	c.438A>T	g.16846A>T	R146S
	IVS4+1G>A	g.16849G>A	Exon skipping/frameshift
Exon 5	553delG	g.17073delG	Frameshift
	c.491_492delTG (578delTG or 576delTG)	g.17096delTG	Frameshift
	584C>T	g.17103C>T	Nonsense
	IVS5+1G>A	g.17110G>A	Frameshift
	c.502+1G>T	g.17110G>T	Frameshift
	IVS5+1insT	g.17110insT	Frameshift
	IVS5+3A>C	g.17112A>C	Splicing/frameshift
Exon 6	IVS6-17T>A	g.17927T>A	Frameshift
	IVS6del-9/-2	g.17934del7	Splice acceptor mutation
	IVS6del-7/-2	g.17936del5	Splice acceptor mutation
	615delGATT/insTATGATCAATC	g.17969delGATT/insTATGATCAATC	Frameshift
	618delTGAT	g.17971delTGAT	Frameshift
	632insC	g.17986insC	Frameshift
	c.547G>T	g.17988G>T	D183Y
Exon 7	642-1delGGTCTA	g.18785delGGTCA	In-frame splicing
	653AA>CAC	g.18802AA>CAC	Frameshift
	675insGG	g.18824insGG	Frameshift
	c.597delC	g.18833delC	Frameshift
	617delTTAT	g.18854delTTAT	Frameshift
	706delT	g.18855delT	Frameshift
	710delG	g.18859delG	Frameshift
	710insA	g.18859insA	Frameshift
	c.638C>A	g.18874C>A	A213D
	745delAA	g.18894delAA	Frameshift
	769C>T	g.18918C>T	Nonsense
	del774C	g.18923delC	Frameshift
	781insT	g.18930insT	Frameshift
	c.708+1G>T (IVS6+1G>T)	g.18945G>T	Exon 7 skipping
Exon 8	c.709-(5-107)del 103	g.20764del 103	Reduced R1a expression
	c.709(-7/-2)del6 (IVS7del -7/-2)	g.20865delTTTTTA	Exon 8 skipping
	799insAA	g.20875insAA	Frameshift
	810 ins A	g.20886 ins A	Frameshift
	c.728del13 (815 del13)	g.20891del13	Frameshift
	845delTC	g.20921delTC	Frameshift
	c.763delAT (850 delAT)	g.20926 delAT	Frameshift
	IVS8+5G>C	g.20937G>C	Splicing/frameshift
Exon 9	873GG>CT or 889GG>CT	g.21918GG>CT	Nonsense
	891insT	g.21936insT	Frameshift
	c.846insA (933insA)	g.21978insA	Frameshift
	c.865G>T	g.21997G>T	G289W
	c.891+3A>G (IVS8 +3A>G)	g.22026A>G	Activation cryptic splice site
Exon 10	997C>T	g.22970C>T	Nonsense
	1007C>G	g.22980C>G	Nonsense
	1038delA	g.23011delA	Frameshift
Exon 11	None described		

*Mutations are listed according to their past and present nomenclature when reported. Genomic location refers to the genomic *PRKAR1A* sequence (RefSeq NG_007093) and the corresponding amino acid sequence change given if known (codon 1 corresponds to translation initiation codon, RefSeq NP_002725).

mutated genes are transcribed and result in mutant or reduced amounts of protein.[259] The PRKAR1A protein is part of the protein kinase A holoenzyme, consisting in two regulatory and two catalytic subunits (see Fig. 7-15A). The tetramer is inactive and requires binding of cAMP to regulatory subunits for catalytic subunits to dissociate and phosphorylate target proteins which in turn will activate downstream events. The two regulatory subunits (R1 and R2) each present two isoforms, alpha and beta, with different tissue-specific patterns of expression. Activity of PKA is dependent upon the availability of free catalytic subunits as well as on the ratio of R1:R2 regulatory subunits, and R1-alpha appears crucial for protection against excessive catalytic activity.[260] In patients with Carney's complex, haploinsufficiency of PRKAR1A due to nonsense-mediated mRNA decay or presence of mutant PRKAR1A proteins, leads to increased basal/stimulated PKA activity in adrenal cells,[155,259,261] which in turn affects downstream signaling. The effects exerted by cAMP-stimulated PKA activity vary in different tissues, from growth promotion in pituitary and thyroid adenomas to differentiation of cardiac cells and inhibition of proliferation in Schwann cells. Of interest, PRKAR1A mutations appear to be more frequent in patients with Carney's complex who develop PPNAD,[261] and specific mutations have been shown to recur in patients with sporadic PPNAD.[262] However, there is no clear genotype-phenotype correlation, and other disease-modifying loci most likely contribute to the clinical presentation. In this context, deletions and amplifications of CNC2 at chromosome 2p16 have also been observed in patients with PRKAR1A mutations.[257]

Interestingly, somatic PRKAR1A mutations have been observed in patients with pigmented adrenal adenoma[139] but none in patients with classic macronodular adrenal hyperplasia.[140] Among other enzymes involved in the cAMP-signaling cascade, phosphodiesterase 11A has recently been linked to both bilateral adrenocortical hyperplasia and dysplasia, and available evidence suggests germline mutations in PDE11A are low-penetrance predisposing factors for these and other tumors.[263] Mutation of another phosphodiesterase, PDE8B, has been detected in a young girl with Cushing's syndrome due to micronodular adrenal hyperplasia.[264]

TREAMENT

Bilateral adrenalectomy is the treatment of choice for PPNAD, since both adrenals are affected. The risk of Nelson's syndrome is nonexistent; plasma ACTH levels may not even rise above the normal range after removal of the adrenal glands.[265] Patients with minimal hypercortisolism have occasionally been treated with unilateral adrenalectomy, and this has proven curative in some[12,77]; in others, however, removal of the remaining adrenal was necessary to contain hypercortisolism.[12,266] In patients submitted to removal of a single adrenal gland, subtle alterations of HPA function, such as disruption of cortisol circadian rhythm, may persist[26,41,267] and lead to progressive development of Cushingoid features over time.[267] Medical adrenalectomy has been obtained in a patient treated with o,p'DDD for some 3 years, followed by remission of hypercortisolism for over 12 years.[12] Brief treatments with low doses of adrenal blocking agents such as ketoconazole may prove beneficial prior to surgery. Spontaneous resolution has also been reported, most notably the first case described by Carney.[12,76]

Carney's Complex

Carney's complex is a hereditary disease with autosomal-dominant inheritance and incomplete penetrance (MIM 160980).

In 1985, some 40 years after the first description of familial PPNAD, Carney and colleagues assembled a series of patients presenting a constellation of rare tumors (see Table 7-4) unlikely to occur together by chance alone, and the term Carney's complex was coined. Various acronyms had been used in the past for patients presenting cardiac and cutaneous lesions (e.g., LAMB, for lentigines, atrial myxomas, blue nevi or NAME, for nevi, atrial myxomas, ephelides), but these terms have been abandoned. Given the significant variability in clinical presentation, the diagnosis of Carney's complex is presumptive if two features are present, definite when three or more occur. Rarely are more than five elements of the complex present. Supplemental criteria for the diagnosis of Carney's complex are an affected first-degree relative or presence of causative mutations, as of now only established for PRKAR1A.

Carney's complex can be likened to multiple endocrine neoplasia syndromes in that tumors arise in two or more endocrine organs. Endocrine and nonendocrine lesions are usually multicentric and affect both sides in paired organs (adrenals, gonads, breasts). It should be recalled that most lesions featured in Carney's complex are usually uncommon occurrences, thus multicentricity, bilateral involvement, recurrence, and (importantly) their presence in the same subject should increase suspicion as to the diagnosis. Other syndromes of multiple endocrine and nonendocrine organ lesions which share some similarity with Carney's complex are Peutz-Jeghers and MAS.

Endocrine Lesions

PPNAD is the most frequent endocrine disorder in Carney's complex, diagnosed in nearly 50% of patients affected by the complex.[12] In order of frequency, testicular tumors are the next most common, followed by pituitary, thyroid, and ovarian lesions.

Three different testicular tumors arising from Sertoli cells, Leydig cells, and adrenal remnants have been reported in patients with Carney's complex. The large-cell calcifying Sertoli cell tumor (LCCSCT) is the most common testicular lesion, arising in some 34% of male patients with Carney's complex.[268] LCCSCTs are usually detected at puberty as solid, calcified masses (5 to 10 mm in diameter), not palpable but easily visualized at sonography. These lesions are benign except for rare cases of malignant metastatic spread. LCCSCTs may also induce hormone-related symptoms such as gynecomastia, owing to the abundant expression of aromatase and increased estrogen production within the tumor. More rarely, the testes harbor steroid-type tumors such as the Leydig cell tumor, characterized by unencapsulated masses of large testosterone-secreting cells, or pigmented nodular adrenal rest tumors, arising close to the rete testis.[12] Testosterone secretion by the testicular tumor may induce sexual precocity. Orchiectomy is the treatment of choice for all testicular lesions in order to avoid hormone-related symptoms and malignant transformation.

Acromegaly and gigantism are part of the initial description made by Carney[26] but rarely occur in more than 10% of patients with the complex, although acromegaly was the leading manifestation of Carney's complex in one sibship.[269] Subclinical alterations of somatotroph function, such as elevated IGF-1 levels and insufficient GH inhibition by glucose, are present in many patients with Carney's complex[270] and have been observed to precede appearance of full-blown acromegaly by several years.[271] PPNAD is usually diagnosed prior to acromegaly; indeed, remission of hypercortisolism has been suggested to "unmask" the GH-secreting tumor.[272] Conversely, micro- and macroadenomas are found in equal proportion, and pathologic specimens may present adenohypophyseal hyperplasia, well-defined adenomas, or multicentric tumors.[269,270] Immunohistochemistry may reveal both GH and prolactin immunoreactivity, thus pointing to mammosomatotroph cells in some patients.[270,271] In this context, prolactin levels may also be increased in patients with Carney's complex, without additional signs of pituitary hyperfunction.[270,273]

Thyroid lesions in patients with Carney's complex range from hyperplasia to carcinoma and Hürthle cell tumor. Although published series are small, given the rarity of the complex, and intensive investigation of affected subjects may lead to an over-representation of these lesions, roughly 1 out of 10 patients with Carney's complex will present thyroid gland abnormalities.[274] These lesions are mostly benign nodules, but malignant follicular or papillary thyroid cancer has been described in a few patients, justifying screening with sonography.

Ovarian cysts were present in two patients in the initial series reported by Carney,[26] and a later study reported the frequent detection of ovarian cysts in both prospective sonograms and autoptic studies.[275] Malignant ovarian lesions, such as endometrioid or mucinous adenocarcinoma, have been described in two patients.[275]

Nonendocrine Lesions

Myxomas may originate in the heart, the skin, and the breast. These mesenchymal tumors, ubiquitous and recurring, are one of the distinctive features of Carney's complex. Cardiac myxomas occurring within Carney's complex present several unique features, most notably the location, multicentricity, and young age of appearance. Myxomas may arise in any of the four cardiac chambers, not just the left atrium, the usual site for sporadic cardiac myxomas, and tend to recur repeatedly. Further, myxomas arise in young adults with Carney's complex, whereas sporadic tumors are most often diagnosed in middle-aged women.[276] Cardiac myxomas, together with metastatic disease, account for the significant excess mortality in patients with Carney's complex.[277] Myxoid fibroadenoma is the most typical breast lesion in patients with Carney's complex and may occur even in male patients.[26] These benign tumors present as bilateral, palpable masses and are usually asymptomatic. In patients presenting with breast myxoid lesions, solid intraductal tumors with features of ductal adenoma have also been detected. Both pathologic examination and mammary gland imaging may indicate malignancy, although none of the ductal adenomas described so far has exhibited malignant behavior.[278] Lastly, skin/mucosal myxomas usually occur in the oropharynx, the eyelids and ears, the trunk (especially around the nipples), the axilla, and the genital tract. Appearance of skin myxomas varies from small sessile papules to large pedunculated lesions.[26]

The so-called "spotty pigmentation" of patients with Carney's complex is due to the abundance of lentigines (increased melanocytes), ephelides (increased melanin production by normal numbers of melanocytes), and blue nevi (accumulation of spindle-shaped melanocytes in the dermis)[279] (Fig. 7-16). Less common are café-au-lait spots and junctional, atypical, or compound nevi. Pigmented lesions may be present at birth or develop shortly thereafter, intensify after puberty, and favor specific sites such as the centrofacial area, the labial border and the lips themselves, the conjunctiva and lachrymal caruncle, the external genitalia, and the anal region.[26] Pigmentations tend to fade with age.

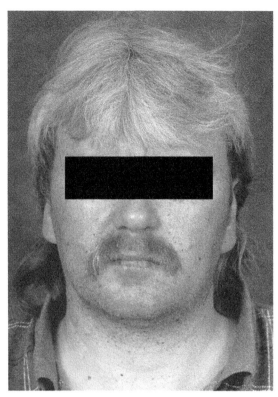

FIGURE 7-16. Patient with Carney's complex. Note multiple lentigines and black spots on the face and neck, in particular on the vermillion border of the lips. (Courtesy Dr. Aidan Carney, Mayo Clinic, Rochester, MN.)

Psammomatous melanotic schwannoma (PMS) is a peripheral nerve sheath tumor characterized by heavy melanin pigmentation and frequent psammoma bodies, features which occur only rarely outside of Carney's complex. PMS arises most frequently in lumbar nerve roots and in the gastrointestinal tract (esophagus, stomach), rarely in the skin, and may give rise to compressive symptoms. Multiple tumors are not uncommon, likewise local recurrences. Although usually benign, PMS may metastasize, most commonly to lung or liver[271] and occasionally represents the cause of death for patients with Carney's complex.[269] Tumors appear dark, circumscribed, with solid or spongy consistency, featuring polygonal epithelium-like cells and spindle cells organized in an organoid pattern with positive S-100 and vimentin staining. The basal lamina is prominent, as are melanosomes.[26] Melanotic cell death may lead to liquor coloring.

Osteochondromyxoma is a congenital mixed mesenchymal tumor of the bone. Pathologically, these lesions are circumscribed, erode surrounding bone and soft tissues, but do not appear to metastasize. Tumors are composed of immature and mature tissue, with cells disposed in solid sheets interspersed by abundant intercellular matrix and mesenchymal, cartilaginous, osseous, and hyaline fibrous tissue.[280] Exeresis of the lesion, when possible, is curative.

The following lesions have been reported in patients with Carney's complex, although whether they are true members of the complex remains to be ascertained: Fallot tetralogy, gastric adenocarcinoma, pilonidal sinus, retroperitoneal malignant fibrous histiocytoma, pheochromocytoma, acoustic neurinoma, maxillary rhabdomyosarcoma, rectal, mammary, ovarian and pancreatic carcinoma, fibrolamellar hepatocellular carcinoma, hepatocellular myxoid uterine leiomyoma, and superficial angiomyxoma.

As mentioned before, clinical presentation varies considerably, and patients usually present at most five features of the complex. Some features develop slowly or are associated with a reduced life expectancy, thus timely detection can provide considerable benefit. Screening procedures for patients and relatives of affected patients should encompass:

- Sequencing of affected *PRKAR1A* and, if no mutation is detected, large gene rearrangements should be excluded
- Cardiac, testes, and thyroid ultrasound
- If schwannomas are suspected, thoracic, abdominal, and pelvic CT scan
- Cortisol circadian rhythm and overnight suppression test (The paradoxical cortisol response to high-dose dexamethasone, while highly suggestive of PPNAD, does not provide absolute diagnostic certainty, and the test should be reserved for later stages in the diagnostic workup.)
- Baseline GH, IGF-1, and prolactin levels; if necessary, assessment of the GH response to a glucose load

Special Clinical Presentations

CHILDHOOD

Cushing's syndrome in children is most often due to adrenocortical neoplasms, with PPNAD and MAS accounting for a scattering of cases.[281] Adrenal cancer is an extremely rare pediatric malignancy (0.3 to 0.4 per million children per year) except for a population in southern Brazil, where this tumor is approximately 10 times more frequent than in the rest of the world (3.4 to 4.2 per million children per year).[282] Tumors arise mostly in preschool children (before 5 years of age) and present a slight female preponderance.[29,282] In contrast to adult adrenocortical tumors, over 80% of childhood adrenal tumors are functional, and cortisol hypersecretion is almost invariably accompanied by enhanced production of androgens and thus virilization. Functioning adrenocortical tumors have even been encountered at birth.[282] Children may present with temporal balding, acne, the appearance of pubic and axillary hair, precocious puberty, increased muscle mass, accelerated height, increased body weight (Fig. 7-17), moon facies, hypertension, and electrolyte imbalances.[29,282] Bone age is usually advanced except in those rare cases of "pure" Cushing's syndrome.[29] Detection of increased 17-ketosteroids or DHEAS is virtually diagnostic for adrenocortical tumor, and imaging procedures such as sonography, CT, or MRI easily reveal its presence.[29,282]

Pathologic classification of tumors on the basis of commonly used algorithms (i.e., Weiss, Hough, van Slooten) does not provide a clear distinction between benign and malignant lesions in childhood adrenal cancer.[283] Indeed, Weiss grade III or IV tumors exhibit an unusually benign course in children,[284] and tumor size, weight, and invasion of adjacent organs appear to be more predictive of malignant behavior than classic histologic features.[284,285] Postsurgical survival ranges between 56% and 70% at the 5-year landmark.[282,284] Treatment with o,p'DDD has been carried out in several children, albeit with significant neurologic side effects and high risk of adrenal insufficiency, whereas reports on efficacy of chemotherapeutic regimens are few.[281,285]

PPNAD and MAS, the other possible causes of hypercortisolism in childhood and adolescence, are usually readily apparent because of the presence of associated features (see specific sections). Bilateral adrenalectomy provides ready relief from symptoms and usually allows catch-up growth.[286]

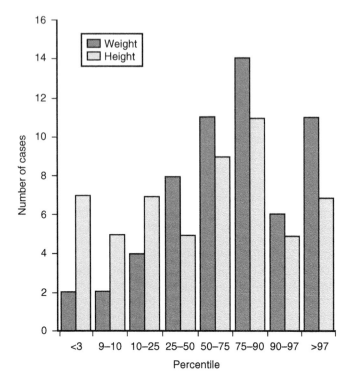

FIGURE 7-17. Distribution of weight and height in 58 children with adrenocortical tumors. (From Sandrini R, Ribeiro RC, de Lacerda L: Childhood adrenocortical tumors, J Clin Endocrinol Metab 82:2028, 1997. © Endocrine Society.)

PREGNANCY

Cushing's syndrome is often associated with oligomenorrhea and anovulation, thus pregnancy very rarely occurs in hypercortisolemic women. However, several cases have been reported with considerable maternal morbidity and high fetal wastage, so prompt diagnosis and correction of hypercortisolism are therefore necessary. Urinary free cortisol is usually clearly elevated in pregnant hypercortisolemic women, and there is little risk of overlap with physiologically increased UFC levels during gestation.[287] By contrast, cortisol suppression after low-dose dexamethasone is impaired during normal pregnancy, and cutoffs for diagnosis of Cushing's syndrome have to be adapted.[81,287] Establishment of the cause of hypercortisolism follows usual procedures, with ACTH levels normally suppressed in adrenal Cushing's syndrome and imaging procedures (sonography or MR) usually enabling visualization of the adrenal lesion.[288] Both malignant and benign lesions, the latter including also AIMAH and PPNAD, have been reported during pregnancy, thus none can be excluded a priori. Interestingly, among patients with Cushing's syndrome diagnosed during gestation, adrenal causes account for over half of reported cases, which is considerably more than in the nonpregnant state.[81] In some cases, cortisol levels increased after βhCG administration, and hypercortisolism resolved spontaneously after delivery,[35,36] suggesting the involvement of aberrant LH/hCG receptors (see heading ACTH-Independent Adrenal Hyperplasia). To what extent these receptors account for the increased frequency of adrenal adenoma and hyperplasia during pregnancy remains to be established. Treatment of hypercortisolism during pregnancy is diversified according to the stage of gestation, with surgical removal of the adrenal lesion preferred during the first half of pregnancy and medical treatment with ketoconazole in the last trimester, although the converse approach also yielded favorable outcome.[289]

Treatment of Adrenal Cushing's Syndrome

Treatment of adrenal Cushing's syndrome has two objectives: removal of the adrenal lesion and containment of hypercortisolism. Adrenal surgery meets both requirements in cortisol-secreting adenomas, PPNAD, and adrenal hyperplasia but is most often only partially resolutive in adrenal cancer. On the other hand, medical therapy is aimed at containing excess cortisol secretion or tumoral progression.

SURGERY

Surgery is straightforward and usually curative in benign adrenal causes of Cushing's syndrome (i.e., adenoma, PPNAD, and AIMAH). Conversely, malignant lesions require extensive resection of the lesion without, however, guaranteeing cure.

Removal of the adrenal adenoma is followed by remission of hypercortisolism, and long-term survival becomes comparable to that of the general population.[104,290] Exceptionally, Cushing's syndrome may recur due to bilateral or ectopic adrenal adenomas[290,291] or, as has also been reported, development of adrenal carcinoma on the same site of a previously resected adrenal adenoma.[117] Alternative surgical approaches, such as percutaneous acetic acid injection, radiofrequency ablation, adrenal arterial embolization, and adrenal-preserving minimally invasive surgery have been attempted with variable success in cortisol-secreting adenomas.[292-295] The drawback of these procedures is the absence of specimens for pathology, thus the preoperative diagnosis has to be certain.

In adrenal cancer, surgery is part of a multimodal approach also comprising chemotherapy and adrenolytic drugs. Only complete resection of the tumor offers potential for cure, although recurrence is not infrequent, sometimes after decades. On the whole, outcome is not encouraging, with less than 40% survival at the 5-year landmark[25] without significant differences between functional and nonfunctional adrenal carcinomas. In hypersecreting malignant tumors, steroid hormone levels (e.g., DHEAS, UFC, estrogen, and 11-deoxycortisol) and plasma ACTH concentrations can be used as markers for residual disease and recurrence. For a detailed discussion of this topic, the reader is referred to Chapter 11.

Surgical procedures evolved from open surgery, via epigastric or subcostal transabdominal access or posterior lumbar extraperitoneal approach, to modern laparoscopic techniques, with a decrease in perioperative morbidity and mortality.[296] This is nowadays the procedure of choice for removal of benign lesions in one or both adrenal glands, except for patients with coagulopathies, previous local surgery, or huge hyperplastic adrenals which necessitate long surgical procedures[296,297] (see also Chapter 15). Adrenal cancer should be operated via laparoscopy only if this ensures wide margin resection of the tumor; most surgeons still prefer transabdominal access because this allows maximal exposure of the tumor and affected organs or vessels, in particular to tumor thrombi in the inferior vena cava, and minimizes the chance of tumor spillage.

Removal of the hyperfunctioning adrenal tissue is followed by a 1- to 2-year period of adrenal insufficiency due to pituitary-mediated inhibition of the normal adrenal gland.[298,299] Steroid replacement therapy has to be administered (hydrocortisone 15 to 25 mg, two or three daily doses) and tapered over time according to recovery of the HPA axis. The latter, as well as the adequacy of steroid dosage, are largely established by clinical assessment rather than biochemical parameters.[300] These include morning serum cortisol concentrations (levels greater than 10 µg/dL) or cortisol response to exogenous ACTH (peak response ≥20 µg/dL). Interestingly, several patients have been reported in whom the HPA axis never fully recovered and replacement therapy could not be discontinued.[16]

Bilateral adrenalectomy is the treatment of choice for AIMAH and PPNAD, with few exceptions (see related sections). Removal of the adrenal glands is easily performed using laparoscopy in PPNAD, whereas open surgery may be required if glands are extremely big in patients with AIMAH.[182,266] Obviously, patients have to be started on lifelong steroid replacement therapy immediately after surgery, and usual precautions for adrenal insufficiency (see Chapter 6) are strenuously recommended; inappropriate treatment of adrenal crisis contributes significantly to mortality in these patients.

MEDICAL THERAPY

Drugs used for containment of hypercortisolism may be classed into three groups: adrenolytic, adrenostatic, and glucocorticoid receptor antagonists. Adrenolytic drugs—that is, compounds that destroy adrenocortical cells in addition to restraining steroid synthesis—are used mainly in adrenocortical cancer, whereas drugs that interfere with steroidogenesis without damaging adrenal cells (i.e., adrenostatic) can be used in any etiology of Cushing's syndrome and also in pituitary-driven or ectopic ACTH-driven hypercortisolism. Lastly, the progesterone and glucocorticoid receptor antagonist mifepristone (RU486) has been employed to relieve symptoms related to severe hypercortisolism in a scattering of cases but has never entered mainstream antiglucocorticoid therapy. The effect of these drugs is not always predictable, thus expert handling, with close monitoring of efficacy and side effects, is necessary.[301] On balance, metyrapone and ketoconazole are the drugs of choice for the medical containment of hypercortisolism, whereas other adrenostatic compounds are little used except for intravenous etomidate in severe Cushing's syndrome. Mitotane (o,p'DDD) is indicated in adrenal cancer.

Medical therapy for illicit receptor–driven hypercortisolism has been discussed previously (see heading ACTH-Independent Adrenal Hyperplasia). On the whole, the use of specific receptor antagonists—while theoretically the most rational approach—is limited by its incomplete efficacy and the ease and feasibility of adrenalectomy. It may be employed in patients with mild hypercortisolism or after unilateral adrenalectomy to delay restrictions imposed by surgical adrenal insufficiency.

Chemotherapy, usually together with mitotane, is used in advanced-stage adrenal cancer, but experience is still limited.[23,25] This and other topics related to oncologic aspects of adrenal cancer are discussed in Chapter 11.

Adrenolytic Drugs

Mitotane

Mitotane, 1,1-(dichlorodiphenyl)-2,2-dichloroethane; o,p'-DDD, derives from the organochloride insecticide DDT (dichlorodiphenyl-trichloroethane) and was first proven to induce adrenal cortical atrophy in 1949 and employed in adrenal cancer some 10 years later. Since then, scores of patients with functioning and nonfunctioning adrenocortical cancer have been treated with this compound, but its efficacy in stalling tumoral progression is unpredictable and often temporary.

Mitotane is a lipophilic compound that requires mitochondrial conversion into its active metabolites, o,p'-dichloroethene (o,p'-DDE) and o,p'-acetic acid (o,p'-DDA). Several facets of mitotane action have been defined, although the exact intracellular mechanisms have yet to be fully elucidated. The most significant action of mitotane is the inhibition of the first step in steroidogenesis, that is, conversion of cholesterol to pregnenolone, with inhibition of 11β-hydroxylase, 18-hydroxylase, and 3β-hydroxysteroid dehydrogenase occurring to a lesser extent.[302] Mitotane also interferes with cortisol metabolism, favoring 6β-hydroxylation over 5β-reduction and accelerating hepatic steroid metabolism.[303] At the same time, mitotane increases the synthesis of several hormone-binding proteins, most notably cortisol-binding globulin, sex hormone–binding globulin, and to a lesser extent thyroxin-binding globulin and vitamin D–binding globulin. The adrenolytic effect is achieved through several mechanisms, specifically, perturbation of lipid microenvironment with lipid accumulation, mitochondrial swelling and lysis, interference with ATPase activity and mitochondrial electron transport, superoxide formation, and covalent binding to proteins. Adrenal cell death occurs in the zonae fasciculata and reticularis as well as in metastases, with relative sparing of the zona glomerulosa. Mitotane also reverses the expression of the chemotherapy resistance gene, P-glycoprotein (*Pgp*), and enhances the efficacy of cytotoxic drugs in vitro.[304] This effect, however, does not appear to translate into greater efficacy of cytotoxic regimens in vivo, and new mitotane analogues with greater suppression of adrenal cell growth and secretion are currently being developed.

Clinical Use. Treatment with mitotane is initiated with 0.5 to 2 g daily and the dosage increased by 1 g every 4 weeks up to maximal daily doses of 4 to 12 g. Given its lipophilic properties, the drug accumulates in adipose tissue and may be discharged up to 2 years after discontinuation.[305] Mitotane has been used in children[282,285] but is contraindicated during pregnancy, owing to its teratogenic effects.[305] The efficacy of mitotane in patients with either functioning or nonfunctioning adrenal cancer is actively debated, with some studies reporting objective tumor regression and lower recurrence rates,[11,306] while others were not equally successful.[7,25] Recent large studies provided new data demonstrating that administration of mitotane after surgery significantly prolonged relapse-free survival in patients with adrenal cancer.[307,308] Serum mitotane levels should reach 14 μg/mL to achieve satisfactory response rates.[309] Once these levels have been reached, usually 3 to 4 months after treatment with increasing doses, mitotane can be tapered down to avoid adverse effects. Combined mitotane-chemotherapy regimens have also been attempted in patients with advanced-stage adrenal cancer and will possibly be validated through prospective, randomized trials.[310] Lastly, in individual patients, long-term treatment (up to 16 years) with low doses of mitotane has proven capable of controlling metastatic disease.[311]

Mitotane controls endocrine hypersecretion in the majority of patients.[25] UFC levels, and in the long run also plasma ACTH, represent the best parameters to monitor the efficacy of mitotane treatment, since secretion of 17-hydroxysteroids is selectively reduced, and serum cortisol may be factitiously increased due to higher CBG levels.

Adverse Effects. Untoward effects represent the main limitation to mitotane administration. Gastrointestinal distress (e.g., diarrhea, nausea, vomiting) may be counteracted by serotonin antagonists and administration at bedtime or meals. Neurologic toxicity symptoms (e.g., dizziness, lethargy, vertigo, speech disturbances, ataxia) usually accompany higher-dosage regimens.[309]

Optic nerve toxicity may result in complete blindness. Additional side effects are fatigue, gynecomastia, skin rashes, and hypoadrenalism. Iatrogenic adrenal insufficiency is counteracted by hydrocortisone and prednisone rather than dexamethasone administration, because the latter is metabolized at a greater rate by the hepatic microsomal machinery.[303] As with adrenostatic compounds, concomitant administration of drugs such as rifampicin, warfarin, and phenytoin, which induce hepatic enzymes, thereby enhancing steroid metabolism, may require upscaling of steroid replacement dosage. Mineralocorticoid insufficiency may occur with long-term mitotane administration. Clinical chemistry evaluation usually reveals increased gamma glutamyl transferase, alkaline phosphatase, aminotransferases (rarely serious enough to require drug withdrawal), hyperlipidemia, hypouricemia, and reduced blood cell counts. Free and total thyroid hormone levels may decrease, but thyrotropin remains within the normal range. Symptomatic hypotestosteronemia requiring replacement therapy may ensue in male patients.[11,312] Most side effects benefit from brief reduction or interruption of mitotane with a simultaneous increase in steroid replacement therapy.

Other anticancer compounds with antiproliferative or adrenolytic effects have been studied, such as gossypol, suramin, octreotide, taxol, paclitaxel, lonidamide, tegafur, and gemcitabine, but none can be recommended for clinical use as yet.

Adrenostatic Drugs

These compounds reduce cortisol secretion by interfering with one or more steps of steroid synthesis (Fig. 7-18). With the exception of ketoconazole, all compounds of this class induce a compensatory ACTH increase which may partially override pharmacologic blockade. Higher drug doses are therefore necessary over time to maintain eucortisolism. If blockade of cortisol synthesis is complete, steroid replacement therapy is required to avoid symptoms of adrenal insufficiency.

In patients with adrenal Cushing's syndrome, steroid synthesis inhibitors are usually employed awaiting surgery or as palliative therapy in adrenal cancer. Amelioration of hypercortisolism may be necessary to stabilize the patient prior to surgery.

Ketoconazole

Since it was discovered that this imidazole derivative, most commonly used as an antimycotic agent, inhibits cytochrome P450 enzymes, ketoconazole has taken center stage in the medical therapy of Cushing's syndrome.[313] Indeed, given its greater tolerability and ease of use, ketoconazole is the most widely used drug to control hypercortisolism.[301,314]

Ketoconazole inhibits several steps of steroidogenesis: in order of potency, the side-chain cleavage complex, 17,20-lyase, 17α-hydroxylase, and 11β-hydroxylase.[315] Ketoconazole also interferes with ACTH-induced cAMP production and is a weak competitor for the glucocorticoid receptor. The inhibition of progestins to androgens conversion by blockade of 17,20-lyase explains the pronounced reduction of DHEA and androstenedione secretion.

Clinical Use. Ketoconazole is usually administered starting with 200 mg daily and progressively increasing to 600 to 800 mg according to adrenal secretory parameters. Higher doses, up to 1200 mg daily, are rarely required. Cimetidine and other antacids interfere with gastric absorption of ketoconazole and thus should not be used together. Ketoconazole reduces UFC levels in patients with adrenal adenoma but is possibly less effective in adrenal carcinoma.[315] Ketoconazole has also been reported to exert cytostatic effects in patients with secreting metastatic adre-

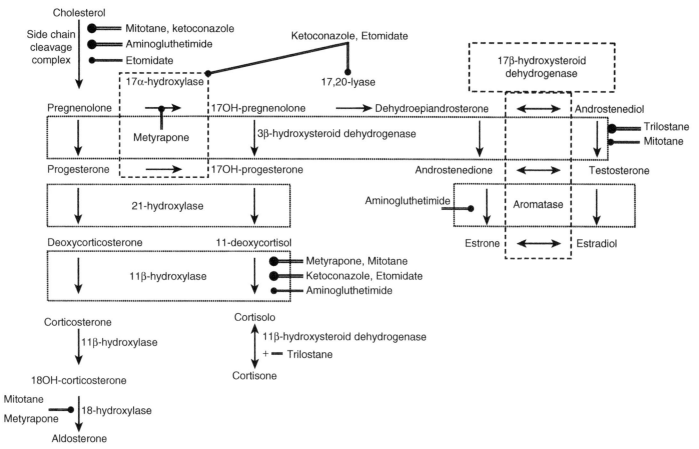

FIGURE 7-18. Blockade of steroidogenic enzymes by adrenolytic and adrenostatic compounds. Sites of major (●━━) and minor (●━) inhibitory as well as stimulatory (+ ━) actions are shown.

nocortical cancer.[316] Of note, notwithstanding the considerable size of the adrenals, low doses of ketoconazole are usually sufficient to obtain eucortisolism in patients with AIMAH. Ketoconazole may safely be used in children and during pregnancy.

Adverse Effects. Ketoconazole is usually well tolerated, with only a minority of patients (less than 5%) reporting adverse effects. These are mostly gastrointestinal (e.g., nausea, vomiting) or dermatologic (e.g., skin rash, pruritus) and disappear after drug suspension. Gynecomastia and impotence, most likely due to reduced androgen synthesis, have occasionally been reported. Hepatic dysfunction (cholestasis, hepatocellular injury) occurs in some 10% of patients treated with ketoconazole and typically resolves after drug discontinuation. If the increase in hepatic transaminases is modest (i.e., less than threefold increase over normal), ketoconazole may be continued with close monitoring of hepatic function. Fatal hepatitis is an exceptional occurrence. Similarly, liver metastases do not preclude the use of ketoconazole in adrenal cancer. Lastly, administration of ketoconazole at appropriate dosage does not necessitate adjunctive steroid replacement therapy.

Another nitroimidazole derivate, fluconazole, has recently been employed in a patient with cortisol-secreting adrenal cancer and achieved normalization of UFC and amelioration of symptoms for nearly 2 years.[317]

Metyrapone

This pyridine derivate—2-methyl-1,2-bis-(3-pyridyl)-1-propanone; SU-4885—inhibits 11β hydroxylase, the enzyme respon-

sible for the final step in cortisol biosynthesis and, to a lesser extent, also 18-, 19-, and 17α-hydroxylases.[318] In addition, metyrapone has been shown to suppress adrenal expression of the ACTH receptor MC2R.[319] Metyrapone is used in both diagnosis and treatment of Cushing's syndrome, although more accurate testing procedures have superseded its use in the former setting (see heading Diagnosis of Adrenal Cushing's Syndrome). Metyrapone is usually administered together with other steroid synthesis inhibitors in patients with malignant lesions. Although efficacious, this compound is not universally available, which limits its use.

Clinical Use. Metyrapone is administered in dosages ranging from 500 mg to 6 g daily, subdivided in three or four doses. Cortisol levels decrease promptly; indeed, one advantage of metyrapone treatment is its rapid cortisol-lowering effect (within 2 hours).[320] Most patients with adrenal lesions respond well as regards both clinical signs and UFC concentrations.[321] Hypoadrenalism may occur, and patients should be started on prednisone replacement. Additional side effects are worsening of hirsutism, acne, hypokalemia, and hypertension secondary to the increase in androgen and mineralocorticoids, as well as rash, nausea, and dizziness. The use of metyrapone in pregnancy is debated, with some reports describing amelioration of hypercortisolism without adverse fetal effects[36] and others reporting worsening of hypertension and preeclampsia.[322] Lastly, administration of metyrapone, together with aminoglutethimide, for 18 months obtained lasting normalization of HPA parameters and disappearance of Cushingoid features in an infant with MAS.[323]

Aminoglutethimide

Aminoglutethimide is an anticonvulsant drug which exerts a potent inhibitory action of P450 side chain–cleavage enzyme. Less relevant is its action on other P450 steroidogenic enzymes, on aromatase, and on the adrenal ACTH receptor.[319] Aminoglutethimide also exerts an antiproliferative effect on adrenocortical cells in vitro.[319]

Clinical Use. Successful palliation of hypercortisolism has been reported in over 60% of patients with adrenal carcinoma treated with aminoglutethimide.[324] Starting dose is 250 mg daily, with progressive increases up to 1 to 2 g daily.[324] Side effects include mild sedation, itchy rash, goiter, and upper gastrointestinal discomfort which may disappear spontaneously during treatment. Hypoadrenalism should be corrected with hydrocortisone rather than dexamethasone, because hepatic clearance of the latter is accelerated. Hypothyroidism may develop due to inhibition of thyroid hormone synthesis.

Trilostane

This androstane-carbonitrile derivative (WIN 24,540) selectively inhibits 3β-hydroxysteroid dehydrogenase and potentiates 11β-hydroxysteroid dehydrogenase type 2, thus yielding increased cortisone:cortisol ratios. Clinical efficacy in containing hypercortisolism is weak, even at high doses up to 1400 mg daily,[44] and is accompanied by gastrointestinal side effects. Hypoadrenalism may ensue.

Etomidate

Etomidate is a short-acting hypnotic drug only effective when administered intravenously. This imidazole derivative potently inhibits 11β-hydroxylase and, to a lesser extent, also 17α-hydroxylase, 17,20-lyase, and side chain–cleavage enzymes.[315] In addition, etomidate markedly inhibits adrenocortical cell proliferation and expression of the ACTH receptor.[319] In vitro, etomidate is the most potent adrenostatic compound compared with other agents.[315,319] It has been used successfully to reduce hypercortisolism in severely ill patients who are unresponsive or unable to ingest oral medications, and this is most likely the only indication for this compound,[301] since sedation often occurs even when infused at nonhypnotic doses (1.2 to 2.5 mg/h). Adrenal insufficiency invariably occurs on etomidate therapy, thus replacement with dexamethasone or hydrocortisone is mandatory.

Glucocorticoid Receptor Antagonist

Mifepristone (RU486)

RU486 is a steroid analogue [17β-hydroxy, 11β-(4-dimethylaminophenyl), 17α-(1-propynyl)-estra-4,9-diene-3-one] that competitively antagonizes binding to glucocorticoid and progesterone receptors and blocks steroid-induced peripheral effects. Administration of RU486 to small series of patients with Cushing's syndrome induced a reversal of clinical manifestations of hypercortisolism, most notably acute psychosis.[325] Dosage of RU486 is usually 5 to 25 mg/kg or 400 to 800 mg daily, with close monitoring to avoid adrenal insufficiency. Detection of the latter rests on indirect biochemical and clinical parameters such as hypoglycemia, hyperkalemia, and nausea, because cortisol levels remain elevated. The absence of a marker of peripheral glucocorticoid activity, the long half-life of the drug, and the difficulty in counteracting its antiglucocorticoid activity all hinder the clinical use of this compound.

REFERENCES

1. Osler W: An acute myxoedematous condition, with tachycardia, glycosuria, melena, mania, and death, J Nerv Ment Dis 26:65–71, 1899.
2. Cushing H: The basophil adenomas of the pituitary body and their clinical manifestations, Johns Hopkins Bull 50:137–195, 1932.
3. Walters W, Wilder RM, Kepler EJ: The suprarenal cortical syndrome with presentation of ten cases, Ann Surg 100:670–688, 1934.
4. Carpenter PC: Diagnostic evaluation of Cushing's syndrome, Endocrinol Metab Clin North Am 17:445–472, 1988.
5. Lindholm J, Juul S, Jørgensen JOL, et al: Incidence and late prognosis of Cushing's syndrome: a population-based study, J Clin Endocrinol Metab 86:117–123, 2001.
6. Demura H, Takeda R, Miyamori I, et al: Cushing's syndrome in Japan with special reference to adrenocortical nodular dysplasia or hyperplasia. In Takeda R, Miyamori I, editors: Controversies in Disorders of Adrenal Hormones: Proceedings of the Open Symposium of Disorders of Adrenal Hormones, New York, 1988, Elsevier Science, pp 3–17.
7. Bertagna X, Orth DN: Clinical and laboratory findings and results of therapy in 58 patients with adrenocortical tumors admitted to a single medical center (1951 to 1978), Am J Med 71:855–875, 1981.
8. Hsing AW, Nam JM, Co Chien HT, et al: Risk factors for adrenal cancer: an exploratory study, Int J Cancer 65:432–436, 1996.
9. National Cancer Institute: Third National Cancer Survey: incidence data. In: Anonymous DHEW Publ. No. (NIH) 75–787, Bethesda, 1975, NCI Monograph, pp 41.
10. Crucitti F, Bellantone R, Ferrante A, et al: The Italian registry for adrenal cortical carcinoma: analysis of a multiinstitutional series of 129 patients, Surgery 119:161–170, 1996.
11. Luton JP, Cerdas S, Billaud L, et al: Clinical features of adrenocortical carcinoma, prognostic factors, and the effect of mitotane therapy, N Engl J Med 322:1195–1201, 1990.
12. Carney JA, Young WF Jr: Primary pigmented nodular adrenocortical disease and its associated conditions, Endocrinologist 2:6–21, 1992.
13. Lacroix A, N'Diaye N, Tremblay J, et al: Ectopic and abnormal hormone receptors in adrenal Cushing's syndrome, Endocrine Rev 22:75–110, 2001.
14. Lieberman SA, Eccleshall TR, Feldman D: ACTH-independent massive bilateral adrenal disease (AIMBAD): a subtype of Cushing's syndrome with major diagnostic and therapeutic implications, Eur J Endocrinol 131:67–73, 1994.
15. Perry RR, Nieman LK, Cutler GB Jr, et al: Primary adrenal causes of Cushing's syndrome, Ann Surg 210:59–68, 1989.
16. Daitsch JA, Goldfarb DA, Novick AC: Cleveland Clinic experience with adrenal Cushing's syndrome, J Urol 158:2051–2055, 1997.
17. Kirk JMW, Brain CE, Carson DJ, et al: Cushing's syndrome caused by nodular adrenal hyperplasia in children with McCune-Albright syndrome, J Pediatr 134:789–792, 1999.
18. Kasperlik-Zaluska AA, Migdalska BM, Zgliczynski S, et al: Adrenocortical carcinoma. A clinical study and treatment results of 52 patients, Cancer 75:2587–2591, 1995.
19. Rockall AG, Babar S, Sohaib SA, et al: CT and MR imaging of the adrenal glands in ACTH-independent Cushing's syndrome, RadioGraphics 24:435–452, 2004.
20. Tenschert W, Baumgart P, Greminger P, et al: Pathogenetic aspects of hypertension in Cushing's syndrome, Cardiology 72(Suppl 1):84–90, 1985.
21. Ross EJ, Linch DC: The clinical response to treatment in adult Cushing's syndrome following remission of hypercortisolaemia, Postgrad Med J 61:205–211, 1985.
22. Pikkarainen L, Sane T, Reunanen A: The survival and well-being of patients treated for Cushing's syndrome, J Intern Med 245:463–468, 1999.
23. Assié G, Antoni G, Tissier F, et al: Prognostic parameters of metastatic adrenocortical carcinoma, J Clin Endocrinol Metab 92:148–154, 2007.
24. Wajchenberg BL, Albergaria Pereira MA, Bilharinho de Mendonça B, et al: Adrenocortical carcinoma. Clinical and laboratory observations, Cancer 88:711–736, 2000.
25. Allolio B, Fassnacht M: Adrenocortical carcinoma: clinical update, J Clin Endocrinol Metab 91:2027–2037, 2006.
26. Carney JA, Gordon H, Carpenter PC, et al: The complex of myxomas, spotty pigmentation, and endocrine overactivity, Medicine 64:270–283, 1985.
27. Invitti C, Pecori Giraldi F, De Martin M, et al: Diagnosis and management of Cushing's syndrome: results of an Italian multicentre study, J Clin Endocrinol Metab 84:440–448, 1999.
28. O'Hare MJ, Monaghan P, Neville AM: The pathology of adrenocortical neoplasia: a correlated structural and functional approach to the diagnosis of malignant disease, Hum Pathol 10:137–154, 1979.
29. Bilharinho de Mendonça B, Lucon AM, Menezes CAV, et al: Clinical, hormonal and pathological findings in a comparative study of adrenocortical neoplasms in childhood and adulthood, J Urol 154:2004–2009, 1995.
30. Fukai N, Hirono Y, Yoshimoto T, et al: A case of estrogen-secreting adrenocortical carcinoma with subclinical Cushing's syndrome, Endocr J 53:237–246, 2006.
31. Adachi J, Hirai Y, Terui K, et al: A report of 7 cases of adrenal tumors secreting both cortisol and aldosterone, Intern Med 42:714–718, 2003.
32. Balakumar T, Perry LA, Savage MO: Adrenocortical adenoma—an unusual presentation with hypersecretion of oestradiol, androgens and cortisol, J Pediatr Endocrinol Metab 10:227–229, 1997.

33. Nieman LK, Biller BMK, Findling JW, et al: Diagnosis of Cushing's syndrome: an Endocrine Society Clinical Practice Guideline, J Clin Endocrinol Metab 93:1526–1540, 2008.

34. Pecori Giraldi F, Ambrogio AG, De Martin M, et al: Specificity of first-line tests for the diagnosis of Cushing's syndrome: assessment in a large series, J Clin Endocrinol Metab 92:4123–4129, 2007.

35. Lacroix A, Hamet P, Boutin J: Leuprolide acetate therapy in luteinizing hormone-dependent Cushing's syndrome, N Engl J Med 341:1577–1581, 1999.

36. Hána V, Dokoupilová M, Marek J, et al: Recurrent ACTH-independent Cushing's syndrome in multiple pregnancies and its treatment with metyrapone, Clin Endocrinol 54:277–281, 2001.

37. Stratakis CA, Sarlis NJ, Kirschner LS, et al: Paradoxical response to dexamethasone in the diagnosis of primary pigmented nodular adrenocortical disease, Ann Intern Med 131:585–591, 1999.

38. Lim LC, Tan LHC, Rajasoorya C: Unravelling the mystery in a case of persistent ACTH-independent Cushing's syndrome, Ann Acad Med Singapore 35:892–896, 2006.

39. Orth DN: Cushing's syndrome, N Engl J Med 332:791–803, 1995.

40. Klose M, Kofoed-Enevoldsen A, Østergaard Kristensen L: Single determination of plasma ACTH using an immunoradiometric assay with high detectability differentiates between ACTH-dependent and -independent Cushing's syndrome, Scand J Clin Lab Invest 62:33–38, 2002.

41. Ruder HJ, Loriaux DL, Lipsett MB: Severe osteopenia in young adults associated with Cushing's syndrome due to micronodular adrenal disease, J Clin Endocrinol Metab 39:1138–1147, 1974.

42. Tillman V, Mägi ML, Metsvaht T: Prenatal Cushing's syndrome secondary to nodular adrenocortical hyperplasia with unsuppressed plasma ACTH levels, J Pediatr Endocrinol Metab 18:1027–1031, 2005.

43. Law A, Hague WM, Daly JG, et al: Inappropriate ACTH concentrations in two patients with functioning adrenocortical carcinoma, Clin Endocrinol 29:53–62, 1988.

44. Komanicky P, Spark RF, Melby JC: Treatment of Cushing's syndrome with trilostane (WIN 24,540), an inhibitor of adrenal steroid biosynthesis, J Clin Endocrinol Metab 47:1042–1051, 1978.

45. Müller OA, Stalla GK, von Werder K: Corticotropin releasing factor: a new tool for the differential diagnosis of Cushing's syndrome, J Clin Endocrinol Metab 57:227–229, 1983.

46. Hensen J, Buhl M, Bähr V, et al: Endocrine activity of the "silent" adrenocortical adenoma is uncovered by response to corticotropin-releasing hormone, Klin Wochenschr 68:608–614, 1990.

47. Crapo L: Cushing's syndrome: a review of diagnostic tests, Metabolism 28:955–977, 1979.

48. Yamaji T, Ishibashi M, Sekihara H, et al: Serum dehydroepiandrosterone sulfate in Cushing's syndrome, J Clin Endocrinol Metab 59:1164–1168, 1984.

49. Terzolo M, Alì A, Osella G, et al: The value of dehydroepiandrosterone sulfate measurement in the differentiation between benign and malignant adrenal masses, Eur J Endocrinol 142:611–617, 2000.

50. Tóth M, Rácz K, Varga I, et al: Plasma dehydroepiandrosterone sulphate levels in patients with hyperfunctioning and non-hyperfunctioning adrenal tumors before and after adrenal surgery, Eur J Endocrinol 136:290–295, 1997.

51. Smals AGH, Kloppenborg PWC, Benraad TJ: Plasma testosterone profiles in Cushing's syndrome, J Clin Endocrinol Metab 45:240–245, 1977.

52. Doerr P, Pirke KM: Cortisol-induced suppression of plasma testosterone in normal adult males, J Clin Endocrinol Metab 43:622–629, 1976.

53. Levine AC, Mitty HA, Gabrilove JL: Steroid content of the peripheral and adrenal vein in Cushing's syndrome due to adrenocortical adenoma and carcinoma, J Urol 140:11–15, 1988.

54. Kikuchi E, Yanaihara H, Nakashima J, et al: Urinary steroid profile in adrenocortical tumors, Biomed & Pharmacother 54(Suppl 1):194–197, 2000.

55. Gröndal S, Erkisson B, Hagenas L, et al: Steroid profile in urine: a useful tool in the diagnosis and follow-up of adrenocortical carcinoma, Acta Endocrinol (Copenh) 122:656–663, 1990.

56. Kelly WF, Barnes AJ, Cassar J, et al: Cushing's syndrome due to adrenocortical carcinoma—a comprehensive clinical and biochemical study of patients treated by surgery and chemotherapy, Acta Endocrinol (Copenh) 91:303–318, 1979.

57. Homoki J, Holl R, Teller WM: Urinary steroid profiles in Cushing's syndrome and tumors of the adrenal cortex, Klin Wochenschr 65:719–726, 1987.

58. Haigh SE, Tevaarwerk JM: A rise in the glomerular filtration rate as the cause of a 'paradoxical' increase in urinary free cortisol during dexamethasone suppression in a patient with an adrenal adenoma: a case report, Clin Endocrinol 15:53–56, 1981.

59. Invitti C, Pecori Giraldi F, Cavagnini F, et al: Unusual association of adrenal angiosarcoma and Cushing's disease, Horm Res 56:124–129, 2001.

60. Barzon L, Sonino N, Fallo F, et al: Prevalence and natural history of adrenal incidentalomas, Eur J Endocrinol 149:273–285, 2003.

61. Mantero F, Terzolo M, Arnaldi G, et al: A survey on adrenal incidentaloma in Italy, J Clin Endocrinol Metab 85:637–644, 2000.

62. Tanabe A, Naruse M, Nishikawa T, et al: Autonomy of cortisol secretion in clinically silent adrenal incidentaloma, Horm Metab Res 33:444–450, 2001.

63. Tsagarakis S, Vassiliadi D, Thalassinos N: Endogenous subclinical hypercortisolism: diagnostic uncertainties and clinical implications, J Endocrinol Invest 29:471–482, 2006.

64. Bardet S, Rohmer V, Murat A, et al: ^{131}I-6β-Iodomethylnorcholesterol scintigraphy: an assessment of its role in the investigation of adrenocortical incidentalomas, Clin Endocrinol 44:587–596, 1996.

65. Reincke M, Niecke J, Krestin GP, et al: Preclinical Cushing's syndrome in adrenal "Incidentalomas": comparison with adrenal Cushing's syndrome, J Clin Endocrinol Metab 75:826–832, 1992.

66. Toniato A, Merante-Boschin I, Opocher G, et al: Surgical versus conservative management for subclinical Cushing syndrome in adrenal incidentalomas: a prospective randomized study, Ann Surg 249:388–391, 2009.

67. Reznek RH, Armstrong P: Imaging in endocrinology: The adrenal gland, Clin Endocrinol 40:561–576, 1994.

68. Goldman SM, Coelho RD, Freire Filho EdO, et al: Imaging procedures in adrenal pathology, Arq Bras Endocrinol Metab 48:592–611, 2004.

69. Bonnin A, Abecassis JP, Broussouloux C, et al: La place de l'examen tomodensitométrique dans l'exploration des surrénales, Ann Endocrinol (Paris) 49:332–336, 1988.

70. Korobkin M, Brodeur FJ, Francis IR, et al: CT time-attenuation washout curves of adrenal adenomas and nonadenomas, Am J Roentgenol 170:747–752, 1998.

71. Prince EA, Yoo DC, DeLellis RA, et al: CT and PET appearance of a pigmented "black" adrenal adenoma in a patient with lung cancer, Clin Radiol 62:1229–1231, 2007.

72. Newhouse JH, Heffess CS, Wagner BJ, et al: Large degenerated adrenal adenomas: radiologic-pathologic correlation, Radiology 210:385–391, 1999.

73. Kouriefs C, Mokbel K, Choy C: Is MRI more accurate than CT in estimating the real size of adrenal tumours? Eur J Surg Oncol 27:487–490, 2001.

74. Fig LM, Gross MD, Shapiro B, et al: Adrenal localization in the adrenocorticotropin hormone-independent Cushing syndrome, Ann Intern Med 109:547–553, 1988.

75. Dunnick NR, Schaner EG, Doppman JL, et al: Computed tomography in adrenal tumors, AJR 132:43–46, 1979.

76. Grant CS, Carney JA, Carpenter PC, et al: Primary pigmented nodular adrenocortical disease: diagnosis and management, Surgery 100:1178–1184, 1986.

77. Doppman JL, Travis W, Nieman LK, et al: Cushing syndrome due to primary pigmented nodular adrenocortical disease: findings at CT and MR imaging, Radiology 172:415–420, 1989.

78. Ilias I, Sahdev A, Reznek RH, et al: The optimal imaging of adrenal tumours: a comparison of different methods, Endocr Relat Cancer 14:587–599, 2007.

79. Lee MJ, Mayo-Smith WW, Hahn JA, et al: State-of-the-art MR imaging of the adrenal gland, Radio Graphics 14:1015–1029, 1994.

80. Outwater EK, Siegelman ES, Huang AB, et al: Adrenal masses: correlation between CT attenuation value and chemical shift ratio at MR imaging with in-phase and opposed-phase sequences, Radiology 200:749–752, 1996.

81. Polli N, Pecori Giraldi F, Cavagnini F: Cushing's syndrome in pregnancy, J Endocrinol Invest 26:1045–1050, 2003.

82. Sarkar SD, Cohen EL, Beierwaltes WH, et al: A new and superior adrenal imaging agent, ^{131}I-6β-iodomethyl-19-Nor-cholesterol (NP-59): evaluation in humans, J Clin Endocrinol Metab 45:353–362, 1977.

83. Gross MD, Shapiro B, Thrall JH, et al: The scintigraphic imaging of endocrine organs, Endocrine Rev 5:221–281, 1984.

84. Yoh T, Hosono M, Komeya Y, et al: Quantitative evaluation of norcholesterol scintigraphy, CT attenuation value, and chemical-shift MR imaging for characterizing adrenal adenomas, Ann Nucl Med 22:513–519, 2008.

85. Gross MD, Wong KK, Rubello D: Scintigraphic imaging of adrenal disease, Minerva Endocrinol 33:1–17, 2008.

86. Reschini E, Baldini M, Cantalamessa L: A black adrenocortical adenoma causing Cushing's syndrome not imaged by radiocholesterol scintigraphy, Eur J Nucl Med 17:185–187, 1990.

87. Barzon L, Zucchetta P, Boscaro M, et al: Scintigraphic patterns of adrenocortical carcinoma: morpho-functional correlates, Eur J Endocrinol 145:743–748, 2001.

88. Thorin-Savouré A, Tissier-Rible F, Guignat L, et al: Collision/composite tumors of the adrenal gland: a pitfall of scintigraphy imaging and hormone assays in the detection of adrenal metastasis, J Clin Endocrinol Metab 90:4924–4929, 2005.

89. Reschini E, Peracchi M: Uptake of ^{75}Se-selenocholesterol by an adrenal cortical carcinoma and its metastases, Eur J Nucl Med 9:291–293, 1984.

90. Lumachi F, Zucchetta P, Marzola MC, et al: Usefulness of CT scan, MRI and radiocholesterol scintigraphy for adrenal imaging in Cushing's syndrome, Nucl Med Commun 23:469–473, 2002.

91. Sels JP, Wouters RM, Lamers R, et al: Pitfall of the accessory spleen, Neth J Med 56:153–158, 2000.

92. Wulffraat NM, Drexhage HA, Wiersinga WM, et al: Immmunoglobulins of patients with Cushing's syndrome due to pigmented adrenocortical micronodular dysplasia stimulate in vitro steroidogenesis, J Clin Endocrinol Metab 66:301–307, 1988.

93. Yu KC, Alexander R, Ziessman HA, et al: Role of preoperative iodocholesterol scintiscanning in patients undergoing adrenalectomy for Cushing's syndrome, Surgery 118:981–987, 1995.

94. Garcia-Mayor RV, Perez Mendez L, Paramo C, et al: Primary adrenocortical nodular dysplasia presented as adrenal adenoma by functional scintigraphy, Clin Nucl Med 18:220–222, 1993.

95. Young WF Jr, du Plessis H, Thompson GB, et al: The clinical conundrum of corticotropin-independent autonomous cortisol secretion in patients with bilateral adrenal masses, World J Surg 32:856–862, 2007.

96. Becherer A, Vierhapper H, Potzi C, et al: FDG-PET in adrenocortical carcinoma, Cancer Biother Radiopharm 16:289–295, 2001.

97. Leboulleux S, Dromain C, Bonniaud G, et al: Diagnostic and prognostic value of 18-fluorodeoxyglucose positron emission tomography in adrenocortical carcinoma: a prospective comparison with computed tomography, J Clin Endocrinol Metab 91:920–925, 2006.

98. Han SJ, Kim TS, Jeon SW, et al: Analysis of adrenal masses by ^{18}F-FDG positron emission tomography scanning, Int J Clin Pract 61:802–809, 2007.

99. Hennings J, Lindhe Ö, Bergström M, et al: [^{11}C]Metomidate positron emission tomography of adrenocortical tumors in correlation with histopathological findings, J Clin Endocrinol Metab 91:1410–1414, 2006.

100. Aiba M, Hirayama A, Iri H, et al: Adrenocorticotropic hormone-independent bilateral adrenocortical macronodular hyperplasia as a distinct subtype of Cushing's syndrome, Am J Clin Pathol 96:334–340, 1991.

101. Saeger W, Reinhard K, Reinhard C: Hyperplastic and tumorous lesions of the adrenals in an unselected autopsy series, Endocr Pathol 9:235–239, 1998.

102. Sasano H, Suzuki T, Irie J, et al: Adrenal cortical disease: international case conference, Endocr Pathol 13:141–148, 2002.

103. Mackay B, El-Naggar A, Ordonez NG: Ultrastructure of adrenal cortical carcinoma, Ultrastruct Pathol 18:181–190, 1994.
104. Välimäki M, Pelkonen R, Porkka L, et al: Long-term results of adrenal surgery in patients with Cushing's syndrome due to adrenocortical adenoma, Clin Endocrinol 20:229–236, 1984.
105. Desai N, Kapoor A, Sing BK, et al: Bilateral adrenal adenomas and persistent leukocytosis: a unique case of Cushing's syndrome, Am J Med 119:e3-e5, 2006.
106. Aiba M, Kawakami M, Ito Y, et al: Bilateral adrenocortical adenomas causing Cushing's syndrome. Report of two cases with enzyme histochemical and ultrastructural studies and a review of the literature, Arch Pathol Lab Med 116:146–150, 1992.
107. N'Diaye N, Hamet P, Tremblay J, et al: Asynchronous development of bilateral nodular adrenal hyperplasia in gastric inhibitory polypeptide-dependent Cushing's syndrome? J Clin Endocrinol Metab 84:2616–2622, 1999.
108. Sofat N, Turner J, Khoo B, et al: An unusual case of Cushing's syndrome: primary pigmented nodular adrenal dysplasia, Int J Clin Pract 54:269–271, 2000.
109. Aiba M, Hirayama A, Iri H, et al: Primary adrenocortical micronodular dysplasia: enzyme histochemical and ultrastructural studies of two cases with a review of the literature, Hum Pathol 21:503–511, 1990.
110. Teding van Berkhout F, Croughs RJM, Kater L, et al: Familial Cushing's syndrome due to nodular adrenocortical dysplasia. A putative receptor-antibody disease? Clin Endocrinol 24:299–310, 1986.
111. Stratakis CA, Carney JA, Kirschner LS, et al: Synaptophysin immunoreactivity in primary pigmented nodular adrenocortical disease: neuroendocrine properties of tumors associated with Carney complex, J Clin Endocrinol Metab 84:1122–1128, 1999.
112. D'Agata R, Malozowski S, Barkan AL, et al: Steroid biosynthesis in human adrenal tumors, Horm Metab Res 19:38–388, 1987.
113. Weiss LM: Comparative histologic study of 43 metastasizing and nonmetastasizing adrenocortical tumors, Am J Surg Pathol 8:163–169, 1984.
114. Hough AJ, Hollifield JW, Page DL, et al: Prognostic factors in adrenal cortical tumors. A mathematical analysis of clinical and morphologic data, Am J Clin Pathol 72:390–399, 1979.
115. van Slooten H, Schaberg A, Smeenk D, et al: Morphologic characteristics of benign and malignant adrenocortical tumors, Cancer 55:766–773, 1985.
116. Sasano H, Suzuki T, Moriya T: Discerning malignancy in resected adrenocortical neoplasms, Endocr Pathol 12:397–406, 2001.
117. Tan HS, Thai AC, Nga ME, et al: Development of ipsilateral adrenocortical carcinoma sixteen years after resection of an adrenal tumour causing Cushing's syndrome, Ann Acad Med Singapore 34:271–274, 2005.
118. Klibanski A, Stephen AE, Greene MF, et al: A 35-year-old pregnant woman with new hypertension, N Engl J Med 355:2237–2245, 2006.
119. Koch CA, Pacák K, Chrousos GP: The molecular pathogenesis of hereditary and sporadic adrenocortical and adrenomedullary tumors, J Clin Endocrinol Metab 87:5367–5384, 2002.
120. Brown FM, Gaffey TA, Wold LE, et al: Myxoid neoplasms of the adrenal cortex: a rare histologic variant, Am J Surg Pathol 24:396–401, 2000.
121. Geramizadeh B, Norouzzadeh B, Bolandparvaz S, et al: Functioning adrenocortical oncocytoma: a case report and review of the literature, Indian J Pathol Microbiol 51:237–239, 2008.
122. Hisamatsu H, Sakai H, Tsuda S, et al: Combined adrenal adenoma and myelolipoma in a patient with Cushing's syndrome: case report and review of the literature, Int J Urol 11:416–418, 2004.
123. Wieneke JA, Thompson LD, Heffess CS: Corticomedullary mixed tumor of the adrenal gland, Ann Diagn Pathol 5:304–308, 2001.
124. Miettinen M: Neuroendocrine differentiation in adrenocortical carcinoma. New immunohistochemical findings supported by electron microscopy, Lab Invest 66:169–174, 1992.
125. Haak HR, Fleuren GJ: Neuroendocrine differentiation of adrenocortical tumors, Cancer 75:860–864, 1995.
126. Geller JL, Azer PC, Weiss LM, et al: Pigmented adrenocortical carcinoma: case report and review, Endocr Pathol 17:297–304, 2006.
127. Midorikawa S, Hashimoto S, Kuriki M, et al: A patient with preclinical Cushing's syndrome and excessive DHEA-S secretion having unilateral adrenal carcinoma and contralateral adenoma, Endocr J 46:59–66, 1999.
128. Venkatesh S, Hickey RC, Sellin RV, et al: Adrenal cortical carcinoma, Cancer 64:765–769, 1989.
129. Gicquel C, Leblond-Francillard M, Bertagna X, et al: Clonal analysis of human adrenocortical carcinomas and secreting adenomas, Clin Endocrinol 40:465–477, 1994.
130. Diaz-Cano SJ, de Miguel M, Blanes A, et al: Clonality as expression of distinctive cell kinetics patters in nodular hyperplasia and adenomas of the adrenal cortex, Am J Pathol 156:311–319, 2000.
131. Bernard MH, Sidhu S, Berger N, et al: A case report in favor of a multistep adrenocortical tumorigenesis, J Clin Endocrinol Metab 88:998–1001, 2003.
132. Stratakis CA, Boikos S: Genetics of adrenal tumors associated with Cushing's syndrome: a new classification for bilateral adrenocortical hyperplasias, Nat Clin Pract Endocrinol Metab 3:748–757, 2007.
133. Kjellman M, Kallioniemi OP, Karhu R, et al: Genetic aberrations in adrenocortical tumors detected using comparative genomic hybridization correlate with tumor size and malignancy, Cancer Res 56:4219–4223, 1996.
134. Fogt F, Vargas MP, Zhuang Z, et al: Utilization of molecular genetics in the differentiation between adrenal cortical adenomas and carcinoma, Hum Pathol 28:518–521, 1998.
135. Riberio RC, Sandrini F, Figueiredo B, et al: An inherited p53 mutation that contributes in a tissue-specific manner to pediatric adrenal cortical carcinoma, Proc Natl Acad Sci U S A 98:9330–9335, 2001.
136. Beuschlein F, Schulze E, Mora P, et al: Steroid 21-hydroxylase mutations and 21-hydroxylase messenger ribonucleic acid expression in human adrenocortical tumors, J Clin Endocrinol Metab 83:2585–2588, 1998.
137. Latronico AC, Reincke M, Bilharinho de Mendonça B, et al: No evidence for oncogenic mutations in the adrenocorticotropin receptor gene in human adrenocortical neoplasms, J Clin Endocrinol Metab 80:875–877, 1995.
138. Syddall HE, Baig A, Malchoff DM, et al: Impaired desensitization of a mutant adrenocorticotropin receptor associated with apparent constitutive activity, Mol Endocrinol 16:2746–2753, 2002.
139. Bertherat J, Groussin L, Sandrini F, et al: Molecular and functional analysis of *PRKAR1A* and its locus (17q22–24) in sporadic adrenocortical tumors: 17q losses, somatic mutations, and protein kinase A expression and activity, Cancer Res 63:5308–5319, 2003.
140. Bourdeau I, Matyakhina L, Stergiopoulos SG, et al: 17q22–24 chromosomal losses and alterations of protein kinase A subunit expression and activity in adrenocorticotrophin-independent macronodular adrenal hyperplasia, J Clin Endocrinol Metab 91:3626–3632, 2006.
141. Vincent-Dejean C, Cazabat L, Groussin L, et al: Identification of a clinically homogeneous subgroup of benign cortisol-secreting adrenocortical tumors characterized by alterations of the protein kinase A (PKA) subunits and high PKA activity, Eur J Endocrinol 158:829–839, 2008.
142. Tissier F, Cavard C, Groussin L, et al: Mutations of beta-catenin in adrenocortical tumors: activation of the Wnt signaling pathway is a frequent event in both benign and malignant adrenocortical tumors, Cancer Res 65:7622–7627, 2005.
143. Munro LM, Kennedy A, McNicol AM: The expression of inhibin/activin subunits in the human adrenal cortex and its tumours, J Endocrinol 161:341–347, 1999.
144. Schulte HM, Mengel M, Heinze M, et al: Complete sequencing and messenger ribonucleic acid expression analysis of the *MEN1* gene in adrenal cancer, J Clin Endocrinol Metab 85:441–448, 2000.
145. Waldmann J, Bartsch DK, Kann PH, et al: Adrenal involvement in multiple endocrine neoplasia type 1: results of 7 years prospective screening, Langenbeck's Arch Surg 392:437–443, 2007.
146. Alzahrani AS, Al-Khaldi N, Shi Y, et al: Diagnosis by serendipity: Cushing syndrome attributable to cortisol-producing adrenal adenoma as the initial manifestation of multiple endocrine neoplasia type 1 due to a rare splicing site *MEN1* gene mutation, Endocr Pract 14:595–602, 2008.
147. Weinstein LS, Shenker A, Gejman OV, et al: Activating mutations of the stimulatory G protein in the McCune-Albright syndrome, N Engl J Med 325:1688–1695, 1991.
148. Boston BA, Mandel S, LaFranchi SH, et al: Activating mutation in the stimulatory guanine nucleotide-binding protein in an infant with Cushing's syndrome and nodular adrenal hyperplasia, J Clin Endocrinol Metab 79:890–893, 1994.
149. Dall'Asta C, Ballarè E, Mantovani G, et al: Assessing the presence of abnormal regulation of cortisol secretion by membrane hormone receptors: in vivo and in vitro studies in patients with functioning and non-functioning adrenal adenoma, Horm Metab Res 36:578–583, 2004.
150. Bugalho MJM, Li X, Rao CV, et al: Presence of a $G_{s\alpha}$ mutation in an adrenal tumor expressing LH/hCG receptor and clinically associated with Cushing's syndrome, Gynecol Endocrinol 14:50–54, 2000.
151. Villares Fragoso MCB, Domenice S, Latronico AC, et al: Cushing's syndrome secondary to adrenocorticotropin-independent macronodular adrenocortical hyperplasia due to activating mutations of the *GNAS1* gene, J Clin Endocrinol Metab 88:2147–2151, 2003.
152. Groen EJ, Roos A, Muntinghe FL, et al: Extra-intestinal manifestations of familial adenomatous polyposis, Ann Surg Oncol 15:2439–2450, 2008.
153. Beuschlein F, Reincke M, Königer M, et al: Cortisol producing adrenal adenoma: a new manifestation of Gardner's syndrome, Endocrine Res 26:783–790, 2000.
154. Casey M, Vaughan CJ, He J, et al: Mutations in the protein kinase A R1α regulatory subunit cause familial cardiac myxomas and Carney complex, J Clin Invest 106:R31-R38, 2000.
155. Kirschner LS, Carney JA, Pack SD, et al: Mutations of the gene encoding the protein kinase A type I-alpha regulatory subunit in patients with the Carney complex, Nat Genet 26:89–92, 2000.
156. Ogo A, Haji M, Ohashi M, et al: Markedly increased expression of cytochrome P-450 17α-hydroxylase ($P\text{-}450_{c17}$) mRNA in adrenocortical adenomas from patients with Cushing's syndrome, Mol Cell Endocrinol 80:83–89, 1991.
157. Hornsby PJ: Physiological and pathological effects of steroids on the function of the adrenal cortex, J Steroid Biochem 27:1161–1171, 1987.
158. Shibata H, Suzuki H, Ogishima T, et al: Significance of steroidogenic enzymes in the pathogenesis of adrenal tumour, Acta Endocrinol (Copenh) 128:235–242, 1993.
159. Sakai Y, Yanase T, Takayanagi R, et al: High expression of cytochrome b_5 in adrenocortical adenomas from patients with Cushing's syndrome associated with high secretion of adrenal androgens, J Clin Endocrinol Metab 76:1286–1290, 1993.
160. Lamberts SWJ, Zuiderwijk J, Uitterlinden P, et al: Characterization of adrenal autonomy in Cushing's syndrome: a comparison between in vivo and in vitro responsiveness of the adrenal gland, J Clin Endocrinol Metab 70:192–199, 1990.
161. Sasano H, Suzuki T, Nagura H, et al: Steroidogenesis in human adrenocortical carcinoma: biochemical activities, immunohistochemistry, and in situ hybridization of steroidogenic enzymes and histopathologic study in nine cases, Hum Pathol 24:397–404, 1993.
162. Barzon L, Masi G, Fincati K, et al: Shift from Conn's syndrome to Cushing's syndrome in a recurrent adrenocortical carcinoma, Eur J Endocrinol 153:629–636, 2005.
163. Sasano H: Localization of steroidogenic enzymes in adrenal cortex and its disorders, Endocr J 41:471–482, 1994.
164. Morita H, Isomura Y, Mune T, et al: Plasma cortisol and cortisone concentrations in normal subjects and patients with adrenocortical disorders, Metabolism 53:89–94, 2004.
165. Mazzocchi G, Aragona F, Malendowicz LK, et al: Cortisol-secreting adrenal adenomas express 11beta-hydroxysteroid dehydrogenase type-2 gene yet possess low 11beta-HSD2 activity, J Investig Med 49:191–194, 2001.
166. Imai T, Sarkar D, Shibata A, et al: Expression of adrenocorticotropin receptor gene in adrenocortical adeno-

mas from patients with Cushing syndrome: possible contribution for the autonomous production of cortisol, Ann Surg 234:85–91, 2001.
167. Reincke M, Beuschlein F, Menig G, et al: Localization and expression of adrenocorticotropic hormone receptor mRNA in normal and neoplastic human adrenal cortex, J Endocrinol 156:415–423, 1998.
168. Penhoat A, Jaillard C, Saez JM: Corticotropin positively regulates its own receptors and cAMP response in cultured bovine adrenal cells, Proc Natl Acad Sci USA 86:4978–4981, 1989.
169. Beuschlein F, Fassnacht M, Klink A, et al: ACTH receptor expression, regulation and role in adrenocortical tumor formation, Eur J Endocrinol 144:199–206, 2001.
170. Ishizuka T, Daidoh H, Morita H, et al: ACTH-induced cortisol secretion is mediated by cAMP and PKC in various adrenocortical adenomas, Endocr J 44:661–670, 1997.
171. Schorr I, Ney RL: Abnormal hormone responses of an adrenocortical cancer adenyl cyclase, J Clin Invest 50:1295–1300, 1971.
172. Hornsby PJ: Regulation of adrenocortical cell proliferation in culture, Endocrine Res 10:259–281, 1984.
173. Mesiano S, Jaffe RB: Developmental and functional biology of the primate fetal adrenal cortex, Endocrine Rev 18:378–403, 1997.
174. Fassnacht M, Hahner S, Hansen IA, et al: N-terminal proopiomelanocortin acts as a mitogen in adrenocortical tumor cells and decreases adrenal steroidogenesis, J Clin Endocrinol Metab 88:2171–2179, 2003.
175. Coll AP, Fassnacht M, Klammer S, et al: Peripheral administration of the N-terminal pro-opiomelanocortin fragment 1–28 to Pomc$^{-/-}$ mice reduces food intake and weight but does not affect adrenal growth or corticosterone secretion, J Endocrinol 190:515–525, 2006.
176. Darbeida H, Durand P: Mechanisms of glucocorticoid enhancement of the responsiveness of ovine adrenocortical cells to adrenocorticotropin, Biochem Biophys Res Commun 166:1183–1191, 1990.
177. Loose DS, Do YS, Chen TL, et al: Demonstration of glucocorticoid receptors in the adrenal cortex: evidence for a direct dexamethasone suppressive effect on the rat adrenal gland, Endocrinology 107:137–146, 1980.
178. Kontula K, Pomoell UM, Gunsalus GL, et al: Glucocorticoid receptors and responsiveness of normal and neoplastic human adrenal cortex, J Clin Endocrinol Metab 60:283–289, 1985.
179. Kirschner MA, Powell RD Jr, Lipsett MB: Cushing's syndrome: nodular cortical hyperplasia of adrenal glands with clinical and pathological features suggesting adrenocortical tumor, J Clin Endocrinol Metab 24:947–955, 1964.
180. Malchoff CD, Rosa J, DeBold RC, et al: Adrenocorticotropin-independent bilateral macronodular adrenal hyperplasia: an unusual cause of Cushing's syndrome, J Clin Endocrinol Metab 68:855–860, 1989.
181. Shinojima H, Kakizaki H, Usuki T, et al: Clinical and endocrinological features of adrenocorticotropic hormone-independent bilateral macronodular adrenocortical hyperplasia, J Urol 166:1639–1642, 2002.
182. Swain JM, Grant CS, Schlinkert RT, et al: Corticotropin-independent macronodular adrenal hyperplasia: a clinicopathologic correlation, Arch Surg 133:541–545, 1998.
183. Verma A, Mohan S, Gupta A: ACTH-independent macronodular adrenal hyperplasia: imaging findings of a rare condition—a case report, Abdom Imaging 33:225–229, 2008.
184. Morioka M, Ohashi Y, Watanabe H, et al: ACTH-independent macronodular adrenocortical hyperplasia (AIMAH): report of two cases and the analysis of steroidogenic activity in adrenal nodules, Endocr J 44:65–72, 1997.
185. Josse RG, Bear R, Kovacs K, et al: Cushing's syndrome due to unilateral nodular adrenal hyperplasia: a new pathophysiological entity? Acta Endocrinol (Copenh) 93:495–504, 1980.
186. Bourdeau I, D'Amour P, Hamet P, et al: Aberrant membrane hormone receptors in incidentally discovered bilateral macronodular adrenal hyperplasia with subclinical Cushing's syndrome, J Clin Endocrinol Metab 86:5534–5540, 2001.
187. Sasao T, Itoh N, Sato Y, et al: Subclinical Cushing syndrome due to adrenocorticotropic hormone-independent macronodular adrenocortical hyperplasia: changes in plasma cortisol levels during long-term follow-up, Urology 55:145x–145xii, 2000.
188. Ohashi A, Yamada Y, Sakaguchi K, et al: A natural history of adrenocorticotropin-independent adrenal macronodular hyperplasia (AIMAH) from preclinical to clinically overt Cushing's syndrome, Endocr J 48:677–683, 2001.
189. Doppman JL, Chrousos GP, Papanicolaou DA, et al: Adrenocorticotropin-independent macronodular adrenal hyperplasia: an uncommon cause of primary adrenal hypercortisolism, Radiology 216:797–802, 2000.
190. Smals AGH, Pieters GF, van Haelst UJ, et al: Macronodular adrenocortical hyperplasia in long-standing Cushing's disease, J Clin Endocrinol Metab 58:25–31, 1984.
191. Bourdeau I, Antonini SRR, Lacroix A, et al: Gene array analysis of macronodular adrenal hyperplasia confirms clinical heterogeneity and identifies several candidate genes as molecular mediators, Oncogene 23:1575–1585, 2004.
192. Lampron A, Bourdeau I, Hamet P, et al: Whole genome expression profiling of glucose-dependent insulinotropic peptide (GIP)- and adrenocorticotropin-dependent adrenal hyperplasias reveals novel targets for the study of GIP-dependent Cushing's syndrome, J Clin Endocrinol Metab 91:3611–3618, 2006.
193. Hermus AR, Pieters GF, Smals AGH, et al: Transition from pituitary-dependent to adrenal-dependent Cushing's syndrome, N Engl J Med 318:966–970, 1988.
194. Hocher B, Bähr V, Dormüller S, et al: Hypercortisolism with non-pigmented micronodular adrenal hyperplasia: transition from pituitary-dependent to adrenal-dependent Cushing's syndrome, Acta Endocrinol (Copenh) 128:120–125, 1993.
195. Vrezas I, Willenberg HS, Mansmann G, et al: Ectopic adrenocorticotropin (ACTH) and corticotropin-releasing hormone (CRH) production in the adrenal gland: basic and clinical aspects, Microsc Res Tech 61:308–314, 2003.
196. Hiroi N, Chrousos GP, Kohn B, et al: Adrenocortical-pituitary hybrid tumor causing Cushing's syndrome, J Clin Endocrinol Metab 86:2631–2637, 2001.
197. Lefebvre H, Duparc C, Chartrel N, et al: Intraadrenal adrenocorticotropin production in a case of bilateral macronodular adrenal hyperplasia causing Cushing's syndrome, J Clin Endocrinol Metab 88:3035–3042, 2003.
198. Feelders RA, Lamberts SWJ, Hofland LJ, et al: Luteinizing hormone (LH)-responsive Cushing's syndrome: the demonstration of LH receptor messenger ribonucleic acid in hyperplastic adrenal cells, which respond to chorionic gonadotropin and serotonin agonists in vitro, J Clin Endocrinol Metab 88:230–237, 2003.
199. Suri D, Alonso M, Weiss RE: A case of ACTH-independent bilateral macronodular adrenal hyperplasia and severe congestive heart failure, J Endocrinol Invest 29:940–946, 2006.
200. Antonini SRR, Baldacchino V, Tremblay J, et al: Expression of ACTH receptor pathway genes in glucose-dependent insulinotrophic peptide (GIP)-dependent Cushing's syndrome, Clin Endocrinol 64:29–36, 2006.
201. Mazzucco TL, Thomas M, Martinie M, et al: Cellular and molecular abnormalities of a macronodular adrenal hyperplasia causing beta-blocker-sensitive Cushing's syndrome, Arq Bras Endocrinol Metab 51:1452–1462, 2007.
202. Hinshaw HT, Ney RL: Abnormal control in the neoplastic adrenal cortex. In McKerns KW, editor: Hormones and Cancer, New York, 1974, Academic Press, pp 309–327.
203. Reznik Y, Allali-Zerah V, Chayvialle JA, et al: Food-dependent Cushing's syndrome mediated by aberrant adrenal sensitivity to gastric inhibitory polypeptide, N Engl J Med 327:981–986, 1992.
204. Lacroix A, Bolté E, Tremblay J, et al: Gastric inhibitory polypeptide-dependent cortisol hypersecretion—a new cause of Cushing's syndrome, N Engl J Med 327:974–980, 1992.
205. Reznik Y, Lefebvre H, Rohmer V, et al: Aberrant adrenal sensitivity to multiple ligands in unilateral incidentaloma with subclinical autonomous cortisol hypersecretion: a prospective clinical study, Clin Endocrinol 61:311–319, 2004.
206. Suzuki S, Uchida D, Koide H, et al: Hyperresponsiveness of adrenal grand to vasopressin resulting in enhanced plasma cortisol in patients with adrenal nodules, Peptides 29:1767–1772, 2007.
207. Mircescu H, Jilwan J, N'Diaye N, et al: Are ectopic or abnormal membrane hormone receptors frequently present in adrenal Cushing's syndrome? J Clin Endocrinol Metab 85:3531–3536, 2000.
208. Groussin L, Perlemoine K, Contesse V, et al: The ectopic expression of the gastric inhibitory polypeptide receptor is frequent in adrenocorticotropin-independent bilateral macronodular hyperplasia, but rare in unilateral tumors, J Clin Endocrinol Metab 87:1980–1985, 2002.
209. Mazzucco TL, Chabre O, Sturm N, et al: Ectopic expression of the gastric inhibitory polypeptide receptor gene is a sufficient genetic event to induce benign adrenocortical tumor in a xenotransplantation model, Endocrinology 147:782–790, 2006.
210. Mazzucco TL, Chabre O, Feige JJ, et al: Aberrant expression of human luteinizing hormone receptor by adrenocortical cells is sufficient to provoke both hyperplasia and Cushing's syndrome features, J Clin Endocrinol Metab 91:196–203, 2006.
211. Miyamura N, Tsutsumi A, Senokuchi H, et al: A case of ACTH-independent macronodular adrenal hyperplasia: simultaneous expression of several aberrant hormone receptors in the adrenal gland, Endocr J 50:333–340, 2003.
212. Louiset E, Contesse V, Groussin L, et al: Expression of serotonin7 receptors and coupling of ectopic receptors to protein kinase A and ionic currents in adrenocorticotropin-independent macronodular adrenal hyperplasia causing Cushing's syndrome, J Clin Endocrinol Metab 91:4578–4586, 2006.
213. Bertherat J, Contesse V, Louiset E, et al: In vivo and in vitro screening for illegitimate receptors in adrenocorticotropin-independent macronodular adrenal hyperplasia causing Cushing's syndrome: identification of two cases of gonadotropin/gastric inhibitory polypeptide-dependent hypercortisolism, J Clin Endocrinol Metab 90:1302–1310, 2005.
214. N'Diaye N, Tremblay J, Hamet P, et al: Adrenocortical overexpression of gastric inhibitory polypeptide receptor underlies food-dependent Cushing's syndrome, J Clin Endocrinol Metab 83:2781–2785, 1998.
215. Lebrethon MC, Avallet O, Reznik Y, et al: Food-dependent Cushing's syndrome: characterization and functional role of gastric inhibitory polypeptide receptor in the adrenal of three patients, J Clin Endocrinol Metab 83:4514–4519, 1998.
216. Swords FM, Aylwin SJB, Perry L, et al: The aberrant expression of the gastric inhibitory polypeptide (GIP) receptor in adrenal hyperplasia: does chronic adrenocorticotropin exposure stimulate up-regulation of GIP receptors in Cushing's disease? J Clin Endocrinol Metab 90:3009–3016, 2005.
217. Antonini SRR, N'Diaye N, Baldacchino V, et al: Analysis of the putative regulatory region of the gastric inhibitory polypeptide receptor gene in food-dependent Cushing's syndrome, J Steroid Biochem Mol Biol 91:171–177, 2004.
218. Baldacchino V, Oble S, Décarie PO, et al: The Sp transcription factors are involved in the cellular expression of the human glucose-dependent insulinotropic polypeptide receptor gene and overexpressed in adrenals of patients with Cushing's syndrome, J Mol Endocrinol 35:61–71, 2005.
219. Tsagarakis S, Tsigos C, Vassiliou V, et al: Food-dependent androgen and cortisol secretion by a gastric inhibitory polypeptide-receptor expressive adrenocortical adenoma leading to hirsutism and subclinical Cushing's syndrome: in vivo and in vitro studies, J Clin Endocrinol Metab 86:583–589, 2001.
220. Albiger N, Occhi G, Mariniello B, et al: Food-dependent Cushing's syndrome: from molecular characterization to therapeutical results, Eur J Endocrinol 157:771–778, 2007.
221. Gwinup G, Steinberg T, King CG, et al: Vasopressin-induced ACTH secretion in man, J Clin Endocrinol Metab 27:927–930, 1967.
222. Perraudin V, Delarue C, Lefebvre H, et al: Vasopressin stimulates cortisol secretion from human adrenocortical tissue through activation of V1 receptors, J Clin Endocrinol Metab 76:1522–1528, 1993.
223. Hensen J, Hader O, Bähr V, et al: Effects of incremental infusions of arginine vasopressin on adrenocorticotro-

pin and cortisol secretion in man, J Clin Endocrinol Metab 66:668–671, 1988.

224. Lacroix A, Tremblay J, Touyz R, et al: Abnormal adrenal and vascular responses to vasopressin mediated by a V1-vasopressin receptor in a patients with adrenocorticotropin-independent macronodular adrenal hyperplasia, Cushing's syndrome, and orthostatic hypotension, J Clin Endocrinol Metab 82:2414–2422, 1997.

225. Perraudin V, Delarue C, De Keyzer Y, et al: Vasopressin-responsive adrenocortical tumor in a mild Cushing's syndrome: in vivo and in vitro studies, J Clin Endocrinol Metab 80:2661–2667, 1995.

226. Daidoh H, Morita H, Hanafusa J, et al: In vivo and in vitro effects of AVP and V1a receptor antagonist on Cushing's syndrome due to ACTH-independent bilateral macronodular adrenocortical hyperplasia, Clin Endocrinol 48:403–409, 1998.

227. Mune T, Murase H, Yamakita N, et al: Eutopic overexpression of vasopressin V1a receptor in adrenocorticotropin-independent macronodular adrenal hyperplasia, J Clin Endocrinol Metab 87:5706–5713, 2002.

228. Vezzosi D, Cartier D, Régnier C, et al: Familial adrenocorticotropin-independent macronodular adrenal hyperplasia with aberrant serotonin and vasopressin adrenal receptors, Eur J Endocrinol 156:21–31, 2007.

229. Louiset E, Contesse V, Groussin L, et al: Expression of vasopressin receptors in ACTH-independent macronodular bilateral adrenal hyperplasia causing Cushing's syndrome: molecular, immunohistochemical and pharmacological correlates, J Endocrinol 196:1–9, 2008.

230. Lee S, Hwang R, Lee J, et al: Ectopic expression of vasopressin V1b and V2 receptors in the adrenal glands of familial ACTH-independent macronodular adrenal hyperplasia, Clin Endocrinol 63:625–630, 2006.

231. Nakamura Y, Son Y, Kohno Y, et al: Case of adrenocorticotropic hormone-independent macronodular adrenal hyperplasia with possible adrenal hypersensitivity to angiotensin II, Endocrine 15:57–61, 2001.

232. Pabon JE, Li X, Lei ZM, et al: Novel presence of luteinizing hormone/chorionic gonadotropin receptors in human adrenal glands, J Clin Endocrinol Metab 81:2397–2400, 1996.

233. Kero J, Poutanen M, Zhang FP, et al: Elevated luteinizing hormone induces expression of its receptor and promotes steroidogenesis in the adrenal cortex, J Clin Invest 105:633–641, 2000.

234. Schoemaker NJ, Teerds KJ, Mol JA, et al: The role of luteinizing hormone in the pathogenesis of hyperadrenocorticism in neutered ferrets, Mol Cell Endocrinol 197:117–125, 2002.

235. Hirata Y, Uchihashi M, Sueoka S, et al: Presence of β-adrenergic receptors on human adrenocortical cortisol-producing adenomas, J Clin Endocrinol Metab 53:953–957, 1981.

236. Lacroix A, Tremblay J, Rousseau G, et al: Propranolol therapy for ectopic β-adrenergic receptors in adrenal Cushing's syndrome, N Engl J Med 337:1429–1434, 1997.

237. Lefebvre H, Contesse V, Delarue C, et al: Effect of the serotonin-4 receptor agonist zacopride on aldosterone secretion from the human adrenal cortex: in vivo and in vitro studies, J Clin Endocrinol Metab 77:1662–1666, 1993.

238. Cartier D, Lihrmann I, Parmentier F, et al: Overexpression of serotonin-4 receptors in cisapride-responsive adrenocorticotropin-independent bilateral macronodular adrenal hyperplasia causing Cushing's syndrome, J Clin Endocrinol Metab 88:248–254, 2003.

239. Mannelli M, Ferruzzi P, Luciani P, et al: Cushing's syndrome in a patient with bilateral macronodular adrenal hyperplasia responding to cisapride: an in vivo and in vitro study, J Clin Endocrinol Metab 88:4616–4622, 2003.

240. Willenberg HS, Stratakis CA, Marx C, et al: Brief report: Aberrant interleukin-1 receptors in a cortisol- secreting adrenal adenoma causing Cushing's syndrome, N Engl J Med 339:27–31, 1998.

241. Hanley N, Williams BC, Nicol M, et al: Interleukin-1 beta stimulates growth of adrenocortical cells in primary culture, J Mol Endocrinol 8:131–136, 1992.

242. Caticha O, Odell WD, Wilson DE, et al: Estradiol stimulates cortisol production by adrenal cells in estrogen-dependent primary adrenocortical nodular dysplasia, J Clin Endocrinol Metab 77:494–497, 1993.

243. Findlay JC, Sheeler LR, Engeland WC, et al: Familial adrenocorticotropin-independent Cushing's syndrome with bilateral macronodular adrenal hyperplasia, J Clin Endocrinol Metab 76:189–191, 1993.

244. Kubo N, Onoda N, Ishikawa T, et al: Simultaneous bilateral laparoscopic adrenalectomy for adrenocorticotropic hormone-independent macronodular adrenal hyperplasia: report of a case, Surg Today 36:642–646, 2006.

245. Kageyama Y, Ishizaka K, Iwashina M, et al: A case of ACTH-independent bilateral macronodular adrenal hyperplasia successfully treated by subtotal resection of the adrenal glands: four-year follow-up, Endocr J 49:227–229, 2002.

246. Iacobone M, Albiger N, Scaroni C, et al: The role of unilateral adrenalectomy in ACTH-independent macronodular adrenal hyperplasia (AIMAH), World J Surg 32:882–889, 2008.

247. Omori N, Nomura K, Omori K, et al: Rational, effective metyrapone treatment of ACTH-independent bilateral macronodular adrenocortical hyperplasia (AIMAH), Endocr J 48:665–669, 2001.

248. Nagai M, Narita I, Omori K, et al: Adrenocorticotropic hormone-independent bilateral adrenocortical macronodular hyperplasia treated with mitotane, Intern Med 38:969–973, 1999.

249. Groussin L, Jullian E, Perlemoine K, et al: Mutations of the PRKAR1A gene in Cushing's syndrome due to sporadic primary pigmented nodular adrenocortical disease, J Clin Endocrinol Metab 27:4324–4329, 2002.

250. Schulz S, Redlich A, Köppe I, et al: Carney complex—an unexpected finding during puerperium, Gynecol Obstet Invest 51:211–213, 2001.

251. Danoff A, Jormark S, Lorber D, et al: Adrenocortical micronodular dysplasia, cardiac myxomas, lentigines, and spindle cell tumors. Report of a kindred, Arch Intern Med 147:443–448, 1987.

252. Young WF Jr, Carney JA, Musa BU, et al: Familial Cushing's syndrome due to primary pigmented nodular adrenocortical disease, N Engl J Med 321:1659–1664, 1989.

253. Stratakis CA, Carney JA, Lin JP, et al: Carney complex, a familial multiple neoplasia and lentiginosis syndrome. Analysis of 11 kindreds and linkage to the short arm of chromosome 2, J Clin Invest 97:699–706, 1996.

254. Oelkers WKH, Bahr V, Hensen J, et al: Primary adrenocortical micronodular adenomatosis causing Cushing's syndrome. Effects of ketoconazole on steroid production and in vitro performance of adrenal cells, Acta Endocrinol (Copenh) 113:370–377, 1986.

255. Bourdeau I, Lacroix A, Schürch W, et al: Primary pigmented nodular adrenocortical disease: paradoxical responses of cortisol secretion to dexamethasone occur in vitro and are associated with increased expression of the glucocorticoid receptor, J Clin Endocrinol Metab 88:3931–3938, 2003.

256. Casey M, Mah C, Merliss A, et al: Identification of a novel genetic locus for familial cardiac myxomas and Carney complex, Circulation 98:2560–2566, 1998.

257. Matyakhina L, Pack SD, Kirschner LS, et al: Chromosome 2 (2p16) abnormalities in Carney complex tumours, J Med Genet 40:268–277, 2003.

258. Horvath A, Bossis I, Giatzakis C, et al: Large deletions of the PRKAR1A gene in Carney complex, Clin Cancer Res 14:388–395, 2008.

259. Greene EL, Horvath A, Nesterova M, et al: In vitro functional studies of naturally occurring pathogenic PRKAR1A mutations that are not subject to nonsense mRNA decay, Hum Mutat 29:633–639, 2008.

260. Amieux PS, Cummings DE, Motamed K, et al: Compensatory regulation of RIalpha protein levels in protein kinase A mutant mice, J Biol Chem 272:3993–3998, 1997.

261. Groussin L, Kirschner LS, Vincent-Dejean C, et al: Molecular analysis of the cyclic AMP-dependent protein kinase A (PKA) regulatory subunit 1A (PRKAR1A) gene in patients with Carney complex and primary pigmented nodular adrenocortical disease (PPNAD) reveals novel mutations and clues for pathophysiology: augmented PKA signaling is associated with adrenal tumorigenesis in PPNAD, Am J Hum Genet 71:1433–1442, 2002.

262. Groussin L, Horvath A, Jullian E, et al: A PRKAR1A mutation associated with primary pigmented nodular adrenocortical disease in 12 kindreds, J Clin Endocrinol Metab 91:1943–1949, 2006.

263. Horvath A, Giatzakis C, Robinson-White A, et al: Adrenal hyperplasia and adenomas are associated with inhibition of phosphodiesterase 11A in carriers of PDE11A sequence variants that are frequent in the population, Cancer Res 66:11571–11575, 2006.

264. Horvath A, Mericq MV, Stratakis CA: Mutation in PDE8B, a cyclic AMP-specific phosphodiesterase in adrenal hyperplasia, N Engl J Med 358:750–752, 2008.

265. Limone P, Maccario M, Vigliani R, et al: Primary pigmented micronodular disease of the adrenals, J Endocrinol Invest 13:171–175, 1990.

266. Powell AC, Stratakis CA, Patronas NJ, et al: Operative management of Cushing syndrome secondary to micronodular adrenal hyperplasia, Surgery 143:750–758, 2008.

267. Sarlis NJ, Chrousos GP, Doppman JL, et al: Primary pigmented nodular adrenocortical disease: re-evaluation of a patient with Carney complex 27 years after unilateral adrenalectomy, J Clin Endocrinol Metab 82:1274–1278, 1996.

268. Washecka R, Dresner MI, Honda SAA: Testicular tumors in Carney's complex, J Urol 167:1299–1302, 2002.

269. Pecori Giraldi F, Fatti LM, Bertola G, et al: Carney's complex with acromegaly as the leading clinical condition, Clin Endocrinol 68:322–324, 2008.

270. Pack SD, Kirschner LS, Pak E, et al: Genetic and histologic studies of somatomammotropic pituitary tumors in patients with the "syndrome of spotty skin pigmentation, myxomas, endocrine overactivity and schwannomas" (Carney complex), J Clin Endocrinol Metab 85:3860–3865, 2000.

271. Watson JC, Stratakis CA, Bryant-Greenwood PK, et al: Neurosurgical complications of Carney complex, J Neurosurg 92:413–418, 2000.

272. Ogo A, Haji M, Natori S, et al: Acromegaly with hyperprolactinemia developed after bilateral adrenalectomy in a patient with Cushing's syndrome due to adrenocortical nodular hyperplasia, Endocr J 40:17–25, 1993.

273. Raff SB, Carney JA, Krugman D, et al: Prolactin secretion abnormalities in patients with the "syndrome of spotty skin pigmentation, myxomas, endocrine overactivity and schwannomas" (Carney complex), J Pediatr Endocrinol Metab 13:373–379, 2000.

274. Stratakis CA, Courkoutsakis NA, Abati A, et al: Thyroid gland abnormalities in patients with the "syndrome of spotty skin pigmentation, myxomas, endocrine overactivity, and schwannomas (Carney complex), J Clin Endocrinol Metab 82:2037–2043, 1997.

275. Stratakis CA, Papageorgiou T, Premkumar A, et al: Ovarian lesions in Carney complex: clinical genetics and possible predisposition to malignancy, J Clin Endocrinol Metab 85:4359–4366, 2000.

276. Edwards A, Bermudez C, Piwonka G, et al: Carney's syndrome: complex myxomas. Report of four cases and review of the literature, Cardiovasc Surg 10:264–275, 2002.

277. Stratakis CA, Kirschner LS, Carney JA: Clinical and molecular features of the Carney complex: diagnostic criteria and recommendations for patient evaluation, J Clin Endocrinol Metab 86:4041–4046, 2001.

278. Carney JA, Toorkey BC: Ductal adenoma of the breast with tubular features. A probable component of the complex of myxomas, spotty pigmentation, endocrine overactivity, and schwannomas, Am J Surg Pathol 15:722–731, 1991.

279. Mateus C, Palangié A, Franck N, et al: Heterogeneity of skin manifestations in patients with Carney complex, J Am Acad Dermatol 59:801–810, 2008.

280. Carney JA, Boccon-Gibod L, Jarka DE, et al: Osteochondromyxoma of the bone, Am J Surg Pathol 25:164–176, 2001.

281. Sutter JA, Grimberg A: Adrenocortical tumors and hyperplasias in childhood—etiology, genetics, clinical presentation and therapy, Ped Endocrinol Rev 4:32–39, 2006.

282. Sandrini R, Riberio RC, DeLacerda L: Childhood adrenocortical tumors, J Clin Endocrinol Metab 82:2027–2031, 1997.

283. Sbragia L, Oliveria-Filho AG, Vassallo J, et al: Adrenocortical tumors in Brazilian children, Arch Pathol Lab Med 129:1127–1131, 2005.

284. Wieneke JA, Thompson LDR, Heffess CS: Adrenal cortical neoplasms in the pediatric population, Am J Surg Pathol 17:867–881, 2003.

285. Teinturier C, Pauchard MS, Brugières L, et al: Clinical and prognostic aspects of adrenocortical neoplasms in childhood, Med Pediatr Oncol 32:106–111, 1999.

286. Storr HL, Chan LF, Grossman AB, et al: Paediatric Cushing's syndrome: epidemiology, investigation and therapeutic advances, Trends Endocrinol Metab 18:167–174, 2007.

287. Odagiri E, Ishiwatari N, Abe Y, et al: Hypercortisolism and the resistance to dexamethasone suppression during gestation, Endocrinol Jpn 35:685–690, 1988.

288. Lindsay JR, Jonklaas J, Oldfield EH, et al: Cushing's syndrome during pregnancy: personal experience and review of the literature, J Clin Endocrinol Metab 90:3077–3083, 2005.

289. Bianco C, Maqueda E, Rubio JA, et al: Cushing's syndrome during pregnancy secondary to adrenal adenoma: metyrapone treatment and laparoscopic adrenalectomy, J Endocrinol Invest 29:164–167, 2006.

290. Imai T, Kikumori T, Funahashi H, et al: Surgical management of Cushing's syndrome, Biomed & Pharmacother 54(Suppl 1):140–145, 2000.

291. Tung SC, Wang PW, Huang TL, et al: Bilateral adrenocortical adenomas causing ACTH-independent Cushing's syndrome at different periods: a case report and discussion of corticosteroid replacement therapy following bilateral adrenalectomy, J Endocrinol Invest 27:375–379, 2004.

292. Minowada S, Fujimura T, Takahashi N, et al: Computed tomography-guided percutaneous acetic acid injection therapy for functioning adrenocortical adenoma, J Clin Endocrinol Metab 88:5814–5817, 2003.

293. Ueno K, Nakajo M, Miyazono N, et al: Transcatheter adrenal arterial embolization of cortisol-producing tumors, Acta Radiol 40:100–103, 1999.

294. Arima K, Yamakado K, Suzuki R, et al: Image-guided radiofrequency ablation for adrenocortical adenoma with Cushing syndrome: outcomes after mean follow-up of 33 months, Urology 70:407–411, 2007.

295. Disick GIS, Munver R: Adrenal-preserving minimally invasive surgery: update on the current status of laparoscopic partial adrenalectomy, Curr Urol Rep 9:67–72, 2008.

296. Porterfield JR, Thompson GB, Young WF Jr, et al: Surgery for Cushing's syndrome: an historical review and recent ten-year experience, World J Surg 32:659–677, 2008.

297. Porpiglia F, Fiori C, Bovio S, et al: Bilateral adrenalectomy for Cushing's syndrome: a comparison between laparoscopy and open surgery, J Endocrinol Invest 27:654–658, 2004.

298. Doherty GM, Nieman LK, Cutler GB Jr, et al: Time to recovery of the hypothalamic-pituitary-adrenal axis after curative resection of adrenal tumors in patients with Cushing's syndrome, Surgery 108:1085–1090, 1990.

299. Schulick RD, Brennan MF: Long-term survival after complete resection and repeat resection in patients with adrenocortical carcinoma, Ann Surg Oncol 6:719–726, 1999.

300. Andrioli M, Pecori Giraldi F, De Martin M, et al: Therapies for adrenal insufficiency, Exp Opin Ther Patents 17:1323–1329, 2007.

301. Pecori Giraldi F, Cavagnini F: Advances in the medical management of Cushing's syndrome, Expert Opin Pharmacother 9:1–11, 2008.

302. Ojima M, Saitoh M, Itoh N, et al: The effects of o,p'-DDD on adrenal steroidogenesis and hepatic steroid metabolism, Nippon Naibunpi Gakkai Zasshi 61:168–178, 1985.

303. Robinson BG, Hales IB, Henniker AJ, et al: The effect of o,p'-DDD on adrenal steroid replacement therapy requirements, Clin Endocrinol 27:437–444, 1987.

304. Bates SE, Shieh CY, Mickely LA, et al: Mitotane enhances cytotoxicity of chemotherapy in cell lines expression a multidrug resistance gene (mdr-1/P-glycoprotein) which is also expressed by adrenocortical carcinomas, J Clin Endocrinol Metab 73:18–29, 1991.

305. Leiba S, Weinstein R, Shindel B, et al: The protracted effect of op'-DDD in Cushing's disease and its impact on adrenal morphogenesis of young human embryo, Ann Endocrinol (Paris) 50:49–53, 1989.

306. Kasperlik-Zaluska AA: Clinical results of the use of mitotane for adrenocortical carcinoma, Braz J Med Biol Res 33:1191–1196, 2000.

307. Terzolo M, Angeli A, Fassnacht M, et al: Adjuvant mitotane treatment for adrenocortical carcinoma, N Engl J Med 356:2372–2380, 2007.

308. Abiven G, Coste J, Groussin L, et al: Clinical and biological features in the prognosis of adrenocortical cancer: poor outcome of cortisol-secreting tumors in a series of 202 consecutive patients, J Clin Endocrinol Metab 91:2650–2655, 2006.

309. van Slooten H, Moolenaar AJ, van Seters AP, et al: The treatment of adrenocortical carcinoma with o,p'-DDD: prognostic implications of serum level monitoring, Eur J Cancer Clin Oncol 20:47–53, 1984.

310. Berruti A, Ferrero A, Sperone P, et al: Emerging drugs for adrenocortical carcinoma, Expert Opin Emerging Drugs 13:497–509, 2008.

311. Ilias I, Alevizaki M, Phlippou G, et al: Sustained remission of metastatic adrenal carcinoma during long-term administration of low-dose mitotane, J Endocrinol Invest 24:532–535, 2001.

312. Daffara F, De Francia S, Reimondo G, et al: Prospective evaluation of mitotane toxicity in adrenocortical cancer patients treated adjuvantly, Endocr Relat Cancer 15:1043–1053, 2008.

313. Sonino N: The use of ketoconazole as an inhibitor of steroid production, N Engl J Med 317:812–818, 1987.

314. Castinetti F, Morange I, Jaquet P, et al: Ketoconazole revisited: a preoperative or postoperative treatment in Cushing's disease, Eur J Endocrinol 158:91–99, 2008.

315. Engelhardt D, Weber MM: Therapy of Cushing's syndrome with steroid biosynthesis inhibitors, J Steroid Biochem Mol Biol 49:261–267, 1994.

316. Contreras P, Rojas A, Biagini L, et al: Regression of metastatic adrenal carcinoma during palliative ketoconazole treatment, Lancet II:151–152, 1985.

317. Riedl M, Maier C, Zettinig G, et al: Long term control of hypercortisolism with fluconazole: case report and in vitro studies, Eur J Endocrinol 154:519–524, 2006.

318. Gower DB: Modifiers of steroid-hormone metabolism: a review of their chemistry, biochemistry and clinical applications, J Steroid Biochem 5:501–523, 1974.

319. Fassnacht M, Hahner S, Beuschlein F, et al: New mechanisms of adrenostatic compounds in a human adrenocortical cancer cell line, Eur J Clin Invest 30:76–82, 2000.

320. Verhelst JA, Trainer PJ, Howlett TA, et al: Short and long-term responses to metyrapone in the medical management of 91 patients with Cushing's syndrome, Clin Endocrinol 35:169–178, 1991.

321. Obinata D, Yamaguchi K, Hirano D, et al: Preoperative management of Cushing's syndrome with metyrapone for severe psychiatric disturbances, Int J Urol 15:361–362, 2008.

322. Connell JMC, Cordiner J, Davies DL, et al: Pregnancy complicated by Cushing's syndrome: potential hazard of metyrapone therapy. Case report, Br J Obstet Gynaecol 92:1192–1195, 1985.

323. Gillis D, Rösler A, Hannon TS, et al: Prolonged remission of severe Cushing syndrome without adrenalectomy in an infant with McCune-Albright syndrome, J Pediatr 152:882–884, 2008.

324. Schteingart DE, Cash R, Conn JW: Aminoglutethimide and metastatic adrenal cancer. Maintained reversal (six months) of Cushing's syndrome, JAMA 198:1007–1010, 1966.

325. Johanssen S, Allolio B: Mifepristone (RU 486) in Cushing's syndrome, Eur J Endocrinol 157:561–569, 2007.

Chapter 8

DEFECTS OF ADRENAL STEROIDOGENESIS

MICHAEL P. WAJNRAJCH and MARIA I. NEW

The human adrenal gland is composed of the cortex and the medulla. The medulla produces bioamines, and the adrenal cortex secretes several classes of steroids (corticosteroids). The adrenal cortex can be considered to be made up of three distinct subunits, each having a characteristic steroid profile. The outermost unit, the zona glomerulosa, produces mineralocorticoids, principally aldosterone (a salt-retaining hormone), which serve to maintain sodium and fluid balance. Glucocorticoids, primarily cortisol, arise from the central zona fasciculata and maintain glucose homeostasis and vascular integrity. The innermost subunit, the zona reticularis, secretes sex steroids (androgens). Disorders of adrenal steroidogenesis may involve overproduction, underproduction, or both the simultaneous overproduction and underproduction of corticosteroids (Fig. 8-1). In this chapter, the following conditions are discussed:

1. Disorders of P450c21 resulting in the 21-hydroxylase deficiency form of congenital adrenal hyperplasia (CAH) (salt-wasting, simple virilizing, and nonclassic forms)
2. Disorders of P450c11, including (a) 11β-hydroxylase deficiency form of CAH (classic and nonclassic forms), (b) corticosterone methyl oxidase (CMO) deficiency types I and II, (c) dexamethasone-suppressible hyperaldosteronism
3. 3β-Hydroxysteroid dehydrogenase (3β-HSD) deficiency form of CAH (classic and nonclassic forms)
4. Disorders of P450c17 activity, including (a) isolated 17α-hydroxylase deficiency, (b) isolated 17,20-lyase deficiency, and (c) combined 17α-hydroxylase deficiency/17,20-lyase deficiency
5. Lipoid CAH: P450scc deficiency and steroidogenic acute response (StAR) deficiency
6. Adrenal failure with male-limited gonadal failure and XY gender reversal: steroidogenic factor-1 deficiency

A summary of the clinical, hormonal, and genetic features of these steroidogenic defects appears in Table 8-1.

The most common adrenal steroidogenic defects are those related to cortisol production; they are collectively referred to as the CAHs. These defects generally are transmitted as autosomal recessive traits, and the genetic errors that cause them have been described. Loss of the negative feedback inhibition of the hypothalamic-pituitary-adrenal (HPA) axis by cortisol induces

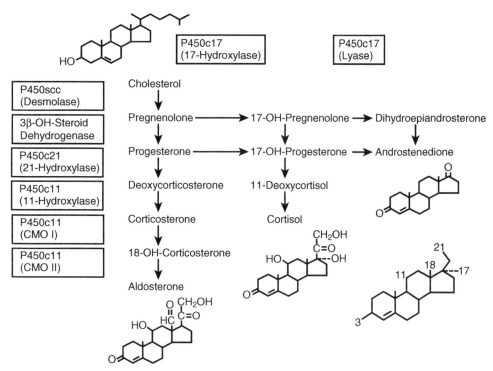

FIGURE 8-1. Adrenal steroidogenesis. Biosynthetic pathways from cholesterol to mineralocorticoids (aldosterone), glucocorticoids (cortisol), and androgens (androstenedione) are shown and the cellular locations of enzyme activities indicated. *CMO,* Corticosterone methyl oxidase; *OH,* hydroxylase. (From White PC, New MI, Dupont B: Medical progress: congenital adrenal hyperplasia, N Engl J Med 316:1519–1524, 1987. © 1987, Massachusetts Medical Society.)

oversecretion of adrenocorticotropic hormone (ACTH) by the anterior pituitary, resulting in adrenal hyperplasia. Specific forms of CAH are identified by the abnormal patterns of glucocorticoid, mineralocorticoid, and sex steroid secretion and by accompanying clinical manifestations, including abnormal fetal genital development, disturbances in sodium homeostasis and blood pressure regulation, and the postnatal consequences of sex steroid imbalance affecting somatic growth and fertility. Molecular genetic analysis is used to confirm the diagnosis. Lifelong, carefully monitored treatment with glucocorticoids and salt-retaining steroids can afford many patients with CAH relatively normal lives despite their potentially life-threatening metabolic defects. However, it is not yet possible to always ensure normal hormonal levels throughout the day, ultimate normal stature, and normal fertility.

Distinction is made between classic forms of disease, defined by significantly reduced enzyme activity manifesting clinically at birth, and nonclassic forms, in which the enzyme defect is less severe and symptoms are not present at birth, and when they do appear are generally milder. The classification of CAH subtypes has significant clinical implications for treatment and prenatal diagnosis, but it should be appreciated that patients exist on a clinical continuum rather than within absolute, discrete, easily defined conditions. Approximately 90% to 95% of cases of classic CAH are due to 21-hydroxylase deficiency,[1] whereas defects in the enzymes 11β-hydroxylase and 3β-HSD account for almost all the rest. 17α-Hydroxylase deficiency and lipoid CAH are rare causes of CAH.

The 21-hydroxylase and 11β-hydroxylase deficiencies, which occur late in cortisol synthesis, cause shunting of accumulated precursor steroids into pathways of androgen biosynthesis, which do not require these enzymes. Because the external genitalia of the fetus are sensitive to androgens,[2] excess androgen

secretion by the adrenal masculinizes the female genitalia, causing genital ambiguity in utero in affected females, but no genital alterations in affected males. Postnatal hyperandrogenism affects both genders.

Inefficient/inadequate cortisol production is common to all forms of CAH; imbalances in salt metabolism and fluid volume are part of what differentiates 21-hydroxylase from 11β-hydroxylase deficiency. In 21-hydroxylase deficiency, inadequate aldosterone synthesis leads to salt wasting and hypovolemia, whereas in 11β-hydroxylase deficiency, an excess of mineralocorticoids (e.g., deoxycorticosterone [DOC]) causes expanded fluid volume and hypertension. The nonclassic forms of 21-hydroxylase and 11β-hydroxylase deficiency do not cause severe hypertension or masculinized genitalia in newborn females.

In the 3β-HSD defect, poor conversion of Δ^5 steroids (pregnenolone, 17-hydroxypregnenolone, and dehydroepiandrosterone [DHEA]) to Δ^4 steroids (progesterone, 17-hydroxyprogesterone [17-OHP], and androstenedione) occurs. The Δ^5 steroid precursors are relatively inactive, but the defective cortisol and aldosterone synthesis causes profound salt wasting. Whereas the lack of potent Δ^4 androgens produces hypovirilization in the male, enormously high levels of relatively inactive Δ^5 androgens, which are converted peripherally to active Δ^4 steroids, may cause masculinization of external genitalia in females.

The nonclassic forms of 21-hydroxylase and 11β-hydroxylase deficiencies may be extremely common (and treatable) causes of hyperandrogenism.[3-8]

In 17α-hydroxylase/17,20-lyase deficiency, blocked production both of 17α-hydroxy (glucocorticoid) and C_{19}/C_{18} (sex) steroids causes pseudohermaphroditism in males and sexual infantilism in females. Shunting of 17α-hydroxylase precursor steroids into the 17-deoxy pathway produces excess mineralo-

Table 8-1. Summary of the Clinical, Hormonal, and Genetic Features of Steroidogenic Defects

Condition	Onset	Abnormality	Genitalia	Mineralocorticoid Effect	Typical Features	Gene
Lipoid CAH	Congenital	StAR Protein	Female, with no sexual development	Salt wasting	All steroid products low	StAR 8p11.2
Lipoid CAH	Congenital	P450scc	Female, with no sexual development	Salt wasting	All steroid products low	CYP11A 15q23-24
Adrenal failure with male-limited gonadal failure and XY sex reversal	Congenital	SF1	Male-limited gonadal failure and XY sex reversal with persistence of müllerian structures	Salt wasting	All steroid products low	NR5A1 9q33
3β-HSD deficiency, classic	Congenital	3β-HSD	Females virilized, males hypovirilized	Salt wasting	Elevated DHEA, 17-pregnenolone, low androstenedione, testosterone, elevated K, low Na, CO_2	HSD3B2 1p13.1
3β-HSD deficiency, nonclassic	Postnatal	3β-HSD	Normal genitalia with mild to moderate hyperandrogenism postnatally	None	Elevated DHEA, 17-pregnenolone, low androstenedione, testosterone	—
17α-OH deficiency	Congenital	P450c17	Normal sexual development	Hyperkalemic low-renin hypertension	Absent androgens and estrogen, elevated DOC, corticosterone	CYP17 10q24.3
17,20-Lyase deficiency	Congenital	P450c17	Infantile female, with no sexual development/ ambiguous	None	Decreased androgens and estrogens	CYP17 10q24.3
Combined 17α-OH/17,20-lyase deficiency	Congenital	P450c17	Infantile female, with no sexual development/ ambiguous	Hyperkalemic low-renin hypertension	Decreased androgens and estrogens	CYP17 10q24.3
Combined 17α-OH/17,20-lyase deficiency	Postnatal	P450c17	Infertility	None	Decreased follicular estradiol and increased progesterone	CYP17 10q24.3
Classic 21-OH deficiency, salt wasting	Congenital	P450c21	Females prenatally virilized, males unchanged	Salt wasting	Elevated 17-OHP, DHEA, and androstenedione, elevated K, low Na, CO_2	CYP21 6p21.3
Classic 21-OH deficiency, simple virilizing	Congenital	P450c21	Females prenatally virilized, males unchanged	None	Elevated 17-OHP, DHEA, and androstenedione, normal electrolytes	CYP21 6p21.3
Nonclassic 21-OH deficiency	Postnatal	P450c21	All with normal genitalia at birth, hyperandrogenism postnatally	None	Elevated 17-OHP, DHEA, and androstenedione on ACTH stimulation	CYP21 6p21.3
Classic CAH 11β-deficiency	Congenital	P450c11B1	Females virilized, males unchanged	Low-renin hypertension	Elevated DOC, 11-deoxycortisol (S) and androgens, low K, elevated Na, CO_2	CYP11B1 8q24.3
Nonclassic CAH 11β-deficiency	Postnatal	P450c11B1	All with normal genitalia at birth, hyperandrogenism postnatally	Normal	Elevated 11-deoxycortisol ± DOC, elevated androgens	CYP11B1 8q24.3
CMO I deficiency	Congenital	P450c11B2	All normal	Severe salt wasting	No aldosterone, low-normal 18-OH-corticosterone, elevated K, low Na, CO_2	CYP11B2 8q24.3
CMO II deficiency	Congenital	P450c11B2	All normal	Mild salt wasting, especially in infancy with spontaneous resolution	Low-normal aldosterone, very elevated 18-OH-corticosterone, elevated K, low Na, CO_2	CYP11B2 8q24.3
Dexamethasone suppressible hyperaldosteronism	Congenital	Chimeric P450c11B1/	All normal	Low-renin hypertension	Elevated aldosterone, elevated Na, CO_2	CYP11B1/ CYP11B2

CAH, Congenital adrenal hyperplasia; CMO, corticosterone methyl oxidase; DHEA, dehydroepiandrosterone; DOC, deoxycorticosterone; 3β-HSD, 3β-hydroxysteroid dehydrogenase; OH, hydroxylase; 17-OHP, 17-hydroxyprogesterone.

corticoids (e.g., DOC) and hypertension. Isolated 17α-hydroxylase deficiency prevents the conversion of mineralocorticoids to glucocorticoids, whereas isolated 17,20-lyase deficiency is a variant of 17α-hydroxylase deficiency in which only androgen synthesis is disturbed, and glucocorticoid and mineralocorticoid levels are relatively unaffected.

Lipoid CAH manifests as the inability to produce any of the steroid products from the primary precursor cholesterol. Accordingly, affected individuals are aldosterone, cortisol, and sex steroid deficient. All affected individuals present as phenotypic females, regardless of genetic gender.

History

The observation of hyperplastic adrenal glands in association with internal female gonads and ductal structures in a phenotypic male appeared in the anatomic literature in 1865 with

De Crecchio's[9] description of his autopsy of a Neapolitan pseudohermaphrodite. Fibiger,[10] Apert,[11] and Gallais[12] amassed case histories involving precocious puberty, hirsutism, pseudohermaphroditism, and obesity in the early 1900s, and attempted to classify them. The term *adrenogenital syndrome* was used for many years to describe conditions characterized by elevated adrenal androgens due to virilizing adrenal tumors or to CAH.

The first comprehensive view of CAH was based on the biochemical discoveries of the 1940s and 1950s.[13] Among the pioneers who subsequently characterized the variants of CAH in the late 1950s and early 1960s were Bongiovanni,[14,15] Eberlein and Bongiovanni,[16] Prader and Siebenmann,[17] Biglieri and colleagues,[18] and New.[19] CAH now is more appropriately referred to by the names of the specific enzyme deficiencies that characterize it.

In 1977, the discovery of the association between the well-studied human leukocyte antigens (HLAs) and the 21-hydroxylase trait opened a window to a new form of definition of CAH through molecular genetics.[20] Since the gene responsible for classic 21-hydroxylase deficiency (found within the HLA complex) was isolated in 1984,[21] knowledge of the specific mutations that cause the different forms of CAH has grown rapidly, much the way that biochemical discoveries of the earlier era led to construction of the scheme for steroidogenesis. Mutations in the genes encoding the steroidogenic enzymes have been confirmed as the basis for all the CAHs. Additionally, steroidogenic defects may be due to mutations in transcription factors or other cofactors (e.g., StAR protein).[22]

Evidence is accumulating that the correlation between the clinical expression of endocrine disease and mutations of the primary structural gene is not perfect. Thus, the role of the clinician in ascertaining physiologic facts remains central to the prospect of future growth in our understanding of the pathogenesis of CAH and the basis for its treatment.

Disorders of 21-Hydroxylase

Three expressions of 21-hydroxylase deficiency have been clinically identified: classic simple virilizing with manifestations of excess androgen secretion; classic salt wasting, which consists of aldosterone deficiency in addition to excess androgen secretion due to the 21-hydroxylase defect in the parallel mineralocorticoid pathway in the zona glomerulosa; and nonclassic, a less severe hyperandrogenic, variably expressed, and allelically distinct form of the disease, in which affected males and females have unambiguous genitalia at birth.

The result of 21-hydroxylase deficiency is that 17-OHP is not converted to 11-deoxycortisol (compound S) in the pathway of cortisol synthesis, resulting in (1) a deficiency of the essential glucocorticoid cortisol (compound F) and (2) overproduction and accumulation of cortisol precursors proximal to the 21-hydroxylation step (17-OHP, progesterone, 17-hydroxypregnenolone, and pregnenolone) as a result of the loss of normal feedback regulation on the hypothalamus and pituitary. The 17-hydroxylated precursors are shunted into the androgen synthesis pathway. Mutations in the 21-hydroxylase enzyme male may also impair aldosterone synthesis, resulting in the salt-wasting form of CAH.

EPIDEMIOLOGY AND POPULATION GENETICS

Results of newborn screening in a number of localities around the world[23-27] yield a worldwide incidence of classic 21-hydroxylase deficiency of approximately 1 in 14,500 live births,

ranging from 1 in 8586[28] to 23,000.[29] It has been estimated that 75% have the salt-wasting phenotype.[30] Applying the Hardy-Weinberg formula for a population at equilibrium gives a computed heterozygote frequency for classic 21-hydroxylase deficiency of 1 in 61 persons. In areas where patient retesting is difficult/inefficient, it may be necessary to lower the treatment threshold to save lives of affected individuals who die before the diagnosis is confirmed and treatment is started.[31]

Nonclassic 21-hydroxylase deficiency, one of the most common autosomal recessive diseases, is more frequent than cystic fibrosis. The frequency is ethnic specific, as first determined by Speiser and colleagues.[32] Incidences are 1 in 27 Ashkenazi Jews, 1 in 40 Hispanics, 1 in 50 Yugoslavs, 1 in 300 Italians, and 1 in 100 in a heterogeneous New York population.[32-34] In an attempt to determine an earliest date for the appearance within the Ashkenazi Jewish population of a founder mutation, DNA analysis was undertaken for representative individuals from the Roman Jewish ghetto, a community already established by the time of the second Diaspora (70 CE). No evidence was seen in Roman Jews of the B14-related nonclassic 21-hydroxylase deficiency mutation, thus suggesting a date after 70 CE for the appearance of this mutation among Ashkenazi Jews.[35] Further genetic characterization of this population in terms of its affinity to the general European population and to other Jewish groups continues.[36] The nonclassic 21-hydroxylase deficiency mutation can be dated to between 70 CE and the second millennium, based on the significantly higher frequency observed in Ashkenazi Jews compared with Sephardic Jews.

CLASSIC 21-HYDROXYLASE DEFICIENCY
Effects of Hyperandrogenism
External Genitalia

Adrenocortical cell differentiation occurs early in embryogenesis, and although the biochemical schedule of steroid synthesis has not been completely elucidated, it is clear that genital development in the fetus takes place in the setting of active fetal adrenal steroid synthesis. Because differentiation of the external genitalia is sensitive to androgen, excess adrenal androgen produces genital ambiguity in females affected by classic 21-hydroxylase deficiency. In utero masculinization consists of mild to pronounced clitoral enlargement, varying degrees of labioscrotal fusion, and a urogenital sinus with the type and degree of virilization proportional to the onset of hyperandrogenism (Figs. 8-2 and 8-3). The 21-hydroxylase form of CAH is the most common

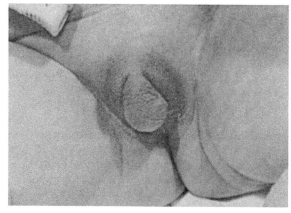

FIGURE 8-2. Ambiguous genitalia in a newborn female with congenital adrenal hyperplasia due to 21-hydroxylase deficiency. Note the enlarged clitoris, the single orifice on the perineum, and scrotalization of the labia majora. (Modified from New MI, Levine LS: Congenital adrenal hyperplasia. In Harris H, Hirschhorn K [eds]: Advances in Human Genetics, vol 4. New York, Plenum, 1973, pp 251–326.)

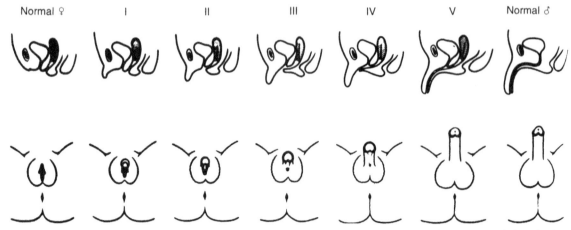

FIGURE 8-3. Prader characterization of the range of genital malformations found in females with classic 21-hydroxylase deficiency. In type I, the only abnormality is enlargement of the clitoris; in type II, partial labioscrotal fusion occurs; in type III, a funnel-shaped urogenital sinus is seen at the posterior end of a small vulva; in type IV, a very small urogenital sinus is found at the base of an enlarged phallus; and in type V, a penile urethra is evident. (From Prader A: Die Haufigkeit der Kongenitalen Adrenogenitalen Syndromes, Helv Paediatr Acta 13:5, 1958.)

cause of genital ambiguity in females. Every phenotypic male with hypospadias and bilateral cryptorchidism should be considered a female with CAH and should be evaluated immediately for classic 21-hydroxylase deficiency.

Although differentiation of male genitalia in utero is not affected, the genitalia of infants of both genders undergo androgen-stimulated growth postnatally. High testosterone levels of adrenal origin cause gonadotropin suppression, which results in the characteristic finding in older boys of a large penis and small testes. Hyperpigmentation of the genitalia of both males and females can also result from high ACTH secretion.

Internal Genitalia

Gonadal differentiation and internal genital morphogenesis are not affected by the enzyme abnormalities of classic steroid 21-hydroxylase deficiency. Because there is no anomalous secretion of antimüllerian hormone (AMH), which is synthesized by the Sertoli cells of the fetal testis, müllerian duct development in the female proceeds normally into the uterus and fallopian tubes.[37] Thus, normal child-bearing capacity exists in females. Wolffian duct stabilization and differentiation normally take place in the context of local testosterone levels in the male, and this process appears to be unaffected by elevated systemic prenatal adrenal androgens.

Growth

Postnatal somatic growth in both genders is markedly affected by the chronic hyperandrogenism of untreated 21-hydroxylase deficiency. High levels of androgens cause accelerated growth in early childhood, producing an unusually tall and often quite muscular child, an "infant Hercules" (Fig. 8-4). This early growth spurt, however, is followed by premature epiphyseal maturation and closure, resulting in a final height that is short relative to that expected on the basis of midparental target height. Exposure to glucocorticoids used in replacement therapy at doses that may exceed the physiologic requirement has been postulated to be another important factor in the poor growth of these patients.[38]

We have previously shown that final height is one of the features of CAH least amenable to glucocorticoid replacement therapy.[39] Analysis of 47 patients with classic CAH separated into two groups defined by the degree of hormonal control failed to

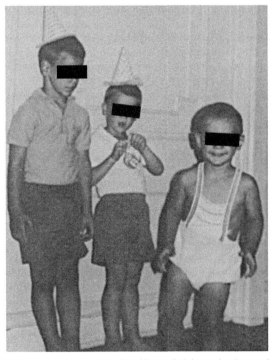

FIGURE 8-4. Untreated congenital adrenal hyperplasia in two brothers: a 4-year-old on the left and a 2-year-old on the right. In the center is their normal 6-year-old brother. (Modified from New MI, Levine LS: Congenital adrenal hyperplasia. In Harris H, Hirschhorn K [eds]: Advances in Human Genetics, vol 4. New York, Plenum, 1973, pp 251–326.)

show a significant difference in height outcome with the use of standard treatment.[40] A pilot study combining recombinant human growth hormone with a gonadotropin-releasing hormone superagonist to improve final height in those patients with CAH with advanced skeletal maturation and poor predicted final adult height demonstrated that this significantly improved final adult height in children with CAH.[41]

Hair and Skin Gland Abnormalities

Facial, axillary, and pubic hair often appears very early; pubarche sometimes occurs in infancy. Adult body odor in children, temporal alopecia, and severe acne are other typical features that are reversible with treatment.

Bone Health

Bone mineral density (BMD) is affected by the competing actions of androgen excess (from undertreatment) and glucocorticoid excess (from overtreatment), which can occur in patients simultaneously. The relative extent of undertreatment and overtreatment determines the net effect on BMD. Two studies found that BMD was lower in young adults with CAH than in controls[42,43]; one of these studies showed a trend toward increased fracture rate of wrist and vertebrae in young women with CAH.[43] Dosing regimens, beginning in the young adult years, clearly must take bone health into consideration.

Fertility

Excess adrenal sex steroids inhibit the pubertal changes in gonadotropin secretion directed by the hypothalamic-pituitary axis, probably via a negative feedback effect at the hypothalamus or the pituitary. This inhibition is reversible by suppression of adrenal androgen production. In most untreated or poorly treated adolescent girls and in some adolescent boys, spontaneous pubertal development does not occur until proper glucocorticoid treatment is instituted. Menstrual irregularity and secondary or even primary amenorrhea with or without hirsutism can occur in untreated and poorly controlled women. An association of virilizing CAH with polycystic ovary syndrome has also been noted.[44,45] Reproductive capacity in females with classic CAH is reduced. Meyer-Bahlburg[46] compared the fertility of women with different forms of classic 21-hydroxylase deficiency. In those women with an adequate introitus and heterosexual activity, he found that fertility was approximately 60% with the simple virilizing form (n = 25), whereas in the salt-wasting form (n = 15), fertility was only 7%.

Traditionally, well-treated patients were thought to have the onset of puberty occur at the expected chronologic age; however, a recent analysis suggests that puberty does in fact occur early than expected—and height is compromised—especially in salt-wasting males.[47] The gonadotropin response to gonadotropin-releasing hormone (gonadotropin-releasing hormone or luteinizing hormone-releasing hormone) is appropriate for age in well-controlled prepubertal and pubertal female patients unless ovarian disease is present. Poor control of the disease in males with classic CAH has been associated with small testes and azoospermia. However, cases of normal testicular maturation and spermatogenesis and fertility in untreated men have been reported.[48] Well-treated males are normally fertile and have normal pubertal development, spermatogenesis, and testicular function. Later in life, males may develop nodular hyperplasia of adrenal rest tissue, causing enlargement of the testes, which may respond to high-dose glucocorticoid treatment. With the use of ultrasonography, several studies have identified testicular "tumors" in many or even most adolescent and adult male patients with CAH (ages 16 to 40 years).[49,50] Tumors ranged in size from 0.2 to 4.0 cm, and in many of these patients, the tumors were palpable. The degree of hormonal control did not correlate with the presence of tumor; indeed, many adequately or even overtreated subjects had identifiable tumors. Genotype was predictive of tumor size, with the most severe mutations correlating with the largest tumors.[49] Leydig cell function also was commonly impaired in these subjects.[50] The adrenal glands of subjects with mutations in the 21-hydroxylase gene, both homozygous and heterozygous, are known to be larger than those of controls. This increased surface area has been associated with an increased risk of adrenal tumor formation, and indeed adrenal "incidentalomas" are more common in these groups.[51] However, a retrospective analysis of "true" adrenal tumors failed to demonstrate an increased incidence of mutations, either germline or somatic.[52]

SALT WASTING

Salt wasting is characterized by hyponatremia, hyperkalemia, metabolic acidosis, inappropriate sodium excretion in the urine, and low serum aldosterone with concomitantly high plasma renin activity (PRA).

Salt wasting results from inadequate secretion of salt-retaining steroids, especially aldosterone. In addition, hormone precursors elevated in 21-hydroxylase deficiency may act as mineralocorticoid antagonists (e.g., 17-hydroxyprogesterone). Newborns are especially prone to the development of a salt-wasting crisis because the sodium-conserving mechanism of their renal tubules is only marginally competent. The adrenal medulla of patients with CAH may be incompletely formed in some patients. Merke and coworkers[53] noted that the epinephrine and metanephrine concentrations of subjects manifesting a salt-wasting crisis were approximately 50% of those of controls; pathologic evaluation of adrenal medullary tissue (removed during adrenalectomy) demonstrated depletion of secretory vesicles.

A single enzyme is responsible for 21-hydroxylation in both the zona fasciculata and the zona glomerulosa. The pathogenetic difference between salt wasting and simple virilizing 21-hydroxylase deficiency may simply be the result of a quantitative difference in enzyme activity caused by conformational changes induced by the specific mutations. In vitro expression studies show that as little as 1% of normal activity of 21-hydroxylase allows adequate aldosterone synthesis to prevent significant salt wasting.[54,55] The issue is complicated by the occasional finding of discordance for salt-wasting expression among siblings with identical mutations in their inherited 21-hydroxylase genes, and by the observed improvement in salt wasting in some individuals over time.[48,56-58] In one case, a girl born with male genitalia and salt wasting, presumably with severe enzyme deficiency, was no longer a salt waster by age 4. Another important case finding was that of a girl with a homozygous deletion of the 21-hydroxylase gene and a history of multiple salt-wasting crises in infancy, who discontinued her therapy in adolescence and was found at that time to be secreting aldosterone.[59]

Salt-Wasting Crisis

Infants with classic CAH of both genders are at risk for hypovolemic and hypoglycemic adrenal crises, typically occurring within the first 4 to 6 weeks of life. Undiagnosed males who lack the genital ambiguity that usually calls attention to the condition in a newborn female are at added risk for shock and death, as evidenced by the higher female-to-male ratio of salt-wasting adults. In females, the degree of genital ambiguity in a newborn does not indicate the likelihood of the potential for salt wasting. Thus, surveillance of infants of both genders in the newborn period for incipient adrenal crisis is essential, and close surveillance should continue after discharge from the hospital. Infants should remain in the hospital after birth for approximately 7 days or until the aldosterone/sodium balance status has been established, although it should be stressed that the first salt-wasting crisis may not occur for several months. In older children and adults, acute adrenal insufficiency can be precipitated by physical exertion or emotional stress, undertreatment, or noncompliance with therapy, or can occur as a result of immunization, infection, trauma, or surgery. The salt-wasting crisis of the newborn period associated with CAH often is confused with pyloric stenosis, which may present at the same age and also often manifests as an ill-appearing newborn with vomiting and dehydration. The salt-wasting crisis associated with CAH (manifesting with hyponatremia, hyperkalemia, and metabolic acidosis) should be differentiated immediately from that of pyloric stenosis (hypokalemia, hypochloremia, and metabolic alkalosis) with the use of routine biochemical tests.

NONCLASSIC 21-HYDROXYLASE DEFICIENCY

Nonclassic 21-hydroxylase deficiency is distinguished from the classic form symptomatically by its age at onset and biochemically by its less severe impairment of steroid 21-hydroxylation; because of these two factors, it does not result in ambiguous genitalia in the newborn female. It often initially manifests just before the age of normal puberty, although it may present at any age after birth. Patients may be homozygous for a mild genetic defect or may have compound heterozygotes for one severe mutation and one mild mutation. Nonclassic 21-hydroxylase deficiency was first defined in the course of family studies of patients with classic CAH. Family members who should have been carriers for 21-hydroxylase deficiency were found to have overt hormonal disturbances that were associated with distinct alleles at the 21-hydroxylase locus. These alleles were determined to be in linkage disequilibrium with the HLA locus on chromosome 6. It thus was found through these studies that the gene locus for 21-hydroxylase lies between HLA-B and HLA-DR.[60]

In addition to linkage of the 21-hydroxylase locus with the neighboring HLA-B and HLA-DR antigen loci, 21-hydroxylase deficiency alleles are found in linkage disequilibrium with other HLA genes or haplotypic combinations that may include specific alleles of the neighboring genes C4A and C4B encoding the fourth component of serum complement.[61] The two most prominent such cases are linkage disequilibrium of the extended haplotype HLA-A3,Bw47,DR7 with the classic salt-wasting form, and HLA-B14,DR1 with nonclassic 21-hydroxylase deficiency.[62]

Clinical Features

The clinical features of nonclassic 21-hydroxylase deficiency range widely, begin at any age, and commonly wax and wane over time. Although genital ambiguity in the newborn period is never a feature of this disorder, the appearance of any of the other signs and symptoms of hyperandrogenism can prompt the patient to seek medical attention, or patients may be identified through family or population screening. Individuals commonly present just before the time of expected pubarche. Underlying biochemical abnormalities are always demonstrable at any age by ACTH stimulation testing, regardless of whether symptoms are evident.[63]

Nonclassic 21-hydroxylase deficiency can result in the premature development of pubic hair (pubarche), which may occur as early as 6 months of age.[64] In one study, nonclassic 21-hydroxylase deficiency was found in 30% of children with premature pubarche,[65] whereas a lower prevalence was reported by another group.[66] Severe cystic acne refractory to oral antibiotics

and retinoic acid has been associated with nonclassic 21-hydroxylase deficiency by some.[67,68] In one young woman, male pattern alopecia was the sole presenting symptom. Menarche in females can be normal or delayed, and secondary amenorrhea or oligomenorrhea is frequent. Final height, as in classic 21-hydroxylase deficiency, is less than predicted based on the midparental target height and linear growth percentiles, even though excess androgen secretion may not have been apparent.[40,50]

A number of women with polycystic ovary disease have been found on ACTH testing to have a primary adrenal defect, for example, nonclassic 21-hydroxylase deficiency, 3β-HSD deficiency, or 11β-hydroxylase deficiency.[45,69-72] The reported prevalence of nonclassic 21-hydroxylase deficiency as a cause of these endocrine symptoms in women ranges from 1.2% to 30%. The scope of the range may relate to differences in the ethnic makeup of the groups studied. Women heterozygous for a 21-hydroxylase gene mutation have been shown to have higher free testosterone levels than controls (i.e., hyperandrogenemia), but, it is important to note, not an increased incidence of hyperandrogenism.[73]

In boys, presenting signs include early beard growth, pubarche, acne, and an accelerated growth spurt. In men, signs of androgen excess are difficult to perceive, and the manifestations of adrenal androgen excess may be limited to short stature or oligospermia and diminished fertility from adrenal sex steroid–induced gonadal suppression.

Fertility in Nonclassic 21-Hydroxylase Deficiency

It has been recognized for 30 years that infertility in women may be reversed by glucocorticoid therapy. In one report, five patients with irregular menses and high 17-keto(oxo)steroids (urinary androgen metabolites) resumed regular menses and demonstrated adequate suppression of 17-ketosteroids and pregnanetriol (a urinary metabolite of 17-OHP) within 2 months after beginning therapy with glucocorticoids alone, suggesting the presence of an adrenal 21-hydroxylating defect.[74] In another report of 18 infertile women with acne and/or facial hirsutism and hormonal criteria consistent with 21-hydroxylase deficiency, seven conceived shortly after initiating prednisone treatment; an additional four women conceived within 2 months of the addition of clomiphene to the prednisone.[75] Hormonal profiles after initiation of therapy were not reported in this study. As mentioned earlier, oligospermia and subfertility have been reported in men with nonclassic 21-hydroxylase deficiency.[76] We recommend screening for nonclassic 21-hydroxylase deficiency during every evaluation for infertility.

Molecular Genetics

The molecular genetics basis of 21-hydroxylase deficiency has been studied extensively. The 21-hydroxylase enzyme is a microsomal cytochrome P-450 enzyme termed P450c21. The structural genes encoding P450c21, CYP21, and a pseudogene, CYP21P, are located on chromosome 6p21.3, adjacent to the genes C4B and C4A, encoding the two isoforms of the fourth component of serum complement in the class III region of the HLA complex.[77,78] CYP21 and CYP21P each contains 10 exons. Their nucleotide sequences are 98% identical in exons and approximately 96% identical in introns.[79]

Many of the mutations known to cause 21-hydroxylase deficiency are apparently the result of either of two types of recombination between CYP21 and CYP21P: (1) chromatid misalignment and unequal crossing over, resulting in large-scale DNA deletions, and (2) gene conversion events that result in the transfer to CYP21 of smaller scale deleterious mutations normally present in the *CYP21P* pseudogene. Seven of the eight possible exonic differences between CYP21 and CYP21P have been observed and confirmed to be causative of 21-hydroxylase deficiency. At least 25 mutations causing 21-hydroxylase deficiency have been identified; one single-nucleotide mutation altering the splicing of an intron is particularly common and is associated with both simple virilizing and salt-wasting phenotypes (Fig. 8-5). Deletions and gene conversion events may be common findings in 21-OHD, owing to the chromosomal arrangement of the gene and pseudogene (i.e., homologous genes in a tandem array),[80,81] and to the presence of multiple chi-like sequences.[82]

Correlation of Genotype With Phenotype

In general, the functional consequence of each DNA alteration corresponds with the clinical severity of the inherited disease: total deletion of the functional gene, stop codon (nonsense) mutations, frameshifts, and several amino acid substitutions (missense mutations) have been shown to result in salt-wasting classic alleles; one nonconservative amino acid substitution has been associated exclusively with simple virilizing disease, and a single conservative amino acid substitution (*V281L*) is the mutation associated with the HLA-B14,DR1 haplotype found so frequently in nonclassic disease.[83]

However, comparison of the clinical characteristics and molecular genetics data in 532 affected individuals at one site reveals that the genotype correctly predicted the phenotype in 89% of cases, a high figure but significantly shy of the 100% that might be expected. Rocha et al.[84] suggested that much of the variability in the external virilization of CAH women is due to the genotype (i.e., number of CAG repeats) of the androgen receptor.[84] This analysis underlines the need for careful ongoing clinical assessment of all persons affected by 21-hydroxylase deficiency.

Diagnosis

The diagnosis of steroidogenic enzyme defects in CAH is made on the basis of (1) clinical findings, (2) biochemical and hormonal values, and (3) molecular genetics analysis of mutations. Hormonal values will establish the diagnosis of an enzyme defect by demonstrating an increased precursor-to-product ratio. The substrate of the enzyme will be markedly increased, whereas the product will be normal or slightly decreased. Molecular genetic analysis of the DNA will demonstrate the specific mutations.

Biochemical Characterization

In classic CAH, baseline serum cortisol levels are at the lower limits of detection or in the low to normal range. Baseline concentrations of serum 17-OHP and adrenal androgens are elevated, with serum 17-OHP levels often several hundred times normal.[85] In nonclassically affected persons, because of pulsatile and diurnal variations in 17-OHP secretion, midmorning and afternoon concentrations may be normal.[86] Of all single measurements, early morning measurement of serum 17-OHP concentration is the most likely to show an elevation. However, we caution against relying on baseline 17-OHP levels to exclude nonclassic 21-hydroxylase deficiency; mild defects may be only minimally elevated, especially in the afternoon, leading to many false-negative diagnoses.

The standard diagnostic procedure for diagnosing all forms of CAH is the 60 minute (synthetic) ACTH stimulation test. At 08:00 hours, when cortisol secretion is at its normal diurnal peak, blood is drawn before and then 60 minutes after intravenous injection of a 0.25 mg bolus of ACTH. A nomogram (Fig. 8-6) that relates baseline to ACTH-stimulated serum concentra-

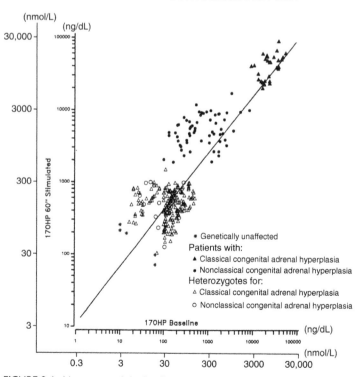

FIGURE 8-6. Nomogram relating baseline to adrenocorticotropic hormone–stimulated serum concentrations of 17-hydroxyprogesterone. Scales are logarithmic. The regression line shown is for all data points. Data points cluster as shown into three nonoverlapping groups: classic (congenital adrenal hyperplasia) and nonclassic forms of 21-hydroxylase deficiency are readily distinguished from each other and from heterozygote/unaffected. Distinguishing unaffected from heterozygote responses is difficult.

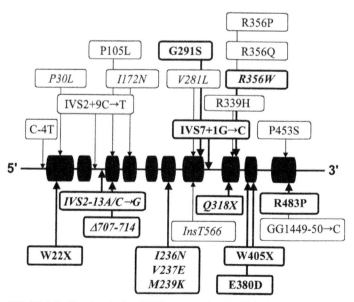

FIGURE 8-5. Mutations in the *CYP21* gene causing the 21-hydroxylase deficiency form of congenital adrenal hyperplasia. Classic alleles are printed in bold, nonclassic in regular type; mutations arising from conversion events are printed in italics.

tions of 17-OHP has been constructed that can be used to identify individuals with classic and nonclassic forms, as well as heterozygote carriers of the 21-hydroxylase deficiency form of CAH.

Neonatal screening via heel-stick capillary blood has been available since 1977[87] and is mandated in many states in the United States. The 17-OHP content of the dried blood, which is sampled on filter paper, analogous to the phenylketonuria test standard for all newborns, can be determined by a qualified laboratory. The value of newborn screening has been demonstrated repeatedly by the finding that most (biochemically proven) affected children were not identified on clinical grounds.[88-90]

The 08:00 hours salivary level of 17-OHP correlates extremely well with serum assays and is highly recommended as a screening test.[86] It is especially useful when venipuncture is difficult.

Diagnosis at Birth

The following data should be collected in the evaluation of a newborn with possible CAH:

1. Karyotype or other genetic analysis should be performed to establish the genetic gender in cases of ambiguous genitalia.
2. ACTH stimulation test: measuring serum 17-OHP concentration before and after ACTH stimulation. This test should NOT be performed during the initial 24 hours of life because samples from this time period are typically elevated in all infants and may yield false-positive results.
3. Aldosterone and plasma renin should be measured during the ACTH test.
4. Urinary sodium and potassium should be measured to assess salt-preserving ability.
5. Evidence of suppression of steroid secretion by glucocorticoid administration should be sought.

Further characterization of DNA by molecular genetic analysis is desirable when available.

Disorders of 11β-Hydroxylase

Steroid 11β-hydroxylase activity in the adrenal cortex is required for the synthesis of both glucocorticoids and mineralocorticoids. It has been shown that distinct isozymes of P450c11 participate in cortisol and aldosterone synthesis in humans.[91] The structure of the two CYP11B genes (nine exons and eight introns) is also identical to that of the *CYP11A* gene, which encodes the cholesterol desmolase protein. The genes for the two CYP11B isozymes are 93% identical in predicted amino acid sequence and 90% identical in the intronic region and are encoded by two vicinal genes on chromosome 8q24.3.[92-94] It is important to note that the upstream regions of the two genes are quite different, suggesting functionally different control. Disorders of the two enzymes may manifest as hypocortisolism (i.e., CAH), hypoaldosteronism, or hyperaldosteronism.

11β-HYDROXYLASE DEFICIENCY CONGENITAL ADRENAL HYPERPLASIA

Abnormal steroid secretion attributed to defective 11β-hydroxylation was first described by Eberlein and Bongiovanni[16] in 1955. It has proved to be the second most common form of CAH (5% to 8% of all cases in the general population).[95] In the cortisol pathway, conversion of 11-deoxycortisol to cortisol is reduced. As a result, 11-deoxysteroids (11-deoxycortisol and

11-DOC) accumulate. The hyperandrogenism resulting from shunting of cortisol precursors is similar to that of 21-hydroxylase deficiency, including genital ambiguity in classically affected females.

Approximately two thirds of patients with 11β-hydroxylase deficiency become hypertensive, with or without hypokalemic alkalosis, sometime early in life. Hypertension does not correlate with the presence or degree of hypokalemia or with the extent of virilization.[96]

In addition to the classic form (i.e., present at birth), milder nonclassic forms of 11β-hydroxylase deficiency have been reported[3-8] and may represent allelic variants, analogous to 21-hydroxylase deficiency. No biochemical defect has been demonstrated consistently in the obligate heterozygote parents of patients with the classic form, either in the baseline state or with ACTH stimulation.[97] As noted earlier, such a biochemical defect can be demonstrated in 21-hydroxylase heterozygotes. As in 21-hydroxylase deficiency, persons with identical 11β-hydroxylase mutations may differ in the severity of their signs and symptoms of androgen and mineralocorticoid excess, suggesting a role for epigenetic or nongenetic factors in the expression of clinical phenotype.[98]

Hypertension in 11β-Hydroxylase Deficiency

Hypertension in 11β-hydroxylase deficiency CAH is commonly attributed to DOC-induced sodium retention, which results in volume expansion. However, it has not been consistently proven that DOC causes hypertension.[91] In 1970, New and Seaman[99] showed that the large amounts of DOC produced in 11β-hydroxylase deficiency are glucocorticoid (dexamethasone) suppressible and therefore originate in the zona fasciculata, rather than in the zona glomerulosa. When DOC is suppressed with dexamethasone treatment, renin levels rise, causing secretion of aldosterone in the zona glomerulosa, in which the 11β-hydroxylase enzyme (P450c11B2) is normal.

Suppression of DOC by glucocorticoid treatment, however, may not lower blood pressure in hypertensive 11β-hydroxylase–deficient patients. Normotensive patients with markedly elevated DOC levels,[100,101] hypertensive patients with normal or only mildly elevated DOC,[102,103] and atypical 11β-hydroxylase–deficient patients with normal PRA[104] present a challenge to the DOC-centered explanation of hypertension. Of course, the lack of response to treatment is a feature of long-standing hypertension of many causes.

Epidemiology

Classic 11β-hydroxylase CAH (due to defects in the *CYP11B1* gene) occurs in approximately 1 in 100,000 births in the general white population.[105] A large number of cases have been reported in Israel. The incidence there now is estimated to be 1 in 5000 to 1 in 7000 births, with a gene frequency of between 1 in 71 and 1 in 83.[106] This unexpected clustering of cases was traced to Jewish families of North African origin, particularly from Morocco and Tunisia. Turkish Jews also have been found to carry the identical 11β-hydroxylase gene mutation with high frequency.[96,105] The incidence of the nonclassic form is not known at present but would be predicted to be considerably higher than the classic form, as in 21-hydroxylase deficiency.

Molecular Genetics

One of the 11β-hydroxylase genes, *CYP11B1,* is expressed at high levels in normal adrenal glands.[93] Transcription of this gene is regulated by cyclic adenosine monophosphate (the second messenger for ACTH). Low levels of transcripts of the second gene, *CYP11B2,* have been detected in normal adrenal with the use of reverse transcriptase polymerase chain reaction. The enzymes encoded by the *CYP11B1* and *CYP11B2* genes have been studied by expressing the corresponding complementary DNA in cultured cells and after actual purification from aldosterone-secreting tumors.[107-109] The high degree of similarity in both gene and protein structures between CYP11B1 and CYP11B2 suggested that the two 11β-hydroxylase genes were members of the same gene family.[93,110]

The isozyme encoded by CYP11B2, termed P450c11B2, 11β-hydroxylates 11-DOC to corticosterone and 11-deoxycortisol to cortisol. It also 18-hydroxylates corticosterone and further oxidizes 18-hydroxycorticosterone to aldosterone, the latter steps referred to as CMO I and CMO II activity, respectively. The CYP11B2 promotor is sensitive to renin/angiotensin. P450c11B2 is also referred to as CMO I/CMO II and as P450c18 and aldosterone synthase.

In contrast, the product of CYP11B1, termed P450c11B1, has strong 11β-hydroxylase activity but 18-hydroxylates only approximately one-tenth as well as P450c11B2. P450c11B1 does not synthesize detectable amounts of aldosterone from 18-hydroxycorticosterone. The CYP11B1 promotor is responsive to ACTH/cyclic adenosine monophosphate.

These data suggest that P450c11B1 predominantly synthesizes cortisol in the zona fasciculata, whereas P450c11B2 predominantly synthesizes aldosterone in the zona glomerulosa. This hypothesis has been confirmed through the study of individuals with defective cortisol or aldosterone synthesis due to deficiencies in 11β-hydroxylase and CMO II activities, respectively.

Mutations in the zona fasciculata enzyme (P450c11B1) result in defective synthesis of cortisol, producing hypertension from precursor (e.g., DOC) accumulation. Mutations in the zona glomerulosa gene *(P450c11B2)* result in defective synthesis of aldosterone and consequent salt wasting. An interesting molecular defect of the 11β-hydroxylase genes results in glucocorticoid-responsive hyperaldosteronism and resultant hypertension (see "Dexamethasone [Glucocorticoid]-Suppressible Hyperaldosteronism").

Almost all affected alleles in the Moroccan-Israeli population carry the same mutation, the substitution of histidine for arginine at codon 448[111] (R448H) in the *CYP11B1* gene. This mutation is incompatible with normal enzymatic activity[112] and appears to represent a founder effect. At least 31 mutations causing 11β-hydroxylase deficiency CAH have been identified and are shown in Fig. 8-7. Mutations are spread across the gene, including at several identified hot spots.[113]

Diagnosis

Elevated serum 11-deoxycortisol (compound S) and DOC, confirmed by marked elevation of their urinary tetrahydrometabolites, is diagnostic. Further confirmation can be found in a complete absence of any 11-oxygenated C_{19} or C_{21} steroids in blood or urine.[114] Diagnosis is made as for 21-hydroxylase deficiency with the additions of baseline and ACTH-stimulated serum 11-deoxycortisol (compound S) and DOC. Further characterization by molecular genetics analysis should be pursued in families anticipating additional children, with prenatal diagnosis now also available. Diagnosis in a newborn is quite difficult because the characteristic hypertension generally does not appear during the newborn period, and distinction from 21-hydroxylase deficiency based on steroid patterns is also problematic at this

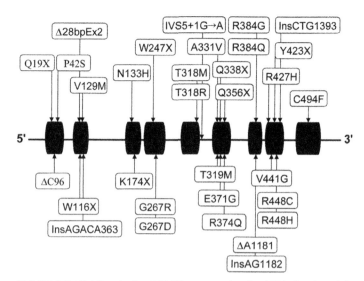

FIGURE 8-7. Mutations in the *CYP11B1* gene causing the 11β-hydroxylase deficiency form of congenital adrenal hyperplasia.

age.[115] Infantile gynecomastia has been described and may offer a clue to the diagnosis.[116] Treatment consists of glucocorticoid replacement. Determination of PRA is the standard test for mineralocorticoid excess. Although a nonelevated DOC is desirable, follow-up usually is accomplished more easily by following the renin (or PRA) level. Conversely, suppressed renin is typically a sign of insufficient control of 11β-hydroxylase deficiency.

CORTICOSTERONE METHYL OXIDASE DEFICIENCY

The conversion of corticosterone to 18-hydroxycorticosterone is referred to as CMO I activity, whereas the subsequent 18-oxidation to aldosterone is known as CMO II activity. In the zona glomerulosa, these steps are catalyzed by distinct domains within a single enzyme, P450c11B2, also referred to as P450c18, aldosterone synthase, and P450aldo. Deficient CMO I activity typically results in (practically) no aldosterone production and phenotypically is more severe than CMO II deficiency. Defects in CMO I activity have been reported but appear to be less common than those of CMO II.[117,118] Defects in both CMO I and CMO II activity are inherited as autosomal recessive conditions, and because cortisol synthesis is not affected in either condition, defects of P450aldo are not considered to be forms of CAH.

Infants with CMO II deficiency are subject to potentially fatal electrolyte abnormalities; in childhood, however, recurrent dehydration, a variable degree of hyponatremia and hyperkalemia, and poor growth are characteristic.[119,120] Adults may be asymptomatic, their affected status coming to light only in the course of family studies of a symptomatic child. CMO II deficiency has been found at an increased frequency among Jews of Iranian origin.[121] Molecular genetic analyses of such families have demonstrated two missense mutations in the *CYP11B2* genes of affected individuals: the replacement of arginine by tryptophan at position 181 (R181W) and the replacement of valine by alanine at position 386 (V386A).[122]

CMO I deficiency is characterized biochemically by essentially unmeasurable aldosterone levels with low or normal 18-hydroxycorticosterone levels. Patients with CMO II deficiency typically have normal (or low) aldosterone levels with elevated 18-hydroxycorticosterone levels (i.e., an elevated serum 18-hydroxycorticosterone-to-aldosterone ratio), along with a low corticosterone-to-18-hydroxycorticosterone ratio. Alternatively, CMO II deficiency can be identified by an elevated ratio of the major metabolites of these steroids (tetrahydro-18-hydroxy-11-dehydrocorticosterone and tetrahydroaldosterone) in urine.[120]

DEXAMETHASONE (GLUCOCORTICOID)-SUPPRESSIBLE HYPERALDOSTERONISM

Dexamethasone-suppressible hyperaldosteronism (DSH; also known as glucocorticoid-remediable aldosteronism) is a rare form of hypertension[123,124] in which aldosterone synthesis appears to be regulated abnormally by ACTH.[125] Dexamethasone-suppressible hyperaldosteronism is characterized by (1) rapid and complete suppression of aldosterone secretion on dexamethasone administration, (2) continued increase in aldosterone with long-term administration of ACTH, (3) suppressed PRA, and (4) a dominant mode of inheritance.[126] Urinary excretion of 18-hydroxycortisol and 18-oxocortisol is increased.[127,128]

Individuals with DSH have been shown to have an intergenic recombination, juxtaposing the promoter of CYP11B1 with the coding sequence of CYP11B2.[129,130] The fusion or chimeric gene creates an alteration in the regulation of synthesis of aldosterone, making the zona glomerulosa sensitive to ACTH rather than to renin-angiotensin, resulting in glucocorticoid-responsive hyperaldosteronism and hypertension.

Disorders of 3β-Hydroxysteroid Dehydrogenase

The enzyme 3β-HSD is necessary for the synthesis of bioactive Δ^4 adrenal and gonadal steroids from the relatively inactive Δ^5 precursors. In addition to 3β-hydroxysteroid dehydrogenation, this enzyme performs 3-oxosteroid isomerization, giving rise to the alternate term of Δ^4/Δ^5 isomerase. 3β-HSD is present not only in the adrenal cortex, gonads, and placenta but also in the liver and in nearly all peripheral tissues. The placental form is distinct from the adrenal/gonadal form. Differences in the levels of 3β-HSD activity in different tissues suggest tissue-specific isoforms or tissue-specific regulation of one or more shared isoforms of this protein.[131-134]

CLASSIC 3β-HYDROXYSTEROID DEHYDROGENASE DEFICIENCY

3β-HSD deficiency is an autosomal recessive form of CAH that was first described by Bongiovanni[135] in 1962. The exact frequency of this rare disorder is unknown. It has been postulated that individuals with defects early in the pathway of steroidogenesis, which severely impair cortisol synthesis (i.e., 3β-HSD and StAR), have poor survival rates.

Owing to reduced 3β-HSD enzyme activity in the gonads, genetic males are incompletely masculinized and exhibit genital ambiguity at birth. In affected females, conversely, very high levels of circulating DHEA converted peripherally to active androgens produce a limited androgen effect. Clitoral enlargement occurs and, rarely, labial fusion. As with the 21-hydroxylase and 11β-hydroxylase enzymes, the severity of the enzyme defect may not be determined on the basis of the appearance of the external genitalia at birth. Deficient steroid production in 3β-HSD deficiency may result in salt wasting, although this clearly is not true in every case.[136,137]

NONCLASSIC 3β-HYDROXYSTEROID DEHYDROGENASE DEFICIENCY

As with nonclassic 21-hydroxylase deficiency, nonclassic 3β-HSD deficiency is an attenuated enzyme defect with no major developmental abnormalities.[69,138] Signs of virilization appear in females after adrenarche or at the time of puberty.

The possibility that nonclassic 3β-HSD deficiency may be a significantly underdiagnosed cause of excess androgen symptoms, including hirsutism and infertility, has been suggested.[139] Review of clinical data on more than 700 women with signs of androgen excess demonstrated decreased 3β-HSD activity in 16%.[140] It has been suggested that nonclassic 3β-HSD deficiency may be more frequent than nonclassic 21-hydroxylase deficiency in women with androgen excess syndrome.[140] In a group of 25 menarchal women with 3β-HSD deficiency, an improvement in regulation of menses and in acne was observed to result from glucocorticoid therapy of at least 3 months' duration.[139] Hirsutism was less well reversed by treatment. Polycystic ovary disease was noted in 50% of these women.

Biochemistry and Molecular Genetics

Two genes encoding 3β-HSD have been localized to chromosome 1p13.1 and cloned.[134,141] These genes, HSD3B1 and HSD3B2, encode the skin-placental form (referred to as the type I isoform) and the adrenal-gonadal form (type II isoform) (Fig. 8-8). These isozymes are 372 and 371 amino acids in length, respectively, and 93.5% similar. A representation of mutations in the 3β-HSD type II gene is shown in Fig. 8-8.[142-144]

Caution should be exercised when the nonclassic form of 3β-HSD deficiency is diagnosed because the diagnostic hormonal profile in this condition has been shown to "disappear" in previously confirmed cases.[69] In addition, the paucity of confirmed mutation analysis/enzyme expression studies has made suspect the diagnosis of nonclassic 3β-HSD deficiency as a genetic disorder.

Diagnosis

The external genitalia of affected newborn males with classic 3β-HSD are incompletely masculinized, and females are

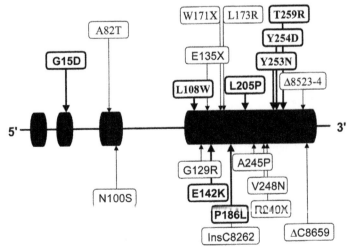

FIGURE 8-8. Mutations in the HSD3B2 gene causing the 3β-hydroxysteroid dehydrogenase/Δ^5/Δ^4 isomerase deficiency form of congenital adrenal hyperplasia. Alleles associated with salt wasting are printed in bold; non–salt-wasting alleles are in regular type.

masculinized to a variable degree. A high ratio of Δ^5-to-Δ^4 steroids, characterized specifically by elevated serum levels of the Δ^5 steroids pregnenolone, 17-hydroxypregnenolone, and DHEA, along with increased excretion of the Δ^5 metabolites pregnenetriol and 16-pregnenetriol in the urine, is diagnostic for this enzyme disorder. These criteria should not be used during the newborn period when Δ^5 steroids are universally elevated, representing a "physiologic 3β-HSD deficiency."[136] The 3β-HSD defect is diagnosed by 60 minute ACTH testing that produces elevations of 2 or more standard deviations above the mean in all the following: (1) serum Δ^5 17-hydroxypregnenolone, (2) DHEA concentration, (3) serum ratios of Δ^5 17-hydroxypregnenolone/17-hydroxyprogesterone, and (4) serum ratios of Δ^5 17-hydroxypregnenolone/cortisol.[137] Using genotypically proven subjects, Lutfallah and colleagues[145] suggested biochemical criteria using ACTH-stimulated 17-hydroxypregnenolone levels alone. In the general population, findings limited to modestly elevated Δ^5 17-hydroxypregnenolone and/or DHEA are nonspecific and do not establish the diagnosis of partial or mild 3β-HSD deficiency. As stated above, although nonclassic 3β-HSD deficiency may represent a true abnormality in endocrine physiology, it has very rarely been shown to have a genetic basis.

To rule out an adrenal or ovarian steroid–producing tumor, a dexamethasone suppression test (0.5 mg every 6 hours for 2 to 3 days) should be performed with subsequent measurement of serum hormone concentrations. An ovarian source of the androgens is excluded by the addition of the progestogen norethindrone acetate (5 mg every 8 hours for 3 days) to the dexamethasone. Both adrenal and ovarian hormones should be suppressed under this regimen. Ovarian sonography and either adrenal computed tomography or magnetic resonance imaging may be performed when there is a high index of suspicion for an adrenal or ovarian tumor, such as rapid progression or failure to suppress steroid production with dexamethasone or dexamethasone and norethindrone. As an aid to diagnosis, one can use published nomograms (Fig. 8-9A and B). Reference data established by Temeck and associates[65] on ACTH-stimulated hormonal values are used for the diagnosis of nonclassic 3β-HSD in children with precocious adrenarche (see Fig. 8-9C and D).

Disorders of 17α-Hydroxylase/17,20-Lyase

A single enzyme (P450c17) catalyzes both the conversion of mineralocorticoids to glucocorticoids (17α-hydroxylase activity) and the conversion of glucocorticoids to sex steroids (17,20-lyase activity). The enzyme P450c17 is encoded by the gene *CYP17,* which is located on chromosome 10q24-25. Abnormal enzyme function can, however, present as isolated 17α-hydroxylase deficiency, isolated 17,20-lyase deficiency, or combined 17α-hydroxylase/17,20-lyase deficiency. Based on the total number of reported cases (in both genders), 17α-hydroxylase with or without 17,20-lyase deficiency appears to be a rare steroidogenic defect.[146]

ISOLATED 17α-HYDROXYLASE DEFICIENCY

The enzyme domain that performs the 17α-hydroxylase activity is functionally distinct from the domain that performs the 17,20-lyase function. Therefore, it is reasonable to expect that isolated deficiency of either function may be found. However, because the product of 17α-hydroxylation is the precursor for 17,20-

lyase action, isolated 17α-hydroxylase deficiency may be difficult to identify because it should present as the more common combined 17α-hydroxylase/17,20-lyase deficiency. Individuals with "pure 17α-hydroxylase deficiency" would be expected to present with hypokalemic hypertension with alkalosis, possibly with normal gender development. These individuals could be identified by expression studies of mutant enzymes in cell culture, and it has been suggested that more than 20% residual 17,20-lyase function would not be apparent. Clinically, at least one such description has been reported,[147] but in reality, these cases represent a quantitative rather than a qualitative difference. Individuals with isolated 17α-hydroxylase deficiency would be phenotypically identical to patients with DSH.

ISOLATED 17,20-LYASE DEFICIENCY

Deficiency of 17,20-lyase activity impedes synthesis of C_{19} sex steroids in the adrenal and gonads[148] without affecting cortisol synthesis in the adrenal gland and therefore is not a form of CAH but is a potential cause of abnormal gender development. Urinary pregnanetriolone, a metabolite of 17-OHP, is increased and increases further after ACTH and human chorionic gonadotropin stimulation. DHEA and testosterone excretion does not increase appreciably. At birth, such individuals all have normal female genitalia, regardless of chromosomal gender, and generally present at adolescence with primary amenorrhea and/or lack of gender development. Other oversecreted steroids (e.g., corticosterone) subserve the glucocorticoid function. It is important to note that one longitudinal study of a 46,XY individual who began receiving estrogen replacement at puberty revealed apparently progressive extinction of 17α-hydroxylating activity from ages 20 to 26.[149] Thus, this patient, who started life with an isolated 17,20-lyase defect, converted to a combined 17α-hydroxylase/17,20-lyase defect at puberty, suggesting the need for continued vigilance in cases of isolated 17,20-lyase deficiency.

COMBINED 17α-HYDROXYLASE/17,20-LYASE DEFICIENCY

A defect in 17α-hydroxylase/17,20-lyase will result in diminished production of cortisol and sex steroids, the production of which requires the 17,20-lyase function. The enzyme defect affects steroid synthesis in both the adrenals and the gonads and reduces production of all androgens and estrogens. Because of high corticosterone (B) levels, patients with P450c17 abnormalities do not manifest adrenal crises and therefore often go undiagnosed, often until evaluated for abnormal pubertal development.[150] In the genetic male, there is pseudohermaphroditism, whereas in the female, infantile genitalia are present.[151] At puberty, gonadotropins increase to very high concentrations, the very low sex steroid production failing to provide adequate regulatory feedback. Breast development may occur in males.[19] In the female at pubertal age, no secondary gender characteristics develop, and primary amenorrhea may be noted. Phenotypically, such subjects may be similar to individuals with androgen insensitivity syndrome. 17,20-Lyase deficiency (isolated or as combined 17α-hydroxylase/17,20-lyase deficiency) occurs approximately 65% as often as androgen insensitivity syndrome.[152]

Nonclassic combined 17α-hydroxylase/17,20-lyase deficiency has been described in a subset of women undergoing evaluation for infertility. These women had normal potassium levels, blood pressure, and female external genitalia but high follicular phase progesterone combined with low estrogen levels.[153]

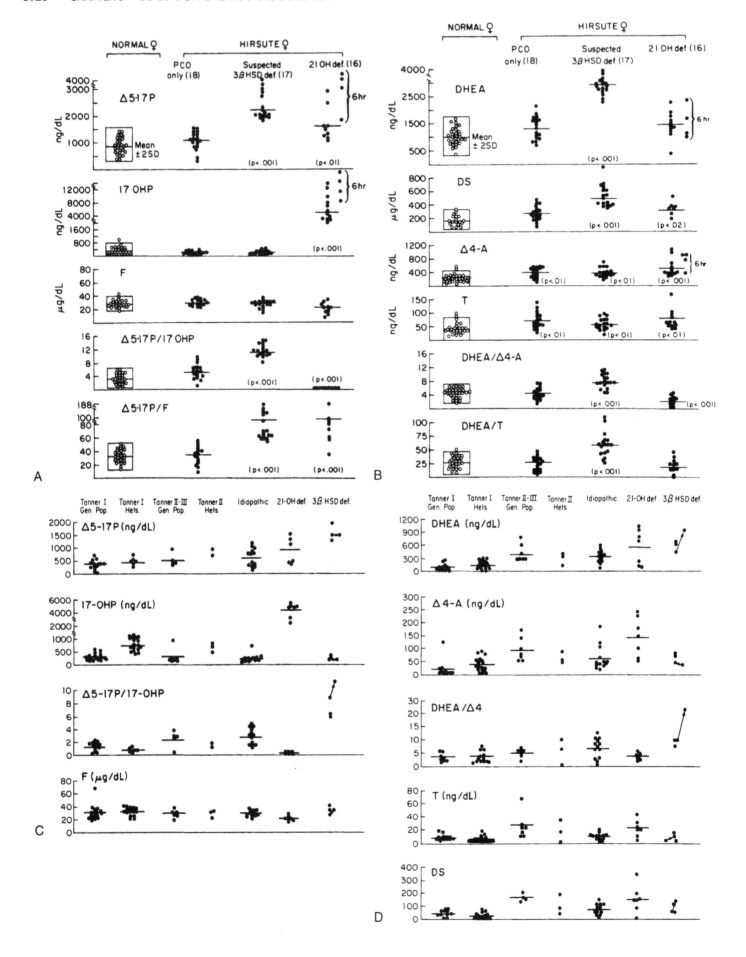

FIGURE 8-9. **A,** Serum 17-hydroxysteroid responses to adrenocorticotropic hormone (ACTH) stimulation (1 hour after a 0.25 mg IV bolus dose) in normal women and women with hirsutism. **B,** Serum androgen levels after ACTH stimulation in normal women and women with hirsutism. **C,** ACTH-stimulated serum 17-hydroxysteroid levels in normal children from the general population and from proven heterozygotes for 21-hydroxylase deficiency and in children with premature pubarche. The children with premature pubarche are classified as idiopathic (no steroidogenic defect) or as patients with 21-hydroxylase deficiency or 3β-hydroxysteroid dehydrogenase (3β-HSD) deficiency. **D,** ACTH-stimulated serum androgen levels in normal children from the general population and from proven heterozygotes for 21-hydroxylase deficiency and in children with premature pubarche. Children with premature pubarche are classified as idiopathic (no steroidogenic defect) or as patients with 21-hydroxylase deficiency or 3β-HSD deficiency. The testosterone (T) levels in males are represented by filled squares. (**A** and **B,** From Pang SY, Lerner AJ, Stoner E, et al: Late-onset adrenal steroid 3 beta-hydroxysteroid dehydrogenase deficiency. I. A cause of hirsutism in pubertal and postpubertal women, J Clin Endocrinol Metab 60:428–439, 1985. © 1985, The Endocrine Society. **C** and **D,** From Temeck JW, Pang S, Nelson C, New MI: Genetic defects of steroidogenesis in premature pubarche, J Clin Endocrinol Metab 64:609–617, 1987. © 1987, The Endocrine Society.)

Hypertension

Hypertension is observed in the 17α-hydroxylase deficiency form of CAH. The serum concentration of DOC is markedly elevated (30 to 60 times normal), but, as in 11β-hydroxylase deficiency,[105] circulating levels of DOC do not correlate entirely with blood pressure values, suggesting that other factors contribute to hypertension in this condition.[154,155] The serum aldosterone level in some individuals is also elevated, but usually the aldosterone is very low, secondary to the volume expansion caused by excess mineralocorticoid secretion and the resultant suppressed renin. Individuals may develop hypertension in childhood.

As in 21-hydroxylase deficiency, sibling pairs expected to have a common genetic defect do not always exhibit the same biochemical findings.[146]

Partial Defects

The heterozygous state has been identified by ACTH stimulation testing[156]; however, a nonclassic form has not been identified. The steroid pattern of some cases of low-renin hypertension without abnormalities of gender[157] raises the possibility that an isolated 17α-hydroxylase deficiency may be a more common cause of low renin hypertension than is currently recognized.[146]

Molecular Genetics

Human complementary DNA corresponding to P450c17 has been characterized,[158] and the single-copy CYP17 gene locus is situated on chromosome 10q24-25.[159] Many structural and gene-regulatory mutations in CYP17 have been identified in patients with combined 17α-hydroxylase/17,20-lyase deficiency (Fig. 8-10). It is interesting to note that phenotypic variation occurs even among mutation-identical subjects.[152] An interesting finding reported by Imai and colleagues[160] is the discovery of a mutation (a four-base duplication) common to two unrelated Canadian Mennonite pedigrees and six families (eight individuals) living in the Friesland region of the Netherlands. This mutation almost certainly represents a founder effect because the Mennonite sect originated in Friesland.

Diagnosis

Testing for 17α-hydroxylase deficiency should be performed in anyone with hypokalemic (low-renin, low-aldosterone) hypertension,[150] whereas 17,20-lyase deficiency (isolated or combined) should be sought in (apparent) females presenting at pubertal age with sexual infantilism. The disorder may be revealed earlier in 46,XY subjects who present in infancy or childhood with a hernia or inguinal mass and the finding of normal male internal structures with female external genitalia. Consideration also

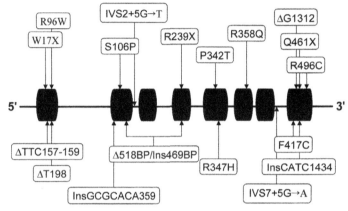

FIGURE 8-10. Mutations in the CYP17 gene causing 17α-hydroxylase/17,20-lyase deficiency.

should be given in women with unexplained infertility. As described previously, the hormonal picture will vary depending on the relative deficiencies of 17α-hydroxylase and 17,20-lyase activities. Plasma levels of corticosterone and 18-hydroxy-DOC and an elevated ratio of 18-hydroxycorticosterone to aldosterone are diagnostic of 17α-hydroxylase deficiency, whereas low androgens to estrogens indicates the addition of 17,20-lyase deficiency.[161] In long-standing untreated cases, refractory hypertension of considerable severity can develop.

COMBINED DISORDERS OF 21- AND 17α-HYDROXYLASE/17,20-LYASE DEFICIENCY

The combination of prenatal androgen excess with postnatal androgen deficiency has been reported. In some of these patients (postnatal), steroid profiles are consistent with combined (partial) 21-hydroxylase and 17α-hydroxylase/17,20-lyase deficiencies. Female newborns may have severe virilization (Prader III or IV), and males may be normal or undervirilized. Many of these subjects also have skeletal and other abnormalities consistent with Antley-Bixler syndrome (type 2). Steroid analysis of such subjects (especially after the neonatal period) typically demonstrates elevation of progesterone, 17-hydroxyprogesterone, and corticosterone. Pregnancies are commonly marked by maternal virilization—with both male and female fetuses—and low (maternal) estriol levels. Mild forms may be detected by the low maternal estriol level, with completely normal ultrasound.[162] Subjects with combined 21-hydroxylase and 17α-hydroxylase/17,20-lyase deficiencies, with or without Antley-Bixler syndrome (type 2), have been shown to have mutations in the P450 oxidoreductase gene, POR.[163,164] P450 oxidoreductase is an important cofactor for electron transfer from nicotinamide adenine dinucleotide phosphate (NADPH) to the 21-hydroxylase and 17α-hydroxylase/17,20-lyase (as well as many other) enzymes.[164] Maternal gestational virilization is likely due to the P450 oxidoreductase effect on P450 aromatase.[163,165]

Adrenal Failure With Male-Limited Gonadal Failure and XY Gender Reversal

LIPOID CONGENITAL ADRENAL HYPERPLASIA

Lipoid CAH is a rare form of CAH that was originally described in 1955 by Prader and associates[17,166] and represents the most extreme form of CAH with only negligible production of all steroids. Massive accumulations of cholesterol in the adrenocortical tissue (but not in the Leydig cells of the testis, where the enzyme is also active) lead to the characteristic fatty appearance of the glands and the descriptive name used for this disorder.

The cholesterol side-chain cleavage enzyme (P450scc, also known as cholesterol desmolase and encoded by CYP11A) catalyzes the conversion of cholesterol to pregnenolone in the first and rate-limiting step in the production of corticosteroids, and therefore was the most logical but not the only genetic candidate proposed for lipoid CAH. Mutations leading to lipoid CAH occur in CYP11A and in the gene coding for the StAR protein, encoded by the StAR gene on chromosome 8p11.2. StAR serves to shuttle cholesterol to the inner mitochondrial membrane, where the P450scc enzyme is located.[22] Mutations in StAR appear to be more common than those in CYP11A.

Affected individuals exhibit hypogonadism, severe fluid and electrolyte disturbances, hyperpigmentation, and susceptibility to infection. They often do not survive infancy. Lipoid CAH is rare in most populations but appears to occur at a somewhat higher frequency and with less severity among Japanese, Koreans, and Palestinian Arabs.[167,168] Phenotypic variability exists, with some patients described as having small adrenal glands without significant intracellular lipid deposits.

Both dominant and recessive mutations have been described in CYP11A. Tajima and colleagues[169] described an apparent somatic mutation present in multiple tissues in the affected subject but not found in either parent. This child was born with normal weight and length and was assigned a female gender. She was clinically unaffected (and untreated) until after 4 years of age, when she developed acute adrenal failure. No uterus was identified, and a karyotype at that time revealed 46,XY. This mutation appears to lead to a protein with essentially no enzymatic activity.

Another child with adrenal insufficiency was found to be a compound heterozygote for mutations in CYP11A. One mutation arose de novo, whereas the other was inherited from the mother, who was clinically unaffected.[170]

Baker et al described two families with mutations in the StAR gene, with a mild phenotype. The affected children presented with adrenal failure at the relatively late age of 2 to 4 years, but with normal genital development; the mutant StAR protein was shown to retain 20% of wild-type activity. They referred to this phenotype as "nonclassical lipoid CAH."[171]

The pathology of lipoid CAH appears to result from two distinct but related events. The first event results from deficient steroid hormone production. The second event is increasing lipid deposition inside the cell, which results in increasing intracellular damage/death. This latter event is theorized to lead to the salt-wasting adrenal crisis that often results in death in infancy.[172] The case report by Tajima and colleagues also would appear to confirm this hypothesis.[169] Histologic examination of a StAR knockout mouse supports this theory, with significant lipid deposits noted in the adrenals and mild accumulation in the testes but none in the ovaries.[173]

Diagnosis

In addition to the absence of any steroids in plasma or urine, high basal concentrations of ACTH and high PRA are found. In 46,XY patients, the genitalia are ambiguous or completely female, whereas 46,XX females have infantile female genitalia (i.e., the gonadal failure is not gender limited).

Individuals with adrenal failure but normal StAR and CYP11A genes have been described. In many such cases, the females are otherwise normal, but the males exhibit gonadal failure and XY gender reversal, analogous to the mutant Drosophila, with a defect in the fushi tarazu factor (FTZF1 or FTZ1). Mutations in several nuclear receptors (including DAX1 and SF1) have been associated with this phenotype. Unlike with the purely steroidogenic causes of male pseudohermaphroditism, these individuals exhibit persistence of the müllerian structures.

Steroidogenic Factor-1 Deficiency

The human homologue of the fushi tarazu factor is the steroidogenic factor-1 (SF1), also known as adrenal 4–binding protein. This protein is a nuclear receptor that regulates the transcription of numerous genes, including AMH, DAX1, CYP11A, CYP11B2, CYP21, and StAR; the gonadotropins; and aromatase[174] and itself is regulated by the upstream stimulatory factor-1[175] and by mitogen-activated protein kinase–dependent phosphorylation.[176,177]

Independent of its steroidogenic actions, SF1 is an active determinant of gender differentiation, chiefly via upregulation of AMH (or müllerian-inhibiting substance),[178] in conjunction with the product of the Wilms tumor gene (WT-1). DAX1 serves to block male differentiation by binding to SF1 and preventing this interaction with AMH.[179] SF1 also combines with SRY and SOX9 in advancing male differentiation of the gonad. Mutations of SF1 (and DAX1) therefore can be associated with persistence of müllerian structures in XY individuals.[180]

The SF1 gene (also known as the nuclear receptor NR5A1) is expressed in adrenal cortex, testicular Leydig cells, ovarian theca and granulosa cells, and the corpus luteum. In the fetus, SF1 is expressed in the mouse urogenital ridge at the earliest stage of gonadal development and in the Sertoli cells, the site of AMH production.

Subjects with mutations in NR5A1 have been described. The first report described a 2-week-old, phenotypically female infant with adrenal failure. She was found to have normal müllerian structures but a 46,XY karyotype. As noted by Achermann and colleagues,[181] the failure of müllerian regression may have been directly due to the loss of SF1-directed AMH production or secondarily through Sertoli cell maldevelopment. A second subject with adrenal failure and XY gender reversal was found to have a homozygous mutation of NR5A1. Both parents (and a sister) were shown to be carriers but were unaffected.[182] In contrast to this, a 46,XX female with a heterozygous mutation of NR5A1 had adrenal failure but normal ovarian function, consistent with the male-limited nature of the gonadal failure but demonstrating that the adrenal requirement is not gender specific.[183] The conclusion that can be drawn from most SF1/NR5A1 mutations is that *SF1* is critical to adrenal gland development but is not critical to ovarian or testicular development. However, reports have described humans with *SF1* mutations with genital abnormalities but normal adrenal function,[184] showing that the above statement is also not absolute.

DSS-AHB Critical Region on the X Chromosome 1

The *DAX1* gene (also called *NR0B1*) is located on the short arm of the X chromosome and, when mutated, leads to X-linked congenital adrenal hypoplasia (also referred to as adrenal hypoplasia, congenita [AHC]), as well as hypogonadotropic hypogonadism. *DAX1* duplication, however, leads to XY-limited gender reversal with ambiguous or completely female phenotypic development, regardless of chromosomal gender.[185]

The DAX1 protein is an important negative modulator of transcription, which decreases *SF1* and *StAR* expression (and therefore general steroid production).[186] *DAX1* also downregulates AMH, leading to müllerian duct development/internal female differentiation. *DAX1* is expressed in the adrenal gland, the gonad, the pituitary, and the hypothalamus; its expression in the developing gonad decreases as testicular differentiation increases but continues in the case of ovarian differentiation.[187] Mutations in *DAX1* (and *SF1*) should be sought in children with unexplained adrenal failure and especially in boys with hypogonadotropic hypogonadism.[188]

Treatment for Steroidogenic Defects

HORMONE REPLACEMENT THERAPY

The fundamental aim of endocrine therapy for CAH is to provide replacement of the deficient hormones. Since 1949, when Wilkins and colleagues[189] and Bartter[190] discovered the efficacy of cortisone therapy for CAH due to 21-hydroxylase deficiency, glucocorticoid therapy has been the cornerstone of treatment for all forms of cortisol deficiency. Glucocorticoid administration replaces the deficient cortisol and suppresses ACTH overproduction; a concomitant reduction in adrenal cortex activity occurs, thereby reducing the production of other adrenal steroids (i.e., precursor by-products) and remission of (most) symptoms over time. Patients with nonclassical 21-hydroxylase deficiency may have resolution of symptoms within 3 months of initiating corticosteroid treatment.[191]

Adrenal suppression in 21-hydroxylase, 11β-hydroxylase, and 3β-HSD deficiency reduces the excess production of androgens, averting further inappropriate virilization, slowing accelerated growth and bone age advancement to a more normal rate, and allowing normal onset of puberty. An improved body habitus is seen with a progressively earlier start of treatment (Fig. 8-11). Individuals with the salt-wasting type of 21-hydroxylase or 3β-HSD deficiency require the administration of a salt-retaining steroid to maintain adequate sodium balance. Suppression of adrenal activity in 11β-hydroxylase and 17α-hydroxylase deficiency normalizes DOC/mineralocorticoid secretion and often results in remission of hypertension. In lipoid CAH and adrenal failure, total hormone replacement is required.

Excessive glucocorticoid administration should be avoided because this produces cushingoid facies, growth retardation, inhibition of epiphyseal maturation, and decreased bone mineral density.

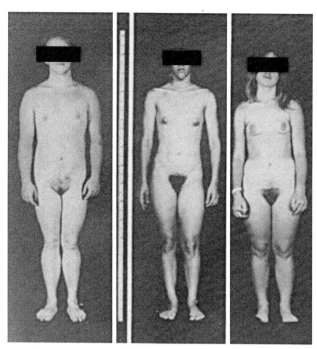

FIGURE 8-11. Habitus of pubertal girls with congenital adrenal hyperplasia due to 21-hydroxylase deficiency. The patient on the left was untreated until age 16 years; the patient in the center was started on treatment at age 9 years; and the patient on the right was treated from age 4 years. Note the progressively more feminine habitus with earlier treatment. (Modified from New MI, Levine LS: Congenital adrenal hyperplasia. In Harris H, Hirschhorn K [eds]: Advances in Human Genetics, vol 4. New York, Plenum, 1973, pp 251–326.)

Hydrocortisone (cortisol) is the corticosteroid of choice for children with all forms of CAH. It is the physiologic hormone and is used most often in the treatment of children because of easy dose adjustment. Oral administration is the preferred and usual mode of treatment, conventionally given in two divided doses: 10 to 15 mg/m² hydrocortisone divided as one third in the morning and two thirds in the evening. We prefer to use the tablet form of hydrocortisone, even in young infants, until stable liquid formulations have been introduced. As noted previously, excessive replacement with glucocorticoids will be detrimental, and although some children may (temporarily) require more than 15 mg/m² per day, individuals have been reported to develop cushingoid features with as little as 16 mg/m² per day of hydrocortisone.

If poor hormonal control with hydrocortisone is noted at the standard dose, the dose may be increased temporarily to 20 (or even 30) mg/m² per day, or the regimen may be changed to a synthetic hormone analogue such as prednisone or dexamethasone. These agents are more potent and longer acting, although their relative glucocorticoid and mineralocorticoid effects differ, and the smaller amounts used make dose adjustment more crucial. Because of individual variations in the activity of hepatic enzymes metabolizing 11-oxosteroids, and thus in plasma clearance and half-life, in some patients, prednisolone (the 11β-hydroxy analogue of prednisone, also called Δ¹ cortisol) is more effective than prednisone (Δ¹ cortisone) as glucocorticoid replacement. Individuals without overt salt wasting have been shown to have elevated renin levels,[192-198] and its fluctuation may correlate with ACTH. Addition of a mineralocorticoid to the therapeutic regimen in individuals with the simple virilizing form of 21-hydroxylase deficiency has been shown to result in improved hormonal control at the same glucocorticoid dose. A longer-term benefit of a reduced glucocorticoid requirement is improved statural growth.[197,198]

In non–life-threatening illness or stress, the glucocorticoid dose should be increased to two or three times the maintenance dose for the duration of the stress. Each family must be given injectable hydrocortisone for emergency use (25 mg for infants, 50 mg for young children, and 100 mg for older children and adults). In the event of a surgical procedure, a total of 5 to 10 times the daily maintenance dose (depending on the nature of the surgical procedure) may be required over the first 24 hours. For elective surgery, we recommend hydrocortisone 100 mg/m² PO at midnight preceding the operation, followed by 100 mg/m² IM on call to the operating room, and then another 100 mg/m² IV drip for every 6 hours of surgery. During the first 24 hours after surgery, the patient should receive 100 mg/m² per day, divided into four doses. Beginning on the second postoperative day, when there are no complications, the dose can be tapered rapidly, dropping to 50 mg/m² per day, and then on the following day, the normal preoperative corticosteroid schedule can be resumed in cases without complications. Appropriate stress doses should be given for complications. Stress doses should not be given in the form of dexamethasone because of the delayed onset of action. Mineralocorticoid doses need not be increased in response to stress.

Patients with the salt-wasting forms of adrenal failure and CAH (21-hydroxylase, 3β-HSD deficiency, and the lipoid form) require mineralocorticoid replacement. The cortisol analogue 9α-fluorohydrocortisone (fludrocortisone, Florinef, 9α-FF) is used for its potent mineralocorticoid activity. Additionally, salt should be allowed ad libitum. In an adrenal crisis, liberal infusions of isotonic saline and parenteral hydrocortisone should be administered at a dose of 100 mg/m²/dose. At this dose, hydrocortisone subserves all necessary mineralocorticoid function.

Several conditions (including those with complete adrenal failure), for example, cholesterol desmolase, StAR, 3β-HSD, and 17α-hydroxylase/17,20-lyase deficiency, also require sex steroid replacement, regardless of the gender of rearing. (Subjects with *SF1* abnormality may require sex steroid replacement, depending on the chromosomal gender.) Sex steroids should be added at the developmentally appropriate time to allow children to optimally resemble their peers. CMO I/CMO II (aldosterone synthase)–deficient individuals will require salt and mineralocorticoid replacement, whereas the hypertension seen in subjects with 11β-hydroxylase or 17α-hydroxylase deficiency may not resolve with glucocorticoid replacement, especially when the hypertension has been long-standing.

It is of the utmost importance for all patients with adrenal insufficiency and those on steroid replacement/suppressive therapy (e.g., for CAH) to wear a Medic-Alert bracelet or medallion listing the medical condition, long-term medications, and standard emergency procedures for the particular diagnosis (e.g., administration of fluids and hydrocortisone). In addition, the patient and family members must be trained in the intramuscular administration of hydrocortisone.

MONITORING TREATMENT

Glucocorticoid doses should be titrated to optimize biochemical control balanced against physiologic parameters (e.g., in a growing child with 21-hydroxylase deficiency, a 17-OHP of between 500 and 1000 ng/dL and suppressed androgens while maintaining a good growth velocity). The goal, with respect to corticosteroid replacement, is to give the minimal dose required for optimal control. Serum 17-OHP and Δ^4 androstenedione

concentrations determined by radioimmunoassay can be used to monitor biochemical control in patients with 21-hydroxylase deficiency.[199-201] In females and prepubertal males (but not in newborn and pubertal males), the serum testosterone level is also a useful index.[200] Combined determinations of PRA, 17-OHP, and serum androgens, as well as clinical assessment of growth and pubertal status, all must be considered when the doses of glucocorticoid and salt-retaining steroid are adjusted for optimal therapeutic control. A combination of hydrocortisone and 9α-FF has proved to be a highly effective treatment modality.[199] Measurement of PRA can be used to monitor efficacy of treatment in most forms of CAH. PRA is elevated in the salt-losing state and is suppressed in the volume-overloaded state. Its normalization indicates improved hormonal control.

Although glucocorticoid treatment has been available since 1950, little agreement has been reached as to which regimen gives the best outcome in terms of height. Recent studies suggest that even the most compliant patient may not achieve a final height compatible with parental stature. It is not known whether this is due to overtreatment, to failure of oral glucocorticoid therapy given twice or even three times daily to suppress excess androgen production, or to simultaneous overtreatment and undertreatment. A simple home-based system to monitor the hormonal status of patients at frequent intervals may improve hormonal control and final growth. Salivary 17-OHP concentration may provide an easy means for monitoring hormone levels on a daily basis.[86] Similar considerations may apply to the preservation of fertility.

MANAGEMENT OF THE CHILD WITH AMBIGUOUS GENITALIA

The newborn with ambiguous genitalia represents a medical emergency. Determination of genetic gender by karyotype and accurate diagnosis of the specific underlying defect are essential for initial management, but these factors do not address questions of gender identity and sexual orientation—questions that often are raised by confused parents at an extremely vulnerable time. It is well established that steroids influence aspects of central nervous system development,[202,203] but the data are controversial regarding specific androgen effects resulting from CAH.[204-206] It has been proposed that a masculinized gender role in girls, with behavioral manifestations such as tomboyishness, results from prenatal androgen excess in CAH. In a controlled play situation, Nordenstrom and colleagues[207] observed that girls with CAH played with masculine toys more than controls, and they demonstrated that the degree of masculine play correlated with the degree of virilization. Girls with CAH were shown to score similarly to control males on tests of spatial cognition.[208] In adult women, Long et al[209] found that self-reported femininity decreased and masculinity increased with prenatal androgen exposure. Similarly considered, behavioral changes resulting from alterations in the androgen milieu are seen in studies on male pseudohermaphrodites with 5α-reductase or 17β-hydroxysteroid dehydrogenase deficiency, who often elect a male gender identity at puberty.[210, 211] However, a great body of psychological studies indicate that in humans, unlike other mammals, the gender of rearing overrides prenatal hormonal effects.[212,213]

When a gender of rearing is assigned to a pseudohermaphrodite, the genetic gender is of less consideration than the physiologic and anatomic character of the genitalia, their potential for development and function, and the psychosocial milieu of the infant. Gender assignment of female pseudohermaphrodites with

21- or 11β-hydroxylase deficiency or 3β-HSD deficiency in the newborn period should be female. In fact, Dessens et al[214] found that gender dysphoria in 46,XX CAH patients was 12.1% when the children were raised as males, compared with 5.2% when they were raised as females.

Wide individual variability has been noted in the presentation of ambiguous genitalia in these patients. When medical treatment is begun early in life, the initially large and prominent clitoris may shrink slightly. As the surrounding structures grow normally, the clitoris becomes much less prominent, and surgical revision may not be required. When clitoral enlargement is conspicuous enough to interfere with parent-child bonding or formation of female gender identity in the patient or raises doubts in the parents about the true gender of the infant, corrective surgery of the genitalia should be carried out as early as possible, and certainly when the child is younger than 2 years of age.[213] Psychoendocrinologically trained psychologists and/or psychiatrists provide a vital component of the treatment regimen because one of the major goals of therapy is to ensure that gender role, gender behavior, and gender identity are isosexual with the gender of assignment.[215,216]

Clitoral surgery must aim to preserve erectile tissue along with the dorsal neurovascular bundle and thus clitoral erotic sensation. It must be determined before menarche that vaginal formation permits adequate outflow of blood, and an early procedure ensuring this may have to be performed in rare cases. Vaginoplasty performed before regular sexual intercourse may require continual mechanical dilatation of the vagina. Surgery before the patient is able to take responsibility for this risks recurrent stenosis, formation of adhesions, and scarring, with a need for further surgery and permanent harm to the vaginal orifice. Too long a delay, conversely, risks harm to the patient's sense of self as a normal female. All these factors are taken into account when the age for the necessary procedure(s) is chosen; this generally is done during the patient's early to middle adolescence. In some patients, mechanical dilatation may be sufficient. In the hands of an experienced surgeon, vaginoplasty can yield excellent results.[217] Because of the normal internal genitalia and gonads in these patients, normal puberty, fertility, and child-bearing are possible with early and proper therapeutic intervention.

Rare cases of late diagnosis of classic 21-hydroxylase, 11β-hydroxylase, and 3β-HSD deficiency with interim misassignment as a male must be dealt with on an individual basis. Corrective surgery to change the gender of assignment is not recommended in a child older than 2 years of age. Primary responsibility should be taken by a psychoendocrinologist in consultation with the family.

For the male pseudohermaphrodite, a male gender assignment is by no means always best. The basic questions include the following: (1) Will the child be able to urinate standing? (2) Will sexual intercourse as a man be possible? If the male pseudohermaphrodite is to be raised as a female, surgical correction of the genitalia and gonadectomy are required. With appropriate therapeutic measures, relatively normal, albeit infertile, female gender development and activity usually ensue in adolescence and adulthood if the parents and the patient are well managed medically and psychologically. Administration of sex steroids is required to induce development of appropriate gender characteristics at puberty. Assigned males who have impaired androgen synthesis will require androgen replacement. Almost all male pseudohermaphrodites to be raised as males require surgery for correction of birth defects of the external genitalia caused by inadequate prenatal masculinization.

The process of assigning and accepting a gender of rearing for a child with ambiguous genitalia is extremely complicated. A team approach that combines the insights of pediatrician, endocrinologist, psychoendocrinologist, surgeon, and the child's parents or guardian is essential. Moreover, it should be anticipated that ongoing counseling will be helpful to most families.

Prenatal Diagnosis

21-HYDROXYLASE DEFICIENCY

Each pregnancy that occurs in a family in which steroid 21-hydroxylase deficiency has been identified has a 25% chance of resulting in an affected newborn. Since 1965, when Jeffcoate and associates[218] correlated a clearly elevated value for amniotic fluid pregnanetriol with the diagnosis of an affected child (confirmed at term), amniotic fluid steroid hormone assay has been done in pregnancies at risk.[219-221] Radioimmunoassay of amniotic fluid for 17-OHP has shown that in all patients affected with the salt-wasting form, the amniotic fluid 17-OHP concentration is unambiguously elevated[222-226]; however, in simple virilizing 21-hydroxylase deficiency, the 17-OHP level may not be elevated above normal.[227] The amniotic fluid Δ^4 androstenedione and testosterone levels also have been measured, but the latter value is less useful because testosterone is normally high in the amniotic fluid of a male fetus.[225,228]

Fetal cells (mostly fibroblasts) in the amniotic fluid may be cultured for DNA analysis. HLA serotyping in conjunction with hormonal assay was begun in 1979[229] but is less sensitive than direct mutation analysis. Specific probes for 21-hydroxylase mutations allow direct and rapid identification of known mutations through the use of polymerase chain reaction (i.e., allele specific). Panels of oligonucleotide probes currently available for use in prenatal diagnosis[230] are expected to identify well more than 95% of current 21-hydroxylase mutations.

According to the population studied, deletions of the active 21-hydroxylase gene (CYP21) occur in from 20% to more than 40% of patients (Northwest United Kingdom)[231,232]; the remaining 60% to 80% of cases represent missense and nonsense mutations, as well as small deletions, sometimes even complicated noncontiguous deletions. These mutations are commonly the result of gene conversions and nonreciprocal transfers of the nucleotide sequence of longer or shorter segments of the pseudogene (CYP21P) to the active gene, with deleterious results.

11β-HYDROXYLASE DEFICIENCY

Levels of 11-deoxysteroids and metabolites in amniotic fluid and maternal urine have been found to be increased in pregnancies with a fetus affected with 11β-hydroxylase deficiency,[233,234] suggesting that prenatal diagnosis of this disorder by hormonal measurement may be feasible,[235] although the reliability of this method has not been reported on by other groups. However, the 11β-hydroxylase genes have been cloned, and many such mutations have been described. Where the mutations are known, prenatal diagnosis by DNA analysis of chorionic villus sampling (CVS) is possible and recommended. Experience with prenatal diagnosis in 11β-hydroxylase deficiency CAH is limited.

Prenatal Treatment

Dexamethasone crosses the placenta without undergoing significant metabolism and therefore has been used in the treatment of various fetal abnormalities. For the fetus at risk of 21- or 11β-hydroxylase deficiency, prophylactic treatment should be started as soon as pregnancy is confirmed.[236-245] Chorionic villus sampling is currently advocated to permit diagnosis in the first trimester and to allow discontinuation of unnecessary steroid treatment in the case of a male fetus or an unaffected female fetus (Fig. 8-12). Initiation of steroid therapy by the sixth or seventh week of gestation should effectively suppress fetal adrenal androgen production in time to allow normal separation of the vaginal and urethral orifices and continued suppression through gestation, to prevent or reduce the degree of clitoromegaly (Fig. 8-13). The current recommendation is dexamethasone at 20 μg/kg of maternal prepregnancy weight, given in three divided doses. To date, no fetus of a mother treated with low-dose dexamethasone has been found to have any congenital malformations other than genital ambiguity. Specifically, no reports have described increases in the number of cases of cleft palate, placental degeneration, or fetal death, all of which are observed in rodent models of in utero exposure to high-dose glucocorticoids.[246,247] Hirvikoski et al.[248] reported that psychoneurological testing in prenatally treated children revealed no differences in psychopathology, behavioral problems, or adaptive functioning. It is interesting to note that children were described by their parents as being more sociable than controls ($P = .042$).[248] We reported a study of all prenatal diagnoses between 1978 and 2002 that confirms the safety and efficacy of this treatment protocol. Of 595 pregnancies evaluated, 126 fetuses were found to be affected, 108 of these with classic

forms and 64 of which were female. In 13 of these cases, the families declined dexamethasone treatment. Female newborns in this cohort were highly virilized at birth, with a mean Prader score of 3.77. Of 51 pregnant women who received treatment, 27 began dexamethasone early (before 9 weeks' gestation) and continued to term. Female newborns in this group were only mildly virilized, with a mean Prader score of 1.04. The remaining 13 pregnant women began treatment late or were treated only partially. Female newborns in this group had an intermediate degree of virilization, with a mean Prader score of 3.00.[245] Statistically significant adverse effects of dexamethasone treatment (relative to the untreated group) included an excess weight gain of 7.1 lb (3.2 kg) and the presence of edema and striae. No correlation was noted between prenatal dexamethasone treatment and fetal demise, birth weight, hypertension, or gestational diabetes mellitus.[245] These data are in close agreement with those of the retrospective analysis of the European Society of Pediatric Endocrinology (ESPE).[249] Normal birth weight and length and normal physical and psychological development were reported in treated fetuses (affected and unaffected) in the French multicenter study[241] and in our series.[245] These studies reflect the experience with prenatal treatment of pregnancies at risk for 21-hydroxylase deficiency; prenatal treatment for pregnancies at risk for 11β-hydroxylase deficiency has been similarly successful and is predicted to have the same outcome and degree of safety.

Dexamethasone treatment should be initiated early in all at-risk pregnancies and maintained until confirmation is obtained

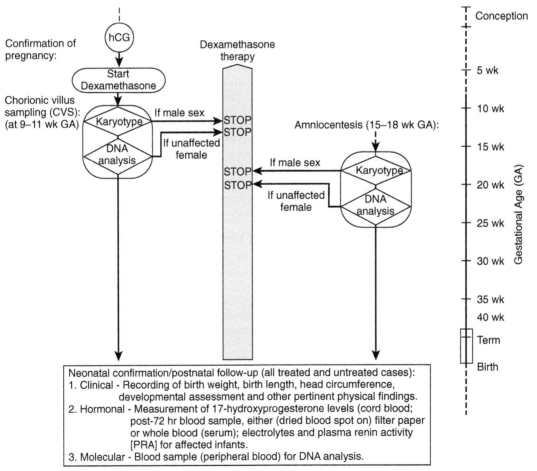

FIGURE 8-12. Protocol for prenatal diagnosis and treatment. *hCG,* Human chorionic gonadotropin. (From Mercado AB, Wilson RC, Cheng KC, et al: Prenatal treatment and diagnosis of congenital adrenal hyperplasia owing to steroid 21-hydroxylase deficiency, J Clin Endocrinol Metab 80:2014–2020, 1995. © 1995, The Endocrine Society.)

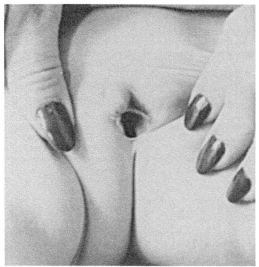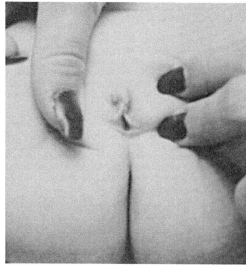

FIGURE 8-13. Untreated *(left)* and prenatally treated *(right)* female newborns. (From Speiser PW, Laforgia N, Kato K, et al: First trimester prenatal treatment and molecular genetic diagnosis of congenital adrenal hyperplasia [21-hydroxylase deficiency], J Clin Endocrinol Metab 70:838–848, 1990. © 1990, The Endocrine Society.)

that such treatment is not necessary, that is, in a genetic male or an unaffected female. This usually can be done by chorionic villus sampling at 9 to 10 weeks, or by amniocentesis at 16 to 18 weeks. The increase in risk for miscarriage after chorionic villus sampling is very low[250] and may be offset by the benefit of early diagnosis (shortened time of exposure to steroid treatment). The pregnant woman must be made aware of the available options and led through these to understand the possible outcomes.

The prognosis for individuals with disorders of adrenal steroidogenesis has improved remarkably over the past 50 years since the introduction of cortisone therapy. Improved glucocorticoid and mineralocorticoid replacement has had a tremendous impact on the quantity and quality of life of affected individuals and their families. Early research on gene therapy for some of these disorders, especially the 21-hydroxylase form of CAH, is promising, and this may become the new standard treatment in years to come.

REFERENCES

1. New MI, White PC, Pang S, et al: The adrenal hyperplasias. In Scriver CR, et al, editors: The Metabolic Basis of Inherited Disease, New York, 1989, McGraw-Hill, pp 1881–1917.
2. Grumbach MM, Conte FA: Disorders of sex differentiation. In Wilson JD, Foster DW, editors: Williams' Textbook of Endocrinology, Philadelphia, 1992, WB Saunders, pp 853–951.
3. Gabrilove J, Sharma D, Dorfman R: Adrenocortical 11B-hydroxylase deficiency and virilism first manifest in the adult woman, N Engl J Med 272:1189–1194, 1965.
4. Newmark D, Dluhy R, Williams G, et al: Partial 11-hydroxylase and 21-hydroxylase deficiencies in hirsute women, Am J Obstet Gynecol 127:594–598, 1977.
5. Cathelineau G, Brerault J, Fiet W: Adrenocortical 11β-hydroxylation defect in adult women with postmenarchal onset of symptoms, J Clin Endocrinol Metab 51:287–291, 1980.
6. Birnbaum M, Rose L: Late onset adrenocortical hydroxylase deficiencies associated with menstrual dysfunction, Obstet Gynecol 63:445–451, 1984.
7. Hurwitz A, Brautbar C, Milwidsky A: Combined 21- and 11β-hydroxylase deficiency in familial congenital adrenal hyperplasia, J Clin Endocrinol Metab 60:631–638, 1985.
8. Clark PA: Nonclassic 11-beta-hydroxylase deficiency: report of two patients and review, J Pediatr Endocr Metab 13:105–109, 2000.
9. De Crecchio L: Sopra un caso di apparenze virile in una donna, Morgagni 7:1951, 1865.
10. Fibiger J: Beiträge zur Kenntnis des weiblichen Scheinzwittertums, Virchows Arch Pathol Anat 181:1–51, 1905.
11. Apert A: Dystrophies en relation avec des lésions de capsules surrénales. Hirsutisme et progeria, Bull Soc Pediatr (Paris) 12:501–518, 1910.

12. Migeon CJ: Diagnosis and treatment of adrenogenital disorders. In DeGroot L, et al, editors: Endocrinology, Philadelphia, 1989, WB Saunders, pp 1676–1704.
13. Wilkins L: Adrenal cortex: virilizing adrenal hyperplasia; virilizing and feminizing tumors; and primary hyperaldosteronism. In Wilkins L, editor: The Diagnosis and Treatment of Endocrine Disorders in Childhood and Adolescence, Springfield, IL, 1965, Charles C Thomas, pp 368–381.
14. Bongiovanni AM: Detection of pregnanediol and pregnanetriol in urine of patients with adrenal hyperplasia: suppression with cortisone: a preliminary report, Bull Johns Hopkins Hosp 92:244–251, 1953.
15. Bongiovanni AM, Root AW: The adrenogenital syndrome, N Engl J Med 268:1283–1289, 1342–1351, 1391–1399, 1963.
16. Eberlein WR, Bongiovanni AM: Congenital adrenal hyperplasia with hypertension: unusual steroid pattern in blood and urine, J Clin Endocrinol Metab 15:1531–1534, 1955.
17. Prader A, Siebenmann RE: Nebenniereninsuffizienz bei kongenitaler Lipoid-hyperplasie der Nebennieren, Helv Paediatr Acta 12:569–595, 1957.
18. Biglieri EG, Herron MA, Brust N: 17-Hydroxylation deficiency in man, J Clin Invest 45:1946–1954, 1966.
19. New MI: Male pseudohermaphroditism due to 17 alpha-hydroxylase deficiency, J Clin Invest 49:1930–1941, 1970.
20. Dupont B, Oberfield SE, Smithwick EM, et al: Close genetic linkage between HLA and congenital adrenal hyperplasia (21-hydroxylase deficiency), Lancet 2:1309–1312, 1977.
21. White PC, New MI, Dupont B: HLA-linked congenital adrenal hyperplasia results from a defective gene encoding a cytochrome P-450 specific for steroid 21-hydroxylation, Proc Natl Acad Sci U S A 81:7505–7509, 1984.

22. Lin D, Sugawara T, Strauss JF, et al: Role of steroidogenic acute regulatory protein in adrenal and gonadal steroidogenesis, Science 267:1828–1831, 1995.
23. Suwa S, Shimozawa K, Kitagawa T, et al: Collaborative study on regional neonatal screening for congenital adrenal hyperplasia in Japan. In Therell BLJ, editor: Advances in Neonatal Screening, New York, 1987, Elsevier, pp 279–286.
24. Wallace AM, Beastall GH, Kennedy R, et al: Congenital adrenal hyperplasia screening in 120,000 Scottish neonates. In Therell BLJ, editor: Advances in Neonatal Screening, New York, 1987, Elsevier, pp 293–295.
25. Sólyom J, Hughes IA: Value of selective screening for congenital adrenal hyperplasia in Hungary, Arch Dis Child 64:338–342, 1989.
26. Pang SY, Wallace MA, Hofman L, et al: Worldwide experience in newborn screening for classical congenital adrenal hyperplasia due to 21-hydroxylase deficiency, Pediatrics 81:866–874, 1988.
27. Cutfield WS, Webster D: Newborn screening for congenital adrenal hyperplasia in New Zealand, J Pediatr 126:118–121, 1995.
28. Cacciari E, Balsamo A, et al: Neonatal screening for congenital adrenal hyperplasia, Arch Dis Child 58:803–806, 1983.
29. Cutfield WS, Webster D: Newborn screening for congenital adrenal hyperplasia in New Zealand, J Pediatr 126:118–121, 1995.
30. Allen DB, Hoffman GL, Fitzpatrick P, et al: Improved precision of newborn screening for congenital adrenal hyperplasia using weight-adjusted criteria for 17-hydroxyprogesterone levels, J Pediatr 130:128–133, 1997.
31. Janejai N, Krasao P, et al: Congenital adrenal hyperplasia: should nationwide screening be implemented in Thailand? Southeast Asian J Trop Med Public Health 34(suppl 3):170–173, 2003.

32. Speiser PW, Dupont B, Rubinstein P, et al: High frequency of nonclassical steroid 21-hydroxylase deficiency, Am J Genet 37:650–667, 1985.
33. Sherman SL, Aston CE, Morton NE, et al: A segregation and linkage study of classical and nonclassical 21-hydroxylase deficiency, Am J Hum Genet 42:830–838, 1988.
34. Dumic M, Brkljacic L, Speiser P, et al: An update on the frequency of nonclassic deficiency of adrenal 21-hydroxylase in the Yugoslav population, Acta Endocrinol (Copenh) 122:703–710, 1990.
35. Bonne-Tamir B, Bodmer JG, Bodmer WF, et al: HLA polymorphism in Israel: an overall comparative analysis, Tissue Antigens 11:235–250, 1978.
36. Kidd KK, Kidd JR, Bonne-Tamir B, et al: Nuclear DNA polymorphisms and population relationships. In Bonne-Tamir B, Adam A, editors: Genetic Diversity among Jews. Diseases and Markers at the DNA Level, London, 1992, Oxford University Press, pp 33–44.
37. Josso N: Antimullerian hormone: new perspectives for a sexist molecule, Endocr Rev 7:421–433, 1986.
38. Klingensmith G, Garcia S, Jones H, et al: Glucocorticoid treatment of girls with congenital adrenal hyperplasia: effects on height, sexual maturation, and fertility, J Pediatr 90:996–1004, 1977.
39. DiMartino-Nardi J, Stoner E, O'Connell A, et al: The effect of treatment of final height in classical congenital adrenal hyperplasia (CAH). In Illig R, Visser HKA, editors: Paediatric Endocrinology, Copenhagen, 1986, Acta Endocrinologica Copenhagen, pp 305–314.
40. New MI, Gertner JM, Speiser PW, et al: Growth and final height in classical and nonclassical 21-hydroxylase deficiency, Acta Paediatr Jpn 30:79–88, 1988.
41. Vogiatzi MG, Lin-Su K, New MI: Treatment with growth hormone and GnRH analogue improves final height in children with congenital adrenal hyperplasia. In Endocrine Society 2003, Philadelphia, 2003, The Endocrine Society.
42. Sciannamblo MR, Cuccato D, Chiumello G, et al: Reduced bone mineral density and increased bone metabolism rate in young adult patients with 21-hydroxylase deficiency, J Clin Endocrinol Metab 91:4453–4458, 2006.
43. Falhammar H, Filipsson H, et al: Fractures and Bone Mineral Density in Adult Women with 21-Hydroxylase Deficiency, J Clin Endocrinol Metab 92:4643–4649, 2007.
44. Barnes RB, Rosenfeld RL, Ehrmann DA, et al: Ovarian hyperandrogynism as a result of congenital adrenal virilizing disorders: evidence for perinatal masculinization of neuroendocrine function in women, J Clin Endocrinol Metab 79:1328–1333, 1994.
45. Lobo R, Goebelsmann U: Adult manifestation of congenital adrenal hyperplasia due to incomplete 21-hydroxylase deficiency mimicking polycystic ovarian disease, Am J Obstet Gynecol 138:720–726, 1980.
46. Meyer-Bahlburg HFL: What causes low rates of childbearing in congenital adrenal hyperplasia? J Clin Endocrinol Metab 84:1844–1847, 1999.
47. Trinh L, Nimkarn S, et al: Growth and pubertal characteristics in patients with congenital adrenal hyperplasia due to 21-hydroxylase deficiency, J Pediatr Endocrinol Metab 20:883–891, 2007.
48. Prader A: Vollkommen männliche äussere Genitalentwicklung und Salzverlustsyndrom bei Madchen mit kongenitalem Adrenogenitalem Syndrom, Helv Paediatr Acta 13:5–14, 1958.
49. Stikkelbroeck NM, Otten BJ, Pasic A, et al: High prevalence of testicular adrenal rest tumors, impaired spermatogenesis, and Leydig cell failure in adolescent and adult males with congenital adrenal hyperplasia, J Clin Endocrinol Metab 86:5721–5728, 2001.
50. Cabrera M, Vogiatzi M, New M: Long term outcome in adult males with classic congenital adrenal hyperplasia, J Clin Endocrinol Metab 86:3070–3080, 2001.
51. Ravichandran R, Lafferty F, McGinniss MJ, et al: Congenital adrenal hyperplasia presenting as massive adrenal incidentalomas in the sixth decade of life: report of two patients with 21-hydroxylase deficiency, J Clin Endocrinol Metab 81:1776–1779, 1996.
52. Beuschlein F, Schulze E, Mora P, et al: Steroid 21-hydroxylase mutations and 21-hydroxylase messenger ribonucleic acid expression in human adrenocortical tumors, J Clin Endocrinol Metab 83:2585–2588, 1998.
53. Merke DP, Chrousos GP, Eisenhofer G, et al: Adrenomedullary dysplasia and hypofunction in patients with classic 21-hydroxylase deficiency, N Engl J Med 343:1362–1368, 2000.
54. Tusie-Luna M, Traktman P, White PC: Determination of functional effects of mutations in the steroid 21-hydroxylase gene (CYP21) using recombinant vaccinia virus, J Biol Chem 265:20916–20922, 1990.
55. Chiou SH, Hu MC, Chung BC: A missense mutation at Ile172-Asn or Arg356-Trp causes steroid 21-hydroxylase deficiency, J Biol Chem 265:3549–3552, 1990.
56. Horner JM, Hintz RL, Luetscher JA: The role of renin and angiotensin in salt-losing, 21-hydroxylase-deficient congenital adrenal hyperplasia, J Clin Endocrinol Metab 48:776–783, 1979.
57. Stoner E, Dimartino-Nardi J, Kuhnle U, et al: Is salt-wasting in congenital adrenal hyperplasia due to the same gene as the fasciculata defect? Clin Endocrinol (Oxf) 24:9–20, 1986.
58. Morel Y, David M, Forest MG, et al: Gene conversions and rearrangements cause discordance between inheritance of forms of 21-hydroxylase deficiency and HLA types, J Clin Endocrinol Metab 68:592–599, 1989.
59. Speiser PW, Agdere L, Ueshiba H, et al: Aldosterone synthesis in salt-wasting congenital adrenal hyperplasia with complete absence of adrenal 21-hydroxylase, N Engl J Med 324:145–149, 1991.
60. Dupont B, Pollack M, Levine L, et al: Congenital adrenal hyperplasia and HLA: joint report from the Eighth International Histocompatibility Workshop. In Terasaki P, editor: Histocompatibility Testing 1980, Los Angeles, 1981, UCLA Tissue Typing Laboratory, pp 693–706.
61. Trowsdale J, Ragoussis J, Campbell RD, et al: Map of the human MHC, Immunol Today 12:443–446, 1991.
62. Dupont B, Virdis R, Lerner AJ, et al: Distinct HLA-B antigen associations for the salt-wasting and simple virilizing forms of congenital adrenal hyperplasia due to 21-hydroxylase deficiency. In Albert ED, Baur M, Mayr W, editors: Histocompatibility Testing 1984, Heidelberg, 1984, Springer-Verlag, p 660.
63. Levine LS, Dupont B, Lorenzen F, et al: Cryptic 21-hydroxylase deficiency in families of patients with classical congenital adrenal hyperplasia, J Clin Endocrinol Metab 51:1316–1324, 1980.
64. Kohn B, Levine LS, Pollack MS, et al: Late-onset steroid 21-hydroxylase deficiency: a variant of classical congenital adrenal hyperplasia, J Clin Endocrinol Metab 55:817–827, 1982.
65. Temeck JW, Pang SY, Nelson C, et al: Genetic defects of steroidogenesis in premature pubarche, J Clin Endocrinol Metab 64:609–617, 1987.
66. Granoff A, Chasalow F, Blethen S: 17-Hydroxyprogesterone responses to adrenocorticotropin in children with premature adrenarche, J Clin Endocrinol Metab 60:409–415, 1985.
67. Lucky A, Rosenfield R, McGuire J, et al: Adrenal androgen hyperresponsiveness to adrenocorticotropin in women with acne and/or hirsutism: adrenal enzyme defects and exaggerated adrenarche, J Clin Endocrinol Metab 62:840–848, 1986.
68. Rose L, Newmark S, Strauss J, et al: Adrenocortical hydroxylase deficiencies in acne vulgaris, J Invest Dermatol 66:324–326, 1976.
69. Pang SY, Lerner AJ, Stoner E, et al: Late-onset adrenal steroid 3 beta-hydroxysteroid dehydrogenase deficiency. I. A cause of hirsutism in pubertal and postpubertal women, J Clin Endocrinol Metab 60:428–439, 1985.
70. Child D, Bullock D, Anderson D: Adrenal steroidogenesis in hirsute women, Clin Endocrinol (Oxf) 12:595–601, 1980.
71. Gibson M, Lackritz R, Schiff I, et al: Abnormal adrenal responses to adrenocorticotropic hormone in hyperandrogenic women, Fertil Steril 33:43–48, 1980.
72. Chrousos G, Loriaux D, Mann D, et al: Late-onset 21-hydroxylase deficiency mimicking idiopathic hirsutism or polycystic ovarian disease, Ann Intern Med 96:143–148, 1982.
73. Knochenhauer ES, Cortet-Rudelli C, Cunningham RD, et al: Carriers of 21-hydroxylase deficiency are not at increased risk for hyperandrogenism, J Clin Endocrinol Metab 82:479–485, 1997.
74. Riddick D, Hammond C: Adrenal virilism due to 21-hydroxylase deficiency in the postmenarchial female, Obstet Gynecol 45:21–24, 1975.
75. Birnbaum M, Rose L: The partial adrenocortical hydroxylase deficiency syndrome in infertile women, Fertil Steril 32:536–541, 1979.
76. Chrousos GP, Loriaux DL, Sherines RJ, et al: Bilateral testicular enlargement resulting from inapparent 21-hydroxylase deficiency, J Urol 126:127–128, 1981.
77. White PC, Grossberger D, Onufer BJ, et al: Two genes encoding steroid 21-hydroxylase are located near the genes encoding the fourth component of complement in man, Proc Natl Acad Sci U S A 82:1089–1093, 1985.
78. Carroll MC, Campbell RD, Porter RR: Mapping of steroid 21-hydroxylase genes adjacent to complement component C4 genes in HLA, the major histocompatibility complex in man, Proc Natl Acad Sci U S A 82:521–525, 1985.
79. White PC, New MI, Dupont B: Structure of the human steroid 21-hydroxylase genes, Proc Natl Acad Sci U S A 83:5111–5115, 1986.
80. Higashi Y, Yoshioka H, et al: Complete nucleotide sequence of two steroid 21-hydroxylase genes tandemly arranged in human chromosome: a pseudogene and a genuine gene, Proc Natl Acad Sci U S A 83:2841–2845, 1986.
81. Harada F, Kimura A, et al: Gene conversion-like events cause steroid 21-hydroxylase deficiency in congenital adrenal hyperplasia, Proc Natl Acad Sci U S A 84:8091–8094, 1987.
82. Amor M, Parker KL, et al: Mutation in the CYP21B gene (Ile-172-Asn) causes steroid 21-hydroxylase deficiency, Proc Natl Acad Sci U S A 85:1600–1607, 1988.
83. Speiser PW, New MI, White PC: Molecular genetic analysis of nonclassic steroid 21-hydroxylase deficiency associated with HLA-B14,DR1, N Engl J Med 319:19–23, 1988.
84. Rocha RO, Billerbeck AE, et al: The degree of external genitalia virilization in girls with 21-hydroxylase deficiency appears to be influenced by the CAG repeats in the androgen receptor gene, Clin Endocrinol (Oxf) 68:226–232, 2008.
85. Bongiovanni AM, Eberlein WR, Goldman AS, et al: Disorders of adrenal steroid biogenesis, Recent Prog Horm Res 23:375–449, 1967.
86. Zerah M, Pang SY, New MI: Morning salivary 17-hydroxyprogesterone is a useful screening test for nonclassical 21-hydroxylase deficiency, J Clin Endocrinol Metab 65:227–232, 1987.
87. Pang S, Hotchkiss J, Drash AL, et al: Microfilter paper method for 17 alpha-hydroxyprogesterone radioimmunoassay: its application for rapid screening for congenital adrenal hyperplasia, J Clin Endocrinol Metab 45:1003–1008, 1977.
88. Therrell BL Jr, Berenbaum SA, et al: Results of screening 1.9 million Texas newborns for 21-hydroxylase-deficient congenital adrenal hyperplasia, Pediatrics 101(4):583–590, 1998.
89. Cavarzere P, Camilot M, et al: Neonatal screening for congenital adrenal hyperplasia in North-Eastern Italy: a report three years into the program, Horm Res 63:180–186, 2005.
90. Gruñieiro-Papendieck L, Chiesa A, et al: Neonatal screening for congenital adrenal hyperplasia: experience and results in Argentina, J Pediatr Endocrinol Metab 21:73–78, 2008.
91. Levine LS, Rauh W, Gottesdiener K, et al: New studies of the 11 beta-hydroxylase and 18-hydroxylase enzymes in the hypertensive form of congenital adrenal hyperplasia, J Clin Endocrinol Metab 50:258–263, 1980.
92. Chua S, Szabo P, Vitek A, et al: Cloning of cDNA encoding steroid 11 beta-hydroxylase (P450c11), Proc Natl Acad Sci U S A 84:7193–7197, 1987.
93. Mornet E, Dupont J, Vitek A, et al: Characterization of two genes encoding human steroid 11 beta-hydroxylase (P-450(11) beta), J Biol Chem 264:20961–20967, 1989.
94. Taymans SE, Pack S, Pak E, et al: Human CYP11B2 (aldosterone synthase) maps to chromosome 8q24.3, J Clin Endocrinol Metab 83:1033–1036, 1998.
95. Rösler A, Leiberman E: Enzymatic defects of steroidogenesis: 11 beta-hydroxylase deficiency congenital adrenal hyperplasia. In New MI, Levine LS, editors: Adrenal Diseases in Childhood: Pathophysiologic and Clinical Aspects, Basel, 1984, S. Karger, pp 47–71.

96. Rösler A, Leiberman E, Sack J: Clinical variability of congenital adrenal hyperplasia due to 11β-hydroxylase deficiency, Horm Res 16:133–141, 1982.
97. Pang S, Levine LS, Lorenzen F, et al: Hormonal studies in obligate heterozygotes and siblings of patients with 11 beta-hydroxylase deficiency congenital adrenal hyperplasia, J Clin Endocrinol Metab 50:586–589, 1980.
98. White PC, Curnow KM, Pascoe L: Disorders of steroid 11 beta-hydroxylase isozymes, Endocr Rev 15:421–438, 1994.
99. New MI, Seaman MP: Secretion rates of cortisol and aldosterone precursors in various forms of congenital adrenal hyperplasia, J Clin Endocrinol Metab 30:361–371, 1970.
100. Gandy HM, Keutmann EH, Izzo AJ: Characterization of urinary steroids in adrenal hyperplasia: isolation of metabolites of cortisol, compound S, and deoxycorticosterone from a normotensive patient with adrenogenital syndrome, J Clin Invest 39:364–377, 1960.
101. Blunck W: Die Beta-ketolischen Cortisol und Corticosteronmetaboliten sowie die 11-oxy-und 11-desoxy-17-ketosteroide im urin von Kindern, Acta Endocrinol 59(Suppl 134):9–112, 1968.
102. Green OC, Migeon CJ, Wilkins L: Urinary steroids in the hypertensive form of congenital adrenal hyperplasia, J Clin Endocrinol Metab 20:929–946, 1960.
103. Glenthoj A, Nielsen MD, Starup J: Congenital adrenal hyperplasia due to 11 beta-hydroxylase deficiency: final diagnosis in adult age in three patients, Acta Endocrinol (Copenh) 93:94–99, 1980.
104. New M, Nemery R, Chow D, et al: The adrenal and hypertension: from cloning to clinic. In Ares-Serona Symposium, New York, 1989, Raven Press.
105. Zachmann M, Tassinari D, Prader A: Clinical and biochemical variability of congenital adrenal hyperplasia due to 11 beta-hydroxylase deficiency. A study of 25 patients, J Clin Endocrinol Metab 56:222–229, 1983.
106. Rösler A: Classic and nonclassic congenital adrenal hyperplasia among non-Ashkenazi Jews. In Bonne-Tamir B, Adam A, editors: New perspectives on genetic markers and diseases among the Jewish people, Oxford, 1992, Oxford University Press, p 488.
107. Kawamoto T, Mitsuuchi Y, Ohnishi T, et al: Cloning and expression of a cDNA for human cytochrome P-450aldo as related to primary aldosteronism, Biochem Biophys Res Commun 173:309–316, 1990.
108. Curnow KM, Tusie-Luna MT, Pascoe L, et al: The product of the CYP11B2 gene is required for aldosterone biosynthesis in the human adrenal cortex, Mol Endocrinol 5:1513–1522, 1991.
109. Ogishima T, Shibata H, Shimada H, et al: Aldosterone synthase cytochrome P-450 expressed in the adrenals of patients with primary aldosteronism, J Biol Chem 266:10731–10734, 1991.
110. Nebert DW, Adesnik M, Coon MJ, et al: The P450 gene superfamily: recommended nomenclature, DNA 6:1–13, 1987.
111. White PC, Dupont J, New MI, et al: A mutation in CYP11B1 (Arg-448-His) associated with steroid 11 beta-hydroxylase deficiency in Jews of Moroccan origin, J Clin Invest 87:1664–1667, 1991.
112. Curnow KM, Slutsker L, Vitek J, et al: Mutations in the CYP11B1 gene causing congenital adrenal hyperplasia and hypertension cluster in exons 6, 7, and 8, Proc Natl Acad Sci U S A 90:4552–4556, 1993.
113. Geley S, Kapelari K, Johrer K, et al: CYP11B1 mutations causing congenital adrenal hyperplasia due to 11 beta-hydroxylase deficiency, J Clin Endocrinol Metab 81:2896–2901, 1996.
114. Eberlein W, Bongiovanni A: Plasma and urinary corticosteroids in the hypertensive form of congenital adrenal hyperplasia, J Biol Chem 223:85–94, 1956.
115. Mimouni M, Kaufman H, Roitman A, et al: Hypertension in a neonate with 11 beta-hydroxylase deficiency, Eur J Pediatr 143:231–233, 1985.
116. Hochberg Z, Schechter J, et al: Growth and pubertal development in patients with congenital adrenal hyperplasia due to 11-beta-hydroxylase deficiency, Arch J Dis Child 139:771–776, 1985.
117. Mitsuuchi Y, Kawamoto K, Ulick S, et al: Congenitally defective aldosterone biosynthesis in humans: inactivation of the P450c18 gene CYP11B2 due to nucleotide deletion in CMO I deficient patients, Biochem Biophys Res Commun 190:864–869, 1993.
118. Portrat-Doyen S, Tourniaire J, Richard O, et al: Isolated aldosterone synthetase deficiency caused by simultaneous E98D and V386A mutations in the CYP11B2 gene, J Clin Endocrinol Metab 83:4156–4161, 1998.
119. Hauffa BP, Sólyom J, Gláz E, et al: Severe hypoaldosteronism due to corticosterone methyl oxidase type II deficiency in two boys: metabolic and gas chromatography-mass spectrometry studies, Eur J Pediatr 150:149–153, 1991.
120. Picco P, Garibaldi L, Cotellessa M, et al: Corticosterone methyl oxidase type II deficiency: a cause of failure to thrive and recurrent dehydration in early infancy, Eur J Pediatr 151:170–173, 1992.
121. Globerman H, Rosler A, Theodor R, et al: An inherited defect in aldosterone biosynthesis caused by a mutation in or near the gene for steroid 11-hydroxylase, N Engl J Med 319:1193–1197, 1988.
122. Pascoe L, Curnow KM, Slutsker L, et al: Mutations in the human CYP11B2 (aldosterone synthase) gene causing corticosterone methyloxidase II deficiency, Proc Natl Acad Sci U S A 89:4996–5000, 1992.
123. New MI, Peterson RE: A new form of congenital adrenal hyperplasia, J Clin Endocrinol Metab 27:300–305, 1967.
124. Sutherland DJ, Ruse JL, Laidlaw JC: Hypertension, increased aldosterone secretion and low plasma renin activity relieved by dexamethasone, CMAJ 95:1109–1119, 1966.
125. Oberfield SE, Levine LS, Stoner E, et al: Adrenal glomerulosa function in patients with dexamethasone suppressible hyperaldosteronism, J Clin Endocrinol Metab 53:158–164, 1981.
126. New MI, Oberfield SE, Levine LS, et al: Demonstration of autosomal dominant transmission and absence of HLA linkage in dexamethasone suppressible hyperaldosteronism, Lancet 1:550–551, 1980.
127. Ulick S, Chu M: Hypersecretion of a new corticosteroid, 18-hydroxycortisol in two types of adrenocortical hypertension, Clin Exp Hypertens A 4:1771–1777, 1982.
128. Gomez-Sanchez C, Montgomery M, Ganguly A, et al: Elevated urinary excretion of 18-oxocortisol in glucocorticoid-suppressible aldosteronism, J Clin Endocrinol Metab 59:1022–1024, 1984.
129. Lifton RP, Dluhy RG, Powers M, et al: A chimaeric 11 beta-hydroxylase/aldosterone synthase gene causes glucocorticoid-remediable aldosteronism and human hypertension, Nature 355:262–265, 1992.
130. Pascoe L, Curnow KM, Slutsker L, et al: Glucocorticoid-suppressible hyperaldosteronism results from hybrid genes created by unequal crossovers between CYP11B1 and CYP11B2, Proc Natl Acad Sci U S A 89:8327–8331, 1992.
131. Lachance Y, Luu-The V, Labrie C, et al: Characterization of human 3β-hydroxysteroid dehydrogenase/D5-D4 isomerase gene and its expression in mammalian cells, J Biol Chem 265:20469–20475, 1990.
132. Lachance Y, Luu-The V, Verreault H, et al: Structure of the human type II 3 beta-hydroxysteroid dehydrogenase/delta 5-delta 4 isomerase (3 beta-HSD) gene: adrenal and gonadal specificity, DNA Cell Biol 10:701–711, 1991.
133. Rhéaume E, Simard J, Morel Y, et al: Congenital adrenal hyperplasia due to point mutations in the type II 3 beta-hydroxysteroid dehydrogenase gene, Nat Genet 1:239–245, 1992.
134. Simard J, Rheaume E, Sanchez R, et al: Molecular basis of congenital adrenal hyperplasia due to 3 beta-hydroxysteroid dehydrogenase deficiency, Mol Endocrinol 7:716–728, 1993.
135. Bongiovanni A: Adrenogenital syndrome with deficiency of 3beta-hydroxysteroid dehydrogenase, J Clin Invest 41:2086–2092, 1962.
136. Bongiovanni AM: Congenital adrenal hyperplasia due to 3β-hydroxysteroid dehydrogenase. In New MI, Levine LS, editors: Adrenal Diseases in Childhood, Basel, 1984, Karger, pp 72–82.
137. Pang S, Levine LS, Stoner E, et al: Non-salt-losing congenital adrenal hyperplasia due to 3 beta-hydroxysteroid dehydrogenase deficiency with normal glomerulosa function, J Clin Endocrinol Metab 56:808–818, 1983.
138. Rosenfield RL, Rich BH, Wolfsdorf JI, et al: Pubertal presentation of congenital delta 5–3 beta-hydroxysteroid dehydrogenase deficiency, J Clin Endocrinol Metab 51:345–353, 1980.
139. Schram P, Zerah M, Mani P, et al: Nonclassical 3 beta-hydroxysteroid dehydrogenase deficiency: a review of our experience with 25 female patients, Fertil Steril 58:129–136, 1992.
140. Zerah M, Schram P, New M: The diagnosis and treatment of nonclassical 3β-HSD deficiency, Endocrinologist 1:75–81, 1991.
141. Lorence MC, Corbin CJ, Kamimura N, et al: Structural analysis of the gene encoding human 3β-hydroxysteroid dehydrogenase/D5,4-isomerase, Mol Endocrinol 4:1850–1855, 1990.
142. Katsumata N, Tanae A, Yasunaga T, et al: A novel missense mutation in the type II 3 beta-hydroxysteroid dehydrogenase gene in a family with classical salt-wasting congenital adrenal hyperplasia due to 3 beta-hydroxysteroid dehydrogenase deficiency, Hum Mol Genet 4:745–746, 1995.
143. Tajima T, Fujieda K, Nakae J, et al: Molecular analysis of type II 3β-hydroxysteroid dehydrogenase gene in Japanese patients with classical 3β-hydroxysteroid dehydrogenase deficiency, Hum Mol Genet 4:969–971, 1995.
144. Morel Y, Mebarki F, Rheaume E, et al: 3β-Hydroxysteroid dehydrogenase: Contribution made by the molecular genetics of 3β-hydroxysteroid dehydrogenase deficiency, Steroids 62:176–184, 1997.
145. Lutfallah C, Wang W, Mason JI, et al: Newly proposed hormonal criteria via genotypic proof for type II 3-beta-hydroxysteroid dehydrogenase deficiency, J Clin Endocrinol Metab 87:2611–2622, 2002.
146. Yanase T, Simpson E, Waterman M: 17 Alpha-hydroxylase/17,20-lyase deficiency: from clinical investigation to molecular definition, Endocr Rev 12:91–108, 1991.
147. Miura K, Yasuda K, Yanase T, et al: Mutation of cytochrome P-45017a gene (CYP17) in a Japanese patient previously reported as having glucocorticoid-responsive hyperaldosteronism: with a review of Japanese patients with mutations of CYP17, J Clin Endocrinol Metab 81:3797–3801, 1996.
148. Zachmann M, Prader A: 17,20-Desmolase deficiency. In New M, Levine L, editors: Adrenal Disease in Childhood, Basel, 1984, Karger.
149. Zachmann M, Kempken B, Manella B, et al: Conversion from pure 17,20-desmolase- to combined 17,20-desmolase/17 alpha-hydroxylase deficiency with age, Acta Endocrinol (Copenh) 127:97–99, 1992.
150. Martin RM, Lin CJ, Costa EMF, et al: P450c17 deficiency in Brazilian patients: biochemical diagnosis through progesterone levels confirmed by CYP17 genotyping, J Clin Endocrinol Metab 88:5739–5746, 2003.
151. Mantero F, Scaroni C, Pasini CV, et al: No linkage between HLA and congenital adrenal hyperplasia due to 17b-hydroxylase deficiency [letter], N Engl J Med 303:530, 1980.
152. Boehmer ALM, Brinkmann AO, Sandkuijl LA, et al: 17-Beta-hydroxysteroid dehydrogenase-3 deficiency: diagnosis, phenotypic variability, population genetics, and worldwide distribution of ancient and de novo mutations, J Clin Endocrinol Metab 84:4713–4721, 1999.
153. Levran D, Ben-Shlomo I, Pariente C, et al: Familial partial 17,20-desmolase and 17alpha-hydroxylase deficiency presenting as infertility, J Assist Reprod Genet 20:21–28, 2003.
154. Ulick S: Diagnosis and nomenclature of the disorders of the terminal portion of the aldosterone biosynthetic pathway, J Clin Endocrinol Metab 43:92–96, 1976.
155. Griffing GT, Wilson TE, Holbrook MM, et al: Plasma and urinary 19-nor-deoxycorticosterone in 17 alpha-hydroxylase deficiency syndrome, J Clin Endocrinol Metab 59:1011–1015, 1984.
156. Wit JM, van Roermund HPC, Oostdik W, et al: Heterozygotes for 17α-hydroxylase deficiency can be detected with a short ACTH test, Clin Endocrinol 28:657–664, 1988.
157. Miura K, Yoshinaga K, Goto K, et al: A case of glucocorticoid-responsive hyperaldosteronism, J Clin Endocrinol Metab 28:1807–1815, 1968.
158. Chung B, Picado-Leonard J, Haniu M, et al: Cytochrome P450c17 (steroid 17 alpha-hydroxylase/17,20 lyase): cloning of human adrenal and testis cDNAs indicates the same gene is expressed in both tissues, Proc Natl Acad Sci U S A 84:407–411, 1987.
159. Matteson K, Picado-Leonard J, Chung B, et al: Assignment of the gene for adrenal P450c17 (steroid 17

alpha-hydroxylase/17,20 lyase) to human chromosome 10, J Clin Endocrinol Metab 63:789–791, 1986.

160. Imai T, Yanase T, Waterman M, et al: Canadian Mennonites and individuals residing in the Friesland region of The Netherlands share the same molecular basis of 17 alpha-hydroxylase deficiency, Hum Genet 89:95–96, 1992.

161. D'Armiento M, Reda G, Kater C, et al: 17a-Hydroxylase deficiency: mineralocorticoid hormone profiles in an affected family, J Clin Endocrinol Metab 56:697–701, 1983.

162. Williamson L, Arlt W, et al: Linking Antley-Bixler syndrome and congenital adrenal hyperplasia: a novel case of P450 oxidoreductase deficiency, Am J Med Genet 140A:1797–1803, 2006.

163. Flück CE, Tajima T, Pandey AV, et al: Mutant P450 oxidoreductase causes disordered steroidogenesis with and without Antley-Bixler syndrome, Nat Genet 36:228–230, 2004.

164. Arlt W, Walker EA, Draper N, et al: Congenital adrenal hyperplasia caused by mutant P450 oxidoreductase and human androgen synthesis: analytical study, Lancet 363:2128–2135, 2004.

165. Shackleton C, Marcos J, Malunowicz EM, et al: Biochemical diagnosis of Antley-Bixler syndrome by steroid analysis, Am J Med Genet (Part A) 128A:223–231, 2004.

166. Prader A, Gurtner HP: Das Syndrom des Pseudohermaphroditismus masculinus bei kongenitaler Nebennierenden-Hyperplasie ohne Androgenüberproduktion (Adrenaler Pseudohermaphroditismus masculinus), Helv Paediatr Acta 10:397–412, 1955.

167. Yoo HW, Kim GH: Molecular and clinical characterization of Korean patients with congenital lipoid adrenal hyperplasia, J Pediatr Endocrinol Metab 11:707–711, 1998.

168. Bose HS, Sato S, Aisenberg J, et al: Mutations in the steroidogenic acute regulatory protein (StAR) in six patients with congenital lipoid adrenal hyperplasia, J Clin Endocrinol Metab 85:3636–3639, 2000.

169. Tajima T, Fujieda K, Kouda N, et al: Heterozygous mutation in the cholesterol side chain cleavage enzyme (P450scc) gene in a patient with 46,XY sex reversal and adrenal insufficiency, J Clin Endocrinol Metab 86:3820–3825, 2001.

170. Katsumata N, Ohtake M, Hojo T, et al: Compound heterozygous mutations in the cholesterol side-chain cleavage enzyme gene (CYP11A) cause congenital adrenal insufficiency in humans, J Clin Endocrinol Metab 87:3808–3813, 2002.

171. Baker BY, Lin L, et al: Nonclassic congenital lipoid adrenal hyperplasia: a new disorder of the steroidogenic acute regulatory protein with very late presentation and normal male genitalia, J Clin Endocrinol Metab 91:4781–4785, 2006.

172. Bose HS, Sugawara T, Strauss JF III, et al: The pathophysiology and genetics of congenital lipoid adrenal hyperplasia, N Engl J Med 335:1870–1878, 1996.

173. Caron KM, Soo S-C, Wetsel WC, et al: Targeted disruption of the mouse gene encoding steroidogenic acute regulatory protein provides insights into congenital lipoid adrenal hyperplasia, Proc Nat Acad Sci U S A 94:11540–11545, 1997.

174. Luo X, Ikeda Y, Parker KL: A cell-specific nuclear receptor is essential for adrenal and gonadal development and sexual differentiation, Cell 77:481–490, 1994.

175. Harris AN, Mellon PL: The basic helix-loop-helix, leucine zipper transcription factor, USF (upstream stimulatory factor), is a key regulator of SF-1 (steroidogenic factor-1) gene expression in pituitary gonadotrope and steroidogenic cells, Mol Endocrinol 12:714–726, 1998.

176. Hammer GD, Krylova I, Zhang Y, et al: Phosphorylation of the nuclear receptor SF-1 modulates cofactor recruitment: integration of hormone signaling in reproduction and stress, Mol Cell 3:521–526, 1999.

177. Tremblay A, Tremblay GB, Labrie F, et al: Ligand-independent recruitment of SRC-1 to estrogen receptor beta through phosphorylation of activation function AF-1, Mol Cell 3:513–519, 1999.

178. Shen W-H, Moore CCD, Ikeda Y, et al: Nuclear receptor steroidogenic factor 1 regulates the Mullerian inhibiting substance gene: a link to the sex determination cascade, Cell 77:651–661, 1994.

179. Nachtigal M, Hirokawa Y, Enyeart-Van HD, et al: Wilms' tumor 1 and Dax-1 modulate the orphan nuclear receptor SF-1 in sex-specific gene expression, Cell 93:445–454, 1998.

180. Sekido R, Lovell-Badge R: Sex determination involves synergistic action of SRY and SF1 on a specific Sox9 enhancer, Nature 453:930–934, 2008.

181. Achermann JC, Ito M, Ito M, et al: A mutation in the gene encoding steroidogenic factor-1 causes XY sex reversal and adrenal failure in humans [letter], Nat Genet 22:125–126, 1999.

182. Achermann JC, Ozisik G, Ito M, et al: Gonadal determination and adrenal development are regulated by the orphan nuclear receptor steroidogenic factor-1, in a dose-dependent manner, J Clin Endocrinol Metab 87:1829–1833, 2002.

183. Biason-Lauber A, Schoenle EJ: Apparently normal ovarian differentiation in a prepubertal girl with transcriptionally inactive steroidogenic factor 1 (NR5A1/SF-1) and adrenocortical insufficiency, Am J Hum Genet 67:1563–1568, 2000.

184. Biason-Lauber A, Schoenle EJ: Apparently normal ovarian differentiation in a prepubertal girl with transcriptionally inactive steroidogenic factor 1 (NR5A1/SF-1) and adrenocortical insufficiency, Am J Hum Genet 67:1563–1568, 2000.

185. McCabe ERB: Sex and the single DAX1: too little is bad, but can we have too much? J Clin Invest 98:881–882, 1996.

186. Zanaria E, Muscatelli F, et al: An unusual member of the nuclear hormone receptor superfamily responsible for X-linked adrenal hypoplasia congenita, Nature 372:635–641, 1994.

187. Swain A, Zanaria E, et al: Mouse Dax1 expression is consistent with a role in sex determination as well as in adrenal and hypothalamus function, Nat Genet 12:404–409, 1996.

188. Lin L, Gu W-X, et al: Analysis of DAX1 (NR0B1) and steroidogenic factor-1 (NR5A1) in children and adults with primary adrenal failure: ten years' experience, J Clin Endocrinol Metab 91:3048–3054, 2006.

189. Wilkins L, Lewis R, Klein R, et al: The suppression of androgen secretion by cortisone in a case of congenital adrenal hyperplasia, Bull Johns Hopkins Hosp 86:249–252, 1950.

190. Bartter F: Adrenogenital syndromes from physiology to chemistry, 1950–1975. In Lee P, editor: Congenital Adrenal Hyperplasia, Baltimore, 1977, University Park Press, pp 9–18.

191. New MI: An update of congenital adrenal hyperplasia, Ann N Y Acad Sci 1038:14–43, 2004.

192. Godard C, Riondel A, Veyrat R: Plasma renin activity and aldosterone secretion in congenital adrenal hyperplasia, Pediatrics 41:883–904, 1968.

193. Simopoulos A, Marshall J, Delea C, et al: Studies on the deficiency of the deficiency of 21-hydroxylation in patients with congenital adrenal hyperplasia, J Clin Endocrinol 32:438–443, 1971.

194. Strickland A, Kotchen T: A study of the renin-aldosterone system in congenital adrenal hyperplasia, J Pediatr 81:962–969, 1972.

195. Dillon M: Plasma renin activity and aldosterone concentrations in children: results in salt-wasting states, Arch Dis Child 50:330, 1975.

196. Edwin C, Lanes R, Migeon C: Persistence of the enzymatic block in adolescent patients with salt-losing congenital adrenal hyperplasia, J Pediatr 95:534, 1979.

197. Rösler A, Levine LS, Schneider B, et al: The interrelationship of sodium balance, plasma renin activity and ACTH in congenital adrenal hyperplasia, J Clin Endocrinol Metab 45:500–512, 1977.

198. Kuhnle U, Rosler A, Pareira JA, et al: The effects of long-term normalization of sodium balance on linear growth in disorders with aldosterone deficiency, Acta Endocrinol (Copenh) 102:577–582, 1983.

199. Winter J: Current approaches to the treatment of congenital adrenal hyperplasia [editorial], J Pediatr 97:81–82, 1980.

200. Korth-Schutz S, Virdis R, Saenger P, et al: Serum androgens as a continuing index of adequacy of treatment of congenital adrenal hyperplasia, J Clin Endocrinol Metab 46:452–458, 1978.

201. Golden M, Lippe B, Kaplan S: Management of congenital adrenal hyperplasia using serum dehydroepiandrosterone sulfate and 17-hydroxyprogesterone concentrations, Pediatrics 61:867–871, 1978.

202. Döhler K: The special case of hormonal imprinting, the neonatal influence of sex, Experientia 42:759–769, 1986.

203. Döhler K, Hancke J, Srivastava S: Participation of estrogens in female sexual differentiation of the brain: Neuroanatomical, neuroendocrine, and behavioral evidence, Prog Brain Res 61:99–117, 1984.

204. Berenbaum SA: Congenital adrenal hyperplasia: intellectual and psychosexual functioning. In Holmes CPS, editor: Psychoneuroendocrinology: Brain, Behavioral, and Hormonal Interactions, New York, 1990, Springer-Verlag, pp 227–260.

205. Nass R, Baker S: Learning disabilities in children with congenital adrenal hyperplasia, J Child Neurol 6:306–312, 1991.

206. Nass R, Heier L, Moshang T, et al: Magnetic resonance imaging in the congenital adrenal hyperplasia population: increased frequency of white-matter abnormalities and temporal lobe atrophy, J Child Neurol 12:181–186, 1997.

207. Nordenstrom A, Servin A, Bohlin G, et al: Sex-typed toy play behavior correlates with the degree of prenatal androgen exposure assessed by CYP21 genotype in girls with congenital adrenal hyperplasia, J Clin Endocrinol Metab 87:5119–5124, 2002.

208. Mueller SC, Temple V, et al: Early androgen exposure modulates spatial cognition in congenital adrenal hyperplasia(CAH),Psychoneuroendocrinology 33:973–980, 2008.

209. Long DN, Wisniewski CJ: Gender role across development in adult women with congenital adrenal hyperplasia due to 21-hydroxylase deficiency, J Pediatr Endocrinol Metab 17:1367–1373, 2004.

210. Herdt G, Davidson J: The Sambia "turnim-man": sociocultural and clinical aspects of gender formation in male pseudohermaphrodites with 5-alpha-reductase deficiency in Papua New Guinea, Arch Sex Behav 17:33–56, 1988.

211. Price P, Wass J, Griffin J, et al: High dose androgen therapy in male pseudohermaphroditism due to 5 alpha-reductase deficiency and disorders of the androgen receptor, J Clin Invest 74:1496–1508, 1984.

212. Money J, Hampson JG, Hampson JL: Hermaphroditism: recommendations concerning assignment of sex, change of sex, and psychologic management, Bull Johns Hopkins Hosp 96:284–300, 1955.

213. Money J, Ehrhardt AA: Differentiation and dimorphism of gender identity from conception to maturity. In Man and Woman, Boy and Girl, Baltimore, 1972, Johns Hopkins University Press.

214. Dessens AB, Slijper FM, et al: Gender dysphoria and gender change in chromosomal females with congenital adrenal hyperplasia, Arch Sex Behav 34:389–397, 2005.

215. Baker S: Psychological management of intersex children. In Josso N, editor: The Intersex Child, Basel, 1981, Karger.

216. Meyer-Bahlburg HFL: Gender identity development in intersex patients, Child Adolesc Psychiatry Clin North Am 2:501–512, 1993.

217. Nihoul-Fekete C: Feminizing genitoplasty in the intersex child. In Josso N, editor: The Intersex Child, Basel, 1981, Karger.

218. Jeffcoate T, Fleigner J, Russell S, et al: Diagnosis of the adrenogenital syndrome before birth, Lancet 2:553–555, 1965.

219. Merkatz IR, New MI, Peterson RE, et al: Prenatal diagnosis of adrenogenital syndrome by amniocentesis, J Pediatr 75:977–982, 1969.

220. New MI, Levine LS: Congenital adrenal hyperplasia. In Harris H, Hirschhorn K, editors: Advances in Human Genetics, New York, 1973, Plenum, pp 251–326.

221. Levine L: Prenatal detection of congenital adrenal hyperplasia. In Milunsky A, editor: Genetic Disorders and the Fetus, New York, 1986, Plenum, pp 369–385.

222. Frasier S, Thorneycroft I, Weiss B, et al: Elevated amniotic fluid concentration of 17 alpha-hydroxyprogesterone in congenital adrenal hyperplasia [letter], J Pediatr 86:310–312, 1975.

223. Nagamani M, McDonough P, Ellegood J, et al: Maternal and amniotic fluid 17 alpha-hydroxyprogesterone levels during pregnancy: diagnosis of congenital adrenal hyperplasia in utero, Am J Obstet Gynecol 130:791–794, 1978.

224. Hughes I, Laurence K: Antenatal diagnosis of congenital adrenal hyperplasia, Lancet 2:7–9, 1979.
225. Pang S, Levine LS, Cederqvist LL, et al: Amniotic fluid concentrations of delta 5 and delta 4 steroids in fetuses with congenital adrenal hyperplasia due to 21 hydroxylase deficiency and in anencephalic fetuses, J Clin Endocrinol Metab 51:223–229, 1980.
226. Hughes I, Laurence K: Prenatal diagnosis of congenital adrenal hyperplasia due to 21-hydroxylase deficiency by amniotic fluid steroid analysis, Prenat Diagn 2:97–102, 1982.
227. Pang S, Pollack MS, Loo M, et al: Pitfalls of prenatal diagnosis of 21-hydroxylase deficiency congenital adrenal hyperplasia, J Clin Endocrinol Metab 61:89–97, 1985.
228. Frasier S, Weiss B, Horton R: Amniotic fluid testosterone: implications for the prenatal diagnosis of congenital adrenal hyperplasia, J Pediatr 84:738–741, 1974.
229. Pollack MS, Maurer D, Levine LS, et al: Prenatal diagnosis of congenital adrenal hyperplasia (21-hydroxylase deficiency) by HLA typing, Lancet 1:1107–1108, 1979.
230. Speiser PW, Dupont J, Zhu D, et al: Disease expression and molecular genotype in congenital adrenal hyperplasia due to 21-hydroxylase deficiency, J Clin Invest 90:584–595, 1992.
231. Werkmeister JW, New MI, Dupont B, et al: Frequent deletion and duplication of the steroid 21-hydroxylase genes, Am J Hum Genet 39:461–469, 1986.
232. Collier S, Sinnott PJ, Dyer PA, et al: Pulsed field gel electrophoresis identifies a high degree of variability in the number of tandem 21-hydroxylase and complement C4 gene repeats in 21-hydroxylase deficiency, EMBO J 8:1393–1402, 1989.
233. Rösler A, Leiberman E, Rosenmann A: Prenatal diagnosis of 11beta hydroxylase deficiency congenital adrenal hyperplasia, J Clin Endocrinol Metab 49:546–551, 1979.
234. Schumert Z, Rosenmann A, Landau H, et al: 11-Deoxycortisol in amniotic fluid: prenatal diagnosis of congenital adrenal hyperplasia due to 11 beta-hydroxylase deficiency, Clin Endocrinol 12:257–260, 1980.
235. Rösler A, Weshler N, Leiberman E, et al: 11β-Hydroxylase deficiency congenital adrenal hyperplasia: update of prenatal diagnosis, J Clin Endocrinol Metab 66:830–838, 1988.
236. David M, Forest MG: Prenatal treatment of congenital adrenal hyperplasia resulting from 21-hydroxylase deficiency, J Pediatr 105:799–803, 1984.
237. Evans M, Chrousos G, Mann D, et al: Pharmacologic suppression of the fetal adrenal gland in utero. Attempted prevention of abnormal external genital masculinization in suspected congenital adrenal hyperplasia, JAMA 253:1015–1020, 1985.
238. Dorr H, Sippell W, Haack D, et al: Pitfalls of prenatal treatment of congenital adrenal hyperplasia (CAH) due to 21-hydroxylase deficiency. Paper presented at the 25th Annual Meeting of the European Society for Paediatric Endocrinology, 1986, Zurich.
239. Forest M, Betuel H, David M: Traitement antenatal de l'hyperplasie congenitale des surrenales par deficit en 21-hydroxylase: Etude multicentrique, Ann Endocrinol 48:31–34, 1987.
240. Speiser PW, Laforgia N, Kato K, et al: First trimester prenatal treatment and molecular genetic diagnosis of congenital adrenal hyperplasia (21-hydroxylase deficiency), J Clin Endocrinol Metab 70:838–848, 1990.
241. Forest MG, David M, Morel Y: Prenatal diagnosis and treatment of 21-hydroxylase deficiency, J Steroid Biochem Mol Biol 45:75–82, 1993.
242. Mercado AB, Wilson RC, Cheng KC, et al: Prenatal treatment and diagnosis of congenital adrenal hyperplasia owing to steroid 21-hydroxylase deficiency, J Clin Endocrinol Metab 80:2014–2020, 1995.
243. Carlson AD, Obeid JS, Kanellopoulou N, et al: Congenital adrenal hyperplasia: update on prenatal diagnosis and treatment, J Steroid Biochem Mol Biol 69:19–29, 1999.
244. New MI, Carlson A, Obeid J, et al: Prenatal diagnosis for congenital adrenal hyperplasia in 532 pregnancies, J Clin Endocrinol Metab 86:5651–5657, 2001.
245. New MI, Carlson A, Obeid J, et al: Update: prenatal diagnosis for congenital adrenal hyperplasia in 595 pregnancies, Endocrinologist 13:233–239, 2003.
246. Goldman A, Sharpior B, Katsumata M: Human foetal palatal corticoid receptors and teratogens for cleft palate, Nature 272:464–466, 1978.
247. Lajic S, Levo A, et al: A cluster of missense mutations at Arg356 of human steroid 21-hydroxylase may impair redox partner interaction, Hum Genet 99:704–709, 1997.
248. Hirvikoski T, Nordenstrom A, et al: Long-term follow-up of prenatally treated children at risk for congenital adrenal hyperplasia: does dexamethasone cause behavioural problems? Eur J Endocrinol 159:309–316, 2008.
249. Forest MG, Dörr HG: Prenatal therapy in congenital adrenal hyperplasia due to 21-hydroxylase deficiency: retrospective follow-up study of 253 treated pregnancies in 215 families, Endocrinologist 13:252–259, 2003.
250. Canadian Collaborative CVS-Amniocentesis Clinical Trial Group: Multicentre randomised clinical trial of chorion villus sampling and amniocentesis: first report, Lancet 333:1–6, 1989.

Chapter 9

ADRENARCHE AND ADRENOPAUSE

IEUAN A. HUGHES and V. KRISHNA CHATTERJEE

Adrenarche
The Fetal Adrenal Gland
Postnatal Adrenal Morphology and Function
Mechanisms of Androgen Secretion at Adrenarche
Extraadrenal Control of Adrenarche
Clinical Facets of Adrenarche
Role of Adrenal Androgens in Adults

Adrenopause
DHEA Replacement in Aging
DHEA and Adrenal Insufficiency

Conclusions

Adrenarche

The adrenal glands are unique components of the endocrine system in displaying morphologic and functional characteristics that change dramatically according to different stages of prenatal and postnatal development. The onset of increased production of dehydroepiandrosterone (DHEA) and dehydroepiandrosterone sulfate (DHEAS) by the zona reticularis of the adrenals between 6 and 8 years of age defines the phenomenon of *adrenarche*. This appears to be a recapitulation of the steroidogenic pattern of the fetal adrenal during the second half of pregnancy, characterized by a massive increase in size of the adrenals relative to other fetal organs. Such a pattern of fetal and childhood adrenarche is observed only in humans and nonhuman primates. The triggers for the onset of adrenarche may differ among primate species such as the human, rhesus macaques (Old World primate), and marmosets (New World primate). The increase in DHEA is a common feature whose study can shed light on zona reticularis function in health and disease.[1]

THE FETAL ADRENAL GLAND

The fetal adrenal develops by the fourth week of gestation as a thickening of the celomic epithelium adjacent to the urogenital ridge.[1] Cells destined to become steroid secreting in both the adrenals and gonads are derived from the same migratory cells from the primitive mesonephros. The fetal adrenal has the capac-

ity to produce steroids by 6 to 8 weeks of gestation, a fact that dictates the need to start dexamethasone early for the prenatal treatment of congenital adrenal hyperplasia (see Chapter 8).

In the fetal adrenal, the structure of the adult adrenal gland—with its three functional zones producing C21 steroids (zona glomerulosa and zona fasciculata for aldosterone and cortisol, respectively) and C19 steroids (zona reticularis for DHEAS principally)—is absent. The bulk of the gland (about 80%) comprises the fetal zone, and the remaining outer (definitive) zone resembles the characteristics of the adult adrenal cortex. Ultrastructural studies offer evidence of a transitional zone between the fetal and definitive zones, which may have some capacity to synthesize cortisol.

Trophic Control of the Fetal Adrenal

Adrenocorticotropic hormone (ACTH) appears to be the principal trophic factor controlling growth and function of the fetal adrenal.[2] Fig. 9-1 illustrates data on combined adrenal weights according to gestational age in normal fetuses compared with anencephaly and congenital adrenal hyperplasia. There is a clear demarcation outside the normal range for anencephaly and congenital adrenal hyperplasia, indicating the ACTH-dependent growth of the fetal adrenal. Biochemical monitoring of treated pregnancies at risk of congenital adrenal hyperplasia shows the ACTH dependence of fetal adrenal steroidogenesis.[3] Growth is mainly by hypertrophy of the fetal zone, which renders the fetal adrenal as large as the kidney by 20 weeks' gestation and 20- to 30-fold larger than the adult adrenal by 30 weeks. The definitive zone grows mainly by hyperplasia and is controlled by a number of growth factors acting in concert with ACTH. These include basic fibroblast growth factor, epidermal growth factor, insulin-like growth factors, transforming growth factors, and the activins.[1]

In concert with the morphologic changes in the fetal adrenal, there is a vast output of steroids in the form of DHEA, pregnenolone, 17OH-pregnenolone, and their respective sulfated conjugates. The steroid output amounts to about 200 mg per day, of which 60% is DHEAS.[4] This C19 fetal steroid is a major substrate for estrogen biosynthesis via the fetoplacental unit (Fig. 9-2). Key enzymes are 16α-hydroxylase to form 16OH-DHEAS in the liver, placental sulfatase to produce free DHEA, and the action of placental P450 aromatase to synthesize the estrogens, estrone, estradiol, and estriol, from their respective C19 androgen substrates. The abundance of C19 steroids, which are normally aromatized by the placenta, is illustrated by the profound virilizing effects on the mother and her female fetus in the presence of an inactivating mutation of the *CYP19* gene.[5]

POSTNATAL ADRENAL MORPHOLOGY AND FUNCTION

A precipitous fall in adrenal weight by about 50% occurs after birth as a result of involution of the fetal zone. The definitive zone remains and is the template for development into the characteristic zones of the adult adrenal cortex. It is proposed that a combination of proliferation and migration of progenitor cells underlies this characteristic tissue zonation.[6] The rapid reduction in adrenal gland size within weeks of birth is an apoptotic process

rather than due to hemorrhage or necrosis.[7] It appears to be independent of ACTH and is induced by the action of activin and transforming growth factor alpha (TGF-α). Involution of the fetal zone is reflected biochemically in a concomitant decrease in DHEAS levels, which remain low until the increase characteristic of adrenarche from ages 6 to 8. There is thickening of the zona reticularis evident by age 3.[8] Longitudinal studies of 24-hour urinary androgen excretion and serum DHEAS concentrations suggest there is already a gradual increase in C19 steroid output from the postnatal adrenal gland from early childhood.[9,10] This recrudescence of the pattern of fetal adrenal steroidogenesis indicates a common mechanism involving modulating factors operating within the adrenals to increase C19 steroid production independent of ACTH.

MECHANISMS OF ANDROGEN SECRETION AT ADRENARCHE

DHEAS is the most abundant endogenous steroid produced within the endocrine system and circulates in micromolar concentrations. The pattern of secretion throughout prenatal and postnatal life is depicted in Fig. 9-3, and the prerequisites for DHEA and DHEAS synthesis are shown in Fig. 9-4.

The initial step in converting cholesterol to pregnenolone is common to all steroid-producing glands and is rate limiting.[11] The key steroidogenic junction is at the step mediated by the P450c17 enzyme and defined as the qualitative regulator of steroidogenesis.[12] This enzyme uniquely performs two catalytic activities called 17α-hydroxylase and 17,20-lyase. It is the latter enzyme activity that preferentially ensures C19 steroid production and, in particular, DHEA synthesis and adrenarche. A number of factors enhance the differential activities of P450c17. These include posttranslational regulation of P450c17 by phosphorylation on serine/threonine residues and the role of electron transfer proteins.[13-15] The principal electron donor to microsomal P450 enzymes, including P450c17, is nicotinamide adenine dinucleotide phosphate (NADPH) cytochrome P450 oxidoreductase. This enzyme cofactor augments both 17α-hydroxylase and 17,20-lyase activities but is not the principal determinant of increased DHEA synthesis. However, mutations in the P450 oxidoreductase gene lead to a biochemical profile reminiscent of

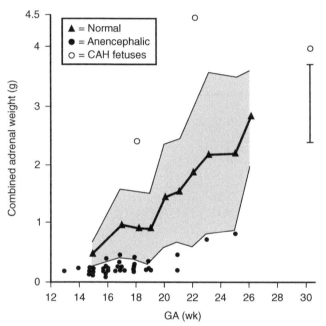

FIGURE 9-1. Combined fetal adrenal weights according to gestational age. (Data from Young MC, Laurence KM, Hughes IA: Relationship between fetal adrenal morphology and anterior pituitary function, Horm Res 32:130–135, 1989.)

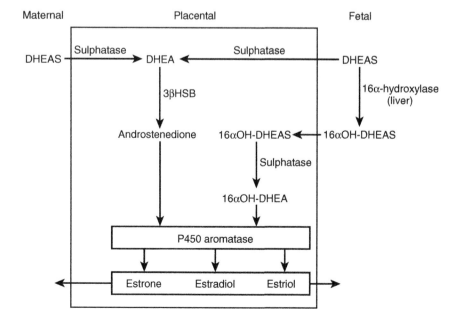

FIGURE 9-2. The fetal-placental-maternal steroid unit.

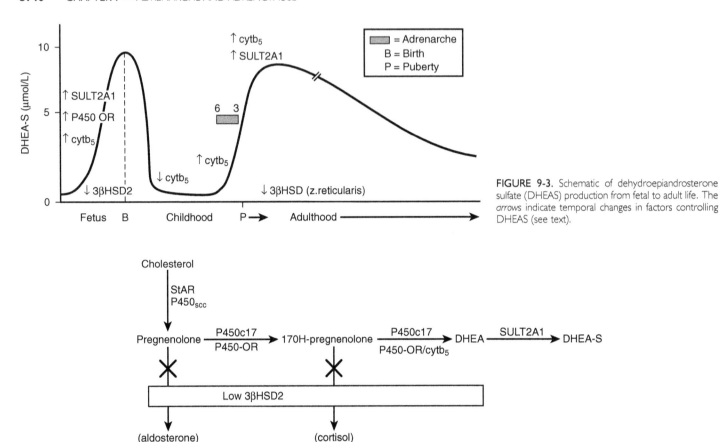

FIGURE 9-3. Schematic of dehydroepiandrosterone sulfate (DHEAS) production from fetal to adult life. The *arrows* indicate temporal changes in factors controlling DHEAS (see text).

FIGURE 9-4. Pathway of dehydroepiandrosterone sulfate (DHEAS) synthesis in fetal adrenal and adult zona reticularis. Also depicted is the effect of low expression of 3β-hydroxysteroid dehydrogenase 2 (3β-HSD2) in these tissues.

combined partial 17α-hydroxylase and 21-hydroxylase deficiencies with virilization in affected girls and undermasculinization in affected boys.[16,17] The Antley-Bixler syndrome, a condition characterized by severe skeletal abnormalities, genital anomalies, and adrenal dysfunction, is also a manifestation of this enzyme deficiency.[18] Enhancement of 17,20-lyase activity is linked specifically to the action of cytochrome b_5 in the presence of adequate P450 oxidoreductase.[12] This effect is far more substantial with Δ^5 substrates such as 170H-pregnenolone as compared with a Δ^4 substrate such as 170H-progesterone. Hence, the predominance of DHEA synthesis. Coupled to the promotion of DHEA synthesis is a relative deficiency of 3β-hydroxysteroid dehydrogenase (HSDB2) in the fetal adrenal and postnatal zona reticularis. This enzyme would normally compete with P450c17 to convert Δ^5 to Δ^4 steroids.[19]

More than 99% of DHEA is sulfated to DHEAS through the action of dehydroepiandrosterone sulfatase (SULT2A1).[20] Sulfated steroids are also unavailable as substrates for HSDB2 activity, thus maintaining the high levels of DHEAS. Immunohistochemical studies in the fetal adrenal and in age-related postnatal adrenal glands have demonstrated a developmental pattern of enzyme and cofactor expression that may explain the intraadrenal control of adrenarche.[21-23] In summary, the pattern of increased DHEAS secretion is associated with increased expression of P450c17, P450 oxidoreductase, cytochrome b_5, SULT2A1, and decreased expression of HSDB2 in the fetal adrenal and again in the postnatal zona reticularis after age 5. In contrast, a reversal of this pattern occurs in the postnatal adrenal gland between infancy and age 5. Expression of cytochrome b_5 and SULT2A1 is maintained beyond the adult age when DHEAS

levels start to decline. The zona reticularis becomes smaller with increasing age, suggesting that the decline in DHEAS levels is associated with a decrease in cell number rather than a change in enzyme content. What factors stimulate the changes in expression of key proteins controlling DHEAS synthesis remain to be determined. HSDB2 has the important function of determining the ratio of Δ^5 and Δ^4 steroid production. A family of orphan nuclear receptors (nerve growth factor–induced clone B [NGF1B]) is expressed in parallel with HSDB2 and directly act on the promoter to up-regulate the *HSD3B2* gene.[24] It is possible that decreased expression of this and other transcriptional regulators of *HSD3B2* at key developmental stages allows the increased production of DHEAS during fetal life and at adrenarche.

EXTRAADRENAL CONTROL OF ADRENARCHE

There is sufficient dissociation between changes in cortisol and DHEAS secretion to indicate that ACTH is not the primary trophic factor responsible for the rise in DHEAS levels at adrenarche. Nevertheless, ACTH may play a permissive role because DHEAS levels are either undetectable or significantly decreased in familial glucocorticoid deficiency associated with ACTH resistance.[25] Corticotropin-releasing factor (CRH) has been suggested as a specific adrenal androgen secretagogue in view of the direct effect of CRH on human fetal adrenal cells in stimulating DHEAS secretion and following CRH infusion in normal men.[26,27] However, the interpretation of such in vivo data is compounded by the concomitant effect of increased ACTH secretion.

Numerous other factors have been postulated to have effects on adrenal androgen secretion, mainly based on in vitro studies using isolated human fetal adrenal cells. These include prolactin, estrogens, TGFs, cytokines, insulin-like growth factors (IGFs), and a fragment of pro-opiomelanocortin (POMC). None has proven to be a specific adrenal androgen secretagogue. Leptin differentially regulates 17,20-lyase activity in an adrenocortical carcinoma cell line that expresses the leptin receptor.[28] There is also an association between DHEAS and leptin levels at the time of adrenarche in obese children.[29] Overall, the adrenarche results from an alteration of expression of CYP17, HSD3B2, CYB5 (cytochrome b_5), and SULT2A1, intertwined with changes in protein kinase A and insulin signaling pathways.

CLINICAL FACETS OF ADRENARCHE

The term adrenarche defines the rise in adrenal androgens (DHEA, DHEAS, and androstenedione) that occurs between 6 and 8 years of age as a result of the modulation of adrenal steroidogenesis previously described; it is thus a biochemical definition for an event that is not usually translated into clinical signs. Adrenarche is often used interchangeably with pubarche, which describes the growth of sexual hair in the suprapubic area and axillae. Adrenal androgens are the stimuli for public and axillary hair growth in females, and hair growth typically starts on the labia. In boys, the distinction is less clear because the growth of pubic and axillary hair is primarily stimulated by the rise in testicular testosterone production. Adrenarche (or pubarche) is considered premature when there is onset of pubic hair growth before age 8 in girls and before age 9 in boys. Because all children have an increase in adrenal androgen production between 6 and 8 years of age, it remains perplexing why hair growth is expressed only in a small minority. Premature adrenarche is more common in girls than boys, and there is an association with low birth weight.[30] However, this sex dimorphism is not apparent in normal children in whom a relationship between lower birth weight and higher adrenal androgen levels is present in both sexes.[31] Children with premature adrenarche are typically taller than average, may have increased body odor and acne, and exhibit a bone age advanced by 1 to 2 years. In a study of girls with premature adrenarche, increased linear growth was already evident in the first 2 years of life and associated with higher IGF-1 levels.[32] The taller stature later is probably the result of increased androgen levels, yet the mini–growth spurt in normal children that also occurs around ages 6 to 8 is probably not a function of adrenarche.[33] Obesity is generally associated with taller stature in childhood, and the body mass index (BMI) tends to be higher in premature adrenarche, but the BMI does not correlate with androgen levels.[29]

Table 9-1 lists the conditions that should be excluded when assessing a child with early pubic hair development and the appropriate investigations to perform in such cases. Imaging using ultrasound or computed tomography (CT) will readily exclude an adrenal tumor. Furthermore, if the cause is an adrenal tumor, signs of virilization are more profound. These signs include clitoromegaly, hirsutism, voice deepening, and in boys, penile growth.[34] The main condition to exclude is late-onset congenital adrenal hyperplasia (CAH) which is found in about 5% of children with early onset of pubic hair. Baseline measurements of 17OH-progesterone, androstenedione, testosterone, and DHEAS are usually sufficiently sensitive and specific to distinguish the two conditions.[35] Further confirmation rests with mutational analysis of the CYP21 gene. Premature adrenarche has generally been regarded as a benign variant with a normal age of menarche in girls and no negative effect on adult height.[36] However, more detailed longitudinal studies of premature adrenarche suggest an increased risk of later ovarian hyperandrogen-

Table 9-1. Causes of Early Pubic Hair and Relevant Investigations

Causes

Premature adrenarche
Late-onset congenital adrenal hyperplasia
Adrenal tumor

Investigations

Adrenal imaging (ultrasound and/or computed tomography)
Bone age
Baseline steroids
 Dehydroepiandrosterone sulfate (DHEAS)
 17OH-progesterone
 Androstenedione
 Testosterone
Adrenocorticotropic hormone (ACTH) stimulation test
 17OH-progesterone
 Cortisol
 Testosterone
 Androstenedione
24-hour urinary steroids

ism in adolescent girls and hyperinsulinism.[37] It is possible that premature adrenarche is a risk factor for later development of the metabolic syndrome in adult life. Daughters of mothers with polycystic ovary syndrome are at higher risk of developing this syndrome, and a significant number exhibit exaggerated adrenarche.[38] The role of sulfotransferases in providing adrenal substrates for androgen production is vividly illustrated by a child with premature adrenarche who subsequently progressed to features of the polycystic ovary syndrome.[39] Investigations showed compound heterozygous mutations in the gene encoding for a sulfate donor required for sulfation of DHEA to DHEAS by DHEA sulfotransferase. The net result is an increase in unconjugated DHEA, which provides the substrate for increased adrenal androgen production. Currently, there is no indication that the use of insulin sensitizers should be considered in a child presenting with typical clinical and biochemical features of premature adrenarche, but it is apposite to counsel parents that affected girls may later experience menstrual disturbances in adolescence. Early intervention after menarche with insulin sensitizers may prevent progression to polycystic ovarian syndrome and reduce the risk of long-term cardiovascular problems.[40]

ROLE OF ADRENAL ANDROGENS IN ADULTS

The physiologic role of adrenal androgens, including DHEAS, is not well understood. The association of adrenarche with pubic and axillary hair development suggests a role for DHEAS as a substrate for androgen synthesis. There is evidence that DHEAS is converted to sex steroids (testosterone, estradiol) in peripheral tissues via several enzymatic steps. Circulating, adrenally derived DHEAS is first converted to DHEA by sulfatase, which is further converted to androstenedione by 3β-hydroxysteroid dehydrogenase (3β-HSD); in turn, androstenedione is modified to testosterone or estradiol by isozymes of 17β-HSD or P450 aromatase, respectively (Fig. 9-5). It has been suggested that such conversion, occurring intracellularly via these enzymes that are widely expressed in many peripheral tissues, constitutes an intracrine mechanism for local generation of sex steroids from DHEA. This mechanism might also account for the observation that DHEA administration can result in androgenic/estrogenic effects without significant changes in circulating levels of these steroids.[41] There is also evidence to suggest that DHEA can act as a neurosteroid to exert effects in the central nervous system. Steroidogenic enzymes mediating DHEA synthesis are expressed in the brain,

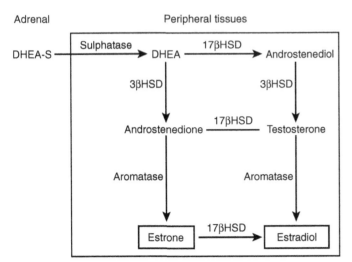

FIGURE 9-5. Pathways by which dehydroepiandrosterone sulfate (DHEAS) is converted intracellularly to sex steroids (testosterone, estradiol) in peripheral target tissues. Elevation in levels of androgen metabolites (e.g., androstanediol glucuronide) following DHEA treatment provides evidence for such peripheral sex steroid synthesis.

and it has effects on neuronal growth and differentiation.[42] DHEA has also been shown to modulate neurotransmitter signaling, acting as an allosteric antagonist at the γ-aminobutyric acid (GABA) receptor but as an agonist at the N-methyl-D-aspartate (NMDA) receptor.[43] DHEA may have a further potential role as an antiglucocorticoid. It has been shown to antagonize glucocorticoid-induced thymic involution or corticosterone-mediated neurotoxicity to hippocampal cells.[44,45]

To date, a specific receptor that mediates the action of DHEA has not been identified, and whether it acts at the cell surface or intracellularly remains to be elucidated. DHEA has been shown to stimulate nitric oxide synthesis in endothelial cells via a specific G protein–coupled membrane receptor[46] and to activate the mitogen-activated protein kinase (MAPK) pathway in vascular smooth muscle cells independently of androgen and estrogen receptors.[47] Microarray studies of human peripheral blood mononuclear cells indicate that DHEA induces a gene expression profile that is distinct from glucocorticoid and testosterone, supporting the notion that it may act via an independent pathway.[48]

Adrenopause

Following peak levels in early adulthood, there is an inexorable decline in DHEA production such that by the age of 80 years, circulating levels are only 10% to 20% of those in young adults,[49] whereas adrenal glucocorticoid and mineralocorticoid synthesis is relatively unchanged. The cause of this age-related decrease in DHEAS levels, termed the *adrenopause,* is not understood, but it is accompanied by involution of the zona reticularis and diminished adrenal 17α-hydroxylase enzyme activity. In both sexes, there is a progressive reduction in DHEA production of about 2% per year,[50] with absolute levels being lower in women than men in the age range of 50 to 89 years.[51] Interestingly, caloric restriction in monkeys attenuates the age-related fall in DHEAS,[52] and smoking has been shown to maintain DHEAS levels in men.[53]

Cross-sectional epidemiologic studies have documented an association between the decline in DHEAS levels and various adverse effects of aging. An inverse relationship has been found between DHEAS levels and cardiovascular disease and mortality in elderly men,[54] but this association was not observed in women.[55] Low DHEAS levels have been correlated with heightened risk of breast cancer in premenopausal women.[56] There is a positive correlation between reduced serum DHEAS levels and lower bone mineral density at the spine, hip, and radius in women 45 to 69 years of age[57] but no such effect in men.[58] In the central nervous system, lower DHEAS levels are associated with depressed mood in older women but not men,[59] and a higher cortisol/DHEA ratio correlates with cognitive decline in both sexes.[60] There are conflicting reports of lower DHEAS levels in Alzheimer's disease.[61,62] DHEAS levels are lower in men with type 2 diabetes mellitus,[63] and insulin-sensitizing drug therapy enhances DHEAS levels, suggesting an inverse relationship with insulin resistance. However, a major caveat of such observational data is that falling DHEAS levels may simply be a marker of the aging process and therefore associated with its morbidities, rather than there being a causal relationship.

DHEA REPLACEMENT IN AGING

Accordingly, studies have sought to show changes in biochemical, metabolic, and neuropsychological parameters following DHEA supplementation in aging. In this context, it is important to note that studies of DHEA administration in nonprimate species (e.g., rodents) are of limited value because there is no rise in DHEAS levels corresponding to human adrenarche, nor an age-related decline in levels of this steroid analogous to the adrenopause.

Pharmacokinetic studies have established appropriate dose ranges for DHEA replacement in human aging: 50 mg of oral DHEA administration in men 49 to 70 years restored circulating DHEAS to young adult levels, whereas 100 mg daily was supraphysiologic.[64] Administration of 25 or 50 mg of DHEA in elderly men and women achieved steady-state physiologic levels in 8 days.[65] Interestingly, the half-life of circulating DHEA was more than 20 hours, similar to its longer-lived sulfated metabolite, suggesting that there may be significant back conversion of DHEAS in vivo. Circulating testosterone and estrogens also rose following DHEA administration, but to levels within the young adult range.

A randomized, double-blind, placebo-controlled trial examined the effect of 50 mg of DHEA treatment for 6 months in 13 men and 17 women 40 to 70 years of age.[66] In addition to restoration of young adult DHEAS levels, there was a marked increase in physical and psychological well-being in both sexes (67% of men and 81% of women), with no change in libido. This effect was only associated with increased insulin-like growth factor 1 (IGF-1) and reduced IGF-binding protein 1 (IGFBP-1) levels, with no change in circulating sex hormone–binding globulin (SHBG), estrogens, or lipids. Extending these observations, the same researchers studied 100 mg of DHEA replacement for 6 months in elderly subjects (9 men, 10 women, aged 50 to 65),[67] showing restoration of circulating DHEAS and the cortisol/DHEAS ratio to young adult levels. There was a decrease in fat mass and enhanced muscle strength in men but not women. Circulating androgens (androstenedione, testosterone, dihydrotestosterone) rose above young adult levels in women but not men, suggesting gender-specific differences in the response to DHEA administration. However, another study of 100 mg DHEA for 3 months in elderly men showed no effect on body composition, serum prostate-specific antigen, or urologic function.[68]

A major randomized, placebo-controlled trial was conducted of 50 mg DHEA replacement for 12 months in 280 men and women aged 60 to 79 years.[69] Although young adult DHEAS levels were restored in both sexes, these researchers observed gender differences with other parameters as well. Serum testosterone and androstanediol glucuronide rose to slightly supraphysiologic levels at 6 months in 21% of women but not in men. Bone mineral density improved at the femoral neck (60- to 69-year age group) and radius (70- to 79-year age group), with a fall in serum collagen telopeptide, selectively in women. Likewise, only women reported an increase in libido, sexual function, and satisfaction. The skin changes seen in both sexes included increased skin hydration, diminished facial pigmentation and epidermal atrophy, and enhanced sebum production (particularly in women over 70). There were no changes in vascular function as assessed by ultrasonographic methods. A placebo-controlled trial evaluated DHEA supplementation for 24 months in 29 men and 27 women over 60 years, showing no effect on body composition, physical performance, insulin sensitivity, or quality of life but an improvement in bone mineral density at the ultradistal radius (women) or femoral neck (men).[70]

Following menopause, testosterone and androstenedione levels fall by 50%, and the decline in DHEAS with aging leads to a further fall in circulating androgens. This knowledge has prompted treatment of postmenopausal women with DHEA as a form of androgen replacement. Treatment of 14 women from the ages of 60 to 70 for 12 months with 10% DHEA cream applied topically successfully raised serum DHEA levels 10-fold.[71] In conjunction with this, increased sebum production and an estrogenic effect on vaginal epithelium was observed. Bone mineral density at the hip was enhanced, with increased osteoblastic (osteocalcin) and decreased osteoclastic (bone alkaline phosphatase, urinary hydroxyproline) marker activity. Other changes included a 10% reduction in skinfold thickness and lower blood glucose and insulin levels, with no adverse effects on the lipid profile.[72] Subjects also reported improved well-being. In contrast, 50 mg DHEA administered orally in 60 perimenopausal women (ages 45 to 55) had less effect. Despite a twofold rise in DHEAS levels, there was no effect on mood, cognition, quality of life, or libido.[73] The addition of DHEA to exercise training in postmenopausal women showed no further benefit in physical performance, insulin sensitivity, or lipid profile.[74]

Exposure to DHEA augments natural killer cell–mediated cytotoxicity in vitro,[75] and DHEA supplementation in postmenopausal women or aging men increases natural killer cell number and function.[76,77] Although DHEA treatment does not influence the immune response to influenza vaccination,[78] future studies of immune function following DHEA replacement which examine better in vivo immunologic correlates of its activity might reveal additional effects. Finally, there may be a pharmacologic role for DHEA in certain contexts. Although short-term (2 weeks' duration) placebo-controlled studies have shown no effect of DHEA treatment on cognitive function in the elderly,[79] a recent study has shown that DHEA therapy for 6 weeks had a significant beneficial effect in major depression.[80]

Based on current evidence, it is clear that DHEA supplementation in aging subjects is effective at restoring circulating levels of this steroid to the levels associated with young adult range and normalizing the cortisol/DHEA ratio. Even though it may raise circulating androgens to slightly supraphysiologic levels in women, this does not appear to be associated with significant adverse androgenic effects (hirsutism, acne, dyslipidemia). Interestingly, some of its beneficial effects—for example, on bone mineral density and sexual function—are either gender-specific or more evident in women, suggesting that the agent may be acting as a precursor for androgen or estrogen biosynthesis. In future studies, especially in postmenopausal women, it would be of interest to compare the efficacy of testosterone replacement directly with DHEA treatment. In both sexes, significant psychological benefit with enhanced well-being has been documented. While these observations may justify short-term treatment, longer-term studies are now required to determine whether, as epidemiologic data suggest, cardiovascular morbidity and mortality, cognitive decline, or cancer risk can be influenced by DHEA replacement.

DHEA AND ADRENAL INSUFFICIENCY

In comparison to aging, circulating DHEAS levels in adrenal failure are very low or undetectable. Such deficiency is observed in secondary as well as primary adrenal insufficiency (Addison's disease), implying that production of this adrenal steroid, like glucocorticoid synthesis, is pituitary dependent. Glucocorticoid and mineralocorticoid deficiencies in adrenal insufficiency are life threatening and require oral replacement therapy, but the associated near-total failure of DHEA synthesis is not usually corrected. Despite optimal therapy with conventional steroids, patients with Addison's disease report persistent fatigue and reduced well-being,[81,82] with specific impairment in subscales of health status.[83,84] These observations have prompted trials of DHEA replacement.

In 10 patients with hypopituitarism, 50 mg of DHEA replacement restored DHEAS, androstenedione, and testosterone to young adult levels, whereas a 200 mg daily dose was supraphysiologic.[85] In young normal subjects in whom endogenous adrenal steroidogenesis had been suppressed with dexamethasone, 50 mg of DHEA daily was also an appropriate dose.[86]

A randomized, double-blind, placebo-controlled trial of 50 mg DHEA replacement was conducted in 24 women with adrenal insufficiency (14 primary, 10 secondary).[87] Physiologic levels of DHEAS and androstenedione were restored, and serum testosterone rose from below to within low-normal range. Following 4 months of therapy, psychological testing showed a significant reduction in scores for depression and anxiety, together with improvement in overall well-being and mood. Patients also reported markedly increased sexual thoughts and interest, with enhanced mental and physical sexual satisfaction. Serum testosterone rose from below to within low-normal range, with a fall in SHBG; 19 subjects developed some cutaneous androgenic side effects. A later study of DHEA replacement in nine women with Addison's disease also reported increased apocrine sweat secretion and acne, with no difference between 50 or 200 mg daily dosage.[88]

In a randomized, placebo-controlled trial in 15 men and 24 women with Addison's disease, the authors observed similar restoration of DHEAS and androstenedione levels in both sexes following 3 months of treatment with 50 mg of DHEA, together with a rise in serum testosterone and fall in SHBG in women but not men.[89] There was an overall trend of enhanced well-being, with particular improvement in self-esteem. Mood and fatigue also improved significantly, with benefit being evident in the evenings. The authors found no effects on cognitive or sexual function. No significant adverse effects were seen in patients. Beneficial psychological effects in males, independent of changes in circulating testosterone, supported the notion of a direct central nervous system effect of DHEA rather than it simply being a substrate for peripheral androgen biosynthesis. DHEA replacement for 12 or 24 weeks in adrenal insufficiency has no effect on vascular and endothelial function[90,91] but is significantly immunomodulatory.[92]

Administration of lower doses (20 to 30 mg) of DHEA for 6 months to 38 women with hypopituitarism was associated with increased axillary or pubic hair, together with improved alertness, stamina, and initiative, as reported by their spouses.[93] A recent study has shown similar benefit in adolescent girls with central adrenal insufficiency.[94] A further benefit in female hypopituitarism is that addition of DHEA treatment reduces the dose of growth hormone replacement required to maintain IGF-1 levels.[95] A longer term, 9-month trial of administering 25 mg of DHEA to 39 women with adrenal insufficiency showed no beneficial effects on subjective health status or sexual function, but the study may have been underpowered.[96,97] In a trial with a larger cohort of over 100 patients with Addison's disease, the authors found that treatment with 50 mg of DHEA for 12 months was associated with beneficial effects in well-being and fatigue, enhancement of lean body mass, and improvement in femoral neck bone mineral density. Adverse androgenic side effects were observed in older females, suggesting that a lower dose of DHEA might be more appropriate in this age group.[83]

Short- and longer-term trials of DHEA replacement in adrenal insufficiency suggest clear benefits regarding mood and well-being, fatigue, sexual function, body composition, and possibly bone mineral density in both women and men. Future studies may ascertain whether certain effects of DHEA (e.g., on sexual function) are most evident in particular subgroups (e.g., in women with premature ovarian failure or of postmenopausal status), whether enhancement of bone and muscle mass by DHEA can be further augmented, and whether effects of DHEA treatment can be influenced by other concurrent conventional hormone replacements.

Conclusions

DHEAS is produced in massive amounts relative to hormones synthesized by other steroid-secreting organs, yet its precise role in normal homeostasis and pathophysiologic states remains a mystery. It has a unique developmental secretory pattern, with control that is different from the standard trophin stimulation characteristic of other classic hormones such as cortisol, sex hormones, and thyroid hormones. DHEAS is a multifunctional hormone, where the primary role may reside outside the classic endocrine system by virtue of the evidence for effects on endothelial cells, immune function, and neuronal activity. It is evident that the precise pathophysiologic states associated with increased or decreased production of a hormone are still not clearly defined in the case of DHEAS.

REFERENCES

1. Abbott DH, Bird IM: Non-human primates as models for human adrenal androgen production: function and dysfunction, Rev Endocr Metab Disord 10:33–42, 2009.
2. Young MC, Laurence KM, Hughes IA: Relationship between fetal adrenal morphology and anterior pituitary function, Horm Res 32:130–135, 1989.
3. Coleman MA, Honour JW: Reduced maternal dexamethasone dosage for the prenatal treatment of congenital adrenal hyperplasia, Br J Obstet Gynaecol 111:176–178, 2004.
4. Rehman KS, Carr BR, Rainey WE: Profiling the steroidogenic pathway in human fetal and adult adrenals, J Soc Gynecol Investig 10:372–380, 2003.
5. Jones ME, Boon WC, McInnes K, et al: Recognizing rare disorders: aromatase deficiency, Nat Clin Pract Endocrinol Metab 3:414–421, 2007.
6. Wolkersdorf G, Bornstein SR: Tissue remodelling in the adrenal gland, Biochem Pharmacol 56:163–171, 1998.
7. Spencer SJ, Mesiano, S, Lee JY, et al: Proliferation and apoptosis in the human adrenal cortex during the fetal and perinatal periods: implications for growth and remodelling, J Clin Endocrinol Metab 84:1110–1115, 1999.
8. Dhom G: The prepubertal and pubertal growth of the adrenal (adrenarche), Beitr Pathol 150:357–377, 1973.
9. Remer T, Manz F: Role of nutritional status in the regulation of adrenarche, J Clin Endocrinol Metab 84:3936–3944, 1999.
10. Palmert MR, Hayden DL, Mansfield MJ, et al: The longitudinal study of adrenal maturation during gonadal suppression: evidence that adrenarche is a gradual process, J Clin Endocrinol Metab 86:4536–4542, 2001.
11. Stocco DM, Clark BJ: Regulation of the acute production of steroids in steroidogenic cells, Endocr Rev 17:221–244, 1996.
12. Miller WL: Androgen biosynthesis from cholesterol to DHEA, Mol Cell Endocrinol 198:7–14, 2002.
13. Zhang L, Rodriguez H, Ohno S, et al: Serine phosphorylation of human P450c17 increases 17,20 lyase activity: implications for adrenarche and for the polycystic ovary syndrome, Proc Natl Acad Sci U S A 92:10619–10623, 1995.
14. Lin D, Black SM, Nagahama Y, et al: Steroid 17a-hydroxylase and 17,20-lyase activities of P450c17: Contributions of serine 106 and P450 reductase, Endocrinology 132:2496–2506, 1993.
15. Lee-Robichaud P, Wright JN, Akhtar ME, et al: Modulation of the activity of human 17a-hydroxylase-17,20-lyase (CYP17) by cytochrome b5: endocrinological and mechanistic implications, Biochem J 308:901–908, 1995.
16. Arlt W, Walker EA, Draper N, et al: Congenital adrenal hyperplasia caused by mutant P450 oxidoreductase and human androgen synthesis: Analytical study, Lancet 363:2128–2135, 2004.
17. Miller WL: P450 oxidoreductase deficiency: a new disorder of steroidogenesis with multiple clinical manifestations, Trends Endocrinol Metab 15:311–315, 2004.
18. Flück CE, Tajima T, Pandey AV, et al: Mutant P450 oxidoreductase causes disordered steroidogenesis with and without Antley-Bixler syndrome, Nat Genet 36:228–230, 2004.
19. Conley AJ, Birm IM: The role of cytochrome P450 17α-hydroxylase and 3β-hydroxysteroid dehydrogenase in the integration of gonadal and adrenal steroidogenesis via the Δ5 and Δ4 pathway of steroidogenesis in mammals, Biol Reprod 56:789–799, 1997.
20. Strott CA: Steroid sulfotransferases, Endocr Rev 17:670–697, 1996.
21. Suzuki T, Sasano H, Takeyama J, et al: Developmental changes in steroidogenic enzymes in human postnatal adrenal cortex: immunohistochemical studies, Clin Endocrinol 53:739–747, 2000.
22. Rainey WE, Carr BR, Sasano H, et al: Dissecting human adrenal androgen production, Trends Endocrinol Metab 13:234–239, 2002.
23. Auchus RJ, Rainey WE: Adrenarche-physiology, biochemistry and human disease, Clin Endocrinol 60:288–296, 2004.
24. Bassett MH, Suzuki T, Sasano H, et al: The orphan nuclear receptor NGF1B regulates transcription of 3β-hydroxysteroid dehydrogenase: implications for the control of adrenal functional zonation, J Biol Chem 279:37622–37630, 2004.
25. Weber A, Clark AJ, Perry LA, et al: Diminished adrenal androgen secretion in familial glucocorticoid deficiency implicates a significant role for ACTH in the induction of adrenarche, Clin Endocrinol 46:431–437, 1997.
26. Smith R, Mesiano S, Cheng EC, et al: Corticotropin-releasing hormone directly and preferentially stimulates Dehydroepiandrosterone sulfate secretion by human fetal adrenal cortical cells, J Clin Endocrinol Metab 83:2916–2920, 1998.
27. Ibanez L, Potau N, Marcos MV, et al: Corticotropin-releasing hormone as adrenal androgen secretagogue, Pediatr Res 46:351–353, 1999.
28. Biason-Lauber A, Zachmann M, Schoenle EJ: Effect of leptin on CYP17 enzymatic activities in human adrenal cells: new insight in the onset of adrenarche, Endocrinology 141:1446–1454, 2000.
29. l'Allemand D, Schmidt S, Rousson V, et al: Associations between body mass, leptin, IGF-1 and circulating adrenal androgens in children with obesity and premature adrenarche, Eur J Endocrinol 146:537–543, 2002.
30. Charkaluk M-L, Trivin C, Brauner R: Premature pubarche as an indicator of how body weight influences the onset of adrenarche, Eur J Pediatr 163:89–93, 2004.
31. Ong KK, Potau N, Petry CJ, et al: Opposing influences of prenatal and postnatal weight gain on adrenarche in normal boys and girls, J Clin Endocrinol Metab 89:2647–2651, 2004.
32. Utrainen P, Voutilainen R, Jääskeläinen J: Girls with premature adrenarche have accelerated early childhood growth, J Pediatr 154:882–887, 2009.
33. Remer T, Manz F: The midgrowth spurt in healthy children is not caused by adrenarche, J Clin Endocrinol Metab 86:4183–4186, 2001.
34. Ribeiro RC, Figueiredo B: Childhood adrenocortical tumours, Eur J Cancer 40:1117–1126, 2004.
35. Armegaud J-B, Charkaluk M-L, Trivin C, et al: Precocious pubarche: distinguishing late-onset congenital adrenal hyperplasia from premature adrenarche, J Clin Endocrinol Metab 94:2835–2840, 2009.
36. Ibanez L, Virdis R, Potau N, et al: Natural history of premature pubarche: an auxological study, J Clin Endocrinol Metab 74:254–257, 1992.
37. Ibanez L, Diaz R, Lopez-Bermejo A, et al: Clinical spectrum of premature pubarche: links to metabolic syndrome and ovarian hyperandrogenism, Rev Endocr Metab Disord 10:63–76, 2009.
38. Maliqueo M, Sir Petermann T, Perez V, et al: Adrenal function during childhood and puberty in daughters of women with polycystic ovary syndrome, J Clin Endocrinol Metab 94:1923–1930, 2009.
39. Noordam C, Dhir V, McNelis C, et al: Inactivating PAPSS2 mutations in a patient with premature adrenarche, N Engl J Med 360:2310–2318, 2009.
40. Ibanez L, Ferrer A, Ong K, et al: Insulin sensitisation early after menarche prevents progression from precocious pubarche to polycystic ovary syndrome, J Pediatr 144:4–6, 2004.
41. Labrie F, Luu-the V, Labrie C, et al: Endocrine and intracrine sources of androgens in women: Inhibition of breast cancer and other roles of androgens and their

precursor dehydroepiandrosterone, Endocr Rev 24:152–182, 2003.

42. Mellon S, Griffin L: Neurosteroids: biochemistry and clinical significance, Trends Endocrinol Metab 13:35–43, 2002.

43. Majewska MD: Neuronal actions of dehydroepiandrosterone. Possible roles in brain development, aging, memory, and affect, Ann N Y Acad Sci 774:111–120, 1995.

44. May M, Holmes E, Rogers W, et al: Protection from glucocorticoid induced thymic involution by dehydroepiandrosterone, Life Sci 46:1627–1631, 1991.

45. Kimonides VG, Spillantini MG, Sofroniew MV, et al: Dehydroepiandrosterone (DHEA) antagonises the neurotoxic effects of corticosterone and translocation of SAPK3 in hippocampal primary cultures, Neuroscience 89:429–436, 1999.

46. Liu D, Dillon JS: Dehydroepiandrosterone activates endothelial cell nitric-oxide synthase by a specific plasma membrane receptor coupled to Gai2,3, J Biol Chem 277:21379–21388, 2002.

47. Williams MR, Ling S, Dawood T, et al: Dehydroepiandrosterone inhibits human vascular smooth muscle cell proliferation independent of ARs and ERs, J Clin Endocrinol Metab 87:176–181, 2002.

48. Maurer M, Trajanoski Z, Frey, G, et al: Differential gene expression profile of glucocorticoids, testosterone, and dehydroepiandrosterone in human cells, Horm Metab Res 33:691–695, 2001.

49. Vermeulen A: Dehydroepiandrosterone sulfate and aging, Ann N Y Acad Sci 774:121–127, 1995.

50. Orentreich N, Brind JL, Rizer RL, et al: Age changes and sex differences in serum dehydroepiandrosterone sulfate concentrations throughout adulthood, J Clin Endocrinol Metab 59:551–555, 1984.

51. Laughlin GA, Barrett-Connor E: Sexual dimorphism in the influence of advanced aging on adrenal hormone levels: The Rancho Bernardo Study, J Clin Endocrinol Metab 85:3561–3568, 2000.

52. Lane MA, Ingram DK, Ball SS, et al: Dehydroepiandrosterone sulfate: a biomarker of primate ageing slowed by calorie restriction, J Clin Endocrinol Metab 82:2093–2096, 1997.

53. Salvini S, Stampfer MJ, Barbieri RL, et al: Effects of age, smoking and vitamins on plasma DHEAS levels: a cross-sectional study in men, J Clin Endocrinol Metab 74:139–143, 1992.

54. Barrett-Connor E, Khaw K-T, Yen SSC: A prospective study of dehydroepiandrosterone sulfate, mortality and cardiovascular disease, New Engl J Med 315:1519–1524, 1986.

55. Barrett-Connor E, Goodman-Gruen D: Dehydroepiandrosterone sulfate does not predict cardiovascular death in postmenopausal women, The Rancho Bernardo Study, Circulation 91:1757–1760, 1995.

56. Helzlsouer KJ, Gordon GB, Alberg AJ, et al: Relationship of prediagnostic serum levels of dehydroepiandrosterone and dehydroepiandrosterone sulfate to the risk of developing premenopausal breast cancer, Cancer Res 52:1–4, 1992.

57. Szathmari M, Szucs J, Feher T, et al: Dehydroepiandrosterone sulphate and bone mineral density, Osteoporos Int 4:84–88, 1994.

58. Greendale GA, Edelstein S, Barrett-Connor E: Endogenous sex steroids and bone mineral density in older women and men: The Rancho Bernardo Study, J Bone Miner Res 12:1833–1843, 1997.

59. Barrett-Connor E, von Muhlen D, Laughlin GA, et al: Endogenous levels of dehydroepiandrosterone sulfate, but not other sex hormones, are associated with depressed mood in older women: the Rancho Bernardo Study, J Am Geriatr Soc 47:685–691, 1999.

60. Kalmijn S, Launer LJ, Stolk RP, et al: A prospective study on cortisol, dehydroepiandrosterone sulfate and cognitive function in the elderly, J Clin Endocrinol Metab 83:3487–3492, 1998.

61. Nasman B, Olsson T, Backstrom T, et al: Serum dehydroepiandrosterone sulfate in Alzheimer's disease and in multi-infarct dementia, Biol Psychiatry 30:684–690, 1991.

62. Schneider LS, Hinsey M, Lyness S: Plasma dehydroepiandrosterone sulfate in Alzheimer's disease, Biol Psychiatry 31:205–208, 1992.

63. Barrett-Connor E: Lower endogenous androgen levels and dyslipidemia in men with non-insulin-dependent diabetes mellitus, Ann Intern Med 117:807–811, 1992.

64. Arlt W, Haas J, Callies F, et al: Biotransformation of oral dehydroepiandrosterone in elderly men: significant increase in circulating estrogens, J Clin Endocrinol Metab 84:2170–2176, 1999.

65. Legrain S, Massien C, Lahlou N, et al: Dehydroepiandrosterone replacement administration: Pharmacokinetic and pharmacodynamic studies in healthy elderly subjects, J Clin Endocrinol Metab 85:3208–3217, 2000.

66. Morales AJ, Nolan JJ, Nelson JC, et al: Effects of replacement dose of dehydroepiandrosterone in men and women of advancing age, J Clin Endocrinol Metab 78:1360–1367, 1994.

67. Morales AJ, Haubrich RH, Hwang JY: The effect of six months treatment with a 100 mg daily dose of dehydroepiandrosterone (DHEA) on circulating sex steroids, body composition and muscle strength in age-advanced men and women, Clin Endocrinol 49:421–432, 1998.

68. Flynn MA, Weaver-Osterholtz D, Sharpe-Timms KL, et al: Dehydroepiandrosterone replacement in aging humans, J Clin Endocrinol Metab 84:1527–1533, 1999.

69. Baulieu EE, Thomas G, Legrain S, et al: Dehydroepiandrosterone (DHEA), DHEA sulfate, and aging: contribution of the DHEAge Study to a sociobiomedical issue, Proc Natl Acad Sci U S A 97:4279–4284, 2000.

70. Nair KS, Rizza RA, O'Brien P, et al: DHEA in elderly women and DHEA or testosterone in elderly men, N Engl J Med 355:1647–1659, 2006.

71. Labrie F, Diamond P, Cusan L, et al: Effect of 12-month dehydroepiandrosterone replacement therapy on bone, vagina and endometrium in postmenopausal women, J Clin Endocrinol Metab 82:3498–3505, 1997.

72. Diamond P, Cusan L, Gomez J-L, et al: Metabolic effects of 12-month percutaneous dehydroepiandrosterone replacement therapy in postmenopausal women, J Endocrinol 150:S43–S50, 1996.

73. Barnhart KT, Freeman E, Grisso JA, et al: The effect of dehydroepiandrosterone supplementation to symptomatic perimenopausal women on serum endocrine profiles, lipid parameters, and health-related quality of life, J Clin Endocrinol Metab 84:3896–3902, 1999.

74. Igwebuike A, Irving BA, Bigelow ML, et al. Lack of dehydroepiandrosterone effect on a combined endurance and resistance exercise program in postmenopausal women, J Clin Endocrinol Metab 93:534–538, 2008.

75. Solerte SB, Fioravanti M, Vignati G, et al: Dehydroepiandrosterone sulfate enhances natural killer cell cytotoxicity in humans via locally generated immunoreactive insulin-like growth factor I, J Clin Endocrinol Metab 84:3260–3267, 1999.

76. Casson PR, Andersen RN, Herrod HG, et al: Oral dehydroepiandrosterone in physiologic doses modulates immune function in postmenopausal women, Am J Obstet Gynecol 169:1536–1539, 1993.

77. Khorram O, Vu L, Yen SS: Activation of immune function by dehydroepiandrosterone (DHEA) in age-advanced men, J Gerontol 52:M1–M7, 1997.

78. Danenberg HD, Ben-Yehuda A, Zakay-Rones Z, et al: Dehydroepiandrosterone treatment is not beneficial to the immune response to influenza in elderly subjects, J Clin Endocrinol Metab 82:2911–2914, 1997.

79. Wolf OT, Kirschbaum C: Wishing a dream came true: DHEA as a rejuvenating treatment? J Endocrinol Invest 21:133–135, 1998.

80. Wolkowitz OM, Reus VI, Keebler A, et al: Double-blind treatment of major depression with dehydroepiandrosterone, Am J Psychiatry 156:646–649, 1999.

81. Reidel M, Weise A, Schurmeyer TH, et al: Quality of life in patients with Addison's disease: effects of different cortisol replacement modes, Exp Clin Endocrinol 101:106–111, 1993.

82. Baker SJK, Hunt PJ, Wass JAH: Assessing the potential for finetuning the management of Addison's disease/steroid replacement therapy, J Endocrinol 155(Suppl):P2, 1997.

83. Gurnell EM, Hunt PJ, Curran SE, et al: Long-term DHEA replacement in primary adrenal insufficiency: a randomised, controlled trial, J Clin Endocrinol Metab 93:400–409, 2008.

84. Hahner S, Loeffler M, Fassnacht M, et al. Impaired subjective health status in 256 patients with adrenal insufficiency on standard therapy based on cross-sectional analysis, J Clin Endocrinol Metab 92:3912–3922, 2007.

85. Young J, Couzinet B, Nahoul K, et al: Panhypopituitarism as a model to study the metabolism of dehydroepiandrosterone (DHEA) in humans, J Clin Endocrinol Metab 82:2578–2585, 1997.

86. Arlt W, Justl H-G, Callies F, et al: Oral dehydroepiandrosterone for adrenal androgen replacement: pharmacokinetics and peripheral conversion to androgens and estrogens in young females after dexamethasone suppression, J Clin Endocrinol Metab 83:1928–1934, 1998.

87. Arlt W, Callies F, van Vlijmen JC, et al: Dehydroepiandrosterone replacement in women with adrenal insufficiency, New Engl J Med 341:1013–1020, 1999.

88. Gebre-Medhin G, Husebye ES, Mallmin H, et al: Oral dehydroepiandrosterone (DHEA) replacement therapy in women with Addison's disease, Clin Endocrinol 52:775–780, 2000.

89. Hunt PJ, Gurnell EM, Huppert FA, et al: Improvement in mood and fatigue after dehydroepiandrosterone replacement in Addison's Disease in a randomized, double blind trial, J Clin Endocrinol Metab 85:4650–4656, 2000.

90. Christiansen JJ, Andersen NH, Sorensen KE, et al: Dehydroepiandrosterone substitution in female adrenal failure: no impact on endothelial function and cardiovascular parameters despite normalization of androgen status, Clin Endocrinol (Oxf) 66:426–433, 2007.

91. Rice SP, Agarwal N, Bolusani H, et al: Effects of dehydroepiandrosterone replacement on vascular function in primary and secondary adrenal insufficiency: a randomized crossover trial, J Clin Endocrinol Metab 94:1966–1972, 2009.

92. Coles AJ, Thompson S, Cox AL, et al: Dehydroepiandrosterone replacement in patients with Addison's disease has a bimodal effect on regulatory (CD4+CD25hi and CD4+FoxP3+) T cells, Eur J Immunol 35:3694–3703, 2005.

93. Johannsson G, Burman P, Wiren L, et al: Low dose dehydroepiandrosterone affects behavior in hypopituitary androgen-deficient women: a placebo-controlled trial, J Clin Endocrinol Metab 87:2046–2052, 2002.

94. Binder G, Weber S, Ehrismann M, et al: Effects of dehydroepiandrosterone therapy on pubic hair growth and psychological well-being in adolescent girls and young women with central adrenal insufficiency: a double-blind, randomized, placebo-controlled phase III trial, J Clin Endocrinol Metab 94:1182–1190, 2009.

95. Brooke AM, Kalingag LA, Miraki-Moud F, et al: Dehydroepiandrosterone (DHEA) replacement reduces growth hormone (GH) dose requirement in female hypopituitary patients on GH replacement, Clin Endocrinol (Oxf) 65:673–680, 2006.

96. Lovas K, Gebre-Medhin G, Trovik ST, et al: Replacement of dehydroepiandrosterone in adrenal failure: no benefit for subjective health status and sexuality in a 9-month, randomized, parallel group clinical trial, J Clin Endocrinol Metab 88:1112–1118, 2003.

97. Arlt W, Allolio B: DHEA. Replacement in adrenal insufficiency, J Clin Endocrinol Metab 88:4001–4002, 2003.

Chapter 10

ADRENAL GLAND IMAGING

MILTON D. GROSS, MELVYN KOROBKIN, HERO K. HUSSAIN, KYUNG J. CHO, and CHUONG BUI

High-resolution imaging affords detailed information concerning adrenal anatomy. Both computed tomography (CT) and magnetic resonance imaging (MRI) demonstrate subtle nuances of adrenal contours and can effectively identify lesions as small as 3 to 5 mm in diameter. When findings are combined with sensitive biochemical tests of adrenocortical and medullary hormones, identification of adrenal gland dysfunction can be made at very early stages in the development of disease. Although present emphasis has shifted to high-resolution, anatomic imaging with CT and MRI, complementary functional tests using radiopharmaceuticals specifically designed to take advantage of unique biochemical characteristics of the adrenal cortex and medulla can be used to diagnostic advantage in many cases.

Adrenal Gland Imaging

Contemporary methods for adrenal gland imaging are listed in Table 10-1. Both ultrasound and arteriography are readily available and have played an important role in the evaluation of adrenal dysfunction, but neither is considered routine for adrenal gland imaging at this time.

CT is currently the primary method of imaging the adrenal gland, both for evaluating patients with abnormal adrenal function and for demonstrating adrenal anatomy in patients with incidentally discovered adrenal masses. MRI can also detect the normal and abnormal adrenal gland with accuracy similar to CT, and frequently is used to help characterize many incidental adrenal masses as adenomas. Because CT is used much more often to evaluate the abdomen for a variety of known or suspected abnormalities unrelated to the adrenal glands, it is the imaging modality with which most incidental adrenal masses are first detected.[1]

COMPUTED TOMOGRAPHY

With the use of modern CT scanners, the normal adrenals can be visualized in virtually 100% of cases. With the advent of helical CT technology, axial slices of 3 to 5 mm can be obtained routinely in patients suspected of adrenal pathology. Oral contrast and intravenous contrast are not necessary for detection of adrenal masses, but are used routinely in abdominal CT.

MAGNETIC RESONANCE IMAGING

Recent advances in MRI technology have improved its ability to demonstrate the normal adrenal glands and small adrenal masses. Most notably, the development of *breath-hold* pulse sequences has dramatically decreased artifacts that limited the utility of adrenal MRI. The traditional advantages of MRI—improved tissue contrast resolution, ability to image in multiple planes, and utility in patients with renal insufficiency and previous idiosyncratic reaction to iodinated contrast material—have always made it a useful alternative to CT. But the image quality of gradient-echo breath-hold scans, use of in-phase and opposed-phrase imaging to detect intracellular lipid in adrenal adenomas, and improved spatial resolution on 3-dimensional dynamic imaging with thin slices, make MRI a truly competitive method with CT for imaging normal and pathologic adrenal glands.

Table 10-1. Adrenal Gland Imaging

Technique	Underlying Principle	Advantages	Disadvantages	Comments	Relative Cost
Ultrasound	Reflection of ultrasound, depicts anatomy	Widely available. No radiation exposure	Limited resolution. Interference by fat and bowel gas	Limited utility	++
Angiography	X-ray attenuation with iodinated contrast, depicts vascular anatomy	Detailed depiction of vascular anatomy	Invasive (arterial puncture). Technically demanding. May cause adrenal hemorrhage or infarction, Risks of contrast reaction	Generally obsolete for adrenal localization	+++
Venous hormone sampling	Direct measurement of adrenal vein hormone levels. X-ray attenuation with iodinated contrast to confirm anatomy and sampling catheter placement	Characterization of hormonal secretory state ± hormone stimulation (gold standard). Can be used to depict venous anatomy	Invasive (venous catheterization). Technically demanding. Multiple hormonal measurements. Radiation exposure. Risk for adrenal hemorrhage, infarction, and contrast reaction	Valuable when noninvasive studies are equivocal. Technically demanding	++++
Computed tomography (CT)	X-ray attenuation, anatomy based (iodinated contrast may be used)	Highest spatial resolution. X-ray attenuation can be quantified as can washout of contrast.	May fail in postoperative or very thin patients. Radiation exposure	Very widely employed	++++
Magnetic resonance imaging (MRI)	Radiofrequency signal by protons in magnetic field following radiofrequency stimulus	High spatial resolution. No ionizing radiation. Some degree of tissue characterization	Limited specificity of tissue characterization. Resolution <CT in routine adrenal imaging applications	Limited advantages over CT. Modes of tissue characterization may be useful.	+++++
Scintigraphy (planar, SPECT, and hybrid SPECT/CT)	Detection of selective radiopharmaceutical uptake by various noninvasive mechanisms	Noninvasive depiction of function and anatomy with hybrid SPECT/CT	Moderate resolution, tracer uptake may be slow (hours to days). Radiation exposure	Complementary to CT and MRI hybrid SPECT/CT useful in functional/anatomic localization	++++
Positron emission tomography/computed tomography (PET/CT)	Detection of positron emitting tracers. Selective uptake by various cellular mechanisms	FDG and other PET agents demonstrate selective accumulation in primary and metastatic malignancy.	Expensive, limited availability of PET radiopharmaceuticals. Radiation exposure	Hybrid PET/CT useful in simultaneous functional/anatomic localization	+++++

FDG, Fluorodeoxyglucose; *SPECT*, single-photon emission computed tomography.

NORMAL ADRENAL ANATOMY

The cross-sectional anatomy of the normal adrenal gland is nearly identical on CT and MRI. The right adrenal lies higher in the abdomen than the left adrenal. It is superior to the upper pole of the right kidney, whereas the left adrenal is anteromedial to the upper pole of the left kidney. The basic morphology of the adrenal glands on transverse axial CT and MRI is that of an inverted V or an inverted Y. In the inverted Y configuration, the anterior limb is shorter and thicker than the posteromedial and posterolateral limbs and sometimes is undetectable, thus the inverted V appearance (Fig. 10-1).

Clinical Utility of CT and MRI

CUSHING'S SYNDROME

Cushing's syndrome results from excess circulating glucocorticoids, which causes characteristic clinical signs and symptoms. It refers to the clinical and metabolic disorder regardless of the underlying cause. The most common cause is iatrogenic steroid administration. Endogenous Cushing's syndrome is due to overproduction of cortisol by the adrenal cortex, caused by (1) excess production of adrenocorticotropic hormone (ACTH) by a pituitary tumor; (2) a steroid-producing adrenal cortical tumor, benign or malignant; or (3) adrenal hyperplasia secondary to an ectopic source of ACTH production. Very rare causes of ACTH-independent bilateral hyperplasia also have been identified.

Strictly speaking, Cushing's disease refers only to bilateral adrenal hyperplasia due to overproduction of ACTH by a pituitary adenoma.

Most cases of Cushing's syndrome (up to 85%) are due to excess ACTH production from a pituitary or ectopic source. The adrenals may be normal on CT or may show diffuse bilateral hyperplasia. A small percentage of patients (12% to 15%) with Cushing's disease demonstrate multiple or, less commonly, single macronodules, varying in size from several millimeters to 7 cm. If macronodular adrenal hyperplasia is characterized by a single dominant nodule, this entity may be confused with a unilateral autonomous adrenal adenoma, leading to performance of an inappropriate unilateral adrenalectomy.[2] Additional small nodules or diffuse overall enlargement of both glands usually is present, however, which together with the biochemical findings, allows the correct diagnosis to be made.

A much rarer form of macronodular adrenal hyperplasia is ACTH-independent disease. Two unique CT and MRI features of this disorder are the large mass of cortical tissue and the size of individual nodules (Fig. 10-2).[3] The size of the nodules can suggest a diagnosis of bilateral metastases or bilateral adenomas, but, in the presence of Cushing's syndrome, the appearance is practically pathognomonic of ACTH-independent macronodular adrenal hyperplasia, and bilateral adrenalectomy is indicated on the basis of clinical and CT findings.

About 15% of cases of ACTH-dependent Cushing's syndrome are due to ectopic ACTH secretion from a nonpituitary source. The most common source of an ectopic ACTH-producing tumor

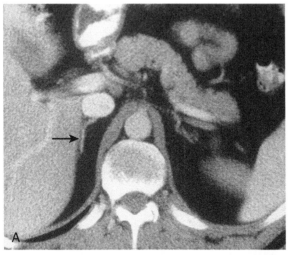

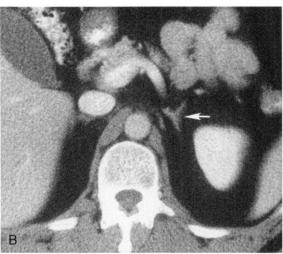

FIGURE 10-1. Computed tomography (CT) appearance of normal adrenal glands. **A,** The cephalad portion of the right adrenal *(arrow)* is seen. **B,** The three limbs of the left adrenal *(arrow)* are shown at this level. (From Korobkin M, Francis IR: Adrenal imaging, Semin Ultrasound CT MR 16:317–330, 1995.)

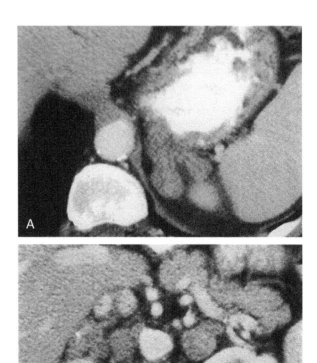

FIGURE 10-2. ACTH-independent macronodular adrenal hyperplasia. **A** and **B** show large nodules bilaterally superimposed on markedly thickened limbs. *ACTH,* Adrenocorticotropic hormone.

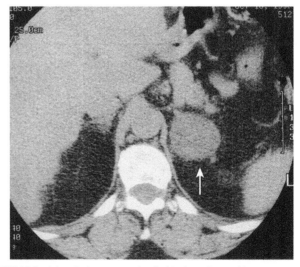

FIGURE 10-3. Adrenal adenoma causing Cushing's syndrome. Homogeneous 4 cm left adrenal mass *(arrow)* has a nonspecific computed tomography (CT) appearance. *L,* Left. (From Korobkin M, Francis I, Kloos R, Dunnick NR: The incidental adrenal mass, RCNA 34:1037–1054, 1996.)

is a small cell carcinoma of the lung. The diagnosis of patients with occult sources of ACTH secretion presents a more difficult diagnostic challenge. Bronchial carcinoid tumors are the most common source of occult, ectopic ACTH secretion, which occurs in about 60% to 80% of cases. In one recent study, five of eight bronchial carcinoid tumors measured between 4 and 10 mm in diameter, and thin section CT was required to evaluate the lungs. Less common sources of ectopic ACTH production include small islet cell tumors of the pancreas, pheochromocytoma, medullary thyroid carcinoma, and thymic carcinoid.

About 30% of cases of Cushing's syndrome are due to an ACTH-independent adrenal cortical neoplasm; about two thirds of these are due to adrenal adenomas and the other one third to adrenal cortical carcinoma. These tumors are easily detectable on both CT and MRI. Adrenal cortical adenomas are nearly always less than 5 cm in diameter, typically 2 to 2.5 cm, and have a nonspecific morphologic appearance (Fig. 10-3). Adrenal cortical carcinomas are typically larger than 5 cm in diameter, often show evidence of necrosis on enhanced CT and MRI scans, and frequently present with spread to adrenal or renal veins or evidence of distant metastatic disease (Fig. 10-4). Carcinomas are usually hypointense relative to liver on T1-weighted images and hyperintense to liver on T2-weighted images.

PRIMARY ALDOSTERONISM

Primary aldosteronism is characterized by moderate to severe hypertension caused by unregulated secretion of aldosterone with elevated levels of serum and urinary aldosterone, hypokalemia, and suppressed plasma renin activity (see also Chapter

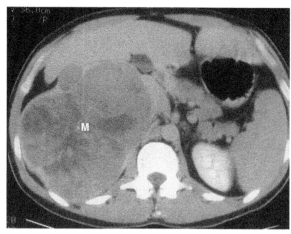

FIGURE 10-4. Adrenal carcinoma causing Cushing's syndrome. Computed tomography (CT) scan shows a huge, inhomogeneous, right adrenal mass (M). (From Korobkin M, Francis IR: Adrenal imaging, Semin Ultrasound CT MR 16:317–330, 1995.)

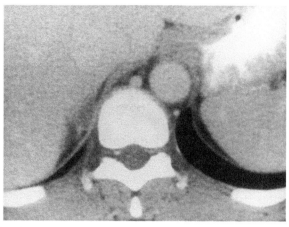

FIGURE 10-5. Computed tomography (CT) demonstration of a 1 cm aldosterone-producing right adrenal adenoma. (From Korobkin M, Francis IR: Adrenal imaging, Semin Ultrasound CT MR 16:317–330, 1995.)

12). A solitary aldosterone-producing adenoma (APA) is present in about 70% of patients, and surgical or laparoscopic adrenalectomy corrects the hypertension and hypokalemia in about 75% to 90% of cases.[4] Most of the remainder have idiopathic hyperaldosteronism (IHA) with bilateral adrenal hyperplasia. Unlike patients with unilateral APA, surgery rarely cures the hypertension and the biochemical abnormalities, and these patients usually are treated medically. It is essential, therefore, to distinguish APA from IHA in primary hyperaldosteronism.

CT is widely used to differentiate between APA and IHA, but the sensitivity and specificity for the diagnosis of an adenoma vary widely in the literature, ranging from 71% to 100% and from 33% to 100%, respectively.[5] If the imaging results are equivocal, adrenal venous sampling is usually recommended. Sensitivity of CT for the diagnosis of APA is lower than for most other adrenal masses because they usually are smaller than 2 cm, and sometimes are smaller than 1 cm, in diameter (Fig. 10-5).

CT evaluation is hampered by the fact that a unilateral aldosteronoma may be associated with non–aldosterone-secreting nodules in the ipsilateral or contralateral gland and can result in a false diagnosis of adrenal hyperplasia.[6] In addition, bilateral hyperplasia may have a predominant unilateral macronodule and may cause an erroneous diagnosis of a unilateral aldosteronoma.

Doppman and colleagues[7] demonstrated that CT cannot reliably differentiate APA from IHA whenever bilateral adrenal nodules are demonstrated. In their series, 6 of 21 patients with APA were incorrectly diagnosed on CT as having IHA. Non–aldosterone-secreting nodules were detected by CT, in addition to the aldosteronoma. Most patients with a unilateral adrenal mass can proceed to unilateral adrenalectomy. Patients with bilateral adrenal nodules, as well as those in whom CT and biochemical evaluations are discordant or equivocal, often undergo bilateral selective adrenal vein sampling for aldosterone levels.[8]

Although most cross-sectional studies of patients with primary aldosteronism have used CT, MRI also can accurately differentiate APA from IHA.[9] Among the 20 patients studied, 10 (50%) had APA and 10 (50%) had IHA. In the detection of APA, MRI had sensitivity of 70%, specificity of 100%, and accuracy of 85%, which is comparable with values reported with CT.[10-12] Traditionally, the diagnosis of IHA by CT or MRI has been made by excluding the presence of an adenoma. A recent study suggests that the diagnosis can be made more directly by measuring the limb size in patients with primary aldosteronism.[5] This CT-based study showed that adrenals were significantly larger in patients with bilateral hyperplasia than in patients with APA or in healthy control subjects. Sensitivity of 100% was achieved when a mean limb width of greater than 3 mm was used to diagnose IHA, and specificity of 100% was achieved when the mean limb width was 5 mm or greater. Therefore, the use of adrenal venous sampling was recommended only when the mean adrenal limb width was between 3 and 5 mm. Even when the radiologist assessed limb thickness visually, the overall results were similar to quantitative measurements.

PHEOCHROMOCYTOMA

Pheochromocytoma (see also Chapter 14) is often called the "10%" tumor, because about 10% are extra-adrenal in location, multiple, inherited, or malignant. Most cases are sporadic, but some are associated with multiple endocrine neoplasia (MEN) syndromes, neurofibromatosis or von Hippel-Lindau disease, or familial pheochromocytoma. Pheochromocytomas secrete the neurotransmitter hormones epinephrine and norepinephrine, which often leads to hypertension, tachycardia, headaches, palpitations, diaphoresis, and chest pains. Some or all of these findings can be present, often in an episodic pattern, but can be absent in about 10% of patients. Diagnosis of pheochromocytoma can be suspected clinically and confirmed by elevated levels of these hormones, particularly their metabolites, in the blood or the urine. Localization of a pheochromocytoma is essential because surgical resection can be curative. CT, MRI, and [131]I (and ^{123}I)-meta-iodobenzylguanidine (MIBG) imaging all have been used to localize pheochromocytomas.

Most pheochromocytomas are readily detected on CT, because they typically measure 2 to 5 cm in diameter. Although some are small and homogeneous in attenuation, many have regions of necrosis or hemorrhage and can have a fluid density on unenhanced CT. For many years, intravenous ionic contrast material was avoided in patients with known or suspected pheochromocytoma because of an effect on catecholamine levels and the fear of inducing a hypertensive crisis.[13] More recently, however, a study using nonionic IV contrast showed no significant increases in catecholamine levels in control subjects or in patients with pheochromocytomas.[14]

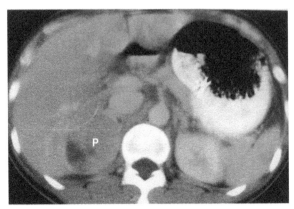

FIGURE 10-6. Intravenous contrast-enhanced computed tomography (CT) shows a right adrenal pheochromocytoma (P) with areas of necrosis. (From Korobkin M, Francis IR: Imaging of adrenal masses, Urol Clin North Am 24:603–622, 1997.)

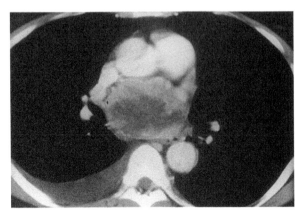

FIGURE 10-8. Intrapericardial extra-adrenal pheochromocytoma. Enhanced computed tomography (CT) shows an inhomogeneous mass in the expected location of the left atrium. MIBG scan was positive in this location. (From Hamilton BH, Francis IR, Gross BH, et al: Intrapericardial paragangliomas [pheochromocytomas]: Imaging features, Am J Roentgenol 168:109–113, 1997.)

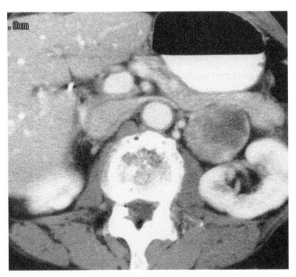

FIGURE 10-7. Retroperitoneal extra-adrenal pheochromocytoma. Enhanced computed tomography (CT) shows an inhomogeneous enhancing mass medial to the left kidney. A normal left adrenal was demonstrated on scans cephalad to this mass.

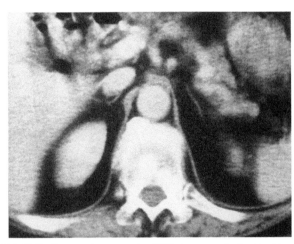

FIGURE 10-9. Computed tomography (CT) shows markedly atrophic adrenal glands in a patient with adrenal insufficiency secondary to idiopathic autoimmune atrophy. (From Korobkin M, Francis IR: Adrenal imaging, Semin Ultrasound CT MR 16:317–330, 1995.)

Contrast-enhanced CT of adrenal pheochromocytoma shows nonspecific homogeneous or, more commonly, inhomogeneous enhancement of a solid mass, similar to the finding in adrenal metastasis or adrenal cortical carcinoma (Fig. 10-6). Most pheochromocytomas have an unenhanced attenuation greater than 10 Hounsfield units (HU), although a recent report described a single case each of pheochromocytoma (9 HU) and medullary hyperplasia (2 HU) with lipid degeneration.[15] Oral contrast opacification of the gastrointestinal tract is essential for the detection of para-aortic tumors in the retroperitoneum (Fig. 10-7), because unopacified bowel at times can simulate a "mass." Although rare, intrapericardial paragangliomas can be detected by dynamic bolus contrast-enhanced CT of the mediastinum (Fig. 10-8). The inhomogeneous mass is usually located adjacent to or involving the left atrium.[16]

On MRI, most pheochromocytomas are hypointense on T1-weighted images and markedly hyperintense on T2-weighted images. Initial reports of MRI of adrenal masses suggested that pheochromocytomas could be distinguished by their marked hyperintensity on T2-weighted images. Considerable overlap with other neoplasms, however, including adrenal cortical car-

cinomas, was demonstrated in up to 33% of cases.[17] The cause of the high T2 signal intensity of pheochromocytomas remains controversial. Most of the initial reports were from mid and low field strength magnets, whereas currently, most MRI magnets have high field strength (1.5 T). The cause may be related to the necrotic or cystic areas so common within these tumors. MRI angiography is useful for demonstrating the presence or absence of intracaval extension of adrenal pheochromocytoma, and MRI is useful in the search for an extra-adrenal paraganglioma from the neck to the bladder.

HYPOADRENALISM

Adrenal insufficiency, or hypoadrenalism, most often is due to autoimmune atrophy, and imaging usually is not useful for diagnosis. The glands are extremely small and may be difficult to identify on CT or MRI[17] (Fig. 10-9). Atrophic glands may be due to chronic granulomatous disease, but these cases usually are associated with adrenal calcification. In patients with adrenal insufficiency due to granulomatous infection caused by tuberculosis, histoplasmosis, or blastomycosis, the acute and subacute phases are manifested as bilateral adrenal enlargement, although

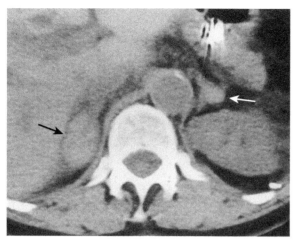

FIGURE 10-10. Adrenal insufficiency secondary to bilateral adrenal hemorrhage. Unenhanced computed tomography (CT) shows a high-attenuation mass in both adrenals *(arrows)* characteristic of acute or subacute hematoma. (From Korobkin M, Francis IR: Adrenal imaging, Semin Ultrasound CT MR 16:317–330, 1995.)

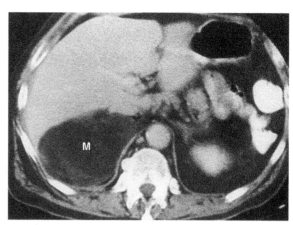

FIGURE 10-11. Myelolipoma. Large, fatty right adrenal mass (M) is seen on this contrast-enhanced computed tomography (CT) examination. (From Korobkin M, Francis IR, Kloos RT, Dunnick NR: The incidental adrenal mass, Radiol Clin North Am 34:1037–1054, 1996.)

often some asymmetry is noted. Inhomogeneous low attenuation within the adrenal mass, best seen on enhanced CT or MRI, is due to caseous necrosis.[18] Unlike patients with adrenal metastases, the enlarged glands in granulomatous adrenalitis typically retain their normal inverted Y contour.[17] Percutaneous biopsy of the adrenals is often necessary to confirm the diagnosis of granulomatous adrenalitis and to identify the organism. Bilateral adrenal calcification from granulomatous disease can be seen in both adrenal hypofunction and normal adrenal function. Demonstration of uninvolved noncalcified adrenal tissue usually indicates normal function.

Bilateral adrenal hemorrhage often is accompanied by adrenal insufficiency, and the detection of bilateral hyperattenuating masses on unenhanced CT can sometimes be the first clue to a clinical diagnosis (Fig. 10-10). Although bilateral adrenal metastases are commonly seen, they usually do not lead to clinically apparent hypoadrenalism. Adrenal insufficiency can be caused by acquired immunodeficiency syndrome (AIDS) and the antiphospholipid antibody syndrome; however, the adrenal anatomy in these diseases can be variable.[19,20]

THE INCIDENTALLY DISCOVERED ADRENAL MASS (INCIDENTALOMA)

The more widespread application of high-resolution anatomic imaging to screen the abdomen for diseases or to stage diseases unrelated to the adrenal has identified a growing number of unexpected adrenal masses or "incidentalomas."[21-24] Given their prevalence in from 4% to 10% of patients studied with CT or MRI for indications other than suspected adrenal disease, novel adaptations to imaging have been made to distinguish frequent, nonhypersecretory, benign adrenal masses from adrenal metastases and adrenocortical carcinoma.[22] The discovery of an adrenal mass presents a diagnostic and, at times, a therapeutic challenge. Because an overwhelming majority of incidentalomas are benign and nonhypersecretory, an aggressive approach to them is not indicated.[21-23] Of course, a solitary adrenal metastasis or an incidentally discovered adrenal carcinoma treated earlier would have a more favorable result. Given the uncertainty in diagnosis of adrenal masses other than cysts and myelolipomas, many diagnostic algorithms and approaches have been offered, making the evaluation of adrenal incidentalomas controversial.[21,25] A

thoughtful approach to such patients must include a biochemical evaluation sufficient to exclude both cortical and medullary hyperfunction and an anatomic and/or functional imaging evaluation sufficient to exclude a malignancy.[21,25-27] The continuing uncertainty about appropriate clinical and imaging management of adrenal incidentalomas was attested to at a National Institutes of Health Consensus Conference on this subject in February 2002.[28]

Specific Imaging Features of Incidentally Discovered Adrenal Masses

Myelolipoma

A myelolipoma is a benign tumor that comprises bone marrow elements. Myelolipomas do not produce hormones and most are detected as incidental findings. Occasionally, large tumors or those undergoing tumor necrosis or spontaneous hemorrhage may cause flank pain.[29,30] Although most are adrenal in location, extra-adrenal myelolipomas have been reported.[31,32] Because they include large amounts of mature fat, most myelolipomas are recognized easily on CT (Fig. 10-11). Elements of soft tissue density are found in varying amounts, and calcification is seen in up to 20% of cases.

The appearance of a myelolipoma on MRI reflects portions of fat and bone marrow elements in the tumor. Fat exhibits high-signal intensity on both T1- and T2-weighted sequences. The bone marrow elements have a low signal intensity on T1-weighted images and a moderate signal intensity on T2-weighted scans.[33,34] Because a confident diagnosis of myelolipoma usually can be made with CT or MRI, most are treated conservatively.

Cyst

Adrenal cysts are uncommon lesions with infrequent reports of their CT appearance. A 3:1 female predilection has been noted, and four types of cysts have been identified on the basis of pathologic classification: endothelial, epithelial, parasitic, and posttraumatic pseudocysts.[35] A recent report of 13 new cystic adrenal masses and review of 26 benign adrenal cysts from the literature included one cystic adrenal cortical carcinoma.[36] Of 37 reviewed benign cysts, 19 had mural and 7 had central calcification, 28 were unilocular, and 7 had high attenuation values. Wall thickness was 3 mm or less in 31 lesions. The authors concluded that a CT finding of a nonenhancing mass with or without wall

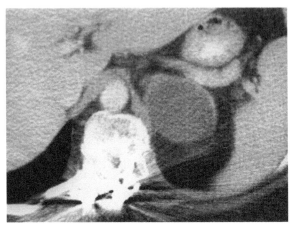

FIGURE 10-12. Adrenal pseudocyst. This homogeneous left adrenal mass measured near-water density (8 HU). The wall is thickened but smooth and less than 3 mm. (From Dunnick NR, Korobkin M: Imaging of adrenal incidentalomas: current status, Am J Roentgenol 179:559–568, 2002.)

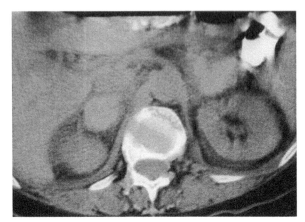

FIGURE 10-13. Adrenal hematoma. Bilateral adrenal masses are seen in this unenhanced computed tomography (CT) examination. High density of masses suggests hematoma. (From Dunnick NR, Korobkin M: Imaging of adrenal incidentalomas: current status, Am J Roentgenol 179:559–568, 2002.)

calcification allows differentiation of an adrenal cyst from an adenoma (Fig. 10-12). A small adrenal cyst with near-water attenuation and a thin (≤3 mm) wall is likely to be benign.

Hemorrhage

Adrenal hemorrhage can be bilateral or unilateral. When bilateral, the cause is usually associated with anticoagulation therapy or a blood dyscrasia; less commonly, it is associated with the stress of surgery, sepsis, or hypotension, and, rarely, it is caused by trauma.[37] Unilateral adrenal hemorrhage usually is caused by blunt abdominal trauma and involves the right gland more often than the left.[38] Adrenal vein thrombosis may cause unilateral adrenal hemorrhage. This may be caused by catheterization performed to collect blood samples from the adrenal vein in patients with suspected adrenal endocrine disease.[39,40] In the absence of catheterization or blunt trauma, unilateral adrenal hemorrhage into a preexisting neoplasm may occur, necessitating surgical exploration if follow-up imaging does not show a nearly normal adrenal gland.

Acute or subacute adrenal hemorrhage typically has an unenhanced attenuation value of 55 to 90 HU (Fig. 10-13). Follow-up studies show diminution in size of the adrenal mass with a gradual decrease in attenuation value.[41] The high attenuation value of a recent adrenal hemorrhage is usually readily apparent on unenhanced CT but is indistinguishable from a solid adrenal neoplasm on contrast-enhanced CT. An adrenal mass detected on contrast-enhanced CT after trauma usually is assumed to be due to a hematoma, but an unrelated adrenal neoplasm can be excluded only by unenhanced CT or serial follow-up CT. Similarly, MRI may indicate hemorrhage by the high signal intensity on T1-weighted scans, reflecting the presence of methemoglobin.[42,43]

Nonspecific Imaging Features of Incidentally Discovered Adrenal Masses

Granulomatous Disease

Tuberculosis, histoplasmosis, and other granulomatous diseases are usually bilateral but often asymmetrical. CT findings are nonspecific and can include soft tissue masses, cystic changes, and/or calcification[44] (Fig. 10-14). Although these are uncom-

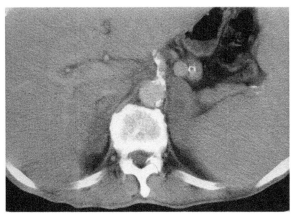

FIGURE 10-14. Histoplasmosis. Both adrenal glands are enlarged but maintain adreniform configuration. (From Dunnick NR, Korobkin M: Imaging of adrenal incidentalomas: current status, Am J Roentgenol 179:559–568, 2002.)

mon adrenal lesions that rarely occur unilaterally, they should be considered in the differential diagnosis of incidental bilateral adrenal masses in the absence of a primary neoplasm or coagulation abnormality. Biopsy is needed to confirm the diagnosis and identify the responsible organism.

Hemangioma

An adrenal hemangioma is a rare benign tumor. Hemangiosarcomas occur but are even less common.[45] Hemangiomas comprise closely adjacent vascular channels lined with a single layer of endothelium.[46] They do not produce adrenal hormones, and most are quite large when found as an incidental finding. On CT, hemangiomas are seen as large, well-defined masses. They have a soft tissue density on unenhanced images and demonstrate inhomogeneous enhancement. Most hemangiomas are calcified as the result of pheboliths within the tumor or previous hemorrhage.[47]

MRI findings include a hypointense appearance relative to the liver on T1-weighted sequences.[48] Central hyperintensity due to hemorrhage may be noted. On T2-weighted images, hemangiomas are hyperintense. Peripheral enhancement that persists on delayed images is characteristic. Tumors are usually removed because of the risk for hemorrhage and inability to exclude malignancy.

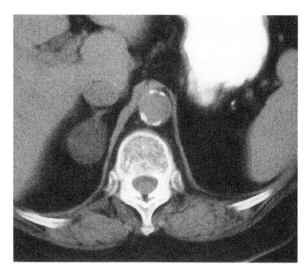

FIGURE 10-15. Lipid-rich adenoma. Right adrenal mass (3 cm) is shown on this unenhanced computed tomography (CT) scan. Attenuation value of −4 HU allows confident diagnosis of benign lesion, either cyst or lipid-rich adenoma. (From Dunnick NR, Korobkin M: Imaging of adrenal incidentalomas: current status, Am J Roentgenol 179:559–568, 2002.)

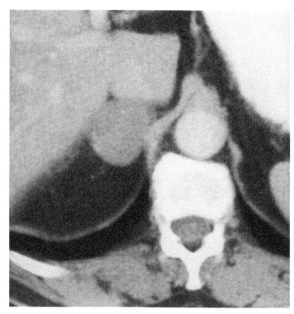

FIGURE 10-16. Adenoma. Right adrenal gland mass (4 cm) is shown on this contrast-enhanced computed tomography (CT) examination. Attenuation value on enhanced scans is not sufficiently characteristic to distinguish benign from malignant causes. (From Dunnick NR, Korobkin M: Imaging of adrenal incidentalomas: current status, Am J Roentgenol 179:559–568, 2002.)

Ganglioneuroma

A ganglioneuroma is a benign tumor composed of Schwann cells and ganglion cells. These tumors occur anywhere along the paravertebral sympathetic plexus, and approximately 20% to 30% arise in the adrenal medulla.[49] Because they do not secrete hormones, most ganglioneuromas are detected as an incidental finding.[50] On CT, ganglioneuromas appear as a solid adrenal mass ranging up to 11 cm in diameter.[49] Extra-adrenal retroperitoneal tumors may be even larger.

Neuroblastoma

Whereas neuroblastoma is the third most common malignant tumor of childhood, it is seen much less frequently in adults. It may occur anywhere along the parasympathetic plexus. Adults are more likely than children to present with disseminated disease.[51] The imaging findings of neuroblastoma in adults are similar to those in children.

Pheochromocytoma

Although most patients with pheochromocytoma present with manifestations of excess catecholamine production, approximately 10% of tumors are silent and are detected by other means such as an imaging study.[52,53] The CT and MRI appearance of pheochromocytomas was described earlier.

Adenoma

Adenoma, the most common adrenal tumor, is reported as occurring in 1.4% to 8.7% of postmortem examinations, depending on the criteria used.[54-56] The incidence is even higher among patients with hypertension or diabetes mellitus.[55-57] Adenomas large enough to be recognized on survey abdominal CT examinations are found in approximately 1% of patients, but identification may be increasing with improvements in CT technology.[58] On CT, adenomas may have the same density as normal adrenal tissue. Because most adenomas contain large amounts of intracytoplasmic lipid, many have a low density, often near that of water on unenhanced examination[59] (Fig. 10-15). Calcification is rare. Adenomas enhance significantly after the intravenous administration of iodinated contrast media (Fig. 10-16). Although the degree of enhancement is not significantly different from that of other adrenal tumors, adenomas show more rapid washout of contrast than do adrenal metastases.[60-62]

The MRI signal characteristics of adenomas are similar to those of normal adrenal tissue. Although the signal intensity of an adenoma tends to be low on T2-weighted sequences, this is not a useful way to distinguish adenomas from metastases, because an overlap of 20% to 30% has been reported with metastases. Chemical shift imaging is used to identify the intracytoplasmic lipid and can distinguish many adenomas from metastases[63,64] (Fig. 10-17).

Carcinoma

Adrenal carcinoma is a rare tumor, with a reported incidence of two cases per million.[65] Patients may present with abdominal pain, a palpable mass, or Cushing's syndrome, as about 50% of these tumors elaborate unregulated amounts of cortisol. Many of these elaborate insufficient amounts of hormone to produce obvious clinical manifestations. Other endocrine manifestations of adrenal carcinoma include Conn's syndrome, virilization, and feminization, but these are very rare. Tumors tend to be very large at the time of presentation (see also Chapter 11).

The CT appearance of an adrenal carcinoma is a large mass. Central necrosis is common, and calcification is seen in 20% to 30% of cases[66,67] (Fig. 10-18A). Enhancement is heterogeneous after intravenous contrast administration. Venous extension of tumor into the left renal vein or the inferior vena cava is common and usually can be identified on contrast-enhanced images[66] (Fig. 10-18B). It is important to define precisely the cephalad extent of the intravenous tumor, as this defines the point where the surgeon can gain vascular control of the tumor.[68] Although this often can be done with CT, MRI may be helpful in problem cases.[69] On MRI, carcinomas are usually heterogeneously hyperintense on both T1- and T2-weighted images, reflecting frequent

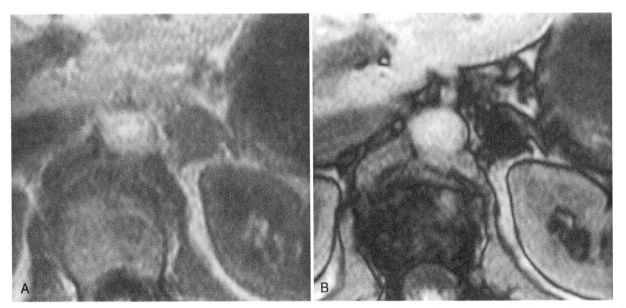

FIGURE 10-17. Adenoma. **A,** Left adrenal mass is seen on this in-phase magnetic resonance image (MRI). **B,** A significant decrease in signal is seen on the out-of-phase MRI. (From Dunnick NR, Korobkin M: Imaging of adrenal incidentalomas: current status, Am J Roentgenol 179:559–568, 2002.)

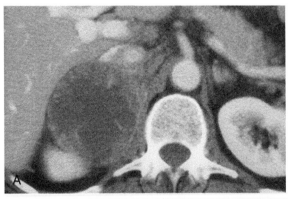

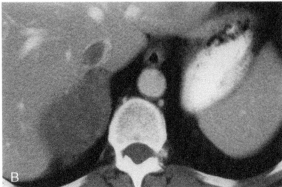

FIGURE 10-18. Adrenal cortical carcinoma. **A,** Contrast-enhanced computed tomography (CT) examination shows 9 cm right adrenal mass. Irregular wall and low-density center indicate necrosis. **B,** More cephalad image in same examination reveals tumor extension into inferior vena cava. (From Dunnick NR, Korobkin M: Imaging of adrenal incidentalomas: current status, Am J Roentgenol 179:559–568, 2002.)

internal hemorrhage and central necrosis. Enhancement is also heterogeneous, revealing nodular areas of intense enhancement and other areas with no enhancement. Intravenous extension of tumor typically is well seen on MRI because of the multiple planes in which data sets can be projected.[69,70]

Lymphoma

Primary lymphoma of the adrenal glands is rare,[71] but secondary involvement when another retroperitoneal lymphoma is present is seen more commonly among patients with non-Hodgkin's lymphoma than among those with Hodgkin's disease.[72] Involvement is often bilateral, and other retroperitoneal disease is usually present. On MRI, lymphoma has a signal intensity lower than that of the liver on T1-weighted images. Lymphoma is typically heterogeneously hyperintense on T2-weighted sequences.

Metastases

The adrenal glands are a common site of metastatic disease, which is found in about 27% of postmortem examinations of patients with malignant neoplasms of epithelial origin.[73] The most common neoplasms with adrenal metastases are carcinomas of the lung and breast, and melanoma.[73,74] Small metastases are often homogeneous on contrast-enhanced CT (Fig. 10-19) or MRI, whereas large metastases often have local regions of heterogeneous appearance due to necrosis or hemorrhage or both (Fig. 10-20). Calcification is rare in adrenal metastases.

ADENOMA OR METASTASIS

Although this section discusses the different methods of CT and MRI that may be used to differentiate a benign (usually adenoma) from malignant (usually metastases) adrenal masses, not all lesions or patients require an evaluation. The prevalence of adrenal adenomas is high, and small, homogeneous adrenal masses discovered incidentally are likely to be adenomas. If a patient shows evidence of metastases elsewhere and the presence of an adrenal metastasis will not alter therapy, further evaluation is not justified.

Evidence has accumulated that unenhanced CT densitometry can be used to accurately differentiate adrenal adenomas from metastases.[75-77] Most adenomas have unenhanced CT attenuation values lower than those of metastases, and the scatterplot data from such studies were used to determine a threshold value that resulted in calculation of the optimal combination of sensitivity and specificity for the diagnosis of adenoma (Fig. 10-21). In an

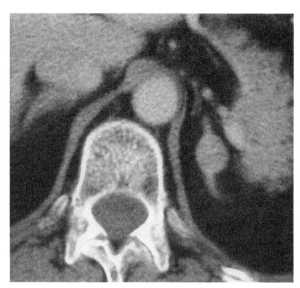

FIGURE 10-19. Metastasis from renal carcinoma in a 31-year-old woman. Small, homogeneous left adrenal mass is seen on this contrast-enhanced computed tomography (CT) examination. (From Dunnick NR, Korobkin M: Imaging of adrenal incidentalomas: current status, Am J Roentgenol 179:559–568, 2002.)

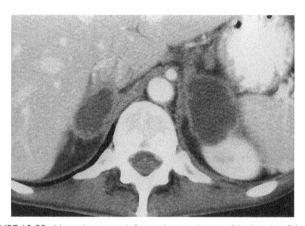

FIGURE 10-20. Necrotic metastasis from adenocarcinoma of the lung in a 34-year-old woman. Bilateral adrenal masses with areas of central necrosis are seen on this contrast-enhanced computed tomography (CT) examination. (From Dunnick NR, Korobkin M: Imaging of adrenal incidentalomas: current status, Am J Roentgenol 179:559–568, 2002.)

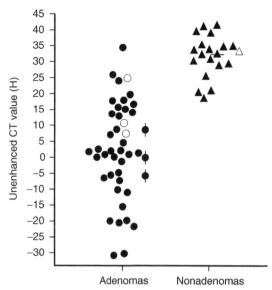

FIGURE 10-21. Scattergram of attenuation values on unenhanced CT of adrenal adenomas and nonadenomas. All masses with H values of less than 18 were adenomas. ●, Nonhyperfunctioning adenomas; O, Cushing adenomas; ◆, primary aldosteronism adenomas; ▲, metastases; △, pheochromocytomas; ◂, cortical carcinomas. (From Korobkin M, Brodeur FJ, Yutzy GG, et al: Differentiation of adrenal adenomas from nonadenomas using CT attenuation values, Am J Roentgenol 166:531–536, 1996.)

oncologic patient with an adrenal mass but no other evidence of distant metastatic disease, the goal of noninvasive diagnostic imaging is to characterize the adrenal mass as an adenoma with high specificity. With the use of pooled data from multiple published studies of calculated accuracies and corresponding threshold values of unenhanced attenuation values, it has been shown that the most optimal sensitivity (71%) and specificity (98%) for the diagnosis of adrenal adenoma results when a threshold attenuation value of 10 HU is chosen on unenhanced CT.[77] Unlike unenhanced attenuation values, however, intravenous contrast-enhanced CT values show too much overlap between adenomas and metastases to allow accurate differentiation between them.[76]

Evidence has accumulated that chemical shift MRI can also be used to differentiate adrenal adenomas from metastases. Taking advantage of the different resonant frequency peaks for the hydrogen atom in water and triglyceride (lipid) molecules, chemical shift MRI results in a decrease in the signal intensity of tissue containing both lipid and water in comparison with tissue containing no lipid.[78] When a breath-hold gradient-echo technique is used, signal intensity loss on opposed-phase versus in-phase images indicates a mixture of lipid and nonlipid tissue that is often present in adrenal adenomas and absent in metastases. Assessment of the chemical shift change can be made via simple visual analysis or by quantitative methods using standard region-of-interest cursor measurements of the mass, and often of an adjacent reference tissue, on in-phase and opposed-phase images. Several different formulas have been proposed to measure the amount of chemical shift change and to determine optimal threshold values by analysis of scatterplot data.[79]

Although some investigators have used these quantitative measurements and formulas to detect the presence of lipid within adrenal adenomas, others have emphasized the advantages of simple visual analysis in detecting relative signal intensity loss on opposed-phase images of adrenal adenomas. The ability to subjectively compensate for motion and other artifacts that are superimposed over an adrenal mass and the identification of local rather than diffuse lipid are two of the advantages cited in favor of visual rather than quantitative analysis of chemical shift changes.[80] Several studies have shown a similar accuracy for detecting intratumoral lipid in adrenal masses when both visual analysis and quantitative methods are used in the same patients,[79-81] but recent observation suggests that quantitative methods may be more sensitive for detecting lipid in an adenoma.[82] The most rigorous assessment of visual analysis of in-phase and opposed-phase imaging of adrenal masses showed a sensitivity of 78% for the detection of lipid within adrenal adenomas with a corresponding specificity of 87%.[80]

Two studies have suggested that unenhanced CT densitometry and chemical shift MRI both detect the presence and amount of lipid within adrenal adenomas. In one study of 47 adrenal masses, which all were imaged with both techniques, good inverse linear correlation was noted on MRI between the CT attenuation value and the amount of chemical shift change.[83] In a histologic/radiologic study of a small number of resected adrenal adenomas that had undergone presurgical CT, chemical shift MRI, or both, good inverse linear correlation was seen between the estimated number of lipid-rich cells and the unenhanced CT attenuation value, and good linear correlation was noted with the relative change in signal intensity on opposed-phase MRI[59] (Figs. 10-22 and 10-23).

However, two more recent publications indicate that chemical shift MRI is more sensitive in detecting sufficient lipid in adenomas with unenhanced CT values between 10 and 30 HU.[82,84]

Standard contrast-enhanced CT images of the adrenal glands are obtained about 60 seconds after bolus intravenous injection of contrast material is begun. Studies suggest that this is the only time when the attenuation values of adenomas and metastases are nearly identical. Adenomas have a much more rapid loss of enhancement, as early as 5 minutes after contrast injection, and attenuation values at 10 or 15 minutes after contrast administration can be used to differentiate adenomas from other masses[62,85] (Fig. 10-24). Although the threshold attenuation value for the diagnosis of an adenoma has varied among series, masses with an attenuation value less than 30 to 40 HU on 15-minute delayed contrast-enhanced CT are almost always adenomas.

Previous reports indicated that the more rapid washout of gadolinium enhancement on MRI of adrenal adenomas could differentiate them from metastases.[91] Subsequent reports could not confirm these results, however, and dynamic gadolinium-enhanced MRI is not used widely for this purpose.[81,86,87]

In addition to the delayed CT attenuation value itself, it is possible to calculate the percentage washout of initial enhancement, which is probably independent of type, amount, and injection rates of contrast administration.[62,88] The optimal threshold enhancement washout at 15 minutes is 60%, resulting in a sensitivity of 88% and a specificity of 96% for the diagnosis of adenoma.[62] Of particular interest is the apparent independence of this rapid enhancement washout from the lipid content of an adenoma. Lipid-poor adenomas, those with unenhanced attenuation values greater than 10 HU on unenhanced CT, have enhancement washout features nearly identical to those of lipid-rich adenomas.[89]

It is easy to calculate the enhancement washout of adrenal masses:

$$\% \text{ enhancement washout} = (E - D)/(E - U) \times 100$$

where E is the enhanced attenuation value, D is the delayed enhanced value, and U is the unenhanced value. For example, if the unenhanced attenuation is 20 HU, the enhanced attenuation is 100 HU, and the 15 minute delayed enhanced attenuation is 40 HU, the percent washout is:

$$(100 - 40)/(100 - 20) = 60/80 \times 100 = 75\%$$

If the threshold value of 60% is used, the mass is likely a lipid-poor adenoma. If there is no unenhanced CT, or the unenhanced attenuation value is unknown, a relative enhancement washout can be calculated as follows:

$$\% \text{ relative enhancement washout} = (E - D)/E \times 100$$

In our department, the optimal threshold value for the relative enhancement washout calculation is 40%, resulting in a sensitivity of 96% and a specificity of 100% for the diagnosis of adenoma. Another study of the accuracy of relative enhancement washout in characterizing adrenal masses reported an optimal threshold of 50%,[90] resulting in a sensitivity and specificity of 100%.

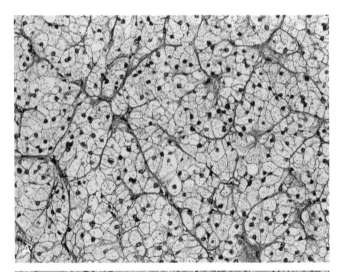
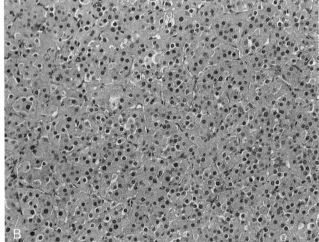
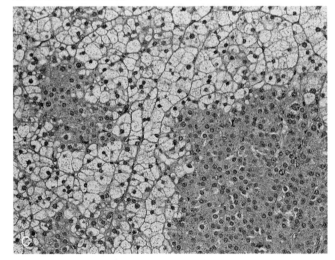

FIGURE 10-22. Histologic specimens from resected adrenal adenomas: **A,** Primarily of lipid-rich clear cells. **B,** Primarily of lipid-poor clear cells. **C,** Of an admixture of clear and compact cortical cells. (Hematoxylin-eosin stain, original magnification, ×200.) (From Korobkin M, Giordano TJ, Brodeur FJ, et al: Adrenal adenomas: relationship between histologic lipid and CT and MR findings, Radiology 200:743–747, 1996.)

In the previous example, the calculation for relative enhancement washout is as follows:

$$(100 - 40)/(100) = 60/100 = 60\%$$

If the threshold value for relative enhancement washout of 40% is used, this calculation again indicates an adenoma.

Assessment of enhancement washout curves for adrenal masses is valid only for lesions with relatively homogeneous attenuation after contrast enhancement. Large regions of low attenuation, probably representing areas of necrosis or hemor-

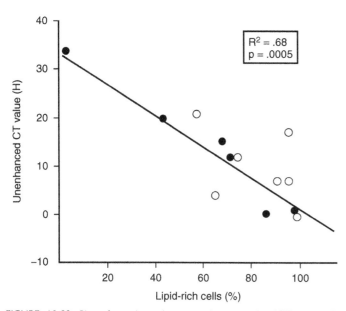

FIGURE 10-23. Plot of unenhanced computed tomography (CT) attenuation number versus the percentage of lipid-rich cells in 13 surgically resected adrenal adenomas. *HU,* Hounsfield units. (From Korobkin M, Giordano TJ, Brodeur FJ, et al: Adrenal adenomas: Relationship between histologic lipid and CT and MR findings, Radiology 200:743–747, 1996.)

rhage, were specifically excluded from evaluation in papers that described and quantitated the washout curves. The calculations apply only to solid tissue with an intact capillary bed. The diagnosis of adrenal adenoma cannot be made in masses that contain prominent regions of necrosis or hemorrhage.

Combining the two independent CT properties of adrenal adenomas—rapid contrast enhancement washout and a propensity for intratumoral lipid—leads to a protocol that spares most adenomas from contrast enhancement. We reported the accuracy of combined unenhanced and delayed enhanced CT densitometry for characterization of adrenal masses.[91] We prospectively studied 166 adrenal masses with unenhanced CT; those with attenuation values greater than 10 HU underwent contrast-enhanced and 15-minute delayed enhanced CT. This protocol correctly characterized 160 of the 166 masses (96%). When the five nonadenomas that were not metastases were excluded, the sensitivity and specificity for characterizing a mass as adenoma versus metastasis were 98% (124/127) and 97% (33/34), respectively. Similar results were subsequently reported with the use of a very similar protocol.[92]

ADENOMA OR CARCINOMA

In patients without a primary extra-adrenal neoplasm, an adrenal mass without specific morphologic features is almost always an adenoma, especially if less than 3 cm in diameter. To obviate the common practice of serial CT imaging over several years to assure a benign lesion in order to show stability in size, we often use the imaging techniques described previously to confirm the findings characteristic of an adenoma. If these features are present, we make a diagnosis of adenoma and do not suggest follow-up imaging. In a recent study of incidentally detected indeterminate, but benign appearing, adrenal masses with no known primary malignancy, all of the 321 lesions studied were confirmed to be benign. Follow-up imaging appears to have a limited role in this common patient cohort.[93]

A unilateral adrenal mass larger than 5 or 6 cm in diameter is considered suspicious for adrenocortical carcinoma, and many

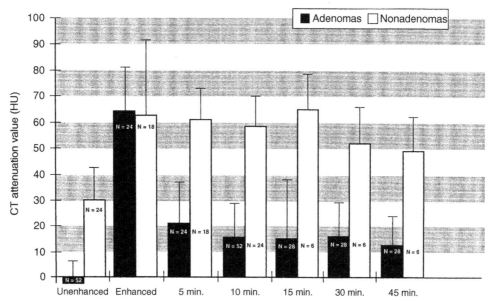

FIGURE 10-24. Bar graph shows mean computed tomography (CT) attenuation value plus 1 standard deviation for adrenal adenomas *(black)* and nonadenomas *(white)* on unenhanced, enhanced, and delayed enhanced scans. (From Korobkin M, Brodeur FJ, Francis IR, et al: CT-time-attenuation washout curves of adrenal adenomas and nonadenomas, Am J Roentgenol 170:747–752, 1998.)

show evidence of metastatic disease. It is important to remember that a large nonhyperfunctioning pheochromocytoma and a large adrenal metastasis can have a CT and MRI appearance identical to that of a carcinoma. In the absence of metastases, the differential diagnosis is usually that of carcinoma versus adenoma. The larger the mass, the greater is the likelihood of carcinoma, although on rare occasions, adenomas can be larger than 5 cm and can have large regions of hemorrhage, necrosis, and calcification.[94] The size criteria for resection of adrenal incidentaloma varies widely, but almost all adrenal masses greater than 6 cm are resected for fear of possible adrenal carcinoma.

Very little is known about chemical shift MRI and CT densitometry of adrenocortical carcinoma. Of the reported series of delayed enhanced CT attenuation values and enhancement washout curves, only one included three cases of adrenal carcinoma, but the carcinomas were included in the data set for nonadenomas, and their locations in the scatterplots of the individual cases were not provided.[85] Adrenal carcinomas greater than 6 cm often have large regions of central necrosis or hemorrhage, invalidating attempts to assess contrast enhancement washout. It is not yet established whether chemical shift MRI, unenhanced CT, or delayed enhanced CT can reliably differentiate adenoma from carcinoma. The answer may depend on the histologic grade of malignancy involved. In one series that included 11 adrenal cortical carcinomas, the absolute and relative enhancement loss on 10 minute delayed imaging of the carcinomas was significantly smaller than for the adenomas and was similar to that for the metastases and the pheochomocytomas.[95] In another series of seven patients with adrenocortical carcinomas, delayed enhanced images at approximately 20 minutes showed a relative percentage of enhancement washout of less than 40%, consistent with malignancy.[96]

Arteriography and Adrenal Vein

HORMONE SAMPLING

If imaging studies are inconclusive, adrenal vein hormone sampling can be performed to distinguish hypersecretory unilateral adenoma from bilateral hyperplasia.[12,16,97-99] Arteriography is used only in a very few selected cases with adrenal lesions or extra-adrenal pheochromocytoma, when additional information about tumor resectability and vascular anatomy is needed. Adrenal venous hormone sampling remains the "gold standard" method for distinguishing unilateral aldosterone-producing adenoma from bilateral adrenal hyperplasia. Transcatheter ethanol injection may be used to treat aldosteronomas and other hypersecretory adrenal adenomas as an alternative to surgery.

ANATOMY

The arterial supply to each adrenal gland comes from three sources: a superior adrenal artery arising from the inferior phrenic artery, the middle adrenal from the aorta, and the inferior adrenal from the renal artery. Each of the arteries divides into multiple small twigs, which course through the cortex centrally into the medulla. The central vein communicates with adrenal capsular veins, which, in turn, communicate with renal capsular veins. On the right, three central veins draining the superior, inferior, and posterior aspects of the gland form a short single common trunk before entering the right posterior aspect of the inferior vena cava (IVC). Rarely, the right adrenal vein may join the right hepatic or renal vein. On the left, the central

adrenal vein courses caudally and joins the inferior phrenic vein just before entering the cranial aspect of the renal vein.

TECHNIQUE

Adrenal Arteriography

The arteriographic technique for examination of the adrenal gland must be meticulous with selective injections of the supplying arteries. Selective arteriography is performed with injection into the celiac, right, and left renal arteries. Superselective angiography then is performed with injection into the inferior phrenic, middle, and inferior adrenal arteries. Because the adrenal arteries are relatively small, contrast medium must be injected gently using the hand-injection technique. The specific risk with adrenal arteriography is rupture of the adrenal arteries with contrast extravasation.

Adrenal Vein Catheterization

Adrenal vein catheterization for venography and sampling is done from a right femoral vein approach. The femoral vein is accessed using the Seldinger technique with a 19- or 21-gauge needle. When simultaneous adrenal venous sampling is to be performed, bilateral femoral punctures or two unilateral femoral vein punctures are made. Two side holes are punched near the tips of the catheters to facilitate aspiration of blood for obtaining biochemical samples. All patients are administered anticoagulants to reduce the risk for adrenal vein thrombosis.

Potential complications of adrenal vein catheterization include intra-adrenal extravasation of contrast, bleeding, and adrenal vein thrombosis. Adrenal hemorrhage can cause severe pain and fever, as well as destruction of adrenal glandular function and hypoadrenalism if both adrenal glands are damaged. Adrenal venography is performed to confirm the catheter position in the adrenal vein after blood has been collected for hormone sampling, and not for the depiction of adrenal anatomy (Fig. 10-25).

ADRENAL VEIN HORMONE SAMPLING

Adrenal vein hormone sampling may be performed sequentially using a single catheter or simultaneously with a catheter in each adrenal vein. Collection of blood samples from the right adrenal vein is done with gravity drainage. Blood sampling from the left adrenal vein and IVC is done with gentle aspiration to reduce adrenal blood dilution by other sources. After baseline sampling, blood samples are obtained at 10 and 20 minutes after intravenous administration of ACTH. In one technique, a bolus of 0.1 mg (10 units) of ACTH is administered, and this is followed by infusion of 0.15 mg (15 units) of ACTH over 5 minutes. ACTH stimulates the release of both cortisol and aldosterone from the normal adrenal gland, and enhances the sensitivity of adrenal venous sampling.

Primary Aldosteronism

Adrenal venous sampling is reserved for patients with primary hyperaldosteronism in whom imaging studies have failed to localize an adenoma or to confirm the presence of bilateral hyperplasia. Determination of aldosterone and cortisol concentrations in the adrenal venous effluent can accurately localize the site of aldosterone excess, distinguishing unilateral from bilateral adrenal disease. Determination of cortisol in each sample not only proves blood collection from the adrenal vein, but also provides a means of compensating for the difference in hormone concentration resulting from catheter placement and dilution of

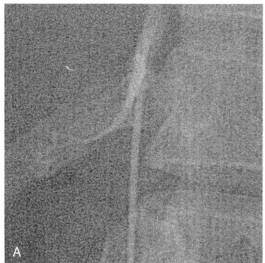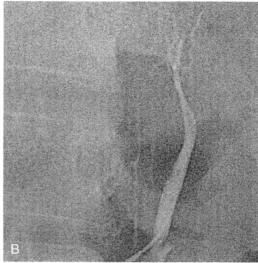

FIGURE 10-25. Bilateral adrenal venograms in a patient with primary hyperaldosteronism. **A,** Right adrenal venogram in the left anterior oblique projection. The intrarenal branches are filled poorly. The main vein enters the posterolateral aspect of the inferior vena cava. **B,** Left adrenal venogram in the anteroposterior projection with the injection of contrast medium via the 3F microcatheter introduced through the 5F reverse hook catheter positioned near the junction of the main adrenal vein and the left renal vein.

Table 10-2. Results of Adrenal Vein Sampling in a Left Adrenal Aldosteronoma

Aldosterone, ng/dL				Cortisol, mg/dL			
Right	Left	IVC	R/L	Right	Left	IVC	R/L
Basal:							
23	580	11	25	23	18	10	1.2
After ACTH:							
10 min							
300	18,118	45	60	1010	496	18.5	2.0
20 min							
430	9403	66	21	967	519	21	1.8

Aldosterone levels in the left adrenal gland are higher than in the right before and after adrenocorticotropic hormone (ACTH) administration. The aldosterone level in the right adrenal vein is similar to the inferior vena cava (IVC) before ACTH stimulation and indicates suppression of the right adrenal. After ACTH stimulation, aldosterone levels in both adrenal veins increase. A 1.1 cm diameter left adrenal aldosterone-secreting adenoma was resected by laparoscopy with subsequent normalization of blood pressure and serum potassium levels.

Table 10-3. Results of Adrenal Vein Sampling in Aldosteronism Due to Bilateral Adrenal Hyperplasia

Aldosterone, ng/dL				Cortisol, μg/dL			
Right	Left	IVC	R/L	Right	Left	IVC	R/L
Basal:							
1233	1222	24	1.0	460	233	13	2.0
After ACTH:							
10 min							
1763	2203	37	0.8	974	606	21	1.6
20 min							
2012	2014	48	1.0	1200	607	25	2.0

Aldosterone levels in both adrenal veins are higher than in the inferior vena cava (IVC). Aldosterone (R/L) ratios are <1.0 before and after adrenocorticotropic hormone (ACTH), and the ratios of aldosterone/cortisol are 2.0, indicative of bilateral hyperfunction and, in this case, bilateral adrenal hyperplasia.

Table 10-4. Results of Adrenal Vein Sampling in Asymmetrical Adrenal Hyperplasia*

Aldosterone, ng/dL				Cortisol, μg/dL			
Right	Left	IVC	R/L	Right	Left	IVC	R/L
Basal:							
1019	514	138	2	18	25	12	0.7
After ACTH:							
10 min							
39,022	2630	114	15	1220	1220	13	1.0
20 min							
51,234	2575	111	20	1300	1210	16	1.1

Aldosterone levels in both adrenal veins are higher than in the inferior vena cava (IVC). Aldosterone (R/L) ratios are 2.0 before and 20 at 20 minutes after adrenocorticotropic hormone (ACTH) stimulation. The left adrenal aldosterone/cortisol ratios after ACTH are lower than the IVC aldosterone/cortisol ratios. A right laparoscopic adrenalectomy demonstrated cortical nodular hyperplasia with a dominant nodule.

*Computed tomography demonstrated a right adrenal mass and NP-59 depicted a pattern of bilateral adrenocortical uptake compatible with hyperplasia.

the adrenal venous effluent. Some centers would also measure catecholamines to confirm catheter placement.

Analysis of the adrenal venous sampling should include calculation of aldosterone ratio, aldosterone/cortisol ratio (A/C ratio), and ratio of the A/C ratios. The A/C ratio is calculated to correct for dilution of samples from the adrenal veins. In unilateral adenoma, differences in concentration of aldosterone are very large because of increased hormone production from the adenoma associated with suppression of the contralateral adrenal gland (Table 10-2). Therefore, the aldosterone ratio is usually greater than 3.0 and the ratio of the A/C ratio is greater than 6.0. In the presence of unilateral disease, the A/C ratio in the normal gland is similar to and often is lower than the IVC A/C ratio. In bilateral adrenal hyperplasia, aldosterone levels and A/C ratios in both adrenal glands are higher than in the IVC before and after ACTH (Table 10-3). In the presence of bilateral adrenal hyperplasia with a dominant nodule, in which CT often depicts a unilateral mass, samples from both adrenal veins demonstrate aldosterone levels and A/C ratios higher than the IVC A/C ratio (Table 10-4).

CATHETER-DIRECTED ABLATION THERAPY FOR ADRENAL ADENOMAS

Nonsurgical methods of treating aldosteronoma include the percutaneous injection of ethanol or acetic acid and the transcatheter arterial infusion of ethanol. Rossi and colleagues[100] injected a mixture of ethanol and iodinated contrast material into a left adrenal adenoma using CT guidance. The patient remained hypertensive despite significant biochemical improvement. Liang and coworkers used a CT-guided percutaneous injection of acetic acid into the adrenal adenomas in two patients with aldosterone-secreting adrenal adenomas and one patient with Cushing's syndrome.[101] Symptoms resolved and subsequent laboratory studies were normal in all patients. Hokotate and colleagues[102] selectively infused ethanol through a microcatheter into the feeding artery of an aldosteronoma. This method was successful in 82% (27/33) of patients. Repeat embolization was performed successfully in one recurrent tumor. No complications were encountered.

Adrenal Scintigraphy

ADRENAL CORTEX

Radiopharmaceuticals for adrenocortical imaging have been available for more than 30 years.[103] Originally based on precursors of cholesterol analogues, newer radiopharmaceutical inhibitors of 11β-hydroxylase, include the positron emission tomography (PET) agents ^{11}C-etiomidate and [11]C-, [18]F-, and more recently ^{123}I-labeled metomidate, allowing single photon emission tomography (SPECT), have been used to image the normal adrenal cortex and a variety of adrenocortical neoplasms.[104] Other PET agents, such as ^{11}C-acetate, an intermediate of aerobic metabolism and [11]C-, and ^{18}F-choline, a precursor component of cell membranes and the glucose analogue, ^{18}F-fluorodeoxyglucose (FDG), have been reportedly used to image the normal adrenal cortex, as well as benign, and, in the case of FDG, malignant adrenal masses.[105-107] At the present time, the radiocholesterol analogue, [131]I-6β-iodomethlynorcholesterol (NP-59), is not available in North America, although it is produced in Europe and Asia, and recent publications have reviewed its use in depicting disorders of the adrenal cortex.[108,109]

CLINICAL APPLICATIONS OF ADRENOCORTICAL SCINTIGRAPHY

Cushing's Syndrome

Anatomic imaging and selective intracranial venous sampling have been especially useful in evaluating the central causes of ACTH-dependent Cushing's syndrome; excessive ACTH secretion from pituitary or ectopic source(s) is the most common cause of Cushing's syndrome, and scintigraphy of the adrenal cortex would not be indicated, in that the cause of glucocorticoid excess is extra-adrenal. The recent introduction of PET with ^{11}C-metomidate (^{11}C-MTO) provides an alternative approach to adrenocortical scintigraphy, and ^{11}C-MTO can be used to differentiate neoplasms of adrenocortical origin (including nonhypersecreting and hypersecreting cortical adenomas, adrenocortical carcinomas, and macronodular hyperplasia) from nonadrenocortical tumors (benign and malignant pheochromocytoma, and metastases to the adrenal) with high specificity and sensitivity; however, ^{11}C-MTO PET does not distinguish benign adrenal neoplasms from adrenocortical carcinomas.[110-114] Maximal adrenal accumulation of ^{11}C-MTO expressed as a weight- and decay-corrected standardized uptake value (SUV) was higher in hypersecreting adrenal adenomas and adrenocortical carcinomas than in normal adrenal cortex, suggesting relative "suppression" of contralateral adrenal 11β-hydroxylase activity. This is the result of uncontrolled adrenal hyperfunction upon hypothalamic and pituitary secretogogues, with a pattern of imaging that is akin to the suppression of radiocholesterol uptake by the normal contralateral adrenal cortex in ACTH-independent Cushing's syndrome from a hypersecreting adrenal adenoma.[111] Alternatively, the glucose analogue, ^{18}F-FDG, has been reported to image both primary and metastatic adrenocortical carcinomas, as well as some adrenocortical adenomas and bilateral adrenal hyperplasia.[112,115-118]

Primary Aldosteronism

The efficacy of adrenal scintigraphy with NP-59 in the evaluation of primary aldosteronism (PA) has been well established, and, with the addition of dexamethasone suppression (DS) of pituitary ACTH secretion and accumulation of radiocholesterol by the inner adrenal cortex, scintigraphy is an accurate means of distinguishing adrenal adenoma from bilateral adrenal hyperplasia.[107]

More recently, PET with ^{11}C-MTO has been used to depict primary aldosteronism due to adrenal adenoma in a small series.[112] Standardized uptake values in adrenal adenomas did not differ greatly from those in the normal adrenal cortex; adenoma/normal cortex SUV ratios ranged from 0.9 to 1.7, with a mean of 1.2, reflecting lack of suppression of 11β-hydroxylase enzyme activity in PA that differs from adenoma/normal adrenal SUV ratios described in Cushing's adenomas and hypersecreting adrenocortical carcinoma, suggesting a role for DS in studies of PA with ^{11}C-MTO.[112]

Incidentally Discovered Adrenal Masses

Functional adrenal imaging using iodocholesterol, metaiodobenzylguanidine (MIBG), or FDG has been demonstrated to have high sensitivity and specificity for characterization of incidentally discovered adrenal masses. As a result of their differing mechanisms of adrenal gland uptake, NP-59, MIBG, and FDG target different physiologic processes, and as a result, each can be used to functionally characterize nonhypersecretory adrenal tumors.[119,120] Maurea et al.[119] demonstrated that iodocholesterol imaging had a positive predictive value of 89% and a negative predictive value of 100% in patients with adrenal adenomas, and that MIBG had positive and negative predictive values of 83% and 100% for confirming an adrenal mass as neuroendocrine, respectively, and FDG differentiated benign from malignant adrenal lesions with 100% sensitivity and specificity. Thus, in using scintigraphy to distinguish nonhyperfunctioning adrenal masses in patients without a history of cancer, iodocholesterol would be the initial radiopharmaceutical of choice, because benign adenomas are the most common incidentally discovered adrenal masses. Should iodocholesterol imaging be normal, MIBG would be used next to identify a nonhypersecreting pheochromocytoma, and if MIBG is nonlocalizing, FDG should follow. In patients with a prior history of malignancy, FDG should be the initial study of choice, followed in sequence by iodocholesterol and MIBG imaging.[119,120]

Fluorodeoxyglucose PET (FDG-PET) can be used to identify adrenocortical carcinomas and metastases to the adrenals from benign adrenal masses (Figs. 10-26 and 10-27). In 50 patients with known or suspected malignancy, FDG-PET had a sensitivity

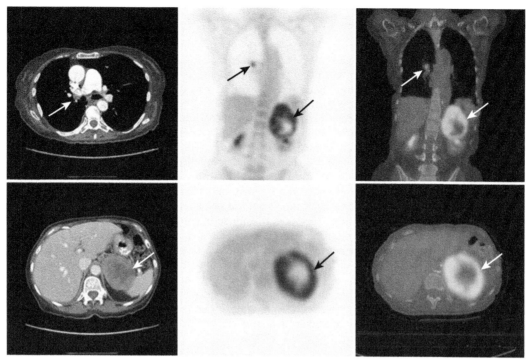

FIGURE 10-26. FDG-PET/CT scan in a 74-year-old woman with non–small cell lung cancer after a right lower lobe resection and chemotherapy. A follow-up PET/CT scan demonstrates metaststic right hilar lymphadenopathy and a large left adrenal metastasis. The adrenal lesion displays intense FDG activity peripherally with a central photopenic area consistent with a metabolically active rim and central tumor necrosis. *CT,* Computed tomography; *FDG,* fluorodeoxyglucose; *PET,* positron emission tomography. (From Gross MD, Avram A, Fig LM, Rubello D: Contemporary adrenal scintigraphy, Eur J Nucl Med Mol Imaging 34:547–557, 2007.)

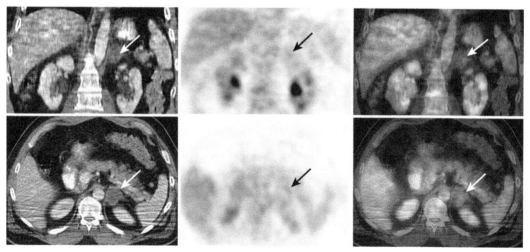

FIGURE 10-27. FDG-PET/CT in a 46-year-old man with a squamous cell carcinoma of the neck after external beam radiation therapy. Restaging PET/CT demonstrates a low-attenuation, non–FDG-avid, 3.7 cm diameter left adrenal nodule consistent with a benign adrenal adenoma. *CT,* Computed tomography; *FDG,* fluorodeoxyglucose; *PET,* positron emission tomography. (From Gross MD, Avram A, Fig LM, Rubello D: Contemporary adrenal scintigraphy, Eur J Nucl Med Mol Imaging 34:547–557, 2007.)

of 100%, a specificity of 94%, and an accuracy of 96% for characterization of adrenal lesions.[121] In another study of 105 patients with adrenal masses, Metser et al.[122] reported that FDG-PET had a sensitivity of 98.5% and a specificity of 92% at a cutoff SUV of 3.1, while the addition of CT to PET resulted in increased specificity to 98%, with all lesions correctly categorized as benign or malignant.

In a study of 21 patients with incidentally discovered hypersecretory and nonhypersecretory masses, ^{11}C-MTO PET identified all lesions of adrenocortical origin, with the highest SUV in adrenocortical carcinomas (SUV 28), followed by hypersecretory adrenal cortical adenomas (SUV 12.7) and nonsecretory adenomas (SUV 12.2); noncortical tumors demonstrated an SUV of 5.7. Fluorodeoxyglucose PET depicted pheochromocytomas and adrenocortical carcinomas, but all nonhypersecreting and most hypersecreting adenomas demonstrated minimal or no appreciable FDG accumulation.[112] Recently, ^{18}F-labeled MTO has been used to image the normal adrenal cortex, and ^{123}I-labeled MTO has shown adrenal accumulation sufficient for SPECT/CT imaging of the adrenal cortex.[123,124]

ADRENAL MEDULLA/ADRENERGIC TUMOR SCINTIGRAPHY

Although radiolabeled catecholamines and analogues were the first compounds evaluated as potential agents for imaging the adrenal medulla, successful imaging did not occur until neuronal blocking agents were considered.[125] The iodobenzylguanidines exhibited avid medulla concentration in experimental animals, and MIBG demonstrated significantly earlier accumulation and favorable target-to-nontarget imaging ratios when compared with other analogues.[125-131] MIBG, labeled with ^{123}I or ^{131}I, has been used to localize tumors of neuroendocrine origin.[114,115,121,145] Various radioisotopes (e.g., [124]I, ^{18}F) and modifications of the parent compound (i.e., aminobenzylguanidine) have been met with success in imaging adrenergic neoplasms.[103]

The mechanism of accumulation of MIBG and analogues by neuroendocrine tissues involves norepinephrine reuptake mechanisms into catecholamine storage vesicles of adrenergic nerve endings and adrenomedullary cells.[132] Uptake of MIBG can be blocked by reserpine, tricyclic antidepressants, and other drugs that affect MIBG accumulation by neuroendocrine tissues, and these must be excluded before MIBG scintigraphy is performed.[127,128] Neither α- nor β-adrenergic blockade interferes with MIBG uptake, and, with the exception of labetolol, which has an inhibitory action on amine uptake, MIBG imaging can be performed during treatment for hypercatecholaminemia.[128,132,133,134]

Hydroxyephedrine (HED), an analogue of norepinephrine, is concentrated into adrenergic nerve terminals by the norepinephrine uptake pathway and may be labeled with ^{11}C for use in PET.[135-137] Other positron-emitting radiopharmaceuticals, such as ^{11}C-epinephrine, the ^{18}F-labeled glucose analogue ^{18}F-fluorodeoxyglucose (FDG), ^{18}F-6-fluorodopamine (^{18}F-DA), and ^{18}F-fluorodihydroxyphenylalanine (^{18}F-DOPA), can be used for adrenal medulla/adrenergic tumor imaging.[103,138-143]

Alternative agents for imaging sympathomedullary neoplasms take advantage of the widespread distribution of somatostatin receptors and the availability of somatostatin analogues with avidity for them.[154,155] ^{123}I-labeled octreotide and ^{111}In-octreotide with the use of diethylenetriaminepentaacetate (DTPA) or tetra-aza-cyclododecane-N,N',N", N-tetra-acetate (DOTA) and

a ^{68}Ga-labeled derivate for PET imaging have been used to image a broad spectrum of somatostatin receptor-expressing neoplasms, including neuroendocrine tumors and pheochromocytomas.[129,143-145] The radiopharmaceutical in most frequent clinical use is the eight amino acid analogue octreotide, which exhibits particular affinity for somatostatin receptor subtypes II and VI.[129,144]

For studies using MIBG, the entire body is imaged with anterior and posterior views from the base of the skull to the bladder. Imaging is performed routinely at 24, 48, and 72 hours after injection with ^{131}I-MIBG.[146] Metaiodobenzylguanidine labeled with ^{123}I provides excellent images as early as 6 hours post injection, and later, 24 hour images.[129] Octreotide imaging requires no prior patient preparation other than discontinuation of other long-acting somatostatin analogues. Imaging usually is performed at 6 and 24 hours post injection with both planar imaging and SPECT (and more recently, hybrid SPECT/CT) of the chest and abdomen.[147] Positron emission tomography with ^{11}C-HED, ^{11}C-epinephrine, ^{18}F-FDG, and ^{18}F-fluorodopamine and ^{18}F-DOPA affords much earlier imaging of pheochromocytomas and other neuroendocrine tumors, within minutes post injection.[129,139,141,142]

CLINICAL APPLICATIONS OF ADRENOMEDULLA SCINTIGRAPHY

Pheochromocytoma

Most pheochromocytomas are sporadic and are found within the adrenal gland.[129,148] MIBG accurately depicts the majority of lesions and, because of the added benefit of whole-body screening afforded by scintigraphy, can identify the not infrequent occurrence of multifocal and/or remote metastatic disease (Fig. 10-28).[132,146,148] MIBG scintigraphy is clinically useful in depicting extra-adrenal pheochromocytomas, because of their small size or close relationship to other structures and potential remote locations from the base of the skull to the pelvis[149,150] (Fig. 10-29). Total body scintigraphy is also valuable in suspected recurrent pheochromocytomas, distant metastases, and in locally recurrent tumor(s). Anatomic imaging procedures may fail to depict recurrence because of distorted anatomy or, in the case of CT, metal clip imaging artifacts. Neither MIBG nor [111]In-

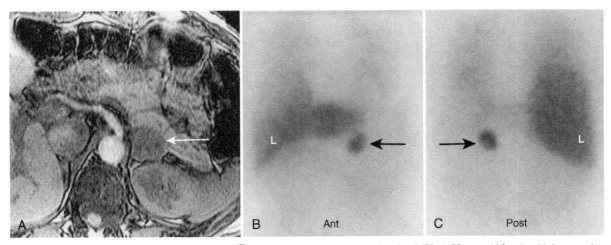

FIGURE 10-28. Left adrenal pheochromocytoma demonstrated by ^{123}I-MIBG and magnetic resonance imaging (MRI). A 50-year-old female with hypertension, a history of neurofibromatosis, elevated plasma catecholamines, and a 3 cm left adrenal mass on MRI. **A,** Abdominal MRI, transverse section, with left adrenal pheochromocytoma *(white arrow).* **B,** Anterior abdominal ^{123}I-MIBG scan with normal liver (L) uptake. The *black arrow* indicates intense, focal tracer uptake in the region of the left adrenal gland. **C,** Posterior abdominal ^{123}I-MIBG scan. The *black arrow* indicates left adrenal pheochromocytoma. *MIBG,* Meta-iodobenzylguanidine. (From Rubello D, Bui C, Casara D, et al: Functional scintigraphy of the adrenal gland, Eur J Endocrinol 147:13–28, 2002.)

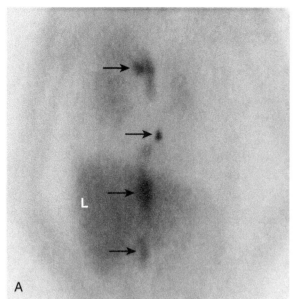

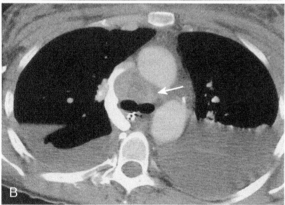

FIGURE 10-29. Malignant, metastatic pheochromocytoma demonstrated by ^{123}I-MIBG and computed tomography (CT) in a 31-year-old woman after bilateral adrenalectomy and persistent hypertension complicated by renal insufficiency and recent development of superior vena cava (SVC) obstruction. **A,** Anterior chest and abdomen scan with normal liver (L) uptake. *Black arrows* depict multiple, abnormal foci of ^{123}I-MIBG in metastatic pheochromocytoma deposits in the mediastinal and para-aortic regions. **B,** Chest CT identifies the superior mediastinal mass responsible for SVC obstruction *(white arrow)*. *MIBG,* Meta-iodobenzylguanidine. (From Rubello D, Bui C, Casara D, et al: Functional scintigraphy of the adrenal gland, Eur J Endocrinol 147:13–28, 2002.)

octreotide is affected by these factors.[108,151] In malignant pheochromocytoma studied with MIBG, the most common sites of metastatic disease are the skeleton, lymph nodes, lung, and peritoneum, and MIBG scintigraphy has been shown to be a sensitive technique for simultaneously evaluating all of these sites; however, more recent studies have suggested that the PET agents ^{18}F-DA and ^{18}F-DOPA may be more sensitive than MIBG in depicting small and remote metastatic disease (Fig. 10-30).[110,139,141,152]

[111]In-octreotide has been shown to have high sensitivity in the evaluation of extra-adrenal pheochromocytoma; however, as a result of the distribution of somatostatin receptors, specificity is limited in malignant and benign neoplasms, as many nonendocrine tumors (e.g., breast cancer, meningioma, Hodgkin's and non-Hodgkin's lymphoma), granulomatous and inflammatory diseases (e.g., sarcoidosis, tuberculosis), and autoimmune diseases (Graves' eye disease, rheumatoid arthritis) express somatostatin receptors and image with octreotide[153,154] (Fig. 10-31).

[111]In-octreotide imaging is useful when MIBG is negative in metastatic pheochromocytoma and with a high clinical suspicion of metastases, or when other neuroendocrine neoplasms are suspected.[129,147,153-156]

Most pheochromocytomas can be imaged with ^{18}F-FDG PET. Shulkin et al.[139] identified 22 of 29 patients with pheochromocytomas with ^{18}F-FDG, and reported that MIBG-negative pheochromocytomas were depicted with FDG, a finding that has been confirmed by others. Discordant results comparing FDG, MIBG, and ^{18}F-DA imaging, were seen in five patients with metastatic pheochromocytoma, and both ^{123}I MIBG and ^{18}F-DA underestimated the extent of disease when compared with CT and MRI. Fluorodeoxyglucose PET depicted lesions not identified by ^{123}I-MIBG or ^{18}F-DA.[158] Fluorodopamine correctly identified 16 patients with metastatic pheochromocytomas in which some metastases did not image with planar ^{131}I-MIBG scans.[159] ^{18}F-DOPA demonstrated better imaging than MIBG in 17 patients with pheochromocytoma, and in a companion study, the combination of MRI and ^{18}F-DOPA PET identified additional lesions that were not appreciated on MRI alone.[142,143] Hydroxyephedrine labeled with ^{11}C has been used with success to image pheochromocytomas. Rapid and early imaging approximately 10 minutes post injection was seen in nine of ten patients.[160] Trampal et al.[161] reported 13 pheochromocytomas that were depicted in 12 patients (sensitivity 92%), with one false-negative and seven true-negative studies (specificity 100%) in patients without pheochromocytomas.

Recommendations for the scintigraphic imaging of pheochromocytomas include consideration of the difficulty involved in predicting the malignant potential of a lesion; thus, localization should include two different imaging modalities: anatomic imaging to assess structural detail (tumor size, vascular and organ invasion) and scintigraphy to survey for metastases. At present, the initial imaging agent of choice is ^{123}I-MIBG (or ^{131}I MIBG, if ^{123}I-MIBG is not available). Should ^{123}I-MIBG be nonlocalizing, if available, PET using ^{18}F-DA or ^{18}F-DOPA should be considered.[157,159,161] In the event that PET radiopharmaceuticals are negative, the tumor may have undergone malignant dedifferentiation with loss of specific uptake transporters. In these instances, imaging with ^{18}F-FDG or ^{111}In-octreotide can be used to identify metastases and guide subsequent therapy.[157,162,163]

Other Clinical Applications

In multiple endocrine neoplasia (MEN) type 2, MIBG has been particularly useful. This autosomal dominant disorder is characterized by parathyroid hyperplasia, medullary carcinoma of the thyroid and adrenal medullary hyperplasia or pheochromocytoma (MEN2A), or medullary carcinoma of thyroid, mucosal ganglioneuromata, and adrenal medullary hyperplasia or pheochromocytoma (MEN2B). MIBG has been used to follow the course of development of disease of the adrenal medulla in this disorder and may facilitate the proper timing of surgical intervention, bilateral adrenalectomy, by functionally characterizing the progression of adrenal medulla hyperplasia to bilateral pheochromocytomas.[164]

Neurofibromatosis is associated with an increased incidence of pheochromocytoma, and because of the difficulty involved in differentiating pheochromocytoma from retroperitoneal neurofibroma, functional imaging with MIBG has utility and efficacy in these patients.[165,167] The role of ^{123}I-MIBG imaging in the detection, staging, and monitoring of responses to therapy, and in the distinction of residual tumor from scar in the management of neuroblastoma, is well established.[173-175] Both ^{131}I and ^{123}I-MIBG

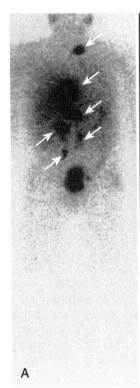

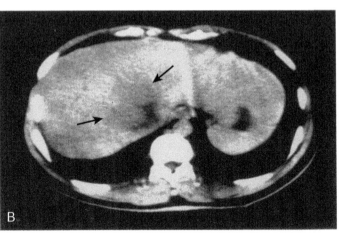

FIGURE 10-30. Anterior whole-body ^{111}In-octreotide **(A)** and transverse abdominal computed tomography **(B)** scans in a patient with metastatic pheochromocytoma. The liver metastasis was the only metastatic deposit *(black arrows)* suspected before the ^{111}In-octreotide scan, which depicted widespread metastatic disease *(white arrows)*. (From Gross MD, Shapiro B: Adrenal scintigraphy. In Khalkhali I, Maublant J, Goldsmith S [eds]: Nuclear Oncology. Philadelphia, Lippincott, Williams & Wilkins, 2000, p 472.)

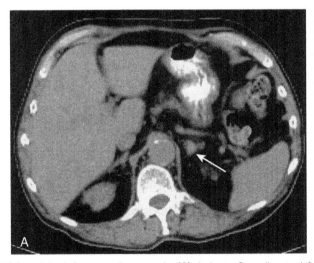
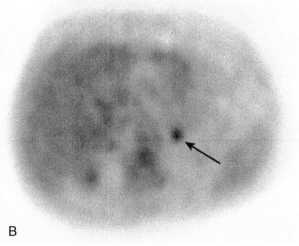

FIGURE 10-31. Abdominal computed tomography **(A)** depicts a <2 cm diameter left adrenal mass *(white arrow)* in a patient with lymphoma in the chest. A corresponding ^{18}F-FDG positron emission tomography (PET) scan **(B)** demonstrates that the mass *(black arrow)* avidly accumulated ^{18}F-FDG, which is compatible with an adrenal metastasis. The PET findings are important as the disease was upstaged from IIA to IIIB. ^{18}F-FDG, ^{18}F-fluorodeoxyglucose.

scintigraphy are superior to bone scintigraphy for the detection of skeletal involvement in neuroblastoma.[168,169]

Carbon-11–labeled HED, ^{11}C-epinephrine, ^{18}F-FDG, and ^{18}F-fluorodopamine have been used to localize neuroblastoma.[138,170] High-quality PET images of these tumors can be obtained as early as 10 minutes after injection and are comparable to SPECT images obtained 24 hours after ^{123}I-MIBG (Fig. 10-32).

Intense uptake and prolonged retention of tracer doses of ^{131}I-MIBG observed in metastatic pheochromocytoma and neuroblastoma have raised the possibility of therapy with this and other related radiopharmaceuticals, which in the case of neuro-

blastoma has become a therapeutic alternative with excellent results.[171-178] In addition, some somatostatin analogues, such as ^{90}Y-DOTA-octreotide, have been used as radiotherapeutic agents for somatostatin receptor-expressing malignant neuroendocrine tumors, including pheochromocytoma.[179]

Summary

The challenge of adrenal imaging lies in understanding the unique and complementary interplay of the anatomic and functionally based imaging modalities. A confirmed diagno-

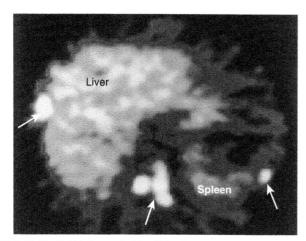

FIGURE 10-32. ^{11}C-Hydroxyephedrine (^{11}C-HED) positron emission tomography (PET) scan in a patient with malignant pheochromocytoma. Multiple areas of increased uptake are seen in the liver, abdomen, and spleen (arrows). (From Gross MD, Shapiro B: Adrenal scintigraphy. In Khalkhali I, Maublant J, Goldsmith S [eds]: Nuclear Oncology. Philadelphia, Lippincott, Williams & Wilkins, 2000, p 472.)

sis of adrenal dysfunction must be the first priority before attempts are made at anatomic or functional localization. The presence of abnormal adrenal anatomy does not invariably confirm abnormal adrenal function; neither does the presence of normal adrenal anatomy exclude abnormal adrenal function. Adrenal physiology and pathophysiology must be considered, so that studies of functional localization are properly performed and correctly interpreted. Regardless of whether the imaging modality is anatomic or functionally based, the imaging approach to a given patient must be flexible and at times must be specifically tailored for a particular disease entity. When conducted in the proper clinical setting and sequence (reasonable suspicion based on clinical features and biochemical studies), CT, MRI, catheter-directed hormone sampling, and novel radiopharmaceutical imaging using hybrid PET/CT and/or SPECT/CT can be expected to have their greatest clinical utility with diagnostic success and to lay the foundation for future advances in adrenal imaging.

REFERENCES

1. Francis IR, Korobkin M, Quint L, et al: Integrated imaging of adrenal disease, Radiology 182:1–13, 1992.
2. Doppman JL, Miller DL, Dwyer AJ, et al: Macronodular adrenal hyperplasia in Cushing disease, Radiology 166:347–352, 1988.
3. Doppman JL, Chrousos GP, Papanicolaou DA, et al: Adrenocorticotropin-independent macronodular adrenal hyperplasia: an uncommon cause of primary adrenal hypercortisolism, Radiology 216:797–1411, 2000.
4. Korobkin M, Francis IR: Adrenal imaging, Semin Ultrasound CT MR 16:317–330, 1995.
5. Lingam RK, Sohaib SA, Vlahos I, et al: CT of primary hyperaldosteronism (Conn syndrome): the value of measuring the adrenal gland, Am J Roentgenol 181:843–849, 2003.
6. Hollack CEM, Prummel MF, Tiel-Van Buul MMC: Bilateral adrenal tumors in primary aldosteronism: localization of a unilateral aldosteronoma by dexamethasone suppression scan, J Intern Med 119:545–548, 1991.
7. Doppman JL, Gill JR, Miller DL, et al: Distinction between hyperaldosteronism due to bilateral hyperplasia and unilateral aldosteronoma: reliability of CT, Radiology 184:677–682, 1992.
8. Blevins LS Jr, Wand GS: Primary aldosteronism: an endocrine perspective, Radiology 184:599–600, 1992.
9. Sohaib SA, Peppercorn PD, Allan C, et al: Primary hyperaldosteronism (Conn syndrome): MR imaging findings, Radiology 214:527–531, 2000.
10. Sheaves R, Goldin J, Reznek RH, et al: Relative value of computed tomography scanning and venous sampling in establishing the cause of primary hyperaldosteronism, Eur J Endocrinol 134:308–313, 1996.
11. Dunnick NR, Leight GS Jr, Roubidoux MA, et al: CT in the diagnosis of primary aldosteronism: sensitivity in 29 patients, Am J Roentgenol 160:321–324, 1993.
12. Ikeda DM, Francis IR, Glazer GM, et al: The detection of adrenal tumors and hyperplasia in patients with primary aldosteronism: comparison of scintigraphy, CT, and MR imaging, Am J Roentgenol 153:301–306, 1989.
13. Raisanen J, Shapiro B, Glazer GM, et al: Plasma catecholamines in pheochromocytoma: effect of urographic contrast media, Am J Roentgenol 143:43–46, 1984.
14. Mukherjee JJ, Peppercorn PD, Reznek RH, et al: Pheochromocytoma: effect of nonionic contrast medium in CT on circulating catecholamine levels, Radiology 202:227–231, 1997.
15. Blake MA, Krishnamoorthy SK, Boland GW, et al: Low-density pheochromocytoma on CT: A mimicker of adrenal adenoma, Am J Roentgenol 181:1663–1668, 2003.

16. Hamilton BH, Francis IR, Gross BH, et al: Intrapericardial paragangliomas (pheochromocytomas): imaging features, Am J Roentgenol 168:109–113, 1997.
17. Francis IR, Korobkin M: Pheochromocytoma, Radiol Clin North Am 34:1101–1112, 1996.
18. McMurry JF Jr, Long D, McClure R, et al: Addison's disease with adrenal enlargement on computed tomographic scans: report of two cases of tuberculosis and review of the literature, Am J Med 77:365–368, 1984.
19. Pedrola G, Casado JL, Lopez E, et al: Clinical features of adrenal insufficiency in patients with acquired immunodeficiency syndrome, Clin Endocrinol (Oxf) 45:97–101, 1996.
20. Caron P, Shabbonier MH, Cambus J-P, et al: Definitive adrenal insufficiency due to bilateral adrenal hemorrhage and primary antiphospholipid syndrome, J Clin Endocrinol Metab 83:1437–1439, 1998.
21. Kloos RT, Gross MD, Francis IR, et al: Incidentally discovered adrenal masses, Endocr Rev 16:460–484, 1995.
22. Barzon L, Boscaro M: Diagnosis and management of adrenal incidentalomas, J Urol 163:398–407, 2000.
23. Bardet S, Rohmer V, Murat A, et al: [131]I-6β-Iodomethylnorcholesterol scintigraphy: an assessment of its role in the investigation of adrenocortical incidentalomas, Clin Endocrinol 44:587–596, 1996.
24. Korobkin M, Francis IR, Kloos RT, et al: The incidental adrenal mass, Radiol Clin North Am 34:1037–1054, 1996.
25. Gross MD, Shapiro B: Clinically silent adrenal masses, J Clin Endocrinol Metab 77:885–888, 1993.
26. Osella G, Terzolo M, Borretta G, et al: Endocrine evaluation of incidentally discovered adrenal masses (incidentalomas), J Clin Endocrinol Metab 79:1532–1539, 1994.
27. Dunnick NR, Korobkin M: Imaging of adrenal incidentalomas: current status, Am J Roentgenol 179:559–568, 2002.
28. Incidentally discovered adrenal mass: National Institutes of Health (NIH) Consensus Conference, Bethesda, MD, February 4–6, 2002.
29. Goldman HB, Howard RC, Patterson AL: Spontaneous retroperitoneal hemorrhage from a giant adrenal myelolipoma, J Urol 155:639, 1996.
30. Russell C, Goodacre BW, van Sonnenberg E, et al: Spontaneous rupture of adrenal myelolipoma: spiral CT appearance, Abdom Imaging 25:431–434, 2000.
31. Sneiders A, Zhang G, Gordon BE: Extra-adrenal perirenal myelolipoma, J Urol 150:1496–1497, 1993.
32. Kammen BF, Elder DE, Fraker DL, et al: Extraadrenal myelolipoma: MR imaging findings, Am J Roentgenol 171:721–723, 1998.

33. Cyran KM, Kenney PJ, Memel DS, et al: Adrenal myelolipoma, Am J Roentgenol 166:395–400, 1996.
34. Rao P, Kenney PJ, Wagner BJ, et al: Imaging and pathologic features of myelolipoma, Radiographics 17:1373–1385, 1997.
35. Cheema P, Cartegena R, Staubitz W: Adrenal cysts: diagnosis and treatment, J Urol 126:396–399, 1981.
36. Rozenblit A, Morehouse HT, Amis SE Jr: Cystic adrenal lesions: CT features, Radiology 201:541–548, 1996.
37. Xarli VP, Steale AA, Davis PJ, et al: Adrenal hemorrhage in the adult, Medicine 57:211–221, 1978.
38. Burks DW, Mirvis SE, Shanmuganathan K: Acute adrenal injury after blunt abdominal trauma: CT findings, Am J Roentgenol 158:503–507, 1992.
39. Bookstein JJ, Conn J, Reuter SR: Intra-adrenal hemorrhage as a complication of adrenal venography in primary aldosteronism, Radiology 90:778–779, 1968.
40. Bayliss RIS, Edwards OM, Starer F: Complications of adrenal venography, Br J Radiol 43:531–533, 1970.
41. Ling D, Korobkin M, Silverman PM, et al: CT demonstration of bilateral adrenal hemorrhage, Am J Roentgenol 141:307–308, 1983.
42. Roubidoux MA: MR imaging of hemorrhage and iron deposition in the kidney, Radiographics 14:1033–1044, 1994.
43. Kawashima A, Sandler CM, Ernst RD, et al: Imaging of nontraumatic hemorrhage of the adrenal gland, Radiographics 19:949–963, 1999.
44. Wilson DA, Muchmore HG, Tisdal RG, et al: Histoplasmosis of the adrenal gland studied by CT, Radiology 150:779–783, 1984.
45. Ferrozzi F, Tognini G, Bova D, et al: Hemangiosarcoma of the adrenal glands: CT findings in two cases, Abdom Imaging 26:336–339, 2001.
46. Honig SC, Klavans MS, Hyde C, et al: Adrenal hemangioma: an unusual adrenal mass delineated with magnetic resonance imaging, J Urol 146:400–402, 1991.
47. Kawashima A, Sandler CM, Fishman EK, et al: Spectrum of CT findings in nonmalignant disease of the adrenal gland, Radiographics 18:393–412, 1998.
48. Krebs TL, Wagner BJ: MR imaging of the adrenal gland: Radiologic-pathologic correlation, Radiographics 18:1425–1440, 1998.
49. Radin R, David CL, Goldfarb H, et al: Adrenal and extra-adrenal retroperitoneal ganglioneuroma: Imaging findings in 13 adults, Radiology 202:703–707, 1997.
50. Johnson GL, Hruban RH, Marshall FF, et al: Primary adrenal ganglioneuroma: CT findings in four patients, Am J Roentgenol 169:169–171, 1997.
51. Feinstein RS, Gatewood OMB, Fishman EK, et al: Computed tomography of adult neuroblastoma, J Comput Assist Tomogr 8:720–726, 1984.

52. St. John Sutton MG, Sheps SG, Lie JT: Prevalence of clinically unsuspected pheochromocytoma: review of a 50-year autopsy series, Mayo Clin Proc 56:354–360, 1981.

53. Lucon AM, Pereira MAA, Mendonca BB, et al: Pheochromocytoma: study of 50 cases, J Urol 157:1208–1212, 1997.

54. Commons RR, Callaway CP: Adenomas of the adrenal cortex, Arch Intern Med 81:37–41, 1948.

55. Kokko JP, Brown TC, Berman MM: Adrenal adenoma and hypertension, Lancet 1:468–470, 1967.

56. Hedeland H, Östberg G, Hökfelt B: On the prevalence of adrenocortical adenomas in an autopsy material in relation to hypertension and diabetes, Acta Med Scand 184:211–214, 1968.

57. Russi S, Blumenthal HT, Gray SH: Small adenomas of the adrenal cortex in hypertension and diabetes, Arch Intern Med 76:284–291, 1945.

58. Aso Y, Homma Y: A survey on incidental adrenal tumors in Japan, J Urol 147:1478–1481, 1992.

59. Korobkin M, Giordano TJ, Brodeur FJ, et al: Adrenal adenomas: relationship between histologic lipid and CT and MR findings, Radiology 200:743–747, 1996.

60. Krestin GP, Friedmann G, Fischbach R, et al: Evaluation of adrenal masses in oncologic patients: dynamic contrast-enhanced MR vs CT, J Comput Assist Tomogr 15:104–110, 1991.

61. Dunnick NR, Korobkin M, Francis I: Adrenal radiology: distinguishing benign from malignant adrenal masses, Am J Roentgenol 167:861–867, 1996.

62. Korobkin M, Brodeur FJ, Francis IR, et al: CT time-attenuation washout curves of adrenal adenomas and nonadenomas, Am J Roentgenol 170:747–752, 1998.

63. Reinig JW, Doppman JL, Dwyer AJ: Adrenal masses differentiated by MR, Radiology 158:81–84, 1986.

64. Outwater EK, Siegelman ES, Radecki PD, et al: Distinction between benign and malignant adrenal masses: Value of T1-weighted chemical-shift MR imaging, Am J Roentgenol 165:579–583, 1995.

65. Hedican SP, Marshall FF: Adrenocortical carcinoma with intracaval extension, J Urol 158:2056–2061, 1997.

66. Dunnick NR, Heaston D, Halvorsen R, et al: CT appearance of adrenal cortical carcinoma, J Comput Assist Tomogr 6:978–982, 1982.

67. Fishman EK, Deutch BM, Hartman DS, et al: Primary adrenocortical carcinoma: CT evaluation with clinical correlation, Am J Roentgenol 148:531–535, 1987.

68. Dunnick NR, Doppman JL, Geelhoed GW: Intravenous extension of endocrine tumors, Am J Roentgenol 135:471–476, 1980.

69. Lee MJ, Mayo-Smith WW, Hahn PF, et al: State-of-the-art MR imaging of the adrenal gland, Radiographics 14:1015–1029, 1994.

70. Schlund JF, Kenney PJ, Brown ED, et al: Adrenocortical carcinoma: MR imaging appearance with current techniques, J Magn Reson Imaging 5:171–174, 1995.

71. Falchook FS, Allard JC: CT of primary adrenal lymphoma, J Comput Assist Tomogr 15:1048–1050, 1991.

72. Paling MR, Williamson BRJ: Adrenal involvement in non-Hodgkin lymphoma, Am J Roentgenol 141:303–305, 1983.

73. Abrams HL, Spiro R, Goldstein N: Metastases in carcinoma: analysis of 1000 autopsied cases, Cancer 3:74–85, 1950.

74. Zornoza J, Bracken R, Wallace S: Radiologic features of adrenal metastases, Urology 8:295–299, 1976.

75. Lee MJ, Hahn PF, Papanicolau N, et al: Benign and malignant adrenal masses: CT distinction with attenuation coefficients, size, and observer analysis, Radiology 179:415–418, 1991.

76. Korobkin M, Brodeur FJ, Yutzy GG, et al: Differentiation of adrenal adenomas from nonadenomas using CT attenuation values, Am J Roentgenol 166:531–536, 1996.

77. Boland GW, Lee MJ, Gazelle GS, et al: Characterization of adrenal masses using unenhanced CT: an analysis of the CT literature, Am J Roentgenol 171:201–204, 1998.

78. Mitchell DG, Crovello M, Matteucci T, et al: Benign adrenocortical masses: diagnosis with chemical shift MR imaging, Radiology 185:345–351, 1992.

79. Mayo-Smith WW, Lee MJ, McNicholas MMJ, et al: Characterization of adrenal masses (<5 cm) by use of chemical shift MR imaging: observer performance versus quantitative measures, Am J Roentgenol 165:91–95, 1995.

80. Outwater EK, Siegelman ES, Radecki PD, et al: Distinction between benign and malignant adrenal masses: value of T1-weighted chemical-shift MR imaging, Am J Roentgenol 165:579–583, 1995.

81. Korobkin M, Lombardi TJ, Aisen AM, et al: Characterization of adrenal masses with chemical shift and gadolinium-enhanced MR imaging, Radiology 197:411–418, 1995.

82. Israel GM, Korobkin M, Wang C, et al: Comparison of unenhanced CT and chemical shift MR imaging in evaluating lipid rich adrenal adenomas, Am J Roentgenol 83:215–219, 2004.

83. Outwater EK, Siegelman ES, Huang AB, et al: Adrenal masses: correlation between CT attenuation value and chemical shift ratio at MR imaging with in-phase and opposed-phase sequences, Radiology 200:749–752, 1996.

84. Haider MA, Ghai S, Jhaveri K, et al: Chemical shift MR imaging of hyperattenuating (>10 HU) adrenal masses: Does it still have a role? Radiology 231:711–716, 2004.

85. Szolar DH, Kammerhuber F: Quantitative CT evaluation of adrenal gland masses: a step forward in the differentiation between adenomas and nonadenomas? Radiology 202:517–521, 1997.

86. Krestin GP, Steinbrich W, Friedmann G: Adrenal masses: evaluation with fast gradient-echo MR imaging and Gd-DTPA-enhanced dynamic studies, Radiology 171:675–680, 1989.

87. Reinig JW, Stutley JE, Leonhardt CM, et al: Differentiation of adrenal masses with imaging: comparison of techniques, Radiology 192:41–46, 1994.

88. Szolar DH, Kammerhuber FH: Adrenal adenomas and nonadenomas: assessment of washout at delayed contrast-enhanced CT, Radiology 207:369–375, 1998.

89. Caoili EM, Korobkin M, Francis IR, et al: Delayed enhanced CT of lipid-poor adrenal adenomas, Am J Roentgenol 175:1411–1415, 2000.

90. Peña CS, Boland GWL, Hahn PF, et al: Characterization of indeterminate (lipid-poor) adrenal masses: Use of washout characteristics at contrast-enhanced CT, Radiology 217:798–802, 2000.

91. Caoili EM, Korobkin M, Francis IR, et al: Combined unenhanced and delayed enhanced CT for characterization of adrenal masses, Radiology 222:629–633, 2002.

92. Blake MA, Kalra MK, Sweeney AT, et al: Distinguishing benig from maligant adrenal masses: Multidetector row CT protocal with 10 minutes delay, Radiology 238:578–585, 2006.

93. Song JH, Chaudhry FS, Mayo-Smith WW: The incidental indeterminate adrenal mass on CT (>10 HU) in patients without cancer. Is further imaging necessary: follow up of 321 consecutive indeterminate adrenal masses, Am J Roentgenol 189:1119–1123, 2007.

94. Newhouse JH, Heffess CS, Wagner GJ, et al: Large degenerated adrenal adenomas: radiologic-pathologic correlation, Radiology 210:385–391, 1999.

95. Szolar DH, Korobkin M, Reittner P, et al: Adrenocortical carcinomas and adrenal pheochromocytomas: mass and enhancement loss evaluation at delayed contrast-enhanced CT, Radiology 234:479–485, 2005.

96. Slattery JM, Blake MA, Kalra MK, et al: Adrenocortical carcinoma: contrast washout characteristics on CT, Am J Roentgenol 187:W21–W24, 2006.

97. Geisinger MA, Zelch MG, Bravo EL, et al: Primary hyperaldosteronism: Comparison of CT, adrenal venography, and venous sampling, Am J Roentgenol 141:299–302, 1983.

98. Young WF Jr, Stanson AW, Grant CS, et al: Primary aldosteronism: adrenal venous sampling, Surgery 120:913–919, 1996.

99. Thakkar RB, Oparil S: Primary aldosteronism: a practical approach to diagnosis and treatment, J Clin Hypertens 3:189–195, 2001.

100. Rossi R, Savastano S, Tommaselli AP, et al: Percutaneous computed tomography–guided ethanol injection in aldosterone-producing adrenocortical adenoma, Eur J Endocrinol 132:302–305, 1995.

101. Liang HL, Pan HB, Lee YH, et al: Small functional adrenal adenoma: treatment with CT-guided percutaneous acetic acid injection: report of three cases, Radiology 213:612–615, 1999.

102. Hokotate H, Inoue H, Baba Y, et al: Aldosteronomas: experience with superselective adrenal arterial embolization in 33 cases, Radiology 227:401–406, 2003.

103. Gross MD, Rubello D, Shapiro B: Is there a future for adrenal scintigraphy? Nucl Med Commun 23:197–202, 2002.

104. Eriksson B, Bergström M, Sundin A, et al: The role of PET in the localization of neuroendocrine and adrenocortical tumors, Ann NY Acad Sci 970:159–169, 2002.

105. Bergström M, Bonasma TA, Bergström E, et al: In vitro and in vivo primate evaluation of carbon-11 etiomidate and carbon-11 metiomidate as potential tracers for PET imaging of the adrenal cortex and its tumors, J Nucl Med 39:982–987, 1998.

106. Shreve P, Kloos RT, Shapiro B, et al: Non-hypersecretory adrenal adenomas show marked uptake and retention of C-11 acetate, J Nucl Med 37:15, 1996.

107. Gross MD, Avram A, Fig LM, et al: Positron emission tomography in the diagnostic evaluation of adrenal tumors, Q J Nucl Med Mol Imaging 51:260–271, 2007.

108. Gross MS, Avram A, Fig LM, et al: Contemporary adrenal scintigraphy, Eur J Nucl Med Mol Imaging 34:547–557, 2007.

109. Avram A, Fig LM, Gross MD: Nuclear imaging of the adrenal gland, Semin Nucl Med 36:212–227, 2006.

110. Pacak K, Eisenhofer G, Goldstein DS: Functional imaging of endocrine tumors: role of positron emission tomography, Endocr Rev 25:568–580, 2004.

111. Minn H, Salonen A, Friberg J, et al: Imaging of adrenal incidentalomas with PET using (11)C-metomidate and (18)F-FDG, J Nucl Med 45:972–979, 2004.

112. Zettinig G, Mitterhauser M, Wadsak W, et al: Positron emission tomography imaging of adrenal masses: 18F-fluorodeoxyglucose and the 11β-hydroxylase tracer 11C-metomidate, Eur J Nucl Med Mol Imaging 31:1224–1230, 2004.

113. Khan TS, Sundin A, Juhlin C, et al: ¹¹C-metomidate imaging of adrenocortical cancer, Eur J Nucl Med Mol Imaging 30:403–410, 2003.

114. Hennings J, Lindhe Ö, Bergström M, et al: [¹¹C]Metomidate positron emission tomography of adrenocortical tumors in correlation with histopathological findings, J Clin Endocrinol Metab 91:1410–1414, 2006.

115. Tenenbaum F, Groussin L, Foehrenbach H, et al: ¹⁸F-fluorodeoxyglucose positron emission tomography as a diagnostic tool for malignancy of adrenocortical tumors? Preliminary results in 13 consecutive patients, Eur J Endocrinol 150:789–792, 2004.

116. Fassnacht M, Kenn W, Allolio B: Adrenal tumors: how to establish malignancy? J Endocrinol Invest 27:387–399, 2004.

117. Rao SK, Caride VJ, Ponn R, et al: F-18 fluorodeoxyglucose positron emission tomography-positive benign adrenal cortical adenoma: Imaging features and pathologic correlation, Clin Nucl Med 29:300–302, 2004.

118. Shimizu A, Oriuchi N, Tsushima Y: High [18F] 2-fluoro-2-deoxy-D-glucose (FDG) uptake of adrenocortical adenoma showing subclinical Cushing's syndrome, Ann Nucl Med 17:403–406, 2003.

119. Maurea S, Klain M, Mainolfi C, et al: The diagnostic role of radionuclide imaging in evaluation of patients with nonhypersecreting adrenal masses, J Nucl Med 42:884–892, 2001.

120. Maurea S, Caraco C, Klain M, et al: Imaging characterization of non-hypersecreting adrenal masses. Comparison between MR and radionuclide techniques, Q J Nucl Med Mol Imaging 48:188–197, 2004.

121. Ilias I, Pacak K: Anatomical and functional imaging of metastatic pheochromocytoma, Ann New York Acad Sci 1018:495–504, 2004.

122. Metser U, Miller E, Lerman H, et al: ¹⁸F-FDG PET/CT in the evaluation of adrenal masses, J Nucl Med 47:32–37, 2006.

123. Wadsak W, Mitterhauser M, Rendl G, et al: [18F]FETO for adrenocortical PET imaging: a pilot study in healthy volunteers, Eur J Nucl Med Mol Imaging 33:669–672, 2006.

124. Hahner S, Stuermer A, Kressl M, et al: [123I]Iodometomidate for molecular imaging of adrenocortical cytochrome P450 family 11β enzymes, J Clin Endocrinol Metab 93:2358–2365, 2008.

125. Korn N, Buswink A, Yu T, et al: A radioiodinated bretylium analog as a potential agent for scanning the adrenal medulla, J Nucl Med 18:87–89, 1977.

126. Boland GW, Goldberg MA, Lee MJ, et al: Indeterminate adrenal mass in patients with cancer: Evaluation at PET with 2[F-18]fluoro-2-deoxy-D-glucose, Radiology 194:131–136, 1995.

127. Wieland DM, Wu JL, Brown LE, et al: Radiolabeled adrenergic neuron blocking agents: adrenal medulla imaging with (^{131}I) iodobenzylguanidine, J Nucl Med 21:349–353, 1980.

128. Wieland DM, Brown LE, Tobes MC, et al: Imaging the primate adrenal medulla with (^{123}I) and (^{131}I) metaiodobenzylguanidine, J Nucl Med 22:358–364, 1981.

129. Rubello D, Bui C, Casara D, et al: Functional scintigraphy of the adrenal gland, Eur J Endocrinol 147:13–28, 2003.

130. Kurtaran A, Traub T, Shapiro B: Scintigraphic imaging of the adrenal glands, Eur J Radiol 41:123–130, 2002.

131. Gross MD, Shapiro B: Radionuclide imaging of the adrenal cortex, Q J Nucl Med 43:224–232, 1999.

132. Sisson JC, Frager MS, Valk TW, et al: Scintigraphic localization of pheochromocytoma, N Engl J Med 305:12–17, 1981.

133. Shapiro B, Wieland DM, Brown LE, et al: ^{131}I-meta-iodobenzylguanidine (MIBG) adrenal medullary scintigraphy: interventional studies. In Spencer RP, editor: Interventional Nuclear Medicine, New York, 1983, Grune & Stratton, pp 451–481.

134. Khafagi FA, Shapiro B, Fig LM, et al: Labetalol reduces iodine-131 MIBG uptake by pheochromocytoma and normal tissues, J Nucl Med 30:481–489, 1989.

135. Rosenspire KC, Haka MS, Jewett DM, et al: Synthesis and preliminary evaluation of (^{11}C) metahydroxyephedrine: a false neurotransmitter agent for heart neuronal imaging, J Nucl Med 31:1328–1334, 1990.

136. Schwaiger M, Kalff V, Rosenspire KC, et al: The noninvasive evaluation of the sympathetic nervous system in the human heart by PET, Circulation 82:457–464, 1990.

137. Shulkin BL, Wieland DM, Schwaiger M, et al: PET scanning with hydroxyepinephrine: an approach to the localization of pheochromocytoma, J Nucl Med 33:1125–1131, 1992.

138. Shulkin BL: PET epinephrine studies of pheochromocytoma, J Nucl Med 36:22P–23P, 1995.

139. Shulkin BL, Koeppe RA, Francis IR, et al: Pheochromocytomas that do not accumulate metaiodobenzylguanidine: Localization with PET and administration of FDG, Radiology 186:711–715, 1993.

140. Pacak K, Eisenhofer G, Carrasquillo JA, et al: 6-[18F]Fluorodopamine positron emission tomographic (PET) scanning for diagnostic localization of pheochromocytoma, Hypertension 38:6–8, 2001.

141. Jajer PL, Chirakal R, Marriott CJ, et al: 6-L-^{18}F-fluorodihydroxyphenylalanine PET in neuroendocrine tumors: basic aspects and emerging clinical applications, J Nucl Med 49:573–586, 2008.

142. Hoegerle S, Nitzsche E, Altehoefer C, et al: Pheochromocytomas: detection with 18F-DOPA whole-body PET—initial results, Radiology 222:507–512, 2002.

143. Hoegerle S, Ghanem N, Altehoefer C, et al: 18F-DOPA positron emission tomography for the detection of glomus tumors, Eur J Nucl Med Mol Imaging 230:689–694, 2003.

144. Krenning EP, Kwekkeboom DJ, Bakker WH, et al: Somatostatin receptor scintigraphy with [^{111}In-DTPA-D-phe^1] and [^{123}I-Tyr^3]-octreotide: the Rotterdam experience with more than 1000 patients, Eur J Nucl Med 20:716–731, 1993.

145. Win Z, Al-Nahhas A, Rubello D, et al: Somatostatin receptor positron emission tomographic imaging with Gallium-68 labeled peptides, Q J Nucl Med Mol Imaging 51:244–250, 2007.

146. Nakajo M, Shapiro B, Copp J, et al: The normal and abnormal distribution of the adrenomedullary imaging agent I-131-metaiodobenzylguanidine (I-MIBG) in man: evaluation by scintigraphy, J Nucl Med 24:672–682, 1983.

147. Gibril F, Reynolds JC, Doppman JL, et al: Somatostatin receptor scintigraphy: Its sensitivity compared with that of other imaging methods in detecting primary and metastatic gastrinomas: a prospective study, Ann Intern Med 125:26–34, 1996.

148. Shapiro B, Wieland DM, Brown LE, et al: ^{131}I-metaiodobenzylguanidine (MIBG) adrenal medullary scintigraphy: Interventional studies. In Spencer RP, editor: interventional Nuclear Medicine, New York, 1983, Grune & Stratton, pp 451–481.

149. Laursen K, Damgaard-Pedersen K: CT for pheochromocytoma diagnosis, Am J Roentgenol 134:277–280, 1980.

150. Shapiro B, Sisson JC, Kalff V, et al: The location of middle mediastinal pheochromocytomas, J Thorac Cardiovasc Surg 87:814–820, 1984.

151. Krenning EP, Bakker WH, Kooij PPM, et al: Somatostatin receptor scintigraphy with ^{111}In-DTPA-D-Phe^1-octreotide in man: metabolism, dosimetry and comparison with ^{123}I-Tyr^3-octreotide, J Nucl Med 33:652–658, 1992.

152. Ilias I, Jorge JY, Carrasquillo JA, et al: Superiority of 6-[^{18}F]-Fluorodopamine positron emission tomography versus [^{131}I]-metaiodobenzylguanidine scintigraphy in the localization of metastatic pheochromocytoma, J Clin Endocrinol Metab 88:4083–4087, 2003.

153. Hoefnagel CA: Metaiodobenzylguanidine and somatostatin in oncology, Eur J Nucl Med 21:568–581, 1994.

154. Reubi JC: Peptide receptors as molecular targets for cancer diagnosis and therapy, Endocr Rev 24:389–427, 2003.

155. Van der Harst E, de Herder WW, Bruining HA, et al: 123(I)Metaiodobenzylguanidine and 111(In)octreotide uptake in benign and malignant pheochromocytoma, J Clin Endocrinol Metab 86:685–693, 2000.

156. Tenenbaum F, Lumbroso J, Schlumberger M, et al: Comparison of radiolabeled octreotide and meta-iodobenzylguanidine (MIBG) scintigraphy in malignant pheochromocytoma, J Nucl Med 36:1–6, 1995.

157. Ilias I, Pacak K: Diagnosis and management of tumors of the adrenal medulla, Horm Metab Res 37:717–721, 2005.

158. Mamede M, Carrasquillo JA, Chen CC, et al: Discordant localization of 2-[18F]-fluoro-2-deoxy-D-glucose in 6-[18F]-fluorodopamine- and [123I]-metaiodobenzylguanidine-negative metastatic pheochromocytoma sites, Nucl Med Commun 27:31–36, 2006.

159. Ilias I, Shulkin B, Pacak K: New functional imaging modalities for chromaffin tumors, neuroblastoma and ganglioneuromas, Trends Endocrinol Metab 16:66–72, 2005.

160. Hay RV, Gross MD: Scintigraphic imaging of the adrenals and neuroectodermal tumors. Chapter 51 In Henkin RE, Bova D, Karesh SM, et al, editors: Nuclear Medicine, ed 2, Philadelphia, 2006, Mosby, pp 820–844.

161. Trampal C, Engler H, Juhlin C, et al: Pheochromocytomas: detection with ^{11}C hydroxyephedrine PET, Radiology 230:423–428, 2004.

162. Eriksson B, Bergström M, Sundin A, et al: The role of PET in the localization of neuroendocrine and adrenocortical tumors, Ann N Y Acad Sci 970:159–169, 2002.

163. Ilias I, Yu J, Carrasquillo JA, et al: Superiority of 6-[^{18}F]-Fluorodopamine positron emission tomography versus [^{131}I]-metaiodobenzylguanidine scintigraphy in the localization of metastatic pheochromocytoma, J Clin Endocrinol Metab 88:4083–4087, 2003.

164. Valk TW, Frager MS, Gross MD, et al: Spectrum of pheochromocytoma in multiple endocrine neoplasia: a scintigraphic portrayal using 131-I-metaiodobenzylguanidine, Ann Intern Med 94:762–767, 1981.

165. Kalff V, Shapiro B, Lloyd R, et al: The spectrum of pheochromocytoma in hypertensive patients with neurofibromatosis, Arch Intern Med 142:2092–2097, 1982.

166. Shulkin BL, Shapiro B: Radioiodinated meta-iodobenzylguanidine in the management of neuroblastoma. In Pochedly C, editor: Neuroblastoma, Boca Raton, FL, 1990, CRC, pp 171–198.

167. Gelfand MJ: Metaiodobenzylguanidine in children, Semin Nucl Med 23:231–242, 1993.

168. Gordon I, Peters AM, Gutman A, et al: Tc-99m bone scans are more sensitive than I-123 MIBG scans for bone imaging in neuroblastoma, J Nucl Med 31:129–134, 1990.

169. Shulkin BL, Shapiro B, Hutchinson RJ: ^{131}I-MIBG and bone scintigraphy for the detection of neuroblastoma, J Nucl Med 33:1735–1740, 1992.

170. Shulkin BL, Wieland DM, Baro ME, et al: PET studies of neuroblastoma with carbon 11-hydroxyephedrine, J Nucl Med 33:220, 1993.

171. Sisson JC, Shapiro B, Beierwaltes WH, et al: Radiopharmaceutical treatment of malignant pheochromocytoma, J Nucl Med 25:197–206, 1984.

172. Shapiro B, Sisson JC, Lloyd RV, et al: Malignant pheochromocytoma: clinical, biochemical and scintigraphic characterization, Clin Endocrinol (Oxf) 20:189–203, 1984.

173. Shapiro B, Copp JE, Sisson JC, et al: 131-I-metaiodobenzylguanidine for the locating of suspected pheochromocytoma: experience in 400 cases (441 studies), J Nucl Med 26:576–585, 1985.

174. Sisson JC, Shapiro B, Beierwaltes WH, et al: Treatment of malignant pheochromocytomas with a new radiopharmaceutical, Trans Assoc Am Physicians 96:209–217, 1983.

175. Shapiro B, Fig LM, Gross MD, et al: Radiochemical diagnosis of adrenal disease, Crit Rev Clin Lab Sci 27:265–298, 1989.

176. Shapiro B, Fig LM: General principles and perspectives of cancer therapy with radiopharmaceuticals, J Nucl Med Allied Sci 34:260–264, 1990.

177. Bravo EL, Tagle R: Pheochromocytoma: state-of-the-art and future prospects, Endocr Rev 24:539–553, 2003.

178. Shapiro B, Fig LM: Medical therapy of pheochromocytoma, Endocrinol Metab Clin North Am 18:443–481, 1989.

179. Pacak K, Linehan WM, Eisenhofer G, et al: Recent advances in genetics, diagnosis, localization and treatment of pheochromocytoma, Ann Intern Med 134:319–329, 2001.

Chapter 11

ADRENOCORTICAL CARCINOMA

BRUNO ALLOLIO and MARTIN FASSNACHT

Epidemiology

Benign adrenal tumors belong to the most common human neoplasias, with a prevalence of >4% in computed tomography (CT) studies[1-3] and an even higher prevalence in autopsy series.[4] In contrast, adrenocortical carcinoma (ACC) is a rare malignancy with an incidence of only 1 to 2 per million population per year,[5,6] leading to 0.2 % of cancer deaths according to U.S. data. However, these data may underestimate the true incidence of ACC. An unusually high incidence of ACC has been found in children in southern Brazil (3.4 to 4.2 per 1 million children versus an estimated worldwide incidence of 0.3 per 1 million children younger than 15 years) related to a founder germline p53 tumor-suppressor gene mutation.[7] ACC is more frequent in women than in men (ratio: 1.5). The incidence shows a maximum around the 4th and 5th decade, but the tumor can appear at any age.[8]

Molecular Pathology

The molecular pathogenesis of adrenocortical tumors is incompletely understood.[9,10] Important insights come from hereditary tumor syndromes associated with the development of ACC. In the Li-Fraumeni syndrome,[11] the frequency of ACC is up to 4%,[12] and 70% of patients with Li-Fraumeni syndrome have germline mutations of the p53 tumor-suppressor gene located at the 7p13 locus.[13] A second variant is caused by a heterozygous germline mutation in the hCHK2 gene.[14] In children in southern Brazil, a specific germline mutation of p53 encoding an R337H amino acid substitution has been demonstrated. This mutation leads to a pH-sensitive and temperature-dependent alteration in the function of the p53 protein.[15] Somatic mutations in the p53 gene have also been found in tumors of patients with sporadic ACC.[16] Another hereditary syndrome associated with ACC is the Beckwith-Wiedemann Syndrome (BWS), a congenital overgrowth syndrome characterized by exomphalos, macroglossia, gigantism, and the development of childhood tumors.[17] BWS has been mapped to the 11p15.5 region and is associated also with Wilms tumor and hepatoblastoma. Genes located at 11p15 and implicated in the pathogenesis of BWS are insulin-like growth factor 2 (IGF-2), H19, and cyclin-dependent kinase inhibitor 1C (CDKN1C, p57^{kip2}). IGF-2 is maternally imprinted, whereas H19 and p57^{kip2} are both paternally imprinted. Uniparental paternal isodisomy for this locus associated with IGF-2 overexpression has been observed in BWS. In sporadic ACC, rearrangement at the 11p15 locus, with overexpression of IGF-2, is frequently observed. These are caused either by duplications of the paternal 11p15 allele or by loss of the maternal allele containing the H19 gene. In fact, increased IGF-2 expression is a hallmark of adrenocortical carcinoma and has been consistently described in a variety of studies, including microarray analyses.[18-21] These observations indicate that IGF-2 overexpression is of particular importance in the pathogenesis of ACC. Accordingly, inhibition of IGF-2 action by blocking the IGF-1 receptor leads to reduced growth of ACC cells in vitro.[22]

An important observation relates to phosphodiesterase 11a (PDE11a) and the genetic predisposition to adrenocortical tumors.[23] PDE11a inactivating germline mutations are more frequent in patients harboring adrenocortical tumors, including

ACC, than in age- and sex-matched controls (odds ratio 3.53), suggesting that PDE11a alterations predispose to adrenocortical tumors.

In sporadic ACC, a variety of somatic mutations have been identified. In both benign and malignant adrenocortical tumors, β-catenin accumulation has been frequently observed, indicating activation of the Wnt-signaling pathway. This is explained in a subset of these tumors by somatic mutations of the β-catenin gene (*CTNNB1*) which may contribute to tumor progression.[24]

No activating mutations were found in the ACTH receptor in adrenal tumors.[25] In fact, in ACC a loss of heterozygosity of the ACTH receptor, with reduced expression of ACTH receptor mRNA, was observed, supporting the view that ACTH is mainly a differentiating factor for adrenocortical cells and that growth-promoting activities of pro-opiomelanocortin (POMC) may reside in the N-terminus of POMC.[26,27]

Chromosomal instability has been described in malignant adrenal tumors, indicating defects in the mitogenic machinery.[28] Using comparative genomic hybridization analysis, a significantly higher number of changes in ACCs compared to adrenocortical adenomas (mean of 7.6 to 14 changes versus 1.1 to 2 changes) have been demonstrated.[29,30] The likelihood of chromosomal changes increased with tumor size. Similarly, loss of heterozygosity (LOH) analysis has found LOHs of 17p13, 11p15, 11q13, 17q22-24, and 2p16 in sporadic ACC.[10] It has been shown that the number of somatic aberrations in ACC also predicts prognosis.[31]

Furthermore, telomere maintenance mechanisms are critical for the malignant phenotype in ACC. It has been demonstrated that telomerase activity is the major mechanism for telomere maintenance, but subsets of ACCs also show evidence of alternative telomere lengthening.[32]

Clinical Presentation

Most patients with ACC (60%) present with signs and symptoms of adrenal steroid excess. Rapidly progressing Cushing's syndrome with or without virilization is the most frequent presentation.[8,33] Androgen-secreting ACCs in women present with hirsutism and virilization, with male-pattern baldness and oligo/amenorrhea of recent onset. Estrogen-secreting tumors in males lead to gynecomastia and testicular atrophy. Rare aldosterone-producing adrenocortical carcinomas present with severe hypertension and profound hypokalemia (mean serum potassium 2.3 ± 0.08 mmol/L).[34] However, low serum potassium is more often the result of excessive cortisol production leading to incomplete renal inactivation by 11-β-dehydrogenase type 2, with consecutive mineralocorticoid excess. Careful search for abnormal adrenal steroid secretion will often reveal increased dehydroepiandrosterone sulfate (DHEAS) concentrations or elevation of androstenedione or 17α-hydroxyprogesterone, thereby confirming the adrenocortical origin of the tumor and defining a marker for follow-up. Using gas chromatography/mass spectroscopy (GC-MS) for sophisticated urinary steroid analysis, hormonal activity can be demonstrated in almost all ACC cases.[35] However, owing to low efficiency of intratumoral steroidogenesis or the exclusive secretion of steroid precursors, tumors may appear clinically as hormonally inactive.

Patients with a nonfunctioning ACC usually present with symptoms of abdominal discomfort (nausea, vomiting, abdominal fullness) or back pain caused by the large tumor mass. In particular, local pain may indicate invasive tumor growth and point to malignancy in a larger adrenal lesion. More frequent and improved abdominal imaging have led to an increasing percentage of ACC being discovered incidentally.[36,37] Nonspecific symptoms like fever, weight loss, and loss of appetite are rare. In fact, patients may carry a large tumor burden without much evidence of systemic disease besides signs and symptoms of hormone excess.

Diagnosis

HORMONAL EVALUATION

Detailed hormonal evaluation is performed prior to surgery for ACC to identify tumor markers for long-term follow-up and to guide perioperative treatment strategies (e.g., replacement of glucocorticoids after removal of a cortisol-secreting ACC).[38] Guidelines for hormonal evaluation in suspected or established ACC have been provided by the ACC Working Group of the European Network for the Study of Adrenal Tumors (ENSAT; www.ensat.org) (Table 11-1). Hormone concentrations are of limited value in predicting malignancy. However, high testosterone in women, or high estradiol in men, or cosecretion of glucocorticoids and sex hormones are indicative of a malignant adrenal lesion. In addition, benign adrenocortical tumors very often show low DHEAS concentrations, whereas highly elevated DHEAS is suggestive of ACC. Similarly, high levels of steroid precursors such as 17α-hydroxyprogesterone or androstenedione are often observed in seemingly hormonally inactive ACCs. Measurement of urinary catecholamine excretion or plasma metanephrines is required prior surgery to exclude pheochromocytoma.

Serum LDH may serve as a marker of disease progression in highly aggressive and metastasized disease.

IMAGING

Imaging plays a key role in the diagnostic workup of patients with suspected adrenal malignancy[39-41] (also discussed in Chapter

Table 11-1. Diagnostic Work-Up in Patients With Suspected or Proven ACC*

Hormonal Work-Up	
Glucocorticoid excess (minimum 3 out of 4 tests)	Dexamethasone suppression test (1 mg, 11:00 PM)
	Excretion of free urinary cortisol (24-h urine)
	Basal cortisol (serum)
	Basal ACTH (plasma)
Sexual steroids and steroid precursors	DHEAS (serum)
	17OH-progesterone (serum)
	Androstenedione (serum)
	Testosterone (serum)
	17β-estradiol (serum, only in men and postmenopausal women)
Mineralocorticoid excess	Potassium (serum)
	Aldosterone/renin ratio (only in patients with arterial hypertension and/or hypokalemia)
Exclusion of a pheochromocytoma	Catecholamine excretion (24-h urine)
	Meta- and normetanephrines (plasma)
Imaging	CT or MRI of abdomen and CT thorax
	Bone scintigraphy (when suspecting skeletal metastases)
	FDG-PET (optional)

*Recommendation of the ACC Working Group of the European Network for the Study of Adrenal Tumors (ENSAT), May 2005.

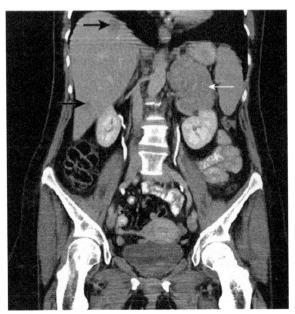

FIGURE 11-1. CT after contrast media of 8.5 cm in homogeneous ACC of the left adrenal gland *(white arrow)* and liver metastases *(black arrows)*. (Image provided by W. Kenn, Dept. of Radiology, University of Würzburg, Germany.)

10). Both size and appearance of an adrenal mass on CT, magnetic resonance imaging (MRI), and 18F-fluorodeoxyglucose positron emission tomography (FDG-PET) are highly relevant to distinguish between benign and malignant lesions. For an adrenal mass >6 cm, the likelihood of ACC increases dramatically.[42] In the German ACC Registry (n = 489), the median tumor size at diagnosis was 11.6 ± 4.7 cm (range 3 to 40 cm). Thus, in many patients, size alone is a strong indicator of malignancy. However, stage I ACC with a diameter of <5 cm has clearly the best prognosis and it is, therefore, important to identify adrenal malignancy as early as possible. Tumors between 3 and 6 cm represent a major diagnostic challenge.

Thin-collimation CT offers high spatial resolution and is fast and widely available. Large size, inhomogeneous appearance, irregular shape, and invasion into surrounding structures indicate malignancy. Frequently, tumor extension into the inferior vena cava, enlarged regional lymph nodes, and other metastases (lung and liver) are already found at presentation of ACC (Fig. 11-1). Measurement of Hounsfield units (HU) in unenhanced CT can often differentiate benign adrenal lesions from malignancy. If the density is <10 HU, diagnosis of adenoma has a sensitivity of 71% and a specificity of 98%, respectively.[43] However, lipid-poor benign adenomas are frequent and show unenhanced HU values >10.[44] In these cases, delayed postcontrast CT yields high sensitivity and specificity.[45,46] Calculating the percentage washout for adrenal masses at 10- to 15-min-delayed enhanced CT, a washout of more than 40% to 50% is highly suggestive of a benign mass, whereas a delayed attenuation of more than 35 HU and a washout of less than 50% suggest malignancy. Delayed enhanced CT is also able to characterize some adrenal masses that cannot be characterized by chemical shift MRI.[47]

Modern MRI of adrenal tumors should include T1- and T2-weighted images plus chemical shift imaging, which consists of in-phase and out-of-phase imaging. Multiplanar MRI is particularly suited to separating adrenal masses from surrounding structures like liver, spleen, pancreas, and kidney. ACCs typically present isointense to liver on T1-weighted images and show an increase in intensity in T2-weighted sequences. Heterogeneity of signals is noted both on T1-weighted and T2-weighted images due to necrosis or hemorrhage. Enhancement after gadolinium is typical, and washout is slow. Modern MRI technology can differentiate benign from malignant adrenal lesions with a sensitivity of 81% to 89% and a specificity between 92% and 99%.[41,48,49] However, the optimum MRI method (T1/T2 relaxation time, chemical shift, fast low angle shot, in vivo proton MR spectroscopy, etc.) for diagnosis of ACC remains a matter of controversy.[37,50,51]

In the past, *adrenal scintigraphy* with [131]I-6β-iodomethyl-norcholesterol (NP59) has been used to characterize adrenal lesions.[52] Benign hypersecretory adenomas show enhanced tracer uptake. However, NP 59 scintigraphy is time consuming and associated with a high radiation dose. In contrast, FDG-PET may be highly valuable in patients with suspected ACC. High uptake of 18F-FDG demonstrates increased glucose metabolism, and with few exceptions indicates malignancy. Thus, FDG-PET may be highly valuable for evaluation adrenal masses that are indeterminate by both CT and MRI. However, some benign adenomas or pheochromocytomas also show uptake of FDG.[41,50,53] Imaging with FDG-PET has the additional advantage of simultaneously detecting metastases at other sites, but metastatic lesions <1 cm (particularly in the lung) are not easily detected by FDG-PET,[54,55] indicating that PET cannot substitute for CT imaging.

None of the imaging methods mentioned can reliably differentiate ACC from a metastasis of other origin or a pheochromocytoma. In this context, a new method for adrenal imaging is promising: 11C-metomidate PET.[56,57] Metomidate specifically binds to adrenal 11β-hydroxylase and aldosterone synthase, so uptake indicates the adrenocortical origin of an adrenal lesion. A potentially more widely available tracer is ^{123}I-iodometomidate for SPECT imaging.[58]

Prior to surgery, high-resolution CT of chest and abdomen should be performed to detect frequent lung and liver metastases. A bone scan is only required if the patient complains of bone pain (see Table 11-1). Fine-needle biopsy of suspected ACC is rarely justified and is associated with the risk of needle-track metastasis. In our view, a biopsy should only be performed if the tumor cannot be removed surgically, and medical therapy needs to be based on clear pathologic evidence.

HISTOPATHOLOGY

The pathologic diagnosis of ACC may be difficult because of the lack of clear-cut morphologic criteria,[59] and in all cases, it is recommended to involve a specialized pathologist.

Weight and size are important criteria for malignancy. Most adenomas have a weight of <50 g, whereas most carcinomas weigh >100 g. The likelihood of an ACC increases steeply with a diameter of more than 6 cm.[60]

The differential diagnosis of carcinomas and adenomas is based largely on morphologic features. Different diagnostic scores[61-63] have been introduced for diagnosis of malignancy. The Weiss system is most widely used and combines nine morphologic parameters, which include three parameters related to structure (description of cytoplasm, diffuse architecture, necrosis), three parameters related to cytology (atypia, atypical mitotic figures, mitotic count), and three related to invasion (veins, sinusoids, and capsule). Further morphologic parameters of importance are broad fibrous bands and hemorrhage. It has been shown that the mitotic index also has prognostic importance.[64,65]

In addition, periadrenal tissue infiltration and vena cava or renal vein invasion carry prognostic significance.[66] Careful assessment of the resection status (R0, R1, R2) is also of great importance in that it may define further treatment strategies. For the same reason, violation of the capsule must be reported.

Important information is also provided by immunohistochemistry. Here, Ki-67 expression can be used both for differentiating benign from malignant tumors and for prognosis in ACC. A cutoff value between adenomas and ACCs varying from 1.5% to 4% has been reported. In patients with ACC, a Ki-67 labeling index of >10% was associated with poor survival in the German ACC registry. Other markers like Melan A, D11, inhibin α, and SF-1 are helpful to define the adrenocortical origin of the tumor, whereas ACC is typically negative for chromogranin A and S100.[59,60,67,68] A number of new markers (LOH at 17p13, IGF-2 overexpression, cyclin E, matrix metalloproteinase-2 [mmp-2], telomerase activity, topoisomerase IIα, and N-cadherin) have been used to separate benign from malignant adrenal lesions. However, currently none of these markers has gained widespread acceptance.

Staging

In 2004, for the first time, a staging system was published by the Union International Contre Cancer (UICC) and the World Health Organization[69] (Table 11-2). Stages I and II describe localized tumors 5 cm or smaller and larger than 5 cm, respectively. Locally invasive tumors or tumors with regional lymph node metastases are classified as stage III, and stage IV consists of tumors invading adjacent organs or presenting with distant metastases. Unfortunately, this staging system, which is largely based on the Macfarlane classification as modified by Sullivan, showed limited prognostic power.[66] Thus, a revised TNM classification was proposed by ENSAT (see Table 11-2). In this staging system, stage III is defined by tumor infiltration in surrounding tissue or in adjacent organs, thrombus in vena cava/renal vein, or positive lymph nodes, whereas stage IV is defined by the presence of distant metastasis. The ENSAT staging system provides a powerful prognostic tool, predicting both disease-free and disease-specific survival in patients with ACC (Fig. 11-2).

Therapy (Fig. 11-3)

SURGERY

Today most patients are diagnosed in stages I to III (see Fig. 11-2). In these stages, complete removal is the single most important therapeutic measure and offers the best chance for cure. All available data indicate that surgery should be performed by a specialized surgeon aware of the pitfalls of surgery for ACC (violation of the capsule, spilling). An R0 resection (resection margins microscopically disease free) is of utmost importance for long-term prognosis. Often surgery needs to be extensive, with en bloc resection of invaded organs. Spillage during surgery is paramount to an upgrade to stage IV[66] and poor prognosis. The presence of a thrombus is compatible with complete resection but occasionally necessitates cardiac bypass technique.[70-72] The use of laparoscopic adrenalectomy for ACC is debated. A higher risk of tumor spillage and local recurrences has been reported.[73-75] However, these reports suffer from a referral bias, and inferiority of laparoscopic surgery for ACC has never been demonstrated.

Table 11-2. Staging Systems for Adrenocortical Carcinoma Proposed by the UICC 2004 and ENSAT 2008[66,69]

Stage	UICC/WHO 2004	ENSAT 2008
I	T1, N0, M0	T1, N0, M0
II	T2, N0, M0	T2, N0, M0
III	T1-2, N1, M0	T1-2, N1, M0
	T3, N0, M0	T3-4, N0-1, M0
IV	T1-4, N0-1, M1	T1-4, N0-1, M1
	T3, N1, M0	
	T4, N0-1, M0	

M0, No distant metastases; M1, presence of distant metastasis; N0, no positive lymph nodes; N1, positive lymph node(s); T1, tumor ≤ 5cm; T2, tumor > 5cm; T3, tumor infiltration in surrounding tissue; T4, tumor invasion in adjacent organs (ENSAT: also venous thrombus in vena cava/renal vein).

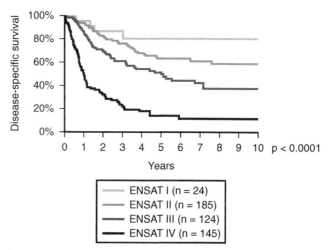

FIGURE 11-2. Disease-specific survival according to tumor stage (ENSAT Classification; see Table 11-2). (Data derived from the German ACC Registry, September 2008.)

While most experts still favor open surgery for ACC, an analysis from the German ACC registry suggests that the long-term outcome in terms of disease-free survival and overall survival is not significantly different between the use of laparoscopic adrenalectomy or open surgery in tumors <10 cm. Probably more important than this technical aspect is the expert status of the surgeon.

Surgery for local recurrence or isolated metastases is frequently used and has been associated in retrospective series with improved survival. However, the value of surgery for metastases always requires careful consideration. In our experience, achieving an R0 resection with removal of metastatic disease leads to improved well-being of the patient, although the disease almost always recurs. As an alternative to surgery, radiofrequency thermal ablation can be used for metastatic lesions smaller than 5 cm.

Tumor debulking in stage IV (metastatic disease) is usually not indicated. In individual cases, it may be used to control hormone excess.

RADIATION THERAPY

The high rate of local relapse after surgery with curative intent suggests that adjuvant tumor-bed irradiation may have therapeutic potential by preventing local relapse, which often precedes metastatic tumor spread. This view is supported by a small study indicating that adjuvant radiotherapy of the tumor bed reduces the rate of local recurrences.[76] Although more data are needed

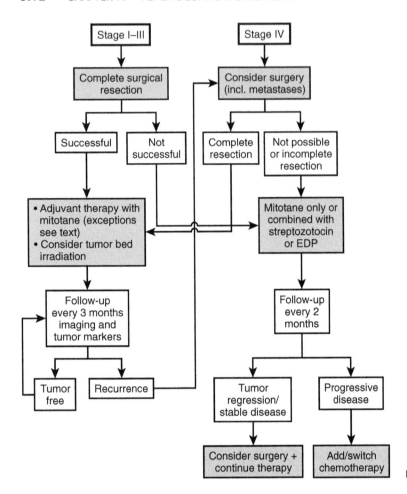

FIGURE II-3. Treatment flow chart for patients with ACC.

to better define the role of radiation therapy in an adjuvant setting, it may be justified to use adjuvant radiotherapy in selected patients. We recommend radiation therapy of the tumor bed in patients with histologically incomplete (R1) resection. In patients with macroscopically visible residual tumor, a second surgical approach by an expert surgeon should be considered first. Another group of patients that may benefit from adjuvant radiotherapy are patients with advanced locoregional disease (stage III), no evidence of distant metastases, and no evidence of residual disease after surgery. A standard fractionation scheme with single doses of 1.8 to 2.0 Gy on 5 days per week for 5 to 6 weeks is recommended. Total doses should not fall below a minimum of 40 Gy and ideally should reach 50 to 60 Gy.

Palliative radiotherapy in symptomatic metastatic lesions is well established for other tumor entities and has also been used in patients with ACC, in particular for bone metastases. Palliative radiotherapy with limited doses may also be effective in unresectable abdominal recurrences causing pain or vascular or intestinal obstruction. For optimum results of radiotherapy in ACC, an experienced radiotherapist using modern treatment concepts with CT planning, high-voltage radiation, and multiple fields is a prerequisite.

MEDICAL THERAPY: MITOTANE

Mitotane (1,1 dichloro-2[o-chlorophenyl]-2-[p-chloro-phenyl] ethane, o,p'-DDD) is an adrenolytic compound with specific adrenocortical activity that was introduced in the treatment of ACC more than 40 years ago by Bergenstal et al.[77] Its precise

mechanism of action is not fully understood.[78] Its therapeutic activity depends on metabolic activation in adrenocortical cells. Mitotane is hydroxylated in the mitochondria and transformed into an acylchloride. The activated metabolites may directly bind to macromolecules, thereby inhibiting their activity and inducing oxidative damage through production of free radicals. Impairment of adrenal steroidogenesis has been reported, and evidence for inhibition of 11β-hydroxylase activity has been demonstrated.

The clinical efficacy of mitotane has long been disputed, and only in 2004 was it approved for advanced ACC by the European Medicine Agency (EMEA). However, there is clear evidence that mitotane can induce significant tumor regression in about 25% of cases with metastasized ACC and achieve control of hypercortisolism in the majority of patients.[78] Complete responses have been described, and long-term survival is seen in the occasional patient. The use of mitotane in an adjuvant setting has been a matter of debate. However, a large retrospective analysis has indicated that adjuvant mitotane holds great potential to prolong disease-free survival and overall survival in ACC.[79] Different from many previous studies, in this investigation, selection bias was largely avoided.

Mitotane is given as tablets (Lysodren; HRA Pharma Paris, Bristol-Myers Squibb New York). Monitoring mitotane blood concentrations is essential for providing optimal efficacy and reducing toxicity. Treatment aims at mitotane concentrations between 14 and 20 mg/L for antitumor response. Higher concentrations may lead to unacceptable toxicity, whereas a response is unlikely at a concentration <14 mg/L. Thus, mitotane has a narrow therapeutic window. However, some patients may respond to lower mitotane concentrations. Owing to the long half-life of mitotane, target levels are often achieved only after weeks to months.[80] This time can be shortened by using high-dose regimens in the early phase of therapy[81]: treatment is initiated with 1.5 g/day and rapidly increased to 5 to 6 g/day until target concentrations have been reached. Most side effects are related to mitotane plasma concentrations, but gastrointestinal side effects like diarrhea seem to be more related to the daily dose. During long-term treatment, the dose of mitotane can usually be reduced, and many patients need only 2 to 3 g/day during long-term therapy. Adverse effects of mitotane treatment are manifold and common.[78] The most troubling side effects involve the central nervous system and include ataxia, confusion, tiredness, and dizziness. In addition, dose-limited gastrointestinal side effects such as nausea, vomiting, anorexia, and diarrhea may occur. Treatment with 5-hydroxytryptamine blockers and loperamide, respectively, may be useful. Because of the long half-life of mitotane, blood levels increase slowly, and adverse effects usually become apparent over time, even if the dose has remained unchanged. In case of significant side effects, drug treatment is interrupted for days or a week, and treatment is restarted with a lower dose. Ingestion of mitotane together with a lipid-rich drink or meal may enhance resorption and increase drug concentrations. Owing to its adrenolytic activity, mitotane treatment induces adrenal insufficiency. Furthermore, mitotane also increases the metabolic clearance of glucocorticoids and increases the concentration of cortisol-binding globulin (CBG).[82] High-dose glucocorticoid replacement (50 to 80 mg hydrocortisone daily) is needed. Insufficient glucocorticoid replacement enhances mitotane intolerance. Aldosterone secretion is less often affected, since mitotane primarily acts on the zona fasciculata and the zona reticularis. However, aldosterone secretion should be monitored, and replacement with fludrocortisone may become necessary with long-term use of mitotane. In addition, mitotane increases sex hormone–binding globulin[82] and often leads to low free-testosterone concentrations in males. With long-term therapy, free–thyroid hormone concentrations decline in the presence of low to low-normal TSH, suggesting secondary hypothyroidism. Mitotane's estrogenic activity may facilitate the development of gynecomastia.

Changes in hepatic gamma-glutamyl transaminase levels are so frequent that their absence questions patient compliance. However, in some cases, serious hepatotoxicity and even liver failure have been observed. Mitotane prolongs bleeding time, and it is advisable to stop mitotane for a minimum of 1 week prior to major surgery. High LDL-cholesterol and/or triglyceride concentrations are regularly observed, and treatment with a statin may be justified.

Despite the plethora of adverse effects of mitotane, most patients can be managed with acceptable toxicity in the long term.[80,83] This is particularly important in an adjuvant setting, because treatment must be given for a minimum of 2 years.

CYTOTOXIC CHEMOTHERAPY

Experience with cytotoxic chemotherapy in ACC is still limited.[38,84] In general, it has been shown that a combination of mitotane with cytotoxic agents is superior to treatment with cytotoxic agents alone.[78] The best results in terms of response rate have been reported for a combination of mitotane with etoposide, doxorubicin, and cisplatin.[85] According to WHO criteria, the overall response rate in 72 patients was 49%, including

Table 11-3. Recommended First-Line Cytotoxic Drug Regimens

Etoposide, doxorubicin, and cisplatin (EDP) plus mitotane (EDP/M) (adapted from ref. 85) every 28 days:
Day 1: 40 mg/m² D
Day 2: 100 mg/m² E
Days 3 + 4: 100 mg/m² E + 40 mg/m² P plus oral mitotane aiming at blood levels between 14 and 20 mg/L
Streptozotocin plus mitotane (Sz/M) (ref. 86):
Induction: days 1-5: 1 g Sz/day
Afterwards: 2 g/d Sz every 21 days plus oral mitotane aiming at blood levels between 14 and 20 mg/L

5 patients with a complete response. A response rate of 36% was reported for a combination of mitotane and streptozotocin.[86] This protocol is more easily administered and may have less toxicity. At the time of this writing, these two cytotoxic regimens (Table 11-3) are directly compared in the first ever phase III trial in ACC (www.firm-act.org). Results will be available in 2011 and will provide a reference cytotoxic drug regimen against which future treatments will be compared. A variety of other protocols have been used in small series of patients.[87] From this experience, it can be concluded that platinum-based therapies are in general more successful than cytotoxic regimens without platinum compounds. For other tumors, it has been shown that expression of ERCC1 plays a key role in the resistance to platinum compounds. In a retrospective series, it has been demonstrated that patients with low or absent expression of ERCC1 in their tumor respond better to treatment with a platinum-based cytotoxic chemotherapy than patients who have tumors with high expression of ERCC1.[88] This observation may be a first step towards an individualized therapy of patients with ACC.

TARGETED THERAPIES

Current success with cytotoxic chemotherapy in ACC is not very satisfactory, with less than 50% of tumors responding to treatment and most of them for only a limited period of time. Thus, new treatment options are of great interest, and the advent of targeted therapies has led to the first small trials incorporating such compounds[89] (www.clinicaltrials.gov). However, combinations of erlotinib plus gemcitabine exhibited only limited efficacy as salvage therapy for patients with advanced ACC.[90] Similarly, in a series from M.D. Anderson in Houston, no response to the EGF receptor antagonist gefitinib was seen in 19 patients with advanced ACC.[91] Furthermore, in 9 patients we saw no response to a combination of bevacizumab plus capecitabine given as salvage treatment, also suggesting that this combination has no relevant activity in advanced ACC. Because ACCs express high levels of IGF-2, which acts via the IGF-1 receptor, blockade of the IGF-1 receptor has been suggested as a promising treatment target in ACC.[20-22] Trials have been initiated, but no results have been published.

Another group of compounds that holds promise for the treatment of solid tumors are multi-tyrosine kinase inhibitors (e.g., sunitinib, sorafenib). Again, the available evidence is still very limited. Occasional tumor responses have been reported for the antiangiogenic compound thalidomide.[92] Thus, an intensive search for improved treatment protocols has been initiated, and it is expected that within the next decade, major changes in the treatment of advanced ACC will take place.

Follow-Up

Close follow-up is particularly important after seemingly complete surgery for ACC stage I to III. Initially, staging is repeated every 3 months for a minimum of 2 years (CT abdomen + chest). Even after 2 years without recurrence, there remains a high risk for relapse. Thus, follow-up is further required, but imaging intervals may increase. Regular surveillance of the patient should continue for a minimum of 5 years.

REFERENCES

1. Grumbach MM, Biller BM, Braunstein GD, et al: Management of the clinically inapparent adrenal mass ("incidentaloma"), Ann Intern Med 138(5):424–429, 2003.
2. Bovio S, Cataldi A, Reimondo G, et al: Prevalence of adrenal incidentaloma in a contemporary computerized tomography series, J Endocrinol Invest 29(4):298–302, 2006.
3. Song JH, Chaudhry FS, Mayo-Smith WW: The incidental adrenal mass on CT: prevalence of adrenal disease in 1,049 consecutive adrenal masses in patients with no known malignancy, AJR Am J Roentgenol 190(5):1163–1168, 2008.
4. Abecassis M, McLoughlin MJ, Langer B, et al: Serendipitous adrenal masses: prevalence, significance, and management, Am J Surg 149(6):783–788, 1985.
5. National-Cancer-Institute: Third national cancer survey: incidence data, DHEW Publ No (NIH) 75-787(NCI monograph):41, 1975.
6. Kebebew E, Reiff E, Duh QY, et al: Extent of Disease at Presentation and Outcome for Adrenocortical Carcinoma: Have We Made Progress? World J Surg 30:872–878, 2006.
7. Ribeiro RC, Sandrini F, Figueiredo B, et al: An inherited p53 mutation that contributes in a tissue-specific manner to pediatric adrenal cortical carcinoma, Proc Natl Acad Sci U S A 98(16):9330–9335, 2001.
8. Koschker AC, Fassnacht M, Hahner S, et al: Adrenocortical carcinoma—improving patient care by establishing new structures, Exp Clin Endocrinol Diabetes 114(2):45–51, 2006.
9. Barlaskar FM, Hammer GD: The molecular genetics of adrenocortical carcinoma, Rev Endocr Metab Disord 8(4):343–348, 2007.
10. Soon PS, McDonald KL, Robinson BG, et al: Molecular markers and the pathogenesis of adrenocortical cancer, Oncologist 13(5):548–561, 2008.
11. Li FP, Fraumeni JF Jr: Soft-tissue sarcomas, breast cancer, and other neoplasms. A familial syndrome? Ann Intern Med 71(4):747–752, 1969.
12. Hisada M, Garber JE, Fung CY, et al: Multiple primary cancers in families with Li-Fraumeni syndrome, J Natl Cancer Inst 90(8):606–611, 1998.
13. Varley JM, McGown G, Thorncroft M, et al: Are there low-penetrance TP53 Alleles? Evidence from childhood adrenocortical tumors, Am J Hum Genet 65(4):995–1006, 1999.
14. Bell DW, Varley JM, Szydlo TE, et al: Heterozygous germ line hCHK2 mutations in Li-Fraumeni syndrome, Science 286(5449):2528–2531, 1999.
15. DiGiammarino EL, Lee AS, Cadwell C, et al: A novel mechanism of tumorigenesis involving pH-dependent destabilization of a mutant p53 tetramer, Nat Struct Biol 9(1):12–16, 2002.
16. Reincke M, Karl M, Travis WH, et al: p53 mutations in human adrenocortical neoplasms: immunohistochemical and molecular studies, J Clin Endocrinol Metab 78(3):790–794., 1994.
17. Maher ER, Reik W: Beckwith-Wiedemann syndrome: imprinting in clusters revisited, J Clin Invest 105(3):247–252, 2000.
18. Gicquel C, Raffin-Sanson ML, Gaston V, et al: Structural and functional abnormalities at 11p15 are associated with the malignant phenotype in sporadic adrenocortical tumors: study on a series of 82 tumors, J Clin Endocrinol Metab 82(8):2559–2565, 1997.
19. Gicquel C, Bertagna X, Gaston V, et al: Molecular markers and long-term recurrences in a large cohort of patients with sporadic adrenocortical tumors, Cancer Res 61(18):6762–6767, 2001.
20. Giordano TJ, Thomas DG, Kuick R, et al: Distinct transcriptional profiles of adrenocortical tumors uncovered by DNA microarray analysis, Am J Pathol 162(2):521–531, 2003.
21. de Fraipont F, El Atifi M, Cherradi N, et al: Gene expression profiling of human adrenocortical tumors using complementary deoxyribonucleic acid microarrays identifies several candidate genes as markers of malignancy, J Clin Endocrinol Metab 90(3):1819–1829, 2005.
22. Almeida MQ, Fragoso MC, Lotfi CF, et al: Expression of IGF-II and its receptor in pediatric and adult adrenocortical tumors, J Clin Endocrinol Metab, 2008.
23. Libe R, Fratticci A, Coste J, et al: Phosphodiesterase 11A (PDE11A) and genetic predisposition to adrenocortical tumors, Clin Cancer Res 14(12):4016–4024, 2008.
24. Gaujoux S, Tissier F, Groussin L, et al: Wnt/ss-catenin and cAMP/PKA signaling pathways alterations and somatic ss-catenin gene mutations in the progression of adrenocortical tumors, J Clin Endocrinol Metab, 2008.
25. Latronico AC, Reincke M, Mendonca BB, et al: No evidence for oncogenic mutations in the adrenocorticotropin receptor gene in human adrenocortical neoplasms, J Clin Endocrinol Metab 80(3):875–877, 1995.
26. Beuschlein F, Fassnacht M, Klink A, et al: ACTH-receptor expression, regulation and role in adrenocortical formation, Eur J Endocrinol 144(3):199–206, 2001.
27. Fassnacht M, Hahner S, Hansen IA, et al: N-terminal pro-opiomelanocortin acts as a mitogen in adrenocortical cells and decreases adrenal steroidogenesis, J Clin Endocrinol Metab 88(5):2171–2179, 2003.
28. Dohna M, Reincke M, Mincheva A, et al: Adrenocortical carcinoma is characterized by a high frequency of chromosomal gains and high-level amplifications, Genes Chromosomes Cancer 28(2):145–152, 2000.
29. Sidhu S, Marsh DJ, Theodosopoulos G, et al: Comparative genomic hybridization analysis of adrenocortical tumors, J Clin Endocrinol Metab 87(7):3467–3474, 2002.
30. Zhao J, Speel EJ, Muletta-Feurer S, et al: Analysis of genomic alterations in sporadic adrenocortical lesions. Gain of chromosome 17 is an early event in adrenocortical tumorigenesis, Am J Pathol 155(4):1039–1045, 1999.
31. Stephan EA, Chung TH, Grant CS, et al: Adrenocortical carcinoma survival rates correlated to genomic copy number variants, Mol Cancer Ther 7(2):425–431, 2008.
32. Else T, Giordano TJ, Hammer GD: Evaluation of telomere length maintenance mechanisms in adrenocortical carcinoma, J Clin Endocrinol Metab 93(4):1442–1449, 2008.
33. Abiven G, Coste J, Groussin L, et al: Clinical and biological features in the prognosis of adrenocortical cancer: poor outcome of cortisol-secreting tumors in a series of 202 consecutive patients, J Clin Endocrinol Metab 91(7):2650–2655, 2006.
34. Seccia TM, Fassina A, Nussdorfer GG, et al: Aldosterone-producing adrenocortical carcinoma: an unusual cause of Conn's syndrome with an ominous clinical course, Endocr Relat Cancer 12(1):149–159, 2005.
35. Arlt W, Hahner S, Libe R, et al: Steroid profiling in the diagnosis and monitoring of adrenocortical cancer—results of the EURINE ACC Study of the European Network for the Study of Adrenal Tumors (ENSAT). Abstracts of the 90th annual meeting of the Endocrine Society (San Francisco):OR40-2, 2008.
36. Mantero F, Terzolo M, Arnaldi G, et al: A survey on adrenal incidentaloma in Italy. Study Group on Adrenal Tumors of the Italian Society of Endocrinology, J Clin Endocrinol Metab 85(2):637–644, 2000.
37. Mansmann G, Lau J, Balk E, et al: The clinically inapparent adrenal mass: update in diagnosis and management, Endocr Rev 25(2):309–340, 2004.
38. Allolio B, Fassnacht M: Clinical review: adrenocortical carcinoma: clinical update, J Clin Endocrinol Metab 91(6):2027–2037, 2006.
39. Fassnacht M, Kenn W, Allolio B: Adrenal tumors: how to establish malignancy? J Endocrinol Invest 27(4):387–399, 2004.
40. Ilias I, Sahdev A, Reznek RH, et al: The optimal imaging of adrenal tumors: a comparison of different methods, Endocr Relat Cancer 14(3):587–599, 2007.
41. Heinz-Peer G, Memarsadeghi M, Niederle B: Imaging of adrenal masses, Curr Opin Urol 17(1):32–38, 2007.
42. Ross NS, Aron DC: Hormonal evaluation of the patient with an incidentally discovered adrenal mass, N Engl J Med 323(20):1401–1405, 1990.
43. Boland GW, Lee MJ, Gazelle GS, et al: Characterization of adrenal masses using unenhanced CT: an analysis of the CT literature, Am J Roentgenol 171(1):201–204, 1998.
44. Hamrahian AH, Ioachimescu AG, Remer EM, et al: Clinical utility of noncontrast computed tomography attenuation value (Hounsfield units) to differentiate adrenal adenomas/hyperplasias from nonadenomas: Cleveland Clinic experience, J Clin Endocrinol Metab 90(2):871–877, 2005.
45. Caoili EM, Korobkin M, Francis IR, et al: Adrenal masses: characterization with combined unenhanced and delayed enhanced CT, Radiology 222(3):629–633, 2002.
46. Szolar DH, Korobkin M, Reittner P, et al: Adrenocortical carcinomas and adrenal pheochromocytomas: mass and enhancement loss evaluation at delayed contrast-enhanced CT, Radiology 234(2):479–485, 2005.
47. Park BK, Kim CK, Kim B, et al: Comparison of delayed enhanced CT and chemical shift MR for evaluating hyperattenuating incidental adrenal masses, Radiology 243(3):760–765, 2007.
48. Korobkin M, Lombardi TJ, Aisen AM, et al: Characterization of adrenal masses with chemical shift and gadolinium-enhanced MR imaging, Radiology 197(2):411–418, 1995.
49. Honigschnabl S, Gallo S, Niederle B, et al: How accurate is MR imaging in characterisation of adrenal masses: update of a long-term study, Eur J Radiol 41(2):113–122, 2002.
50. Al-Hawary MM, Francis IR, Korobkin M: Non-invasive evaluation of the incidentally detected indeterminate adrenal mass, Best Pract Res Clin Endocrinol Metab 19(2):277–292, 2005.
51. Faria JF, Goldman SM, Szejnfeld J, et al: Adrenal masses: characterization with in vivo proton MR spectroscopy—initial experience, Radiology 245(3):788–797, 2007.
52. Gross MD, Shapiro B, Francis IR, et al: Scintigraphic evaluation of clinically silent adrenal masses, J Nucl Med 35(7):1145–1152, 1994.
53. Caoili EM, Korobkin M, Brown RK, et al: Differentiating adrenal adenomas from nonadenomas using (18)F-FDG PET/CT: quantitative and qualitative evaluation, Acad Radiol 14(4):468–475, 2007.
54. Mackie GC, Shulkin BL, Ribeiro RC, et al: Use of [18F]fluorodeoxyglucose positron emission tomography in evaluating locally recurrent and metastatic adrenocortical carcinoma, J Clin Endocrinol Metab 91(7):2665–2671, 2006.
55. Leboulleux S, Dromain C, Bonniaud G, et al: Diagnostic and prognostic value of 18-fluorodeoxyglucose positron emission tomography in adrenocortical carcinoma: a prospective comparison with computed tomography, J Clin Endocrinol Metab 91(3):920–925, 2006.
56. Khan TS, Sundin A, Juhlin C, et al: 11C-metomidate PET imaging of adrenocortical cancer, Eur J Nucl Med Mol Imaging 30(3):403–410, 2003.
57. Hennings J, Lindhe O, Bergstrom M, et al: [11C]metomidate positron emission tomography of adrenocortical tumors in correlation with histopathological findings, J Clin Endocrinol Metab 91(4):1410–1414, 2006.
58. Hahner S, Stuermer A, Kreissl M, et al: [123 I]Iodometomidate for molecular imaging of adrenocortical cytochrome P450 family 11B enzymes, J Clin Endocrinol Metab 93(6):2358–2365, 2008.

59. Volante M, Buttigliero C, Greco E, et al: Pathological and molecular features of adrenocortical carcinoma: an update, J Clin Pathol 61(7):787–793, 2008.
60. Saeger W: Histopathological classification of adrenal tumors, Eur J Clin Invest 30(Suppl 3):58–62, 2000.
61. Weiss LM, Medeiros LJ, Vickery AL Jr: Pathologic features of prognostic significance in adrenocortical carcinoma, Am J Surg Pathol 13(3):202–206, 1989.
62. Hough AJ, Hollifield JW, Page DL, et al: Prognostic factors in adrenal cortical tumors. A mathematical analysis of clinical and morphologic data, Am J Clin Pathol 72(3):390–399, 1979.
63. van Slooten H, Schaberg A, Smeenk D, et al: Morphologic characteristics of benign and malignant adrenocortical tumors, Cancer 55(4):766–773, 1985.
64. Stojadinovic A, Ghossein RA, Hoos A, et al: Adrenocortical carcinoma: clinical, morphologic, and molecular characterization, J Clin Oncol 20(4):941–950, 2002.
65. Assie G, Antoni G, Tissier F, et al: Prognostic parameters of metastatic adrenocortical carcinoma, J Clin Endocrinol Metab 92(1):148–154, 2007.
66. Fassnacht M, Johanssen S, Quinkler M, et al: Limited prognostic value of the 2004 UICC staging classification for adrenocortical carcinoma: proposal for a revised TNM classification, Cancer 2008 [in press].
67. Saeger W, Fassnacht M, Chita R, et al: High diagnostic accuracy of adrenal core biopsy: results of the German and Austrian adrenal network multicenter trial in 220 consecutive patients, Hum Pathol 34(2):180–186, 2003.
68. Sasano H, Suzuki T, Moriya T: Recent advances in histopathology and immunohistochemistry of adrenocortical carcinoma, Endocr Pathol 17(4):345–354, 2006.
69. DeLellis RA, Lloyd RV, Heitz PU, et al: World Health Organization Classification of Tumors. Pathology and Genetics of Tumors of Endocrine Organs. IARC Press, Lyons, France, 136, 2004.
70. Mingoli A, Nardacchione F, Sgarzini G, et al: Inferior vena cava involvement by a left side adrenocortical carcinoma: operative and prognostic considerations, Anticancer Res 16(5B):3197–3200, 1996.
71. Hedican SP, Marshall FF: Adrenocortical carcinoma with intracaval extension, J Urol 158(6):2056–2061, 1997.
72. Dackiw AP, Lee JE, Gagel RF, et al: Adrenal cortical carcinoma, World J Surg 25(7):914–926, 2001.
73. Gonzalez RJ, Shapiro S, Sarlis N, et al: Laparoscopic resection of adrenal cortical carcinoma: a cautionary note, Surgery 138(6):1078–1085; discussion 85–86, 2005.
74. Kebebew E, Siperstein AE, Clark OH, et al: Results of laparoscopic adrenalectomy for suspected and unsuspected malignant adrenal neoplasms, Arch Surg 137(8):948–951; discussion 52–53, 2002.
75. Schlamp A, Hallfeldt K, Mueller-Lisse U, et al: Recurrent adrenocortical carcinoma after laparoscopic resection, Nat Clin Pract Endocrinol Metab 3(2):191–195; quiz 1 following 5, 2007.
76. Fassnacht M, Hahner S, Polat B, et al: Efficacy of adjuvant radiotherapy of the bed on local recurrence of adrenocortical carcinoma, J Clin Endocrinol Metab 91(11):4501–4504, 2006.
77. Bergenstal D, Lipsett M, Moy R, et al: Regression of adrenal cancer and suppression of adrenal function in men by o,p′-DDD, Transactions of American Physicians 72:341, 1959.
78. Hahner S, Fassnacht M: Mitotane for adrenocortical carcinoma treatment, Curr Opin Investig Drugs 6(4):386–394, 2005.
79. Terzolo M, Angeli A, Fassnacht M, et al: Adjuvant mitotane treatment in patients with adrenocortical carcinoma, N Engl J Med 356(23):372–380, 2007.
80. Terzolo M, Pia A, Berruti A, et al: Low-dose monitored mitotane treatment achieves the therapeutic range with manageable side effects in patients with adrenocortical cancer, J Clin Endocrinol Metab 85(6):2234–2238, 2000.
81. Faggiano A, Leboulleux S, Young J, et al: Rapidly progressing high o,p′DDD doses shorten the time required to reach the therapeutic threshold with an acceptable tolerance: preliminary results, Clin Endocrinol (Oxf) 64(1):110–113, 2006.
82. Nader N, Raverot G, Emptoz-Bonneton A, et al: Mitotane has an estrogenic effect on sex hormone-binding globulin and corticosteroid-binding globulin in humans, J Clin Endocrinol Metab 91(6):2165–2170, 2006.
83. Dickstein G, Shechner C, Arad E, et al: Is there a role for low doses of mitotane (o,p′-DDD) as adjuvant therapy in adrenocortical carcinoma? J Clin Endocrinol Metab 83(9):3100–3103, 1998.
84. Fareau GG, Lopez A, Stava C, et al: Systemic chemotherapy for adrenocortical carcinoma: comparative responses to conventional first-line therapies, Anticancer Drugs 19(6):637–644, 2008.
85. Berruti A, Terzolo M, Sperone P, et al: Etoposide, doxorubicin and cisplatin plus mitotane in the treatment of advanced adrenocortical carcinoma: a large prospective phase II trial, Endocr Relat Cancer 12(3):657–666, 2005.
86. Khan TS, Imam H, Juhlin C, et al: Streptozocin and o,p′DDD in the treatment of adrenocortical cancer patients: long-term survival in its adjuvant use, Ann Oncol 11(10):1281–1287, 2000.
87. Allolio B, Hahner S, Weismann D, et al: Management of adrenocortical carcinoma, Clin Endocrinol (Oxf) 60:273–287, 2004.
88. Ronchi CL, Sbiera S, Adam P, et al: ERCC1 expression in adrenocortical cancer: relationship with baseline characteristics and response to platinum-based chemotherapy, Endocr Relet Cancer, in press, 2009.
89. Kirschner LS: Emerging treatment strategies for adrenocortical carcinoma: a new hope, J Clin Endocrinol Metab 91:14–21, 2006.
90. Quinkler M, Hahner S, Wortmann S, et al: Treatment of advanced adrenocortical carcinoma with erlotinib plus gemcitabine, J Clin Endocrinol Metab 93(6):2057–2062, 2008.
91. Samnotra V, Vassilopoulou-Sellin R, Fojo AT: A phase II trial of gefitinib monotherapy in patients with unresectable adrenocortical carcinoma (ACC), Proc Ann Soc Clin Oncol:abstract no 15527, 2007.
92. Chacon R, Tossen G, Loria FS, et al: CASE 2. Response in a patient with metastatic adrenal cortical carcinoma with thalidomide, J Clin Oncol 23(7):1579–1580, 2005.

Chapter 12

PRIMARY MINERALOCORTICOID EXCESS SYNDROMES AND HYPERTENSION

ROBERT M. CAREY and SHETAL H. PADIA

Aldosterone
Primary Aldosteronism
Aldosterone-Producing Adrenal Carcinoma
Glucocorticoid-Remediable Aldosteronism

Mineralocorticoids Other Than Aldosterone
17α-Hydroxylase Deficiency
11β-Hydroxylase Deficiency
Deoxycorticosterone Excess States
Corticosterone Excess States
Congenital Apparent Mineralocorticoid Excess Syndrome
Acquired Apparent Mineralocorticoid Excess Syndrome
Ectopic ACTH Syndrome
Glucocorticoid Resistance States
Primary (Essential) Hypertension
Exogenous Mineralocorticoid States

Aldosterone, the most important mineralocorticoid hormone, is synthesized by the adrenal zona glomerulosa and plays a pivotal role in normal body fluid and electrolyte balance. Increased aldosterone production induces sodium retention and potassium loss. By definition, disorders in which aldosterone excess results from activation of the renin-angiotensin system are classified as secondary aldosteronism. This chapter focuses on the primary abnormalities of aldosterone hypersecretion, on a number of related conditions in which mineralocorticoids other than aldosterone produce similar clinical and biochemical characteristics, and on a syndrome with primary ion transport abnormalities at the distal nephron that can mimic primary aldosteronism.

Aldosterone

PRIMARY ALDOSTERONISM

Jerome W. Conn's classic paper[1] initially describing primary aldosteronism was published in 1955. The patient had hypertension, excessive renal potassium wasting, severe hypokalemia, metabolic alkalosis, and neuromuscular symptoms associated with increased levels of a sodium-retaining hormone that was subsequently identified as aldosterone. The clinical and bio-chemical abnormalities were abolished after removal of a unilateral benign adrenal adenoma, introducing a paradigm shift in the study of the role of adrenal mineralocorticoids in hypertension. Over the ensuing decade, many similar cases were discovered. In 1964, Conn and colleagues reviewed the features of 145 cases.[2] The diagnosis of primary aldosteronism was greatly facilitated by the development of methods for the measurement of plasma renin activity (PRA), which was determined to be suppressed in primary aldosteronism[3,4] but elevated in secondary aldosteronism, as represented, for example, by various edema-forming states or malignant or renovascular hypertension.[5]

In primary aldosteronism, aldosterone secretion is increased (Fig. 12-1), leading to increased sodium reabsorption at the renal cortical collecting duct followed by extracellular fluid volume expansion and consequent suppression of renin secretion. Distal nephron exchange of sodium for potassium and hydrogen ions often lead to hypokalemic metabolic alkalosis. Reduced circulating and/or cellular potassium concentrations may oppose the increase in aldosterone secretion but usually are not effective in normalizing it.

Following the original description, identical clinical and biochemical features were discovered in patients with bilateral disease without adrenal tumors. The spectrum of primary aldosteronism as currently recognized is listed in Table 12-1, together with estimates of the prevalence of its different subtypes. In addition to these disorders, the clinical diagnosis of primary aldosteronism should be distinguished from administration of exogenous mineralocorticoids (e.g., fludrocortisone) or drugs or substances previously thought to be mineralocorticoids but now known to act indirectly via inhibition of 11β-hydroxysteroid dehydrogenase (11β-HSD) (e.g., licorice, carbenoxolone) or secretion of excess mineralocorticoids other than aldosterone (e.g., deoxycorticosterone [DOC]).[6]

Definition of Primary Aldosteronism

As stated in the 2008 Endocrine Society Clinical Practice Guideline,[7] primary aldosteronism is defined as a group of disorders in which aldosterone production is inappropriately high, relatively autonomous, and independent of the renin-angiotensin system, and in which aldosterone secretion is not suppressed by sodium loading. Hypokalemia was formerly included as a part of the definition of primary aldosteronism. However, in recent studies in unselected hypertensive populations, most patients

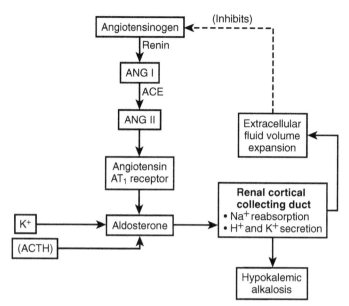

FIGURE 12-1. Schematic representation of the renin-angiotensin-aldosterone system in primary aldosteronism. Aldosterone secretion is increased independently of the renin-angiotensin system. Aldosterone increases sodium (Na^+) reabsorption at the renal cortical collecting duct in exchange for potassium (K^+) and hydrogen (H^+) ions. Reabsorbed Na^+ increases extracellular fluid volume, inhibiting renin production and secretion. For this reason, angiotensin peptide synthesis is suppressed. K^+, normally a stimulator of aldosterone production, is reduced, leading to partial reduction of autonomous aldosterone secretion. Reduced activity of the renin-angiotensin system and K^+ denoted by gray.

Table 12-1. Forms of Primary Aldosteronism and Their Prevalence Rates

Disorder	Prevalence, %
Aldosterone-producing adenoma (APA)	33
Bilateral idiopathic adrenal hyperplasia (IHA)	63
Primary (unilateral) adrenal hyperplasia	<1
Aldosterone-producing adrenocortical carcinoma	<1
Ectopic (nonadrenal) aldosterone-producing adenomas	Rare
Familial hyperaldosteronism (FH)	
Type I (FH I)—Glucocorticoid-remediable hyperaldosteronism	0.5
Type II (FH II)—Adrenocorticotropic hormone (ACTH)-independent familial hyperaldosteronism	3-4

with primary aldosteronism have been normokalemic. Rarely, patients with primary aldosteronism are normotensive, and very rarely normal levels of plasma and urinary aldosterone have been reported.[8,9]

Prevalence of Primary Aldosteronism

Conn[10] originally believed that approximately 20% of patients with essential hypertension might have the syndrome that he had originally reported. At the time, this was thought to be a gross overestimate of prevalence. Later, Conn adjusted his estimated prevalence to approximately 10% of hypertensive individuals—a prediction that has been substantiated approximately 40 years later. Until the early to mid 1980s, when routine measurement of the aldosterone:renin ratio was introduced, most authors suggested that the prevalence of primary aldosteronism was less than 1% in unselected hypertensive populations.[11-14] For example, Lewin and colleagues[13] identified only 3 of 5485 patients with possible primary aldosteronism. A slightly higher prevalence (0.4%) was found in 3783 patients with moderately severe,

nonmalignant hypertension in Glasgow.[14] Other investigators, however, found a significantly higher prevalence when studying selected populations, especially when aldosterone:renin ratios were employed for screening all patients with hypertension and not simply those with hypokalemia (2% to 12%).[15-18]

Use of the plasma aldosterone concentration (PAC):plasma renin activity (PRA) ratio as a screening test followed by aldosterone suppression confirmatory testing to make the definitive diagnosis has led to much higher prevalence rates of primary aldosteronism in patients from five continents.[17] With use of these methods, the prevalence of primary aldosteronism now is generally accepted as 5% to 13% of all patients with hypertension.[17-26]

Cause of Primary Aldosteronism

In addition to aldosterone-producing adenoma (APA) as described by Conn, six subtypes of primary aldosteronism have been described (see Table 12-1). With the exception of glucocorticoid-remediable aldosteronism (GRA) (also termed familial hyperaldosteronism type I [FH-I], dexamethasone-suppressible aldosteronism, or glucocorticoid-remediable hyperaldosteronism), the precise molecular origin of primary aldosteronism has not been determined.

GRA is an autosomal dominant disorder that is responsible for less than 1% of cases of primary aldosteronsim.[27] GRA is characterized by the early onset of moderate to severe hypertension, premature cerebrovascular accidents, variable hypokalemia (most patients are normokalemic), aldosterone excess with suppression of PRA, and excess production of the hybrid steroids 18-hydroxycortisol (18-OH-F) and 18-oxocortisol (18-oxo-F).[27] GRA is caused by a novel gene duplication (i.e., a chimeric gene) resulting from unequal crossing over between the promoter sequence of the $CYP11\beta1$ gene encoding 11β-hydroxylase and the coding sequence of the $CYP11\beta2$ gene encoding aldosterone synthase.[27,28] This gene duplication allows ectopic expression of the aldosterone synthase enzyme in the adrenal zona fasciculata, where it is not normally expressed, explaining the adrenocorticotropic hormone (ACTH)-dependent aldosterone overproduction and the increased levels of cortisol hybrid steroids.[27,28] The steroid secretion pattern found in GRA is compared with the normal pattern in Fig. 12-2. The fact that patients with GRA are frequently normokalemic despite clear aldosterone excess is consistent with findings of recent studies involving patients with other forms of primary aldosteronism, most of whom are also normokalemic.[17,26] Because of similarities between GRA and angiotensin-unresponsive aldosterone-producing adenomas (APAs) (the primary regulation of aldosterone is provided by ACTH), investigators have tested whether the chimeric gene found in GRA is present in APA, but it is not.[29] An abnormality of aldosterone synthase expression or activity has not been reported in APA or IHA.

A different form of familial primary aldosteronism, which also has an autosomal dominant inheritance pattern and may have a monogenic basis, is familial hyperaldosteronism type II (FH-II).[30] In this disorder, aldosterone is not suppressible by glucocorticoids, and no hybrid gene mutation occurs. FH-II can present with APA or adrenocortical hyperplasia. In the extensive experience of the Brisbane, Australia group, FH-II is more common (3% to 4%) than FH-I, and the diagnosis is made at an older age than for FH-I. No difference in age, gender, biochemical parameters, or aldosterone or renin levels has been documented between FH-II and sporadic primary aldosteronism. The molecular basis for FH-II is unclear. However, linkage analysis in large

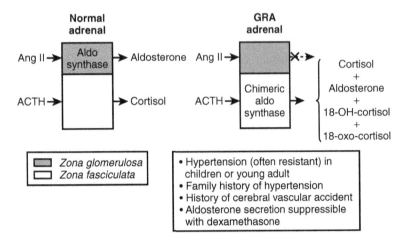

FIGURE 12-2. Schematic depiction of the pathophysiology and major clinical manifestations of glucocorticoid-remediable alsteronism (GRA). *Dashed arrow* indicates response absent.

families has recently shown an association with chromosome region 7p22.[30,31] Possible candidate genes at this locus include *PPKAR1β* encoding the 1-β regulatory subunit of protein kinase A. A related gene encoding the 1-α regulatory subunit, *PPKR1α* is mutated in the Carney complex, another familial condition associated with adrenal cortisol-producing tumors.

Idiopathic hyperaldosteronism (IHA), the most common form of primary aldosteronism, is characterized by bilateral adrenal hyperplasia. The cause of IHA is unknown. Adrenals may be normal or may display diffuse, micronodular, or macronodular hyperplasia. Available evidence suggests that the aldosterone overproduction is angiotensin II dependent and may result at least in part from hypersensitivity of the zona glomerulosa to angiotensin II.[32,33] The positive interrelationship of plasma aldosterone to angiotensin II suggests that IHA may be a form of secondary rather than primary hyperaldosteronism. Padfield and associates[33] suggested that IHA is part of a continuum with low renin essential hypertension (LREH). However, the fact that aldosterone secretion is at least partially autonomous of the renin-angiotensin system in IHA, as demonstrated by failure of normal suppression during sodium loading (despite profound suppression of renin), argues against this possibility. Wisgerhoff and associates[34,35] first documented the exaggerated angiotensin II–induced aldosterone response in both IHA and LREH. Witzgall and colleagues[36] later confirmed increased aldosterone hypersensitivity to angiotensin II and in separate experiments determined that there was increased but ineffective dopaminergic inhibition of aldosterone secretion in both IHA and LREH. However, another group failed to confirm this observation.[37]

The role of angiotensin II in stimulating aldosterone secretion in IHA is supported by the ability of captopril and other angiotensin-converting enzyme (ACE) inhibitors to reduce plasma aldosterone in this condition. The source of the circulating angiotensin II, the synthesis of which is interrupted by converting enzyme inhibition, is unclear in the presence of low PRA. This observation has raised the possibility of an abnormality of the intra-adrenal (local tissue) renin-angiotensin system independent of the systemic circulation. Fallo and coworkers[38] examined the effects of captopril on aldosterone responses to potassium infusion in IHA and APA. Before captopril, potassium stimulated an increase in aldosterone in both groups. After captopril, the response was significantly blunted in IHA but not in APA. These observations suggested that the intra-adrenal renin-angiotensin system may play a role in the aldosterone response to potassium in IHA. However, direct in vitro evidence for this hypothesis is lacking.

Klemm and colleagues[39] reported an increase in renin gene expression in angiotensin-responsive APAs (which biochemically behave similarly to IHA in that aldosterone production is responsive to angiotensin) but not in angiotensin-unresponsive APAs compared with normal tissue. Renin gene expression was also increased in adrenal cortex surrounding some angiotensin-responsive APAs, suggesting that the defect in tissue renin gene expression may not be confined to the tumor.

Although several investigators have attempted to implicate pituitary peptides other than ACTH, especially pro-opiomelanocortin derivatives, no consistent evidence for this hypothesis has been forthcoming in the pathophysiology of IHA.[40]

Essentially nothing is known about the cause of primary adrenal hyperplasia (PAH) in which both adrenal glands or, more rarely, one adrenal gland shows micronodular or macronodular hyperplasia and produces a clinical and biochemical picture very similar to that of angiotensin-unresponsive APA.[41,42]

Recently, another variety of familial primary aldosteronism featuring "non–glucocorticoid-remediable aldosteronism" was described in a father and two daughters.[43] The patients all had increased circulating levels of 18-oxocortisol and 18-hydroxycortisol, steroids reflecting oxidation by both 17-hydroxylase and aldosterone synthase and administration of dexamethasone failed to suppress aldosterone secretion. Bilateral adrenal hyperplasia was found at surgery and, in contrast to IHA, bilateral adrenalectomy corrected the hypertension.[43] Genetic information has not been reported for these patients.

Until 2008, no animal models of IHA were available for study. Davies and colleagues[44] have now established an animal model of nontumorigenic primary aldosteronism via deletion of TWIK-related acid-sensitive K (TASK)-1 and TASK-3 channels in mice. This deletion removes an important adrenal background K^+ currrent, which results in marked depolarization of zona glomerulosa cell membrane potential. Double–TASK channel knockout mice exhibited overproduction of aldosterone, suppressed renin, lack of salt suppressibility of aldosterone secretion, and failure of angiotensin type-1 (AT_1) receptor blockade to lower aldosterone to control levels. Thus, these mice exhibit a phenotype similar to that of IHA.[44] The interesting possibility that human IHA is related to mutations in TASK channel genes awaits future investigation.

Pathobiology of Primary Aldosteronism

Three major pathologic disorders are associated with primary aldosteronism: adenoma, hyperplasia, and carcinoma.

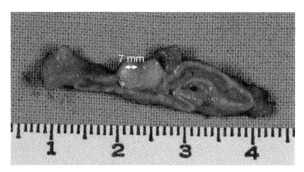

FIGURE 12-3. Typical aldosterone-producing adrenal adenoma removed from a patient with a 24-year history of resistant hypertension. (From Ref. 111.)

Adrenocortical Adenoma

Adenoma, which is found in approximately 60% of patients with primary aldosteronism, was once considered to be the most common abnormality. However, with the current use of PA:PRA ratios for case detection, IHA is now the most common subtype (63%). This change in subtype prevalence is almost certainly related to the less florid clinical and biochemical manifestations of IHA compared with APA, together with the current ability of sensitive screening methods to detect patients with IHA.

Adrenal adenomas occur somewhat more frequently in the left than in the right adrenal.[2,45] Adenomas usually measure less than 2 cm in diameter, and have a golden yellow color (Fig. 12-3). On light microscopy, four cell types have been identified: small and large hybrid cells with features of both zona glomerulosa and zona fasciculata cells, and others with zona glomerulosa or zona fasciculata characteristics.[46] Electron microscopy has shown that most of the mitochondria possess tubular cristae similar to those found in the cells of the zona glomerulosa. If the patient has been exposed to spironolactone therapy, spironolactone bodies may be seen.[46,47] It is interesting to note that zona glomerulosa hyperplasia often accompanies APA in the surrounding cortex.[46] In unusual circumstances, multiple adenomas or an adenoma with associated macronodular hyperplasia or smaller satellite nodules can be found. These findings, which are similar to those of multiple endocrine neoplasia, have suggested that genetic mutations affecting regulation of adrenocortical cell growth and differentiation may serve as the basis for at least some cases of primary aldosteronism.[48] It is interesting that a patient with bilateral adenomas with two types of adenoma cells associated with both primary aldosteronism and Cushing's syndrome has also been reported.[49]

Idiopathic Hyperaldosteronism

In IHA, the zona glomerulosa usually demonstrates diffuse or focal hyperplasia with normal ultrastructure but may be macroscopically normal.[47,50] Associated nodules may be microscopic or may be as large as 2 cm in diameter, and their ultrastructure is typical of clear cells of zona fasciculata origin. In keeping with this observation, in vitro the nodules produce cortisol but not aldosterone. Immunohistochemistry for aldosterone synthase has demonstrated intense staining in the zona glomerulosa and outer zona fasciculata in IHA. The compact cells in APA also stain for aldosterone synthase.[51]

Adrenal pathologic findings may be important to the outcome resulting from unilateral adrenalectomy. Ito and colleagues[52] studied 37 patients with primary aldosteronism: 23 had unilateral solitary adenomas (Group 1), 3 had unilateral multiple adenomas (Group 2), and 11 had adenomas with multiple macroscopic or microscopic nodules (Group 3). Postoperative changes in the renin-angiotensin-aldosterone system were similar, but marked differences in blood pressure responses were noted, as half of Group 3 remained hypertensive at 1 year. The authors suggested that adrenal nodules might result from longstanding hypertension. Glands with nodules almost invariably show arteriopathy of the capsular vessels, which may lead to focal ischemia and atrophy, with the better perfused cells becoming hyperplastic, leading to nodule formation.[53]

Adrenal Carcinoma

Adrenal carcinoma is a rare cause of primary aldosteronism. Histologically, carcinomas may be difficult to distinguish from adenomas, but almost invariably, carcinomas are larger (>3 cm in diameter) and include areas of necrosis and pleomorphic nuclei.[46] Calcification, commonly found in carcinomas, may be detected by magnetic resonance imaging (MRI), computed tomography (CT) scanning, or ultrasonography.

Ectopic Aldosterone-Secreting Adenoma

Ectopic aldosterone-secreting adenoma is an extremely rare cause of primary aldosterone excess.[53-57] Rarely, cases of primary aldosteronism have been reported in association with malignant ovarian tumors.[53-56] After excision of the tumor, biochemical abnormalities and hypertension may resolve or improve. Recurrence of the ectopic tumor can produce a return of the syndrome.[54]

Clinical Presentation of Primary Aldosteronism

The clinical features of primary aldosteronism have been extensively described (Table 12-2).[58-62] Most patients are asymptomatic. Some are discovered to be hypokalemic on routine investigation of hypertension, whereas others may have symptoms of hypokalemia such as muscle weakness, very occasional muscle paralysis, or more commonly, polyuria, polydipsia, nocturia (secondary to nephrogenic diabetes insipidus), paresthesias, and, rarely, tetany.[63] Chinese patients have a high prevalence of hypokalemic periodic paralysis.[64]

Conn et al.[65] found an intriguing sex difference in the prevalence of paresthesias and tetany in patients with primary aldosteronism; that is, females are more likely than males to develop paresthesias or to present with tetany. Tetany results from reduced ionized calcium accompanied by hypokalemic alkalosis. Plasma total calcium and magnesium levels are normal, however, and treatment consists of potassium repletion, not administration of calcium or magnesium.

Malignant hypertension originally was thought not to occur in primary aldosteronism.[2] However, this was found to be erroneous, and many cases have now been reported.[66,67] The diagnosis of primary aldosteronism can be missed in malignant hypertension because PRA may not be suppressed. On the other

Table 12-2. Clinical Manifestations of Primary Aldosteronism

Hypertension due to extracellular fluid volume expansion and sympathetic activation
Hypokalemia, metabolic alkalosis, and cardiac arrhythmias
Renal dysfunction
Nephrogenic diabetes insipidus
Muscle weakness
Paresthesias and tetany; magnesium deficiency
Flaccid paralysis

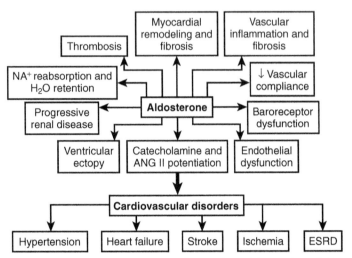

FIGURE 12-4. Schematic representation of the detrimental tissue actions of aldosterone leading to cardiovascular disorders. *ESRD,* End-stage renal disease.

Table 12-3. Cardiovascular Disease and Events in Primary Aldosteronism

Striking increase in the relative risk of
- Stroke (4.2×)
- Myocardial infarction (6.5×)
- Atrial fibrillation (12.1×)

Increased left ventricular hypertrophy (LVH) and diastolic dysfunction
Increased stiffness of large arteries
Widespread tissue fibrosis
Increased remodeling of resistance vessels

hand, normotensive aldosteronism has been documented.[68,69] Normotensive primary aldosteronism is most likely to occur in families with familial hyperaldosteronism (FH-I or FH-II), as affected individuals may be detected at an early, preclinical stage of the disease process by means of genetic family screening programs.[70]

In primary aldosteronism, the normal circadian pattern of blood pressure appears to be preserved with nocturnal dipping,[71] but the magnitude of the nighttime decrease is reduced.[72] However, blood pressure variability may be reduced in primary aldosteronism compared with essential hypertension,[73] possibly as a result of protection of baroreflex function, or as a consequence of the salt-loaded state with extracellular fluid volume expansion.

Originally, primary aldosteronism was thought to be a relatively benign disorder with low morbidity and mortality. Studies conducted during the past decade, however, have provided new insights into the role of aldosterone in tissue damage (inflammation, fibrosis, and remodeling) (Fig. 12-4).[74] Many studies have shown that patients with primary aldosteronism are at higher risk than other patients with hypertension for target organ damage, especially involving the heart, kidneys, and blood vessels (Table 12-3).[75-83] When matched for age, blood pressure, and duration of hypertension, patients with primary aldosteronism have greater left ventricular mass measurements compared with other patients with hypertension.[77] In patients with APA, both left ventricular wall thickness and mass regress markedly within a year of unilateral adrenalectomy. Patients who present with APA or IHA have an increased number of cardiovascular events when compared with an age-, gender- and blood pressure–matched population with essential hypertension.[75] In

primary aldosteronism, a striking increase in the relative risks for stroke (4.2%), myocardial infarction (6.5%), and atrial fibrillation (12.1%) has been noted.[75] Patients with primary aldosteronism have enhanced diastolic dysfunction when compared with hypertensive individuals without increased aldosterone production. Circulating aldosterone also produced a negative effect on various parameters of cardiac structure and function even in nonhypertensive subjects with GRA compared with age- and gender-matched control subjects.[83] After matching for age, body mass index, cholesterol, triglycerides, and glucose levels, arterial wall stiffness was found to be increased in primary aldosteronism compared with essential hypertension.[79] Hyperaldosteronism has been associated with widespread tissue fibrosis and increased remodeling of resistance vessels.[74]

Patients with primary aldosteronism have increased renal dysfunction compared with those with essential hypertension. In the relatively large Primary Aldosteronism Prevalence in Hypertensives (PAPY) Study from Italy, patients with APA or IHA had higher urinary microalbumin excretion compared with those with essential hypertension.[80,81] Also, prevalence of the metabolic (insulin resistance) syndrome is increased in patients with primary aldosteronism compared with those with essential hypertension.[82]

Epidemiology of Primary Aldosteronism

Primary aldosteronism occurs in patients of all ages, including children. In children, growth failure may be the presenting feature. As in children with other causes of hypokalemia such as Bartter's syndrome, growth failure may be the presenting feature. Patients with APA are usually younger than those with IHA.[66,84] However, primary aldosteronism in children younger than 16 years is usually due to adrenal hyperplasia. Among reported children with adrenal adenoma causing primary aldosteronism, most are female.

At any age, adenomas are more common in females than in males.[2,45] IHA has been found by some to be equally common in males and females[46] and by others to be more common in males.[84]

Diagnosis of Primary Aldosteronism
General Considerations

In 2008, The Endocrine Society published a clinical guideline on the detection, diagnosis, and treatment of primary aldosteronism with specific recommendations for diagnostic workup.[7] Sequential steps recommended for workup include (1) case detection (screening), (2) confirmation of the diagnosis, and (3) subtype classification.[7]

The approach to the diagnosis of primary aldosteronism differs from center to center. In some centers, the only patients investigated are those with hypokalemia and hypertension. As discussed above, most patients with this syndrome are normokalemic. Thus, a large fraction of patients with primary aldosteronism will not be detected if this approach is taken. In other centers, all hypertensive patients are screened for this diagnosis. Favoring this approach, the cost involved in screening is relatively small compared with the cost of lifelong drug therapy and the potential benefit derived from surgical cure or specific medical treatment.

Clinical criteria and methods for screening for primary aldosteronism are summarized in Fig. 12-5. All patients with the combination of hypertension and hypokalemia (spontaneous or diuretic induced) should be screened. Other recommendations

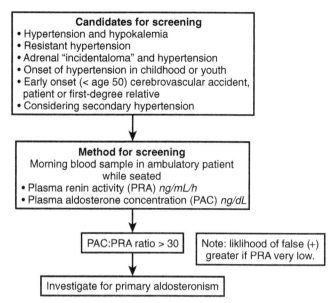

FIGURE 12-5. Algorithm for case detection (screening) in primary aldosteronism.

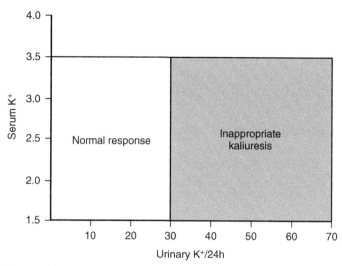

FIGURE 12-6. Relationship of urinary potassium (K^+) excretion to serum K^+ in normal subjects and patients with primary mineralocorticoid excess states, who have inappropriate kaliuresis.

for screening include young patients with hypertension, patients with early onset of cerebrovascular accident (<age 50), patients with a positive family history of early stroke in a first-degree relative, patients with hypertension and adrenal incidentalomas,[85] those whose blood pressure is difficult to control (resistant hypertension), and those in whom the diagnosis of secondary hypertension is being entertained for other reasons.[7]

Primary hyperaldosteronism is especially common among patients with resistant hypertension. Resistant hypertension is defined as blood pressure that remains above goal despite concurrent use of three antihypertensive agents of different classes, or that requires a minimum of four agents to achieve therapeutic goal.[86] In evaluations by several different investigators, the prevalence of primary hyperaldosteronism has been consistently reported to be about 20% among subjects with resistant hypertension.[86] In support of hyperaldosteronism as a common cause of resistant hypertension, aldosterone antagonists have been shown to provide significant additional blood pressure reduction when added to existing multidrug regimens in patients whose blood pressure remains uncontrolled.[86]

At Mayo Clinic, an average of 12 patients per annum were diagnosed with primary aldosteronism from 1960 to 1991. However, with intensive screening, the number of patients with this diagnosis increased 10-fold over the subsequent 8 years.[58] In the past, the tipoff for thinking of the disease was the measurement of serum potassium in a hypertensive patient. The presence of hypokalemia (serum potassium <3.6 mmol/L) in an untreated hypertensive patient demanded further investigation of the renin-angiotensin-aldosterone system. As was previously discussed, it is also worthwhile to investigate patients who have diuretic-induced hypokalemia.[87] It is worth keeping in mind that circulating potassium levels may be elevated by red blood cell hemolysis and/or by the use of a tourniquet with muscle pumping.[88] In an otherwise hypokalemic patient, normokalemia may be induced by low sodium intake because urinary potassium excretion is directly related to the distal nephron sodium load in conditions of mineralocorticoid excess.[89,90] If 24-hour urinary sodium excretion is less than 100 mmol, hypokalemia may be provoked by increasing sodium intake (e.g., NaCl 6 g/day for 5 days) and then repeating the serum potassium measure-

ment. Under these circumstances, some patients with normokalemic primary aldosteronism will become frankly hypokalemic. Twenty years ago, plasma or serum potassium was thought to have a sensitivity of 75% to 90% in the diagnosis of primary aldosteronism.[15,91] Current data from centers employing aldosterone:PRA ratios for case detection suggest that this figure should be reduced to less than 50%. The precise prevalence of normokalemic primary aldosteronism in an untreated hypertensive population is currently unknown but now appears to be much higher than was previously appreciated. Bravo and associates[92] reported 80 patients with primary aldosteronism, 27.5% of whom had normal serum potassium. In another study,[66] 11% of patients with primary aldosteronism were normokalemic. Many other laboratories have confirmed these findings.[15,85] Thus, even before the aldosterone:renin ratio was introduced as the screening test of choice, between 7% and 38% of patients with primary aldosteronism had basal circulating potassium levels greater than 3.6 mmol/L. After screening with the ratio was introduced, 60% to 70% of patients with primary aldosteronism were reported as being normokalemic.

In general, hypokalemia secondary to mineralocorticoid excess is associated with inappropriate renal loss of potassium (kaliuresis). The degree of kaliuresis depends on daily potassium intake, but potassium excretion usually exceeds 30 mmol/24 hour in hypokalemic patients with primary aldosteronism (Fig. 12-6). In addition, enhanced distal nephron sodium-hydrogen exchange leads to increased hydrogen ion excretion, usually as ammonium ion, which is responsible for the relatively mild metabolic alkalosis observed in these patients. Although it is not understood, some patients with GRA have alkalosis but are persistently normokalemic.

In primary aldosteronism, plasma sodium levels usually are in the upper part of the normal range or are slightly elevated owing to resetting of the hypothalamic osmostat. As with other biochemical parameters, this abnormality may be more marked in patients with an adenoma than in those with hyperplasia.[66] Total exchangeable sodium is increased in patients with primary aldosteronism caused by an adenoma but is usually normal in those with idiopathic adrenal hyperplasia.[32] A similar situation exists for total exchangeable potassium, with reduced levels in patients with an adenoma but not in those with hyperplasia.[32] Whether differences also occur between IHA and the angiotensin-responsive variety of adenoma (which biochemically mimics IHA in other ways, including responsiveness of aldosterone to angiotensin II and normalcy of "hybrid steroid" [18-hydroxy-cortisol and 18-oxo-cortisol] levels[93]) has yet to be determined.

Assessment of the Renin-Angiotensin-Aldosterone Axis

Plasma and Urinary Aldosterone. The fundamental abnormality of primary aldosteronism is excessive production of aldosterone, which is independent of the renin-angiotensin system and occurs in the face of suppressed PRA. Various factors, including the effects of antihypertensive drug therapy on the renin-angiotensin system and the inhibiting effect of hypokalemia directly on aldosterone secretion, may render the diagnosis difficult.

If serum potassium is <3.0 mmol/L, potassium supplementation should be administered and normokalemia established before aldosterone is measured.[94,95] However, even when hypokalemia is corrected, plasma aldosterone levels may still sometimes be at the upper part of the normal range among patients with primary aldosteronism, even in those with APA. An acceptable alternative to plasma aldosterone measurement is the 24-hour urinary aldosterone excretion rate, which quantifies its acid-labile conjugate aldosterone-18-glucuronide.[96] Although urinary aldosterone quantifies only approximately 15% of the aldosterone secreted, it provides a reliable index of aldosterone secretion in the absence of severe renal dysfunction. Assays to measure urinary tetrahydro-aldosterone (15% to 40% of metabolites) are employed less commonly. As with the measurement of plasma aldosterone, the urinary aldosterone excretion rate may be normal in primary aldosteronism, especially in the presence of significant hypokalemia.[94,95] Other reasons for normal urinary aldosterone excretion in patients with primary aldosteronism include renal failure, incomplete collection of urine, and variability in rates of hepatic metabolism of aldosterone. Some patients, including some with apparently isolated 11-deoxycorticosterone (DOC) excess, have periodic aldosterone hypersecretion.[97,98] Unlike plasma aldosterone, the urinary aldosterone excretion rate decreases with age.[99] Therefore, it is important to use an age-related normal reference range. Also, for interpretation, a plasma aldosterone concentration (PAC) of 1 ng/dL translates into 27.7 pmol/L in Système International d'Unités (SI units).

Plasma Renin Activity. The renin-angiotensin system usually is assessed by measuring PRA, which reflects the quantity of circulating active renin. This assay depends on the generation of angiotensin I in vitro in the patient's plasma, which is quantified by radioimmunoassay. The validity of the assay as an index of renin secretion depends on the adequacy of renin substrate (angiotensinogen) in the patient's plasma, but this is only rarely a problem. In primary aldosteronism, PRA is usually low or undetectable in contrast to the elevated levels found in secondary aldosteronism. However, PRA alone lacks specificity as a screening test for primary aldosteronism because it does not distinguish primary aldosteronism from low renin essential hypertension (LREH), which occurs in approximately 25% of patients with essential hypertension. Renin secretion is stimulated by assumption of erect posture or by sodium/volume depletion (as with diuretic treatment) and is suppressed in situations in which β-adrenergic input to the juxtaglomerular (JG) cells is abrogated (as in treatment with a β-adrenergic receptor blocker). Renin production also decreases during the aging process and in

patients with chronic renal failure, owing to reduction in functioning JG cells and salt and water retention. In addition, renin secretion has a diurnal variation with highest levels in the morning. Therefore, to correctly interpret the test and PRA values, it is necessary to know the time of day and the patient's age, posture, medical treatment, renal function, and, if possible, dietary sodium intake. Sodium intake can be estimated by concurrent measurement of 24-hour urinary sodium excretion rate and PRA. Also for interpretation, a PRA level of 1 ng/mL/hr in conventional units translates to 12.8 pmol/L/min in SI units.

Aldosterone-Renin Ratio. Introduced by Hiramatsu and colleagues[100] in 1981, the aldosterone:renin ratio is recognized worldwide as the most reliable means of screening for primary aldosteronism.[48,100-102] As indicated previously, this approach has uncovered a surprisingly large number of hypertensive patients with primary aldosteronism.

McKenna and colleagues[102] found that a single elevated aldosterone:renin ratio associated with an elevated or normal plasma aldosterone value correctly diagnosed primary aldosteronism in 10 patients—5 with hyperplasia and 5 with APA. The only problem in this study with false-positive results involved patients with chronic renal failure.[102] Secondary aldosteronism was characterized by elevated plasma aldosterone values together with a normal ratio.

In patients being considered for primary aldosteronism, screening can be accomplished by measuring a morning (8:00 to 10:00 AM) random PAC and PRA (see Fig. 12-5). This test may be performed while the patient is taking antihypertensive agents (except for spironolactone and eplerenone) and does not require postural stimulation.[22,103-106] As was mentioned earlier, hypokalemia reduces the secretion of aldosterone and should be corrected before testing is begun. Patients are encouraged to maintain a liberal dietary sodium intake while undergoing screening to prevent stimulation of renin (and a false-negative ratio) induced by dietary sodium restriction. Mineralocorticoid receptor antagonists spironolactone and eplerenone and high-dose amiloride are the only medications that absolutely interfere with interpretation of the aldosterone:renin ratio and should be discontinued for 5 to 6 weeks before testing is begun.[106] β-Adrenoceptor blocking drugs, renal impairment, and old age can produce false-positive ratios as the result of renin suppression, whereas diuretics, ACE inhibitors, angiotensin receptor blockers, and dihydropyridine calcium channel blockers can produce false-negatives.

Antihypertensive agents that can be used to control blood pressure during a workup for primary aldosteronism are listed in Table 12-4. The α₁-adrenoceptor blockers (prazosin, doxazosin, and terazosin), hydralazine, slow-release verapamil, and α-methyl-DOPA all have minimal effects on the aldosterone:renin ratio in patients with primary aldosteronism and can thus be employed. Slow-release verapamil (120 mg twice daily) is usually well tolerated (unless constipation develops). Side effects from hydralazine are rare if low doses (e.g., 12.5 mg twice daily) are given initially, increasing in a stepwise fashion (e.g., dose increments every 2 weeks) as required, and combination treatment with slow-release verapamil prevents the reflex tachycardia that can occur with "unopposed" use of a direct vasodilator, such as hydralazine. With the above agents, it is usually possible to control severe hypertension satisfactorily after withdrawal of other drug therapy during the process of diagnostic workup.[7]

Nonsteroidal antiinflammatory drugs, by promoting salt and water retention (suppressing renin) and hyperkalemia (stimulating aldosterone secretion), are frequently associated with false-

Table 12-4. Clinical Considerations for Screening for Primary Aldosteronism Using the Plasma Aldosterone Concentration:Plasma Renin Activity Ratio (ARR)

If results not diagnostic, and if hypertension (HT) can be controlled with other meds, withdraw meds that may affect the ARR for at least 2 weeks:
- Beta-adrenergic blockers, central alpha-2 agonists, nonsteroidal antiinflammatory drugs
- Angiotensin-converting enzyme (ACE) inhibitors, angiotensin receptor blockers (ARBs), renin inhibitors, dihydropyridine calcium channel antagonists
- Potassium-wasting diuretics

If necessary to maintain HT control:
- Hydralazine (with verapamil slow-release, to avoid reflex tachycardia)
- Prazosin, doxazosin, terazosin
- α-Methyl-DOPA

Table 12-5. Comparison of the Four Accepted Confirmation Tests for the Diagnosis of Primary Aldosteronism With Normal and Abnormal Values

Oral sodium loading test: Increase dietary Na^+ intake to 300 mmol/d × 3 days; verify by 24 hour urine Na^+ excretion; slow-release KCl to maintain normokalemia
- Abnormal: Urinary aldosterone excretion > 12 mg/24 hours
- Normal: Urinary aldosterone secretion ≤ 12 mg/24 hours

Intravenous saline suppression test: 2 L normal saline IV over 4 hours; measure PAC at baseline and at 4 hours
- Abnormal: PAC ≥ 15 ng/dL (baseline) and ≥ 10 ng/dL at 4 hours
- Indeterminate: PAC 5 to 10 ng/dL at 4 hours
- Normal: PAC < 5 ng/dL at 4 hours

Fludrocortisone suppression test: 4 days high Na^+ diet + slow-release NaCl 30 mEq TID + fludrocortisone acetate 100 mcg q6h
- Abnormal: PAC > 6 ng/dL on day 4 (upright, 10 AM)
- Normal: PAC ≤ 6 ng/dL

Captopril challenge test: Captopril 25 to 50 mg orally in seated patient
- Abnormal: Absence of suppression of PAC by 30% from baseline
- Normal: Suppression of PAC by 30% from baseline

IV, Intravenous; *Na+,* sodium; *PAC,* plasma aldosterone concentration; *TID,* three times daily.

positive ratios and should be withheld for several weeks before testing, if possible.

Interpretation of the PAC:PRA ratio for case detection purposes is relatively straightforward (see Table 12-3). Values ≥30 (when PAC is expressed as ng/dL and PRA as ng/mL/hr; conventional units); or equivalent to 750 when PAC is reported as pmol/L (SI units) and PRA in conventional units; or equivalent to 60 when PAC and PRA are expressed as SI units are generally accepted as positive for primary aldosteronism, with a range of 20 to 40 for most centers.[7] It is important to point out that the lower limit of detection varies among the different PRA assays, and these variations can have a dramatic effect on the PAC:PRA ratio. Very low PRA values can increase the ratio when the PAC value is perfectly normal. To avoid this potential error, some groups have designated a minimal PAC value (≥15 ng/dL) necessary to interpret the ratio.[7,58] Thus, when PAC is ≥15 ng/dL, then PAC:PRA ≥20 is considered positive.[58] A high PAC:PRA ratio constitutes a positive screening test for primary aldosteronism, but it is important to realize that screening should be followed by an aldosterone suppression test to confirm the diagnosis prior to subtype classification.[7,58]

Establishment of the Diagnosis of Primary Aldosteronism

Instead of proceeding directly from a positive screening test to subtype classification, it is strongly recommended that patients undergo one of four aldosterone suppression tests (see below) to definitively confirm or exclude the diagnosis of primary aldosteronism (Table 12-5).[7] Three of these are salt-loading tests that can be conducted by increasing dietary sodium intake, infusing saline, or administering exogenous mineralocorticoid, or through combinations of these approaches. The rationale behind these tests is that in normal subjects, volume expansion with saline suppresses plasma aldosterone, whereas in primary aldosteronism, further volume expansion does not have the same suppressive action on aldosterone secretion. The fourth test depends on inhibition of aldosterone secretion by an ACE inhibitor. Detailed methods for performing these tests have been reviewed recently.[7] At present, evidence is insufficient to allow recommendation of any one of these tests over any of the others.[7] It has been recommended that pharmacologic agents with minimal or no effect on the renin-angiotensin-aldosterone system (see Table 12-4; discussed above) be employed to control blood pressure during confirmatory testing, if possible. Whether or not medications that affect the renin-angiotensin-aldosterone system are discontinued, however, spironolactone and eplerenone clearly interfere with these tests and must be discontinued 5 to 6 weeks before testing in all cases.

Fludrocortisone Suppression Test. In 1967, Biglieri and associates[97] demonstrated that 11-deoxycorticosterone (DOC) acetate administration for 3 days failed to suppress urinary aldosterone excretion in APA but suppressed aldosterone secretion both in normal subjects and in two patients with primary aldosteronism in whom no tumor was found at surgery (probable idiopathic adrenal hyperplasia). This observation suggested that exogenous mineralocorticoid administration might be of value in the diagnosis and differential diagnosis of primary aldosteronism. Subsequent studies, however, reported that some patients with IHA also failed to suppress aldosterone secretion.[15,107] Extracellular fluid volume expansion with a combination of a high-sodium diet and oral fludrocortisone, over a 4-day period, is now regarded as a reliable means of definitively confirming or excluding the diagnosis of primary aldosteronism.[108,109] The reliability of the test is dependent upon the maintenance of normokalemia by potassium chloride supplementation (otherwise, hypokalemia may result in a fall in aldosterone concentrations and a false-negative test) and the demonstration of adequate suppression of PRA (to <1 ng/mL/hr). Additional details regarding the fludrocortisone suppression test have been published.[7,110,111] The Brisbane group has established that PAC >6 ng/dL at 10 AM on day 4 of salt loading and fludrocortisone confirms the diagnosis if PRA is <1 ng/mL/hr.[111] Some centers conduct this test in the ambulatory clinic; others require a few days of hospitalization.

Oral Sodium Loading Test. Failure of suppression of the urinary aldosterone excretion rate in patients on a high-sodium diet (>200 mEq/d) is a valid confirmatory test of primary aldosteronism.[58,92,112] After 3 days on high oral sodium intake, a normal individual is expected to suppress aldosterone excretion to <12 μg/24 hr. In contrast, patients with primary aldosteronism do not suppress urinary aldosterone excretion rates to <12 μg/24 hr, provided that serum potassium concentration is maintained in the normal range by potassium chloride supplementation during the salt-loading period.[58,112]

Intravenous Saline Suppression Test. Another valid confirmatory test is to measure plasma aldosterone concentration after intravenous saline infusion (2 L normal saline over 4 hr).[113] This approach has been used successfully to discriminate between patients with essential hypertension and those with primary aldosteronism. Patients with essential hypertension demonstrate suppression of plasma aldosterone to <5 ng/dL; those with primary aldosteronism do not suppress plasma aldosterone to <10 ng/dL; those with aldosterone suppression to 5 to 10 ng/dL fall into the indeterminate range and may require retesting at a later time. The protocol for this test is to measure basal plasma aldosterone with the patient in the recumbent position at 8:00 AM. Subsequently, after 2 L of normal saline is infused over 4 hours, plasma aldosterone concentration is measured again. None of the above salt-loading tests (with or without exogenous mineralocorticoid) should be performed in patients with severe uncontrolled hypertension, severe renal insufficiency, heart failure, cardiac arrhythmia, or severe hypokalemia.[7]

Captopril Challenge Test. In normal subjects on normal sodium intake, oral administration of an ACE inhibitor (e.g., captopril) reduces plasma aldosterone levels. This reduction does not occur in patients with primary aldosteronism. The usual test involves giving captopril 25 mg orally and measuring plasma aldosterone levels 2 hours later. In patients with primary aldosteronism, the 2 hour level remains >15 ng/dL in contrast to the decrease in normal subjects.[114] Not all investigators have found this approach valuable.[115,116] Muratani and colleagues[116] studied 19 patients with primary aldosteronism and 72 with essential hypertension. Captopril was administered after overnight recumbency. The test was 93% specific and had a 79% predictive value. However, higher specificity (97%) and predictive values (90%) were obtained via analysis of the pre-captopril plasma aldosterone:PRA ratios.

The effect of dietary sodium intake on the captopril challenge test was investigated by Naomi and coworkers.[117] The authors used a higher dose of captopril (50 mg) and found that results of the test were unaffected by altering the sodium intake. They analyzed the PAC:PRA ratios in blood samples taken 90 minutes after oral captopril was given at 9:00 AM and after 1 hour of recumbency. Using a ratio greater than 20 for the diagnosis of primary aldosteronism, they found that the test had 95% sensitivity and 92% specificity. Numerous cases of false-negative or equivocal results were reported with the captopril challenge test.[7]

Dexamethasone Suppression Test. Patients with GRA respond to confirmatory tests of the renin-angiotensin-aldosterone system in a manner similar to that of patients with APA. These two conditions can be distinguished, however, by the patient's response to exogenous glucocorticoid administration. With the patient in the upright position in the morning, plasma aldosterone concentration below 5 ng/dL after overnight dexamethasone administration (1.0 mg at midnight and 0.5 mg at 6:00 AM) has been reported as a cutoff point to separate patients with GRA from those with IHA or APA.[118] The distinction between GRA and other forms of primary aldosteronism becomes clearer with long-term glucocorticoid therapy. Long-term dexamethasone (e.g., 2 mg/d for 3 weeks) in GRA (but not in other forms of primary aldosteronism) leads to recovery of the suppressed renin-angiotensin system, normalization of plasma potassium and aldosterone, reduction of blood pressure (usually to normal), and restoration of responsiveness of the zona glomerulosa to angiotensin II.[119-121]

The need for dexamethasone suppression testing in GRA has now been largely supplanted by the introduction of genetic testing, which is 100% sensitive and specific.[28,121]

Diagnosis of Primary Aldosteronism During Pregnancy

The diagnosis of primary aldosteronism during pregnancy may be problematic because of the high circulating levels of progesterone, which inhibits the renal collecting duct effect of aldosterone on sodium transport. For example, administration of exogenous aldosterone 500 μg during the last month of pregnancy did not affect urinary sodium or potassium excretion, whereas the same dose administered postpartum induced marked sodium reabsorption and increased potassium excretion.[88]

Primary Aldosteronism Subtype Classification

After the diagnosis of primary aldosteronism has been confirmed using one of the four confirmatory tests discussed above, unilateral disease (usually due to APA) needs to be differentiated from bilateral disease (usually due to hyperplasia), rare aldosterone-producing carcinomas, and the extremely rare tumors responsible for ectopic production of aldosterone (see Table 12-1).

Adrenal Venous Sampling

Adrenal venous sampling is considered the "gold standard" for differentiation of unilateral from bilateral disease.[7,58,123] Adrenal vein catheterization is technically difficult, and even an experienced radiologist may be unable to enter the right adrenal vein because of its exit at a right angle directly into the inferior vena cava. Complications may occur (especially adrenal hemorrhage or extravasation of contrast medium into the adrenal parenchyma, which can lead to loss of function), but these are uncommon if adrenal venography is avoided. For this reason, adrenal venography is contraindicated except that a small amount of contrast medium usually can be infused safely to localize the catheter tip.

On the side of the tumor, aldosterone:cortisol ratios measured in blood collected from the adrenal veins are significantly higher than those found in the inferior vena cava, whereas on the contralateral side, aldosterone secretion from the zona glomerulosa is suppressed. Hence, the aldosterone:cortisol ratios on the side contralateral to an APA are not higher than peripheral[124,125] (see example in Fig. 12-7). Because of the problems involved in adrenal vein catheterization, it is critical to measure both aldosterone and cortisol to determine whether the catheter is placed correctly in the adrenal vein. Some authors have administered ACTH to try to improve the test.[85] This approach overcomes the problems of intermittent aldosterone secretion and differences in endogenous ACTH when left and right adrenal vein samples are being obtained at different times. Also, ACTH has been thought to selectively stimulate aldosterone production from APAs compared with hyperplastic tissue. Others, however, have found that ACTH infusion leads to overproduction of aldosterone by the contralateral gland, in addition to stimulation of aldosterone secretion from the APA, leading to a false-positive diagnosis of IHA. Even if it is not possible to enter the right adrenal vein, interpretation of aldosterone:cortisol ratios in the left adrenal vein and in the inferior vena cava sometimes can still provide enough information to localize the side of unilateral aldosterone secretion from an APA.[124]

Fig. 12-8 depicts the ratios of plasma aldosterone (A) to cortisol (C) from the raw values of the adrenal venous sampling example in Fig. 12-7. Commonly employed criteria for the diagnosis of unilateral aldosterone hypersecretion (Table 12-6) are as follows: (1) unilateral hypersecretion is confirmed when the A:C ratios from the high side are more than fourfold greater than those on the contralateral low side; (2) unilateral hypersecretion is not present when the A:C ratios are less then threefold greater on the high side than those on the low side; (3) A:C values between 3 and 4 (high to low side) are considered indeterminate.[7]

Time (min)	Left		Right		IVC	
	A	C	A	C	A	C
−5	2352	297	125	404	61	18
0	2038	227	120	342	62	20
20	1820	271	170	231	110	27
40	8046	359	190	358	224	115

▨ ACTH | Aldosterone ng/dL; cortisol µg/dL

FIGURE 12-7. Example of plasma aldosterone (A) and cortisol (C) concentrations from the adrenal veins and inferior vena cava (IVC) during an adrenal venous sampling procedure in a patient with confirmed primary aldosteronism. Values at −5 and 0 min are baseline values in the absence of exogenous adrenocorticotropic hormone (ACTH); values in the shades box are 20 and 40 min after a bolus dose of synthetic ACTH (Cosyntropin 250 µg intravenously). The catheter was positioned correctly in both the right and left adrenal veins, as demonstrated by the >10-fold increase in plasma cortisol concentrations in the right and left adrenal veins as compared with those in the IVC. ACTH at 40 min increased aldosterone concentration in the left but not the right adrenal vein. The patient appears to have a left adrenal aldosterone-producing adenoma.

Time (min)	Left	Right	IVC
	A:C	A:C	A:C
−5	7.9	0.3	3.4
0	8.9	0.3	3.1
20	6.7	0.7	4.1
40	22.4	0.5	5.1

▨ ACTH

FIGURE 12-8. Aldosterone:cortisol ratios calculated from the raw data in Fig. 12-7. The diagnosis of left aldosterone-producing adenoma is confirmed by comparison of the ratios of aldosterone versus cortisol. Ratios on the left are elevated as compared with those on the right, which are suppressed below the ratios in the IVC. Because the ratios on the left were greater than fourfold those on the right, the diagnosis of left unilateral aldosterone hypersecretion can be made.

Young and coworkers[123,125] have reviewed their experience at the Mayo Clinic with adrenal venous sampling (AVS). In a prospective study of 34 patients with primary aldosteronism, 15 had a normal CT scan or minimal thickening of one adrenal limb, 6 had unilateral microadenomas, 9 had bilateral nodules, and 4 had atypical unilateral macroadenomas. Both adrenal veins were catheterized in 33 of 34 patients. Six (40%) of the patients with normal or minimal thickening on CT scan had unilateral adrenal aldosterone production. All 6 patients with microadenomas had unilateral production. Four of 9 patients with bilateral adrenal masses had a unilateral source of aldosterone, as did 3 of the 4 with atypical macroadenomas. These results, if validated by operative pathologic findings and the therapeutic benefit of unilateral adrenalectomy, indicate that a highly significant number of patients would have erroneous diagnoses if based entirely on CT findings.[125] Young[58] suggested that the age of the patient should be taken into account when one is considering the need for AVS. Thus, if a unilateral hypodense nodule is seen on CT scanning in a patient with confirmed primary aldosteronism and the patient is younger than 40 years, the Mayo Clinic would proceed directly to surgery. If, however, the patient is older than 40, AVS would be performed.

Table 12-6. Criteria for Interpretation of the Results of Adrenal Venous Sampling for Subtype Classification in Primary Aldosteronism

Calculate aldosterone:cortisol ratios for IVC and each adrenal vein = "cortisol-corrected aldosterone ratios" (CCARs).
AV cortisol should be ≈10-fold higher than IVC value if the catheter is positioned correctly.
Unilateral disease: CCAR > 4 (high to low side)
Bilateral disease: CCAR < 3 (high to low side)
Indeterminate: CCAR 3 to 4

AV, Adrenal vein; *IVC,* inferior vena cava.

Adrenal Scintigraphy

[131]I-labeled or ^{75}Se-6-seleno-methylnorcholesterol can be used to image the adrenals and to distinguish between APA and IHA. However, these tests have largely been supplanted by the adrenal venous sampling procedure. Dexamethasone pretreatment and an improved scanning agent, [I[131]I]-iodomethyl-19-norcholesterol, have improved the accuracy of diagnosis compared with that of the initially used [^{131}I]19-iodocholesterol.[126-129] Previous treatment with spironolactone may interfere with this test (this medication should be stopped for 6 weeks). The dose of dexamethasone employed has usually been greater than that required to suppress ACTH (i.e., 1 mg four times daily). Lugol's iodine solution or saturated solution of potassium iodide (SSKI) should be given before radioisotope administration to block thyroid uptake.

The criteria used to make the distinction between APA and IHA are important. In one study of 30 patients with APA and 20 patients with IHA, the authors analyzed [^{131}I]-iodomethyl-19-norcholesterol uptake at 5 days and found that nearly one half of the patients with APA had bilateral uptake, and that nearly one fourth of patients with IHA had marked asymmetrical uptake.[126] Thus, this test would not have been useful in distinguishing APA from IHA. The authors suggested that it was necessary to observe the pattern of adrenal imaging and that, during dexamethasone administration, early unilateral or early bilateral (i.e., <5 days) uptake was the primary indication of the diagnosis.[126]

In reviewing the literature, Young and Klee[130] suggested that the accuracy (i.e., percentage of correct diagnoses) of iodocholesterol scintigraphy was 72% versus 73% for CT scanning and 95% for adrenal venous sampling in which both adrenal veins were correctly sampled. In other reports, however, less satisfactory results for adrenal scintigraphy were reported. Pagny and coworkers,[129] in 160 patients with primary aldosteronism, found that scintigraphy was accurate in only 53% of 51 examinations, whereas CT scanning was accurate in 82% of 85 examinations. However, scintigraphic scanning does have the potential advantage over other imaging techniques of correlating function with anatomic abnormality.

Adrenal carcinomas causing Cushing's syndrome usually fail to take up iodocholesterol by the tumor or by the suppressed normal adrenals. However, in mineralocorticoid excess associated with adrenal carcinoma, uptake of iodocholesterol has been reported in both the primary tumor and its metastases.[131]

Computed Tomography and Magnetic Resonance Imaging of Adrenals

In general, neither adrenal CT nor MRI is accurate in distinguishing between APA and IHA.[58] In many institutions, CT or MRI is employed at an early stage of workup in an attempt to solve the subtype diagnosis in a patient with confirmed primary aldoste-

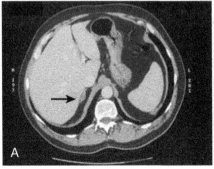 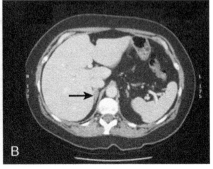

FIGURE 12-9. A, Right aldosterone-producing adenoma (APA). **B,** Idiopathic hyperaldosteronism (IHA) with bilateral aldosterone hypersecretion. Computed tomography (CT) scans of two patients with confirmed primary aldosteronism demonstrating the inability to differentiate between APA and IHA with bilateral aldosterone secretion. Both diagnoses were confirmed with adrenal venous sampling. (From Ref. 111.)

ronism. In contrast to CT technology in the past, modern CT with 3 mm contiguous sections can accurately detect tumors down to 7 mm in diameter.[132-135] Retrospective changes in CT scanning in primary aldosteronism were studied by Balkin and associates,[132] who reviewed the value of CT in 34 patients with primary aldosteronism divided into two groups: those undergoing CT between 1977 and 1980 (Group 1) and those undergoing CT between 1981 and 1983 with a high-resolution GE-8800 scanner (Group 2). The results of CT scanning were compared with those of other diagnostic methods, including AVS, findings at surgery, and response to unilateral adrenalectomy. CT was not very sensitive (48%) but was highly specific (91%) with many false-negative results. Comparison of Group 1 versus Group 2 showed no significant improvement in specificity (92%) but a definite improvement in sensitivity (58%) (Group 1: sensitivity, 42%; specificity, 90%). Even with this improvement, however, a substantial number of tumors can still go undetected with modern CT scanning. An example of the inability to differentiate APA from IHA on the basis of CT scanning results is provided in Fig. 12-9.

Few direct comparisons of CT and MRI results in identifying adrenal lesions are available.[129,132,134] In one series, CT scanning provided the correct diagnosis in 82% of cases of APA, and MRI in 100%.[129] Ou and colleagues[133] compared five methods of localization in 22 patients with operative confirmation of APA. Correct localization of the lesion was obtained in 95% by CT, 100% by MRI, 80% by dexamethasone suppression/[131]I-19-cholesterol scintiscan, 78% by adrenal venography, and 100% by adrenal venous sampling. The authors advocated adrenal CT as the best means of localizing an adenoma on the basis of comfort, safety, and cost. They suggested that adrenal venous sampling should be reserved for patients with confirmed primary aldosteronism with inconclusive lateralization by CT, MRI, and/or radioisotopic scintiscan.

Rossi and collaborators[134] conducted a prospective comparison of CT and MRI in 27 patients with suspected primary aldosteronism, 13 of whom had unilateral APA. The diagnosis was confirmed at surgery and by pathologic examination. MRI correctly identified all cases of APA but provided false-positive results in five cases (one with idiopathic hyperaldosteronism with bilateral nodular hyperplasia and four with essential hypertension, including two with nonfunctioning adenomas). The sensitivity of MRI was 100%, the specificity 64%, and the overall diagnostic accuracy 81%. In contrast, the sensitivity of CT was 62%, specificity 77%, and diagnostic accuracy 69%. These results underscore the dangers of relying totally on a morphologic approach that may fail to detect small tumors or that may produce false-positives in patients with nonfunctioning adrenal adenomas. Because such incidental tumors may be present in approximately 20% of patients with essential hypertension, the risk is substantial.

In a series of 29 patients studied by Dunnick and associates,[135] the sensitivity of CT scanning was 82%. They recommended that a positive CT scan would indicate ipsilateral adrenalectomy but that if no mass were found, adrenal venous sampling should be conducted. However, Stowasser and colleagues[111] found that CT scanning detected an adrenal mass lesion in only 50% of 111 patients with surgically proven APA and in only 25% of those with APAs smaller than 1 cm in diameter, which accounted for almost half of the APAs removed. CT was frankly misleading in 12 patients in whom CT demonstrated a definite or probable mass lesion in one adrenal, but who showed lateralization of aldosterone production to the other side on adrenal venous sampling. The inability of CT to distinguish APAs from many nonfunctioning "incidentalomas" is expected in view of the fact that these lesions may be indistinguishable on gross and histologic examination. Therefore, adrenal venous sampling should be performed in all patients with primary aldosteronism (other than those found to have GRA by genetic testing), irrespective of the CT findings.

In addition to the morphologic diagnosis, attempts have been made to use CT attenuation values to distinguish adenomas from other lesions such as metastases, adrenal carcinoma, and pheochromocytoma. Korobkin and colleagues[136] demonstrated that the mean attenuation value of unenhanced CTs of adenomas was significantly lower than for nonadenomas.

With the highly sensitive screening test for primary aldosteronism, most APAs are identified when smaller than 10 to 20 mm in diameter; therefore they can escape detection with even the latest generation CT or MRI. Furthermore, an adrenal nodule in a patient with primary aldosteronism can be an APA, or it can be a macronodule in a patient with IHA. These observations strongly suggest that a negative imaging test does not exclude a surgically curable form of primary aldosteronism, and that adrenal imaging by itself is inadequate to distinguish APA from IHA. For all of these reasons, adrenal venous sampling is critical in determining appropriate therapy for patients with primary aldosteronism who have a high probability of APA and who seek a surgical cure.[7,58]

Treatment for Primary Aldosteronism

Treatment depends on the cause of the primary aldosteronism, the medical condition of the patient, and various other factors such as adverse drug effects. In general, patients with unilateral disease (APA and unilateral adrenal hyperplasia) are recommended to have surgical treatment, whereas medical treatment with aldosterone antagonists and other drugs is offered to patients with bilateral disease (Fig. 12-10).

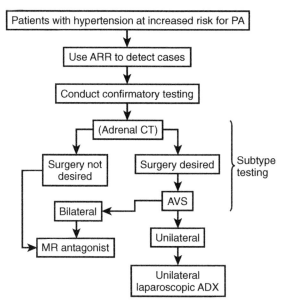

FIGURE 12-10. Summary algorithm for establishing and treating primary aldosteronism. *ADX,* Adrenalectomy; *ARR,* aldosterone:renin ratio; *AVS,* adrenal venous sampling; *CT,* computed tomographic scan; *MR,* mineralocorticoid receptor.

Surgical Treatment

In a patient with APA who is a candidate for surgery, the recommended treatment is unilateral laparoscopic adrenalectomy.[7] Treatment for patients with spironolactone before surgery is often useful, because patients tend to have a smoother perioperative course with better control of blood pressure and plasma potassium levels, and treatment can result in significant improvement in clinical status (including reductions in left ventricular mass and improved left ventricular function) and fitness for surgery. Relatively low doses of spironolactone (12.5 to 50 mg daily) are usually sufficient for reducing blood pressure, provided that several weeks is provided to afford a therapeutic response. Low doses are less likely to induce side effects (gynecomastia, reduced libido, menstrual irregularity, and hyperkalemia) that are common among patients treated with much higher doses.

Laparoscopic adrenalectomy is now the standard approach for the removal of adrenal tumors. Terachi and colleagues[137] reported on a series of 100 such operations (APA, 41 patients; Cushing's syndrome, 15; nonfunctioning adenoma, 22; myelolipoma, 3; pheochromocytoma, 7; complicated adrenal cyst, 3). The mean ± standard deviation (SD) operative time was 240 ± 76 minutes. Only three operations had to be converted to open surgery. The authors concluded that laparoscopic adrenalectomy via the transperitoneal anterior approach is as efficacious as open surgery but is associated with shorter convalescence.[137] Similar results have been reported by Rutherford and associates[138] in a series of 67 successful adrenalectomies, but the operation times were considerably shorter (124 ± 47 minutes).

Nakada and colleagues[139] compared unilateral adrenalectomy versus enucleation of the adenoma (22 unilateral vs. 26 enucleation). Both methods had similar effects on blood pressure, plasma potassium, PRA and plasma aldosterone, cortisol, and ACTH. However, 5 years after surgery, the enucleation group showed significantly greater PRA and plasma aldosterone responses to sodium deprivation and diuretics than did patients who underwent unilateral adrenalectomy. On this basis, they suggest that enucleation may be preferred. However, this approach has the potential to result in suboptimal correction of

primary aldosteronism because it relies on the assumption that the removed adenoma is the correct and sole source of aldosterone excess.[140] As was noted earlier, multiple satellite nodules and/or hyperplastic tissue surrounding the extirpated adenoma can contribute to continuing hypersecretion of aldosterone.

Following surgery for APA, blood pressure usually decreases progressively over a period of weeks to months. In the report of Itoh and associates[141] of 60 patients with primary aldosteronism, 60% were normotensive at 1 month after surgery and 76% by the second year. By the fifth year, 70% remained normotensive. This is very similar to the 69% long-term cure rate for unilateral adrenalectomy for APA based on 694 cases from 20 reports. Itoh and associates[141] found that the best predictor of blood pressure at 2 months was the duration of hypertension before surgery. At 6 months and 1 year, the adrenal histology was predictive. By the fifth year, the most important predictor was a family history of hypertension.[141] Comparison of surgery versus long-term spironolactone suggests that surgery for APA is more likely to lead to normalization of blood pressure.[142] Furthermore, patients undergoing surgery for APA consistently report marked improvement in quality of life to a degree that is more apparent than with spironolactone.

Factors associated with resolution of hypertension in the postoperative period include having one or no first-degree relatives with hypertension and preoperative use of two or fewer antihypertensive agents.[143] Other factors that may play a role include duration of hypertension less than 5 years, higher preoperative PAC:PRA ratio, higher urinary aldosterone secretion, and preoperative response to spironolactone.[7] The most common reasons for persistent hypertension after adrenalectomy are coexistent essential hypertension and older age and/or longer duration of hypertension.[7]

Medical Treatment

A low-sodium diet (less than 80 mEq of sodium per day) is a useful adjunct to pharmacologic therapy. After spironolactone treatment is initiated, correction of hypokalemia is rapid, but blood pressure control may take several weeks. The response of the renin-angiotensin-aldosterone system to treatment with spironolactone may help in difficult diagnostic problems to distinguish between APA and IHA. In patients with APA treated with spironolactone, no increase in plasma or urinary aldosterone was noted, even though normalization of plasma potassium and an increase in PRA occurred.[144] In contrast, in IHA, a twofold to threefold increase was noted in both plasma and urinary aldosterone. In patients who developed adverse effects on spironolactone, the drug of choice is eplerenone (50 mg twice daily). Eplerenone is a mineralocorticoid receptor antagonist that is less potent than spironolactone and usually needs to be given as 50 mg twice daily. Unlike spironolactone, eplerenone does not interfere with the androgen receptor.[145-147] Therefore, eplerenone may be the drug of choice in men in need of long-term mineralocorticoid receptor blocker therapy. Amiloride (2.5 to 20 mg daily), an aldosterone-independent antagonist of renal tubule (cortical collecting duct) sodium transport, also may be employed. The antihypertensive effect is generally less potent than that of spironolactone.

Patients with IHA should be treated medically. Of 99 patients with IHA treated by unilateral or bilateral adrenalectomy, only 19 (19%) were cured.[85,148-151] The usual approach to medical treatment of IHA is to start with spironolactone or eplerenone. Despite improvement in electrolyte status, the blood pressure response is often suboptimal, and additional drugs are required.

These may include amiloride and calcium channel blocking agents such as nifedipine.

The effects of calcium channel blocking drugs have been reported in both APA and IHA. In 10 patients with primary aldosteronism (five with APA, five with IHA), nifedipine, given as both short- and long-term (4 weeks) treatment, lowered blood pressure, normalized serum potassium, and reduced plasma aldosterone in both groups.[152] These results contrasted with those of nitrendipine given to three patients with APA and three with IHA for 4 weeks (40 to 60 mg/d).[153] Opocher and colleagues[154] studied the effects of verapamil infusion on aldosterone levels in 11 patients with primary aldosteronism (five with IHA, six with APA). These investigators found that aldosterone levels decreased in IHA but not in APA. The lack of effect of calcium channel blocking drugs in APA on aldosterone has been observed by others.[155]

The mechanism of action of calcium channel blocking drugs in primary aldosteronism is unclear. Given the sensitivity of the adrenal zona glomerulosa to angiotensin II in IHA and the key role of an angiotensin II–induced increase in intracellular calcium in stimulating aldosterone secretion, it might be anticipated that the drugs might affect aldosterone secretion in IHA. Kramer and associates[156] suggested an alternative mechanism that could be relevant to both IHA and APA. Extracellular fluid volume expansion leads to the secretion of an endogenous inhibitor of sodium-potassium adenosine triphosphatase (Na/K-ATPase), high levels of which have been found in primary aldosteronism. Ouabain, a known inhibitor of Na/K-ATPase, when administered to normal subjects not only inhibits the enzyme but also increases peripheral vascular resistance. These investigators found that this effect could be blocked by nifedipine.

ACE inhibitors have been shown to be effective in IHA. Enalapril lowered blood pressure and aldosterone secretion and improved plasma potassium levels.[157] As was already discussed, this effect may be due to blockade of the intra-adrenal renin-angiotensin system in IHA.

Drugs that block the synthesis of aldosterone have also been investigated. Trilostane, an inhibitor of 3β-hydroxysteroid dehydrogenase (3β-HSD), has been shown to lower blood pressure in both APA and IHA.[158] However, very little experience with the long-term use of this compound has been documented. The adrenolytic drug mitotane is of value in aldosterone-secreting carcinomas.[159] In the future, inhibitors of aldosterone synthase may become available.

In GRA, exogenous glucocorticoid is highly effective in controlling hypertension. It is not necessary to completely suppress ACTH to achieve normal blood pressure, and the lowest dose that maintains normal blood pressure should be given.[7] Treatment leads within 2 weeks to a return of plasma potassium, aldosterone, and PRA levels to normal with reduction of blood pressure. Spironolactone, amiloride, and triamterene are alternatives or can be added to improve blood pressure control.

ALDOSTERONE-PRODUCING ADRENAL CARCINOMA

Aldosterone-producing carcinoma is a relatively rare cause of primary aldosteronism, with a prevalence of approximately 3% to 5% of aldosterone-producing tumors.[160] However, these figures probably represent a gross overestimate, given the recent evidence of increased prevalence of primary aldosteronism.[159,161-164] The prognosis for adrenal carcinoma is poor, with a median survival rate of 14 months and a 5 year survival rate of 24%.[165] The diagnosis may be suspected from the clinical

presentation because the tumors may secrete cortisol or adrenal androgens, or both, in addition to aldosterone. However, supine plasma aldosterone, the plasma aldosterone response to standing, and plasma cortisol at 9:00 AM may be similar to those found in patients with APA.[160] The 24-hour urinary free cortisol excretion rate may be elevated, as urinary 17-ketosteroids sometimes are, reflecting increased adrenal androgen production. The presence of an adrenal tumor greater than 3 cm in diameter with associated biochemistry of primary aldosteronism should alert the clinician to the possibility of adrenal carcinoma. Benign APAs are rarely larger than 2 cm in diameter. The presence of calcification in an adrenal tumor should suggest the possibility of adrenal carcinoma because calcification is not observed in APA.[160] Unlike cortisol-secreting adrenal carcinomas, aldosterone-producing carcinomas may take up the labeled cholesterol adrenal scanning agent [131I]iodomethyl-19-norcholesterol, which may also localize metastases.[131]

Treatment consists of adrenalectomy, which is not curative but may be palliative. Mitotane has produced some benefit.[159]

GLUCOCORTICOID-REMEDIABLE ALDOSTERONISM

First described by Sutherland and coworkers,[166] GRA is a rare autosomal dominant disorder. Fallo[167] noted only 51 cases reported up to 1990. However, this is probably a gross underestimate because it is likely that many cases have remained undiagnosed. The most common feature of the syndrome is hypertension, often found in asymptomatic children or young adults. Patients often have resistant hypertension. The presence of hypokalemia has suggested the possibility of mineralocorticoid excess. However, many patients with this syndrome are normokalemic despite marked aldosterone excess with suppression of the renin-angiotensin system.[28,168,169] Total body exchangeable sodium and potassium in milder cases are not typical of the picture found in Conn's syndrome.[169]

GRA results from a chimeric gene that combines the regulatory sequences of the 11β-hydroxylase gene with the coding region of the aldosterone synthase gene[28] (see Fig. 12-1). This results in the expression of aldosterone synthase in the zona fasciculata and produces a novel ACTH regulatory system. Thus, in contrast to the normal zona glomerulosa, which is suppressed by chronic ACTH excess (e.g., as in 17α-hydroxylase deficiency), ACTH is the dominant control mechanism of aldosterone secretion in GRA. Chronic exogenous ACTH given to patients with GRA results in persistent elevation in aldosterone secretion.[170]

The diagnosis, differential diagnosis, and treatment for GRA have been considered in the section on primary aldosteronism. An International Registry for Glucocorticoid-Remediable Aldosteronism has been established at Brigham and Women's Hospital at Harvard Medical School, which offers a genetic screening test that is 100% sensitive and specific. A polymerase chain reaction–based method has been introduced that allows very rapid diagnosis, even in neonates.

Mineralocorticoids Other Than Aldosterone

17α-HYDROXYLASE DEFICIENCY

17α-Hydroxylase deficiency is a rare, autosomal recessive disorder originally described by Biglieri and colleagues[171] in 1966. The estimated incidence is approximately 1 in 50,000 individuals,[172] and the disease affects both adrenal and gonadal glands. Genetic mutations have been demonstrated in the gene encoding cytochrome P450c17, causing 17α-hydroxylase/17,20-lyase deficiency.[173,174] Consequent defects in cortisol synthesis and compensatory secretion of ACTH stimulate the synthesis of 11-deoxycorticosterone (DOC) and corticosterone (B) by the zona fasciculata. High concentrations of DOC lead to hypertension, hypokalemia, and suppression of the renin-angiotensin-aldoterone system. Most patients have low aldosterone levels, because high concentrations of DOC stimulate sodium and water reabsorption, thereby resulting in decreased aldosterone biosynthesis. However, normal or high aldosterone values have been reported in some cases.[175] In the gonads, lack of 17α-hydroxylase and 17,20-lyase activity results in pseudohermaphroditism in males and primary amenorrhea in females.[176] The plasma steroid profile characteristically demonstrates elevations in DOC, 18-OH-DOC, B, and 18-OH-B, with decreased levels of 17α-hydroxyprogesterone, 11-deoxycortisol, cortisol, and aldosterone. The differential diagnosis of hypertension, hypokalemia, low plasma renin activity, and low plasma aldosterone levels also includes Liddle's syndrome, 11β-hydroxysteroid dehydrogenase deficiency type 2, exogenous mineralocorticoid administration, 11β-hydroxylase deficiency, and isolated DOC or B excess. In adults, the combination of gonadal failure with mineralocorticoid excess suggests 17α-hydroxylase deficiency, although in children, the diagnosis may be less clear. However, 11β-hydroxylase deficiency is accompanied by excess production of adrenal androgens, and thus virilization of young females and pseudoprecocious puberty in young males is usually observed.

Treatment for 17α-hydroxylase deficiency consists of both glucocorticoid and sex steroid replacement therapy. Dexamethasone is commonly used in doses ranging from 0.25 to 1.5 mg/d to suppress ACTH secretion and consequently DOC and B secretion. Suppression of DOC is usually rapid, but the renin-angiotensin-aldosterone system may take months to recover, so glucocorticoid therapy initially may produce symptoms of acute mineralocorticoid deficiency that requires treatment. Over the long term, most patients do not need continued mineralocorticoid replacement therapy.

In females, estrogen replacement therapy can be given for induction of secondary sex characteristics, although in older women, debate about optimal duration of estrogen exposure is ongoing. In males without signs of virilization, bilateral orchidectomy, surgical creation of a vagina, and estrogen replacement therapy are options.

The hypokalemic hypertension usually responds to glucocorticoid therapy[177] but may persist if the diagnosis is delayed.[178] Mineralocorticoid receptor antagonists[178] and/or calcium channel blockers[178,179] may be added to the regimen for refractory hypertension.

11β-HYDROXYLASE DEFICIENCY

11β-Hydroxylase deficiency is a rare cause of mineralocorticoid hypertension and is transmitted as an autosomal recessive disorder. It is accompanied by hyperandrogenism and contributes to 8% to 16% of cases of congenital adrenal hyperplasia.[180] Deficiency of 11β-hydroxylase activity results in failure of conversion of deoxycorticosterone (DOC) to corticosterone (B) and deoxycortisol to cortisol. Lack of cortisol synthesis releases the negative feedback inhibition on ACTH production, which, in turn, stimulates production of DOC and adrenal androgens. Clinically, this disorder presents with variable degrees of virilization and hyper-

tension. In one series, about half of the patients presented as neonates.[180] Females demonstrated clitoromegaly, labial fusion, or formation of a urogenital sinus, and males presented with penile enlargement. The other 50% were diagnosed in childhood or early adolescence owing to symptoms of sexual precocity. Hypertension accompanies the hyperandrogenism in about ⅔ of patients[181,182] and usually occurs in early childhood, but it has been documented in infancy.[183] The hypertension is thought to result from excess DOC, but the level of blood pressure does not necessarily correlate with plasma DOC levels or degree of virilization.[180,184] At an early age, because both disorders present with virilization, the distinction between 21-hydroxylase and 11β-hydroxylase deficiency can be made by measurement of plasma renin activity (PRA). PRA is usually elevated in 21-hydroxylase deficiency and suppressed in 11β-hydroxylase deficiency as the result of elevations in DOC. In neonates, the diagnosis of 11β-hydroxylase deficiency is established on the basis of high basal or ACTH-stimulated levels of 11-deoxycortisol, whereas in early adolescence, ACTH-stimulated 11-deoxycortisol values are often required.

Therapy is directed at providing glucocorticoid replacement in sufficient doses to reduce ACTH secretion, thereby reducing the stimulus for excess DOC and adrenal androgen production. As with 17α-hydroxylase deficiency, initial therapy with glucocorticoids may lead to acute mineralocorticoid insufficiency, because the zona glomerulosa can be atrophic. However, with long-term treatment, the renin-angiotensin-aldosterone axis recovers. The hypertension associated with 11β-hydroxylase deficiency usually responds to glucocorticoid therapy, but if it is refractory, mineralocorticoid receptor antagonists or calcium channel blockers can be used.

DEOXYCORTICOSTERONE EXCESS STATES

In contrast to aldosterone, DOC secretion is regulated primarily by ACTH. DOC overproduction causing mineralocorticoid excess may be primary[185] (caused by adrenal adenomas, malignancy, or hyperplasia) or secondary, depending on the amount of excess ACTH secretion. In patients with primary hyperdeoxycorticosteronism due to pure DOC-producing adenomas, hypertension and hypokalemia are accompanied by suppressed urinary and plasma aldosterone levels. Treatment is identical to that provided for those patients with aldosterone-producing adenomas and involves mineralocorticoid receptor blockade therapy before unilateral adrenalectomy. After surgery, the contralateral adrenal gland can be stimulated by ACTH to produce normal levels of cortisol, but DOC production is blunted.[186] The dissociation between cortisol and DOC, both of which are steroids in the 17-deoxy pathway, suggests that a factor other than ACTH may control DOC secretion.[186]

Adrenal carcinomas that produce DOC exclusively are uncommon. Patients have symptoms of hypertension and hypokalemia, but because these tumors can be quite large,[187] they may present with symptoms associated with rapidly enlarging adrenal masses or metastases. Some of them secrete androgens and estrogens in addition to DOC, and, if corticosterone is also secreted, plasma ACTH and cortisol levels may be low. As with other forms of adrenal carcinoma, the prognosis is usually poor, although some long-term benefit has been derived from adrenalectomy.[188,189]

Patients with primary hyperaldosteronism due to APAs can have elevations in DOC.[185] In contrast, patients with IHA often have normal DOC levels.[185] Isolated DOC excess has been reported in patients with low-renin essential hypertension, but aldosterone secretion is not suppressed in this setting.[185] Patients with all types of Cushing's syndrome, whether ACTH dependent or independent, may demonstrate increased levels of DOC.

CORTICOSTERONE EXCESS STATES

Corticosterone-producing adrenal tumors are extremely rare and usually are carcinomas.[190,191] Hypertension and hypokalemia are observed in the context of elevated plasma corticosterone but suppressed aldosterone and renin levels. As was discussed elsewhere, patients with 17α-hydroxylase deficiency and APAs may demonstrate increased corticosterone levels, but these levels are rarely elevated in patients with hyperaldosteronism due to bilateral adrenal hyperplasia.

CONGENITAL APPARENT MINERALOCORTICOID EXCESS SYNDROME

The syndrome of congenital apparent mineralocorticoid excess was originally described in 1979 by New and colleagues.[175] Two children with hypertension, hypokalemia, and suppressed renin and aldosterone levels were found to have elevated urine cortisol:cortisone ratios, suggesting a defect in the inactivation of cortisol.[175] 11β-Hydroxysteroid dehydrogenase type 2 (11β-HSD2) is the enzyme that normally converts cortisol to cortisone, a steroid that does not bind to the mineralocorticoid receptor (Fig. 12-11). Its actions are physiologically important because cortisol binds with a similar affinity as aldosterone to the mineralocorticoid receptor, and plasma cortisol concentrations are approximately 100-fold higher than plasma aldosterone concentrations.[192] Thus, cortisol would be the primary mineralocorticoid if it were not converted by 11β-HSD2 to cortisone at aldosterone-sensitive sites. The syndrome of congenital apparent mineralocorticoid excess is due to deficiency of 11β-HSD2. The persistence of cortisol resulting from deficiency in 11β-HSD2 leads to a marked elevation in mineralocorticoid activity.

Clinically, most patients with apparent mineralocorticoid excess due to 11β-HSD2 deficiency have been described in childhood. They present with symptoms of hypertension, muscle weakness, impaired growth, and polyuria with polydipsia (secondary to nephrogenic diabetes insipidus).[193,194] Laboratory abnormalities that suggest the diagnosis include hypokalemia, metabolic alkalosis, suppressed PRA and aldosterone, hypercal-

ciuria, and evidence of renal insufficiency. The diagnosis is confirmed by measuring a 24-hour urine free cortisol:urine free cortisone ratio.[195] A normal ratio ranges from 0.3 to 0.5,[26] but when 11β-HSD2 is not functioning properly, urine free cortisol values are quite high, yielding ratios of 5 to 18.[195,196] Genetic testing can be performed to secure the diagnosis.

The differential diagnosis of congenital apparent mineralocorticoid excess syndrome includes other mineralocorticoid excess syndromes in which aldosterone secretion is low. These include the two hypertensive forms of congenital adrenal hyperplasia (17α-hydroxylase and 11β-hydroxylase deficiency), Liddle's syndrome, DOC-producing tumors, ectopic ACTH secretion, and licorice or carbenoxolone ingestion. All of these conditions, except for the last two, can be excluded on the basis of results of the 24-hour urine cortisol:cortisone ratio.[195] A careful history of licorice or carbenoxolone ingestion can aid in the differential diagnosis.

Therapy is aimed at reducing endogenous cortisol production and blocking mineralocorticoid effects. Some authors advocate treatment with dexamethasone, which has a higher affinity for glucocorticoid rather than mineralocorticoid receptors, to suppress endogenous cortisol production.[197] Although dexamethasone treatment may result in improvements in blood pressure, other medications usually are required to normalize blood pressure and reduce hypokalemia.[178,192] Amiloride or triamterene, by reducing epithelial channel sodium reabsorption, or aldosterone receptor antagonists are usually necessary to control blood pressure and restore normokalemia.[198] Higher doses of aldosterone receptor antagonists such as spironolactone are used to block the mineralocorticoid effects of cortisol in this setting, but side effects such as gynecomastia may limit optimal dose titration. If hypercalciuria or nephrocalcinosis is present, the addition of a thiazide diuretic is also warranted.[192,199] Cure has been reported in one patient after transplantation of a kidney with normal 11β-HSD2 activity.[200]

ACQUIRED APPARENT MINERALOCORTICOID EXCESS SYNDROME

Licorice

The ingestion of licorice or licorice-like compounds such as carbenoxolone can result in hypertension and hypokalemia accompanied by low plasma aldosterone and renin levels.[201-203] Licorice contains a steroid, glycyrrhetinic acid, which inhibits 11β-HSD2,[204] the same enzyme that is deficient in congenital apparent mineralocorticoid excess syndrome (see Fig. 12-11). Doses as low as 75 mg of glycyrrhetinic acid, which corresponds to ingestion of about 50 g of licorice a day, are enough to cause a significant rise in blood pressure if consumed for 2 weeks or longer.[205] Initially, because symptoms could be reversed by mineralocorticoid receptor antagonists, the thought was that glycyrrhetinic acid directly activated the mineralocorticoid receptor. However, the affinity of the active component of licorice for the mineralocorticoid receptor was found to be only 10^{-4} that of aldosterone.[206] Furthermore, it became clear that licorice produced sodium retention only when the adrenal glands were present, or when glucocorticoid replacement therapy was given.[207,208] Higher doses of glucocorticoids, such as 2 mg of dexamethasone per day, actually produced natriuresis in subjects taking the active component of licorice.[203] Taken together, the similarities between congenital apparent mineralocorticoid excess and ingestion by subjects of large quantities of licorice led to the notion that licorice may be an exogenous inhibitor of

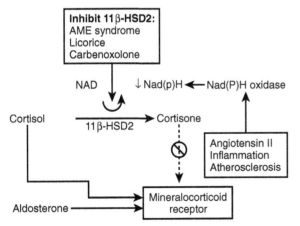

FIGURE 12-11. Schematic representation of the role of 11β-hydroxysteroid dehydrogenase (11β-HSD2) in metabolizing cortisol, which activates the mineralocorticoid receptor, to cortisone, which does not. A cofactor in this reaction is nicotine adenine dinucleotide (NAD). Inflammatory processes in tissues such as the kidney can activate NAD(P)H oxidase, thereby depleting the availability of NAD and inhibiting cortisol:cortisone metabolism.

11β-HSD2 activity. These effects were confirmed by MacKenzie and colleagues when they gave normal subjects 500 mg/day of glycyrrhetinic acid and measured plasma urinary cortisol and cortisone.[204] Although plasma cortisol values remained unchanged, urinary cortisol values increased significantly with glycyrrhetinic acid treatment. Plasma and urinary cortisone values decreased, indicating inhibition of the conversion of cortisol to cortisone during glycyrrhetinic acid treatment. In vitro studies later confirmed that the inhibition of 11β-HSD2 activity by glycyrrhetinic acid was dose dependent.[209]

Carbenoxolone

Carbenoxolone is a hemisuccinate derivative of glycyrrhetinic acid. It was developed originally as an antiulcer drug but was found to cause sodium retention, hypertension, hypokalemia, and suppression of the renin-angiotensin-aldosterone system. Carbenoxolone also inhibits 11β-HSD2 activity (see Fig. 12-11), but there are differences between it and glycyrrhetinic acid. When normal volunteers were given 300 mg of carbenoxolone a day for 2 weeks, sodium retention and hypokalemia occurred, but unlike with licorice ingestion, the hypokalemia was not associated with kaliuresis.[210] Furthermore, although the plasma half-life of cortisol was increased by carbenoxolone, no effect on the urinary cortisol:cortisone ratio was observed, and plasma cortisone values were not reduced by treatment. The reason for these discrepancies remains unclear. One possibility is that carbenoxolone inhibits both the dehydrogenase (11β-HSD2) and reductase forms (11β-HSD1) of the enzyme. The renal isoform is the major dehydrogenase that converts cortisol to cortisone, whereas the primary isoform in the liver and adipose tissue is the reductase form, which converts cortisone to cortisol. Normal subjects given cortisone acetate without carbenoxolone showed lower plasma cortisol levels than those subjects given cortisone acetate plus carbenoxolone, suggesting an effect of carbenoxolone on the reductase isoform of the enzyme (11β-HSD1).[210] Whereas licorice ingestion causes sodium retention and hypertension only in glucocorticoid-replete states,[207,208] carbenoxolone can potentiate the sodium-retaining properties of DOC and aldosterone in adrenalectomized animals.[211] Thus, when the hypertension induced by carbenoxolone is considered, sites and mechanisms of action other than the kidney 11β-HSD2 isoform may be important in mediating its effects.

ECTOPIC ACTH SYNDROME

Hypertension, hypokalemia, and metabolic alkalosis can be found in patients with ectopic ACTH syndrome. The symptoms are less common in patients with pituitary-dependent or ACTH-independent Cushing's syndrome.[212-216] The mechanism by which ectopic ACTH syndrome causes mineralocorticoid excess symptoms is not completely understood but may be the result of a combination of effects. One hypothesis is that cortisol secretion may be so high in ectopic ACTH syndrome that it exceeds the metabolic capacity of 11β-HSD2.[213,216] Indeed, in several patients with ectopic ACTH production, plasma and urine ratios of cortisol:cortisone metabolites are up to two times higher than normal,[213,215] suggesting that ACTH or ACTH-related steroids may inhibit 11β-HSD2. Furthermore, Ulick and colleagues[213] have demonstrated that urinary metabolites of aldosterone are low, while those of DOC are high in patients with ectopic ACTH syndrome. The increased cortisol:cortisone ratio is no better a predictor of hypokalemia than are increased DOC levels in these patients.[215] Thus, the hypertension and hypokalemia observed in this setting may be accounted for by a combination of increased secretion of cortisol and DOC, with decreased inactivation of cortisol by 11β-HSD2.

GLUCOCORTICOID RESISTANCE STATES

Patients with glucocorticoid resistance often present with hypertension and/or signs of androgen excess. Both total and free plasma cortisol levels are increased, as are urinary cortisol values. However, in contrast to patients with Cushing's syndrome, none of the clinical physical stigmata of cortisol excess are present. Patients with glucocorticoid resistance fail to suppress cortisol with low-dose dexamethasone. ACTH levels are increased, resulting in increased adrenal androgen, corticosterone, and DOC secretion.

Familial glucocorticoid resistance is inherited as an autosomal recessive or dominant disorder characterized by mutations in the glucocorticoid receptor gene.[217,218] Glucocorticoid receptor defects include decreased glucocorticoid binding affinity caused by a point mutation in the steroid-binding domain (*Val641* mutant), defective nuclear binding caused by a point mutation in the DNA-binding domain, and decreased receptor number. However, some patients with evidence of glucocorticoid resistance do not have any mutations in the glucocorticoid receptor, but rather in glucocorticoid action.[219]

The mechanism of hypertension in glucocorticoid resistance is likely multifactorial.[215] One possibility is that excess DOC and corticocosterone secretion, similar to that observed in 17α-hydroxylase deficiency, contributes to the hypertension. An additional explanation includes the possibility that the capacity of 11β-HSD2 to convert excess cortisol to cortisone is exceeded[213] (much as it may be in ectopic ACTH syndrome), thereby giving cortisol access to unoccupied mineralocorticoid receptors. It also is possible that the excess ACTH seen in glucocorticoid resistance induces a partial deficiency of 11β-HSD2. Because of compensatory increases in ACTH and cortisol secretion, patients with familial glucocorticoid resistance do not usually experience symptoms of adrenal insufficiency. Glucocorticoid resistance can be confirmed by the response to high-dose as compared with low-dose dexamethasone.[220] Excess androgens and mineralocorticoid effects can be ameliorated by the daily administration of up to 3 mg of dexamethasone.

PRIMARY (ESSENTIAL) HYPERTENSION

Approximately 25% of patients with primary hypertension have low-renin hypertension[221] and derive greater blood pressure reduction with mineralocorticoid antagonism than with other antihypertensive drugs.[222,223] This observation suggests that such patients may have excessive mineralocorticoid activity, but plasma aldosterone levels have actually been found to be normal.[224,225] The plasma aldosterone, however, is less readily suppressed by salt loading, and those patients with normal renin levels show higher than normal aldosterone:PRA and aldosterone:angiotensin II ratios. Other steroids with known mineralocorticoid activity, such as 18-OH-DOC, 19-nor-DOC, and 17α,20-dihydroxyprogesterone, are also normal in patients with essential hypertension. It is possible, though, that they affect blood pressure through mechanisms other than those mediated by the mineralocorticoid receptor.

The role of 11β-HSD2 has been studied in patients with primary hypertension. In approximately ⅓ of patients, the half-life of labeled cortisol is prolonged, suggesting partial 11β-HSD2 deficiency.[226,227] However, mineralocorticoid excess in patients with impaired 11β-HSD2 activity, as judged by plasma electrolytes, PRA, and aldosterone levels, has not been demonstrated.

Salt-sensitive individuals also have evidence of impaired 11β-HSD2 activity as measured by increased urinary cortisol:cortisone ratios. Studies have evaluated a microsatellite within intron 1 of the 11β-HSD2 gene and have demonstrated an association with salt sensitivity,[228,229] wherein short microsatellite alleles were more common in salt-sensitive compared with salt-resistant subjects. Similar observations were made in African American compared with Caucasian subjects,[230] in keeping with the predisposition to low-renin hypertension in this ethnic group.

EXOGENOUS MINERALOCORTICOID STATES

Exogenous mineralocorticoid excess is usually seen in patients with Addison's disease or patients who have undergone bilateral adrenalectomy, who receive excessive doses of adrenal steroid replacement therapy. Large doses of aldosterone, DOC, 9α-fludrocortisol, 9α-fluoroprednisolone[231] (a steroid in nasal spray used for chronic rhinitis and for the treatment of eczema), or hydrocortisone can result in initial sodium retention, hypokalemia, and decreased PRA and aldosterone secretion. The production of hypertension depends on high salt intake. The initial symptoms abate after mineralocorticoid escape occurs, normalizing sodium retention and restoring hypokalemia. Because aldosterone, DOC, 9α-fludrocortisol, and 9α-fluoroprednisolone are not substrates for 11β-HSD2, initial effects are mediated by their actions at the mineralocorticoid receptor. Large doses of hydrocortisone, however, are likely to overload the capacity of the 11β-HSD2, resulting in increased activation of the mineralocorticoid receptor.

Activating Mutations of the Mineralocorticoid Receptor

A gain-of-function mutation (S810L) in the mineralocorticoid receptor that causes early-onset hypertension that is exacerbated in pregnancy has been described.[232] The mutation results in constitutive activation of the mineralocorticoid receptor and changes the specificity of the receptor so that activation by progesterone and other steroids that lack a 21-hydroxyl group becomes possible. Normally, steroids that lack the 21-hydroxyl group act as mineralocorticoid receptor antagonists, thus providing a potential explanation for the amelioration of Conn's syndrome during pregnancy.[233] The S810L mutation results in a gain of van der Waals interaction between helix 3, which substitutes for the normal 21-hydroxyl interaction, and helix 3 in the wild-type receptor.[232]

Disorders of the Renal Tubular Epithelium That Mimic Primary Mineralocorticoid Excess

Liddle's Syndrome

The principal cells of the cortical collecting tubule contribute to net sodium reabsorption and serve as the primary site of potassium secretion in the kidney. Aldosterone, after combining with the cytosolic mineralocorticoid receptor, increases both the number of open sodium channels in the apical membrane of principal cells and the number of basolateral Na/K-ATPase pumps.[234,235] The reabsorption of cationic sodium makes the lumen electronegative, thereby creating a favorable gradient for the secretion of potassium into the lumen. Normally, increased intracellular sodium downregulates the activity of the apical sodium ion channels, while increased export of intracellular sodium (via increased basolateral Na/K-ATPase pump activity) ensures that apical sodium channels remain open.[236] Amiloride closes apical sodium channels, leading to natriuresis and potassium retention.[237] The amiloride-sensitive epithelial sodium channel (ENaC) consists of three subunits: α, β, and γ. In Liddle's syndrome, activity of ENaC is enhanced as the result of varying mutations in a short segment of the cytoplasmic tail of the β or γ subunits.[238-243] Expression of mutated genes in the *Xenopus* oocyte is associated with a significant increase in apical sodium reabsorption and loss of inhibition of ENaC activity by increased levels of intracellular sodium.[236,238,241] Some of the defects also prevent downregulation of ENaC through the loss of interaction with an intracellular protein lipase, leading to an increase in the number of open channels in the apical membrane.[244,245]

Patients with Liddle's syndrome typically present in youth, with excess sodium retention, hypertension, and varying degrees of hypokalemia. These effects are not mediated by increased levels of circulating aldosterone or other mineralocorticoids. The syndrome is transmitted in autosomal dominant fashion,[246,247] and in one kindred, the average serum potassium of 18 affected family members was 3.6 mEq/L.[246] Thus, hypokalemia is not a necessary component of the diagnosis of Liddle's syndrome. The differential diagnosis includes other mineralocorticoid excess syndromes in which aldosterone secretion is low, such as the two hypertensive forms of congenital adrenal hyperplasia (17α-hydroxylase and 11β-hydroxylase deficiency), congenital apparent mineralocorticoid excess syndrome, DOC-producing adrenal tumors, ectopic ACTH secretion, licorice or carbenoxolone ingestion, and familial glucocorticoid resistance. The lack of hyperandrogenism in Liddle's syndrome helps to differentiate it from 11β-hydroxylase deficiency and familial glucocorticoid resistance, and the normal urinary cortisol:cortisone ratio helps rule out congenital apparent mineralocorticoid excess syndrome, licorice ingestion, and ectopic ACTH secretion. Additionally, patients with Liddle's syndrome do not respond to spironolactone therapy,[246] because increased sodium reabsorption is not mediated by aldosterone or other mineralocorticoids. The lack of response also distinguishes it from 11β-HSD2 deficiency. Therapy for Liddle's syndrome involves the use of potassium-sparing diuretics such as amiloride or triamterene,[239,246] which directly close apical membrane sodium channels in principal cells.

REFERENCES

1. Conn JW: Primary aldosteronism: a new clinical syndrome, J Lab Clin Med 45:6–17, 1955.
2. Conn JW, Knopf RF, Nesbit RM: Clinical characteristics of primary aldosteronism from an analysis of 145 cases, Am J Surg 107:159–172, 1964.
3. Brown J, Davies DL, Lever AF, et al: Plasma renin in a case of Conn's syndrome with fibrinoid lesions: Use of spironolactone in treatment, Br Med J 2:1636–1637, 1964.
4. Conn JW, Cohen EL, Rovner DR: Suppressed plasma renin activity in primary aldosteronism, JAMA 190:213–221, 1964.
5. Helmer OM: Renin activity in blood from patients with hypertension, CMAJ 90:221–225, 2000.
6. Brown J, Davies DL, Robertson JIS, et al: Plasma renin concentration in human hypertension. I: relationship between renin, sodium and potassium, Br Med J 2:144–148, 1965.
7. Funder JW, Carey RM, Fardella C, et al: Case detection, diagnosis, and treatment of patients with primary aldosteronism: an Endocrine Society. Clinical Practice Guideline, J Clin Endocrinol Metab 93:3266–3281, 2008.
8. Nomura K, Han DC, Jibiki K, et al: Primary aldosteronism with normal aldosterone levels in blood and urine, Acta Endocrinol (Copenh) 110:522–525, 1985.
9. Hiramatsu K, Takahashi K, Arimori S: A case report of aldosterone producing adenoma with masked hyperaldosteronemia, Tokai J Exp Clin Med 11:87–89, 1986.
10. Conn JW: Plasma renin activity in primary aldosteronism, JAMA 190:222–225, 1964.
11. Beevers DG, Nelson CS, Padfield PL, et al: The prevalence of hypertension in an unselected population, and the frequency of abnormalities of potassium, angioten-

sin II and aldosterone in hypertensive subjects, Acta Clin Belg 29:276–280, 1974.

12. Berglund C, Andersson O, Wilhelmsen L: Prevalence of primary and secondary hypertension: studies in a random population sample, Br Med J 2:554–556, 1976.

13. Lewin A, Blaufox MD, Castle H, et al: Apparent prevalence of curable hypertension in the hypertension detection and follow-up program, Arch Intern Med 145:424–427, 1985.

14. Sinclair AM, Isles CG, Brown I, et al: Secondary hypertension in a blood pressure clinic, Arch Intern Med 147:1289–1293, 1987.

15. Streeten DH, Tomycz N, Anderson GH: Reliability of screening methods for the diagnosis of primary aldosteronism, Am J Med 67:403–413, 1979.

16. Grim CE, Weinberger MH, Higgins JT, et al: Diagnosis of secondary forms of hypertension, JAMA 237:1331–1335, 1977.

17. Mulatero P, Stowasser M, Loh KC, et al: Increased diagnosis of primary aldosteronism, including surgically correctable forms, in centers from five continents, J Clin Endocrinol Metab 89:1045–1050, 2004.

18. Gordon RD, Stowasser M, Tunny TJ, et al: High incidence of primary aldosteronism in 199 patients referred with hypertension, Clin Exp Pharmacol Physiol 21:315–318, 1994.

19. Gordon RD, Ziesak MD, Tunny TJ, et al: Evidence that primary aldosteronism may not be uncommon: 12% incidence among antihypertensive drug trial volunteers, Clin Exp Pharmacol Physiol 20:296–298, 1993.

20. Loh KC, Koay ES, Khaw MC, et al: Prevalence of primary aldosteronism among Asian hypertensive patients in Singapore, J Clin Endocrinol Metab 85:2854–2859, 2000.

21. Fardella CE, Mosso L, Gomez-Sanchez C, et al: Primary hyperaldosteronism in essential hypertensives: prevalence, biochemical profile, and molecular biology, J Clin Endocrinol Metab 85:1863–1867, 2000.

22. Schwartz GL, Turner ST: Screening for primary aldosteronism in essential hypertension: diagnostic accuracy of the ratio of plasma aldosterone concentration to plasma renin activity, Clin Chem 51:386–394, 2005.

23. Lim PO, Dow Brennan G, Jung RT, et al: High prevalence of primary aldosteronism in the Tayside hypertension clinic population, J Hum Hypertens 14:311–315, 2000.

24. Mosso L, Carvajal C, Gonzalez A, et al: Primary aldosteronism and hypertensive disease, Hypertension 42:161–165, 2003.

25. Hamlet SM, Tunny TJ, Woodland E, et al: Is aldosterone/renin ratio useful to screen a hypertensive population for primary aldosteronism? Clin Exp Pharm Physiol 12:249–252, 1985.

26. Rossi GP, Bernini G, Caliumi C, et al: A prospective study of the prevalence of primary aldosteronism in 1,125 hypertensive patients, J Am Coll Cardiol 48:2293–3000, 2006.

27. McMahon GT, Dluhy RG: Glucocorticoid-remediable aldosteronism, Cardiol Rev 12:44–48, 2004.

28. Lifton RP, Dluhy RG, Powers M, et al: A chimaeric 11 beta-hydroxylase/aldosterone synthase gene causes glucocorticoid-remediable aldosteronism and human hypertension, Nature 355:262–265, 1992.

29. Carroll J, Dluhy R, Fallo F, et al: Aldosterone-producing adenomas do not contain glucocorticoid-remediable aldosteronism chimeric gene duplications, J Clin Endocrinol Metab 81:4310–4312, 1996.

30. Stowasser M, Gunasekera TG, Gordon RD: Familial varieties of primary aldosteronism, Clin Exp Pharmacol Physiol 28:1087–1090, 2001.

31. Jeske YW, So A, Lelemen L, et al: Examination of chromosome 7p22 candidate genes RBaK, PMS2 and GNA12 in familial hyperaldosteronism type 2, Clin Exp Pharmacol Physiol 35:380–385, 2008.

32. Davies DL, Beevers DC, Brown JJ, et al: Aldosterone and its stimuli in normal and hypertensive man: are essential hypertension and primary hyperaldosteronism without tumor the same condition? J Endocrinol 81:79–91, 1979.

33. Padfield PL, Brown JI, Davies D, et al: The myth of idiopathic hyperaldosteronism, Lancet 2:83–84, 1981.

34. Wisgerhoff M, Carpenter PC, Brown RD: Increased adrenal sensitivity to angiotensin II in idiopathic hyperaldosteronism, J Clin Endocrinol Metab 47:938–943, 1978.

35. Wisgerhoff M, Brown RD: Increased adrenal sensitivity to angiotensin II in low-renin essential hypertension, J Clin Invest 61:1456–1462, 1978.

36. Witzgall H, Lorenz R, Von Werder K, et al: Dopamine reduces aldosterone and 18-hydroxycorticosterone response to angiotensin II in patients with essential low-renin hypertension and idiopathic hyperaldosteronism, Clin Sci 68:291–299, 1985.

37. Jungmann E, Althoff PH, Rosak C, et al: Endogenous dopaminergic inhibition of aldosterone and prolactin secretion is apparently not increased in primary aldosteronism, Horm Metab Res 18:138–140, 1986.

38. Fallo F, Boscaro M, Sonino N, et al: Effect of naloxone on the adrenal cortex in primary aldosteronism, Am J Hypertens 1:280–282, 1988.

39. Klemm SA, Ballantine DM, Gordon RD, et al: The renin gene and aldosterone-producing adenomas, Kidney Int 46:1591–1593, 1994.

40. Miyamori I, Koshida H, Matsubara T, et al: Pituitary peptides other than ACTH may not be aldosterone secretagogue in primary aldosteronism, Exp Clin Endocrinol 95:323–329, 1990.

41. Chen LG, Lee TI, Lin HD, et al: Primary aldosteronism due to unilateral adrenal hyperplasia: a case report, Chung Hua I Hsueh Tsa Chih (Taipei) 59:114–120, 1997.

42. Otsuka F, Otsuka-Misunaga F, Koyama S, et al: Hormonal characteristics of primary aldosteronism due to unilateral adrenal hyperplasia, J Endocrinol Invest 21:531–536, 1998.

43. Geller DS, Zhang J, Wisgerhof MV, et al: A novel form of human Mendelian hypertension featuring nonglucocorticoid-remediable aldosteronism, J Clin Endocrinol Metab 93:3117–3123, 2008.

44. Davies LA, Hu C, Guagliardo NA, et al: TASK channel deletion in mice causes primary hyperaldosteronism, Proc Natl Acad Sci U S A 105:2203–2208, 2008.

45. Ferriss JB, Beevers DG, Brown JJ, et al: Clinical, biochemical and pathological features of low-renin ("primary") hyperaldosteronism, Am Heart J 95:375–388, 1978.

46. Neville AM, O'Hare MJ: Histopathology of the human adrenal cortex, Clin Endocrinol Metab 14:791–820, 1985.

47. Kuramoto H, Kumazawa J: Ultrastructural studies of adrenal adenoma causing primary aldosteronism, Virchows Arch A Pathol Anat Histopathol 407:271–278, 1985.

48. Gordon RD, Klemm SA, Tunny TJ, et al: Primary aldosteronism: hypertension with a genetic basis, Lancet 340:159–161, 1992.

49. Nagae A, Murakami E, Hiwada K, et al: Primary aldosteronism with cortisol overproduction from bilateral multiple adrenal adenomas, Jpn J Med 30:26–31, 1991.

50. Neville AM, Symington T: Pathology of primary aldosteronism, Cancer 19:1854–1868, 1966.

51. Matsuda A, Beniko M, Ikota A, et al: Primary aldosteronism with bilateral multiple aldosterone-producing adrenal adenomas, Intern Med 35:970–975, 1996.

52. Ito Y, Fujimoto Y, Obara T, et al: Clinical significance of associated nodular lesions of the adrenal in patients with aldosteronoma, World J Surg 14:330–334, 1990.

53. Dobbie JW: Adrenocortical nodular hyperplasia: the ageing adrenal, J Pathol 99:1–18, 1969.

54. Jackson B, Valentine R, Wagner G: Primary aldosteronism due to a malignant ovarian tumour, Aust N Z J Med 16:69–71, 1986.

55. Kulkarni JN, Mistry RC, Kamat MR, et al: Autonomous aldosterone-secreting ovarian tumor, Gynecol Oncol 37:284–289, 1990.

56. Todesco S, Terribile V, Borsatti A, et al: Primary aldosteronism due to a malignant ovarian tumor, J Clin Endocrinol Metab 41:809–819, 1975.

57. Flanagan MJ, McDonald JH: Heterotopic adrenocortical adenoma producing primary aldosteronism, J Urol 98:133–139, 1967.

58. Young WF Jr: Primary aldosteronism: renaissance of a syndrome, Clin Endocrinol 66:607–618, 2007.

59. Melby JC: Diagnosis and treatment of primary aldosteronism and isolated hypoaldosteronism, Clin Endocrinol Metab 14:977–995, 1985.

60. Biglieri EG, Kater CE, Arteaga EA: Mineralocorticoid hypertension due to hyperaldosteronism and hyperdeoxycorticosterone, J Hypertens Suppl 4:S61–S65, 1986.

61. Biglieri EG, Irony I, Kater CE: Identification and implications of new types of mineralocorticoid hypertension, J Steroid Biochem 32:199–204, 1989.

62. Mantero F, Armanini D, Biason A, et al: New aspects of mineralocorticoid hypertension, Horm Res 34:175–180, 1990.

63. Stewart PM: Mineralocorticoid hypertension, Lancet 353:1341–1347, 1999.

64. Ma JT, Wang C, Lam KS, et al: Fifty cases of primary hyperaldosteronism in Hong Kong Chinese with a high frequency of periodic paralysis. Evaluation of techniques for tumour localisation, Q J Med 61:1021–1037, 1986.

65. Conn JW, Knopf RF, Nesbit R: Primary aldosteronism: present evaluation of its clinical characteristics and the results of surgery. In Banlieu EE, Robin P, editors: Aldosterone, Oxford, 1968, Blackwell Scientific, p 327.

66. Ferriss JB, Brown JJ, Fraser R, et al: Primary hyperaldosteronism, Clin Endocrinol Metab 10:419–452, 1981.

67. Murphy BF, Whitworth JA, Kincaid-Smith P: Malignant hypertension due to an aldosterone producing adrenal adenoma, Clin Exp Hypertens [A] 7:939–950, 1985.

68. Snow MH, Nicol P, Wilkinson R, et al: Normotensive primary aldosteronism, Br Med J 1:1125–1126, 1976.

69. Zipser RD, Speckart PF: "Normotensive" primary aldosteronism, Ann Intern Med 88:655–656, 1978.

70. Gordon RSM: Familial forms broaden horizons in primary aldosteronism, Trends Endocrinol Metab 9:220–227, 1998.

71. Imai Y, Abe K, Munakata M, et al: Circadian blood pressure variations under different pathophysiological conditions, J Hypertens Suppl 8:S125–S132, 1990.

72. Middeke M, Kluglich M, Holzgreve H: Circadian blood pressure rhythm in primary and secondary hypertension, Chronobiol Int 8:451–459, 1991.

73. Munakata M, Aihara A, Imai Y, et al: Decreased blood pressure variability at rest in patients with primary aldosteronism, Am J Hypertens 11:828–838, 1998.

74. Funder JW: The role of aldosterone and mineralocorticoid receptors in cardiovascular disease, Am J Cardiovasc Drugs 7:151–157, 2007.

75. Milliez P, Girerd X, Plouin PF, et al: Evidence for increased rate of cardiovascular events in patients with primary aldosteronism, J Am Coll Cardiol 45:1243–1248, 2005.

76. Rossi GP, Sacchetto A, Visentin P, et al: Changes in left ventricular anatomy and function in hypertension and primary aldosteronism, Hypertension 27:1029–1045, 1996.

77. Tanabe A, Naruse M, Naruse K, et al: Left ventricular hypertrophy is more prominent in patients with primary aldosteronism than in patients with other types of secondary hypertension, Hypertens Res 20:85–90, 1997.

78. Rossi GP, Di Bello V, Fanzaroli C, et al: Excess aldosterone is associated with alterations in myocardial texture in primary aldosteronism, Hypertension 40:23–27, 2002.

79. Strauch B, Petrak O, Wichterle D, et al: Increased arterial wall stiffness in primary aldosteronism in comparison with essential hypertension, Am J Hypertens 19:909–914, 2006.

80. Rossi GP, Bernini G, Desideri G, et al: Renal damage in primary aldosteronism: results of the PAPY Study, Hypertension 48:232–238, 2006.

81. Sechi LA, Novello M, Lapenna R, et al: Long-term renal outcomes in patients with primary aldosteronism, JAMA 295:2638–2645, 2006.

82. Fallo F, Veglio F, Bertello C, et al: Prevalence and characteristics of the metabolic syndrome in primary aldosteronism, J Clin Endocrinol Metab 91:454–459, 2006.

83. Stowasser M, Sharman J, Leano R, et al: Evidence for abnormal left ventricular structure and function in normotensive individuals with familial hyperaldosteronism type I, J Clin Endocrinol Metab 90:5070–5076, 2005.

84. Weinberger MH, Grim CE, Hollifield JW, et al: Primary aldosteronism: diagnosis, localization, and treatment, Ann Intern Med 90:386–395, 1979.

85. Young WF Jr: Clinical practice: the incidentally discovered adrenal mass, N Engl J Med 356:601–610, 2007.

86. Calhoun DA, Jones D, Textor S, et al: Resistant hypertension: diagnosis, evaluation and treatment, Hypertension 51:1403–1419, 2008.
87. Stowasser M, Klemm SA, Tunny TJ, et al: Response to unilateral adrenalectomy for aldosterone-producing adenoma: effect of potassium levels and angiotensin responsiveness, Clin Exp Pharmacol Physiol 21:319–322, 1994.
88. Brown JJ, Chinn RH, Davies DL: Falsely high potassium values in patients with hyperaldosteronism, Br Med J 2:18–20, 1970.
89. Christlieb AR, Espiner EA, Amsterdam EA, et al: The pattern of electrolyte excretion in normal and hypertensive subjects before and after saline infusions. A simple electrolyte formula for the diagnosis of primary aldosteronism, Am J Cardiol 27:595–601, 1971.
90. Relman A, Schwartz W: The effect of DOCA on electrolyte balance in normal man and its relation to sodium chloride intake, Yale J Biol Med 24540–24558, 1952.
91. Noth RH, Biglieri EG: Primary hyperaldosteronism, Med Clin North Am 72:1117–1131, 1988.
92. Bravo EL, Tarazi RC, Dustan HP, et al: The changing clinical spectrum of primary aldosteronism, Am J Med 74:641–651, 1983.
93. Gordon RD, Gomez-Sanchez CE, Hamlet SM, et al: Angiotensin-responsive aldosterone-producing adenoma masquerades as idiopathic hyperaldosteronism (IHA: adrenal hyperplasia) or low-renin essential hypertension, J Hypertens Suppl 5:S103–S106, 1987.
94. Cain JP, Tuck ML, Williams GH, et al: The regulation of aldosterone secretion in primary aldosteronism, Am J Med 53:627–637, 1972.
95. Herf SM, Teates DC, Tegtmeyer CJ, et al: Identification and differentiation of surgically correctable hypertension due to primary aldosteronism, Am J Med 67:397–402, 1979.
96. Edwards C, Landon J: Corticosteroids. In Lorraine JA, Bell EJ, editors: Hormone Assays and Their Clinical Application. New York, 1976, Churchill Livingstone, pp 519–579.
97. Biglieri EG, Slaton PE Jr, Kronfield SJ, et al: Primary aldosteronism with unusual secretory pattern, J Clin Endocrinol Metab 27:715–721, 1967.
98. Brown JJ, Fraser R, Love DR, et al: Apparently isolated excess deoxycorticosterone in hypertension. A variant of the mineralocorticoid-excess syndrome, Lancet 2:243–247, 1972.
99. Hegstad R, Brown RD, Jiang NS, et al: Aging and aldosterone, Am J Med 74:442–448, 1983.
100. Hiramatsu K, Yamada T, Yukimura Y, et al: A screening test to identify aldosterone-producing adenoma by measuring plasma renin activity. Results in hypertensive patients, Arch Intern Med 141:1589–1593, 1981.
101. Hamlet SM, Tunny TJ, Woodland E, et al: Is aldosterone/renin ratio useful to screen a hypertensive population for primary aldosteronism? Clin Exp Pharmacol Physiol 12:249–252, 1985.
102. McKenna TJ, Sequeira SJ, Heffernan A, et al: Diagnosis under random conditions of all disorders of the renin-angiotensin-aldosterone axis, including primary hyperaldosteronism, J Clin Endocrinol Metab 73:952–957, 1991.
103. Gallay BJ, Ahmad S, Xu L, et al: Screening for primary aldosteronism without discontinuing hypertensive medications: plasma aldosterone-renin ratio, Am J Kidney Dis 37:699–705, 2001.
104. Nishizaka MK, Pratt-Ubunama M, Zaman MA, et al: Validity of plasma aldosterone-to-renin activity ratio in African American and white subjects with resistant hypertension, Am J Hypertens 18:805–812, 2005.
105. Giacchetti G, Ronconi V, Lucarelli G, et al: Analysis of screening and confirmatory tests in the diagnosis of primary aldosteronism: need for a standardized protocol, J Hypertens 24:737–745, 2006.
106. Seifarth C, Trenkel S, Schobel H, et al: Influence of antihypertensive medication on aldosterone and renin concentration in the differential diagnosis of essential hypertension and primary aldosteronism, Clin Endocrinol 57:457–465, 2002.
107. Arteaga E, Klein R, Biglieri EG: Use of the saline infusion test to diagnose the cause of primary aldosteronism, Am J Med 79:722–728, 1985.
108. Biglieri EG, Stockigt JR, Schambelan M: A preliminary evaluation for primary aldosteronism, Arch Intern Med 126:1004–1007, 1970.
109. Padfield PL, Allison ME, Brown JJ, et al: Response of plasma aldosterone to fludrocortisone in primary hyperaldosteronism and other forms of hypertension, Clin Endocrinol (Oxf) 4:493–500, 1975.
110. Gordon RD: Diagnostic investigations in primary aldosteronism. In Zanchetti A, editor: Clinical Medicine Series on Hypertension, London, 2001, McGraw-Hill, pp 101–114.
111. Stowasser M, Gordon RD, Rutherford JC, et al: Diagnosis and management of primary aldosteronism, J Renin Angiotensin Aldosterone Syst 2:156–169, 2001.
112. Vaughan NJ, Jowett TP, Slater JD, et al: The diagnosis of primary hyperaldosteronism, Lancet 1:120–125, 1981.
113. Kem DC, Weinberger MH, Mayes DM, et al: Saline suppression of plasma aldosterone in hypertension, Arch Intern Med 128:380–386, 1971.
114. Lyons DF, Kem DC, Brown RD, et al: Single dose captopril as a diagnostic test for primary aldosteronism, J Clin Endocrinol Metab 57:892–896, 1983.
115. Muratani H, Abe I, Tomita Y, et al: Is single oral administration of captopril beneficial in screening for primary aldosteronism? [Published erratum appears in Am Heart J 112:357, 1986], Am Heart J 112:361–367, 1986.
116. Muratani H, Abe I, Tomita Y, et al: Single oral administration of captopril may not bring an improvement in screening of primary aldosteronism, Clin Exp Hypertens [A] 9:611–614, 1987.
117. Naomi S, Umeda T, Iwaoka T, et al: Effects of sodium intake on the captopril test for primary aldosteronism, Jpn Heart J 28:357–365, 1987.
118. Grim C, Ganguly A, Weinberger MH: A rapid method to differentiate glucocorticoid-suppressible hyperaldosteronism from other causes of primary aldosteronism with an anomalous postural response of plasma aldosterone. In New MI, editor: Dexamethasone-Suppressible Hyperaldosteronism. Serono Symposium Review. Philadelphia, 1986, JB Lippincott, pp 69–78.
119. Oberfield SE, Levine LS, Stoner E, et al: Adrenal glomerulosa function in patients with dexamethasone-suppressible hyperaldosteronism, J Clin Endocrinol Metab 53:158–164, 1981,
120. Woodland E, Tunny TJ, Hamlet SM, et al: Hypertension corrected and aldosterone responsiveness to renin-angiotensin restored by long-term dexamethasone in glucocorticoid-suppressible hyperaldosteronism, Clin Exp Pharmacol Physiol 12:245–248, 1985.
121. Ganguly A, Grim CE, Weinberger MH: Anomalous postural aldosterone response in glucocorticoid-suppressible hyperaldosteronism, N Engl J Med 305:991–993, 1981.
122. Deleted in proofs.
123. Young WF Jr, Stanson AW, Thompson GB, et al: Role for adrenal venous sampling in primary aldosteronism, Surgery 136:1227–1235, 2004.
124. Iwaoka T, Umeda T, Naomi S, et al: Localization of aldosterone-producing adenoma: venous sampling in primary aldosteronism, Endocrinol Jpn 37:151–157, 1990.
125. Young WF Jr, Stanson AW, Grant CS, et al: Primary aldosteronism: adrenal venous sampling, Surgery 120:913–919, 1996.
126. Gross MD, Shapiro B, Freitas JE: Limited significance of asymmetric adrenal visualization on dexamethasone-suppression scintigraphy, J Nucl Med 26:43–48, 1985.
127. Miles JM, Wahner HW, Carpenter PC, et al: Adrenal scintiscanning with NP-59, a new radioiodinated cholesterol agent, Mayo Clin Proc 54:321–327, 1979.
128. Sarkar SD, Cohen EL, Beierwaltes WH, et al: A new and superior adrenal imaging agent, 131I-6beta-iodomethyl-19-nor-cholesterol (NP-59): evaluation in humans, J Clin Endocrinol Metab 45:353–362, 1977.
129. Pagny JY, Chatellier G, Raynaud A, et al: Localization of primary hyperaldosteronism, Ann Endocrinol (Paris) 49:340–343, 1988.
130. Young WF Jr, Klee GG: Primary aldosteronism. Diagnostic evaluation, Endocrinol Metab Clin North Am 17:367–395, 1988.
131. Shenker Y, Gross MD, Grekin RJ, et al: The scintigraphic localization of mineralocorticoid-producing adrenocortical carcinoma, J Endocrinol Invest 9:115–120, 1986.
132. Balkin PW, Hollifield JW, Winn SD, et al: Primary aldosteronism: computerized tomography in preoperative evaluation, South Med J 78:1071–1073, 1985.
133. Ou YC, Yang CR, Chang CL, et al: Comparison of five modalities in localization of primary aldosteronism, Chung Hua I Hsueh Tsa Chih (Taipei) 53:7–12, 1994.
134. Rossi GP, Chiesura-Corona M, Tregnaghi A, et al: Imaging of aldosterone-secreting adenomas: a prospective comparison of computed tomography and magnetic resonance imaging in 27 patients with suspected primary aldosteronism, J Hum Hypertens 7:357–363, 1993.
135. Dunnick NR, Leight GS Jr, Roubidoux MA, et al: CT in the diagnosis of primary aldosteronism: sensitivity in 29 patients, Am J Roentgenol 160:321–324, 1993.
136. Korobkin M, Brodeur FJ, Yutzy GG, et al: Differentiation of adrenal adenomas from nonadenomas using CT attenuation values, Am J Roentgenol 166:531–536, 1996.
137. Terachi T, Matsuda T, Terai A, et al: Transperitoneal laparoscopic adrenalectomy: experience in 100 patients, J Endourol 11:361–365, 1997.
138. Rutherford JC, Stowasser M, Tunny TJ, et al: Laparoscopic adrenalectomy, World J Surg 20:758–760, 1996.
139. Nakada T, Kubota Y, Sasagawa I, et al: Therapeutic outcome of primary aldosteronism: adrenalectomy versus enucleation of aldosterone-producing adenoma, J Urol 153:1775–1780, 1995.
140. Ishidoya S, Ito A, Sakai K, et al: Laparoscopic partial versus total adrenalectomy for aldosterone producing adenoma, J Urol 174:40–43, 2005.
141. Itoh N, Kumamoto Y, Akagashi K, et al: Study of the predictive factors of postoperative blood pressure in cases with primary aldosteronism, Nippon Naibunpi Gakkai Zasshi 67:1211–1218, 1991.
142. Horky K, Widimsky J Jr, Hradec E, et al: Long-term results of surgical and conservative treatment of patients with primary aldosteronism, Exp Clin Endocrinol 90:337–346, 1987.
143. Sawaka AM, Young WF Jr, Thompson GB, et al: Primary aldosteronism: factors associated with normalization of blood pressure after surgery, Ann Intern Med 135:258–261, 2001.
144. Kater CE, Biglieri EG, Schambelan M, et al: Studies of impaired aldosterone response to spironolactone-induced renin and potassium elevations in adenomatous but not hyperplastic primary aldosteronism, Hypertension 5:V115–V121, 1983.
145. Burgess ED, Lacourciere Y, Ruilope-Urioste LM, et al: Long-term safety and efficacy of the selective aldosterone blocker eplerenone in patients with essential hypertension, Clin Ther 25:2388–2404, 2003.
146. Weinerger MH, Roniker B, Krause SL, et al: Eplerenone, a selective aldosterone blocker, in mild to moderate hypertension, Am J Hypertens 15:709–716, 2002.
147. Pitt B, Remme W, Zannad F, et al: Eplerenone, a selective aldosterone blocker, in patients with left ventricular dysfunction after myocardial infarction, N Engl J Med 348:1309–1321, 2003.
148. Baer L, Sommers SC, Krakoff LR, et al: Pseudo-primary aldosteronism: an entity distinct from primary aldosteronism, Circ Res 27:203–220, 1970.
149. Gunnels JC Jr, Bath NM, Sode J, et al: Primary aldosteronism, Arch Intern Med 120:568–574, 1968.
150. Priestley JT, Ferris DOP, ReMine WH, et al: Primary aldosteronsim: surgical management and pathologic findings, Mayo Clin Proc 43:761–775, 1968.
151. Rhamy RK, McCoy RM, Scott HW Jr, et al: Primary aldosteronsim: experience with current diagnostic criteria and surgical treatment in fourteen patients, Ann Surg 167:718–727, 1968.
152. Nadler JL, Hsueh W, Horton R: Therapeutic effect of calcium channel blockade in primary aldosteronism, J Clin Endocrinol Metab 60:896–899, 1985.
153. Stimpel M, Ivens K, Wambach G, et al: Are calcium antagonists helpful in the management of primary aldosteronism? J Cardiovasc Pharmacol 12(Suppl 6):S131–S134, 1988.
154. Opocher G, Rocco S, Murgia A, et al: Effect of verapamil on aldosterone secretion in primary aldosteronism, J Endocrinol Invest 10:491–494, 1987.
155. Bursztyn M, Grossman E, Rosenthal T: The absence of long-term therapeutic effect of calcium channel blockade in the primary aldosteronism of adrenal adenomas, Am J Hypertens 1:88S–90S, 1988.
156. Kramer HJ, Glanzer K, Sorger M: The role of endogenous inhibition of Na-K-ATPase in human hypertension—sodium pump activity as a determinant of

peripheral vascular resistance, Clin Exp Hypertens [A] 7:769–782, 1985.

157. Griffing GT, Melby JC: The therapeutic use of a new potassium-sparing diuretic, amiloride, and a converting enzyme inhibitor, MK-421, in preventing hypokalemia associated with primary and secondary hyperaldosteronism, Clin Exp Hypertens [A] 5:779–801, 1983.

158. Winterberg B, Vetter W, Groth H, et al: Primary aldosteronism: treatment with trilostane, Cardiology 72(Suppl 1):117–121, 1985.

159. Tenschert W, Maurer R, Vetter H, et al: Primary aldosteronism by carcinoma of the adrenal cortex, Klin Wochenschr 65:428–432, 1987.

160. Farge D, Pagny JY, Chatellier G, et al: Malignant adrenal cortex carcinoma revealed by an isolated picture of primary hyperaldosteronism, Arch Mal Coeur Vaiss 81:83–87, 1988.

161. Farge D, Chatellier G, Pagny JY, et al: Isolated clinical syndrome of primary aldosteronism in four patients with adrenocortical carcinoma, Am J Med 83:635–640, 1987.

162. Arteaga E, Biglieri EG, Kater CE, et al: Aldosterone-producing adrenocortical carcinoma. Preoperative recognition and course in three cases, Ann Intern Med 101:316–321, 1984.

163. Salassa TM, Weeks RE, Northcutt RC, et al: Primary aldosteronism and malignant adrenocortical neoplasia, Trans Am Clin Climatol Assoc 86:163–172, 1975.

164. Isles CG, MacDougall IC, Lever AF, et al: Hypermineralocorticoidism due to adrenal carcinoma: Plasma corticosteroids and their response to ACTH and angiotensin II, Clin Endocrinol (Oxf) 26:239–251, 1987.

165. Ludvik B, Niederle B, Roka R, et al: Malignant aldosteronoma in the differential diagnosis of Conn syndrome, Acta Med Austr 15:117–120, 1988.

166. Sutherland DJ, Ruse JL, Laidlaw JC: Hypertension, increased aldosterone secretion and low plasma renin activity relieved by dexamethasone, CMAJ 95:1109–1119, 1966.

167. Fallo D: Dexamethasone-suppressible hyperaldosteronism. In Biglieri EG, editor: Endocrine Hypertension, New York, 1990, Raven Press, pp 87–97.

168. Fallo F, Sonino N, Armanini D, et al: A new family with dexamethasone-suppressible hyperaldosteronism: aldosterone unresponsiveness to angiotensin II, Clin Endocrinol (Oxf) 22:777–785, 1985.

169. Grim CE, Weinberger MH: Familial, dexamethasone-suppressible, normokalemic hyperaldosteronism, Pediatrics 65:597–604, 1980.

170. Gill JR Jr, Bartter FC: Overproduction of sodium-retaining steroids by the zona glomerulosa is adrenocorticotropin-dependent and mediates hypertension in dexamethasone-suppressible aldosteronism, J Clin Endocrinol Metab 53:331–337, 1981.

171. Biglieri EG, Herron MA, Brust N: 17-Hydroxylation deficiency in man, J Clin Invest 45:1946–1954, 1966.

172. Miller WL: Steroid 17alpha-hydroxylase deficiency—not rare everywhere, J Clin Endocrinol Metab 89:40–42, 2004.

173. Matteson KJ, Picado-Leonard J, Chung BC, et al: Assignment of the gene for adrenal P450c17 (steroid 17 alpha-hydroxylase/17,20 lyase) to human chromosome 10, J Clin Endocrinol Metab 63:789–791, 1986.

174. Picado-Leonard J, Miller WL: Cloning and sequence of the human gene for P450c17 (steroid 17 alpha-hydroxylase/17,20 lyase): similarity with the gene for P450c21, DNA 6:439–448, 1987.

175. Ulick S, Levine LS, Gunczler P, et al: A syndrome of apparent mineralocorticoid excess associated with defects in the peripheral metabolism of cortisol, J Clin Endocrinol Metab 49:757–764, 1979.

176. Yanase T, Simpson ER, Waterman MR: 17 alpha-hydroxylase/17,20-lyase deficiency: from clinical investigation to molecular definition, Endocr Rev 12:91–108, 1991.

177. Peter M, Sippell WG, Wernze H: Diagnosis and treatment of 17-hydroxylase deficiency, J Steroid Biochem Mol Biol 45:107–116, 1993.

178. Mantero F, Opocher G, Rocco S, et al: Long-term treatment of mineralocorticoid excess syndromes, Steroids 60:81–86, 1995.

179. Kater CE, Biglieri EG: Disorders of steroid 17 alpha-hydroxylase deficiency, Endocrinol Metab Clin North Am 23:341–357, 1994.

180. Zachmann M, Tassinari D, Prader A: Clinical and biochemical variability of congenital adrenal hyperplasia due to 11 beta-hydroxylase deficiency. A study of 25 patients, J Clin Endocrinol Metab 56:222–229, 1983.

181. de Simone G, Tommaselli AP, Rossi R, et al: Partial deficiency of adrenal 11-hydroxylase. A possible cause of primary hypertension, Hypertension 7:204–210, 1985.

182. White PC, Curnow KM, Pascoe L: Disorders of steroid 11 beta-hydroxylase isozymes, Endocr Rev 15:421–438, 1994.

183. Mimouni M, Kaufman H, Roitman A, et al: Hypertension in a neonate with 11 beta-hydroxylase deficiency, Eur J Pediatr 143:231–233, 1985.

184. Rosler A, Leiberman E, Sack J, et al: Clinical variability of congenital adrenal hyperplasia due to 11 beta-hydroxylase deficiency, Horm Res 16:133–141, 1982.

185. Biglieri EG, Irony I, Kater CE: Identification and implications of new types of mineralocorticoid hypertension, J Steroid Biochem 32:199–204, 1989.

186. Irony I, Biglieri EG, Perloff D, et al: Pathophysiology of deoxycorticosterone-secreting adrenal tumors, J Clin Endocrinol Metab 65:836–840, 1987.

187. Mussig K, Wehrmann M, Horger M, et al: Adrenocortical carcinoma producing 11-deoxycorticosterone: a rare cause of mineralocorticoid hypertension, J Endocrinol Invest 28:61–65, 2005.

188. Makino K, Yasuda K, Okuyama M, et al: An adrenocortical tumor secreting weak mineralocorticoids, Endocrinol Jpn 34:65–72, 1987.

189. Powell-Jackson JD, Calin A, Fraser R, et al: Excess deoxycorticosterone secretion from adrenocortical carcinoma, Br Med J 2:32–33, 1974.

190. Aupetit-Faisant B, Battaglia C, Zenatti M, et al: Hypoaldosteronism accompanied by normal or elevated mineralocorticosteroid pathway steroid: a marker of adrenal carcinoma, J Clin Endocrinol Metab 76:38–43, 1993.

191. Fraser R, James VH, Landon J, et al: Clinical and biochemical studies of a patient with a corticosterone-secreting adrenocortical tumour, Lancet 2:1116–1120, 1968.

192. Quinkler M, Stewart PM: Hypertension and the cortisol-cortisone shuttle, J Clin Endocrinol Metab 88:2384–2392, 2003.

193. Chemaitilly W, Wilson RC, New MI: Hypertension and adrenal disorders, Curr Hypertens Rep 5:498–504, 2003.

194. Palermo M, Quinkler M, Stewart PM: Apparent mineralocorticoid excess syndrome: an overview, Arq Bras Endocrinol Metabol 48:687–696, 2004.

195. Palermo M, Shackleton CH, Mantero F: Urinary free cortisone and the assessment of 11 beta-hydroxysteroid dehydrogenase activity in man, Clin Endocrinol (Oxf) 45:605–611, 1996.

196. Palermo M, Delitala G, Mantero F: Congenital deficiency of 11beta-hydroxysteroid dehydrogenase (apparent mineralocorticoid excess syndrome): diagnostic value of urinary free cortisol and cortisone, J Endocrinol Invest 24:17–23, 2001.

197. Stewart PM, Corrie JE, Shackleton CH, et al: Syndrome of apparent mineralocorticoid excess. A defect in the cortisol-cortisone shuttle, J Clin Invest 82:340–349, 1988.

198. Speiser PW, Riddick LM, Martin K, et al: Investigation of the mechanism of hypertension in apparent mineralocorticoid excess, Metabolism 42:843–845, 1993.

199. Dave-Sharma S, Wilson RC, Harbison MD, et al: Examination of genotype and phenotype relationships in 14 patients with apparent mineralocorticoid excess, J Clin Endocrinol Metab 83:2244–2254, 1998.

200. Palermo M, Cossu M, Shackleton CH: Cure of apparent mineralocorticoid excess by kidney transplantation, N Engl J Med 339:1787–1788, 1998.

201. Epstein MT, Espiner EA, Donald RA, et al: Liquorice toxicity and the renin-angiotensin-aldosterone axis in man, Br Med J 1:209–210, 1977.

202. Epstein MT, Espiner EA, Donald RA, et al: Effect of eating liquorice on the renin-angiotensin aldosterone axis in normal subjects, Br Med J 1:488–490, 1977.

203. Farese RV Jr, Biglieri EG, Shackleton CH, et al: Licorice-induced hypermineralocorticoidism, N Engl J Med 325:1223–1227, 1991.

204. MacKenzie MA, Hoefnagels WH, Jansen RW, et al: The influence of glycyrrhetinic acid on plasma cortisol and cortisone in healthy young volunteers, J Clin Endocrinol Metab 70:1637–1643, 1990.

205. Sigurjonsdottir HA, Franzson L, Manhem K, et al: Liquorice-induced rise in blood pressure: a linear dose-response relationship, J Hum Hypertens 15:549–552, 2001.

206. Armanini D, Karbowiak I, Funder JW: Affinity of liquorice derivatives for mineralocorticoid and glucocorticoid receptors, Clin Endocrinol (Oxf) 19:609–612, 1993.

207. Girerd RJ, Rassaert CL, Dipasquale G, et al: Endocrine involvement in licorice hypertension, Am J Physiol 198:718–720, 1960.

208. Molhuysen JA, Gerbrandy J, de Vries LA, et al: A liquorice extract with deoxycortone-like action, Lancet 2:381–386, 1950.

209. Monder C, Stewart PM, Lakshmi V, et al: Licorice inhibits corticosteroid 11 beta-dehydrogenase of rat kidney and liver: in vivo and in vitro studies, Endocrinology 125:1046–1053, 1989.

210. Stewart PM, Wallace AM, Atherden SM, et al: Mineralocorticoid activity of carbenoxolone: contrasting effects of carbenoxolone and liquorice on 11 beta-hydroxysteroid dehydrogenase activity in man, Clin Sci (Lond) 78:49–54, 1990.

211. Morris DJ, Souness GW: The 11 beta-OHSD inhibitor, carbenoxolone, enhances Na retention by aldosterone and 11-deoxycorticosterone, Am J Physiol 258:F756–F759, 1990.

212. Liddle GW, Givens JR, Nicholson WE, et al: The ectopic ACTH syndrome, Cancer Res 25:1057–1061, 1965.

213. Ulick S, Wang JZ, Blumenfeld JD, et al: Cortisol inactivation overload: a mechanism of mineralocorticoid hypertension in the ectopic adrenocorticotropin syndrome, J Clin Endocrinol Metab 74:963–967, 1992.

214. Vingerhoeds AC, Thijssen JH, Schwarz F: Spontaneous hypercortisolism without Cushing's syndrome, J Clin Endocrinol Metab 43:1128–1133, 1976.

215. Walker BR, Campbell JC, Fraser R, et al: Mineralocorticoid excess and inhibition of 11 beta-hydroxysteroid dehydrogenase in patients with ectopic ACTH syndrome, Clin Endocrinol (Oxf) 37:483–492, 1992.

216. Mechanick JI, Morris JC: Clinical case seminar: Hypokalemia in a 52-year-old woman with non-small cell lung cancer, J Clin Endocrinol Metab 80:1769–1773, 1995.

217. Charmandari E, Kino T, Chrousos GP: Familial/sporadic glucocorticoid resistance: clinical phenotype and molecular mechanisms, Ann N Y Acad Sci 1024:168–181, 2004.

218. Lamberts SW, Koper JW, Biemond P, et al: Cortisol receptor resistance: the variability of its clinical presentation and response to treatment, J Clin Endocrinol Metab 74:313–321, 1992.

219. Huizenga NA, de Lange P, Koper JW, et al: Five patients with biochemical and/or clinical generalized glucocorticoid resistance without alterations in the glucocorticoid receptor gene, J Clin Endocrinol Metab 85:2076–2081, 2000.

220. Brandon DD, Markwick AJ, Chrousos GP, et al: Glucocorticoid resistance in humans and nonhuman primates, Cancer Res 49(8 Suppl):2203s–2213s, 1989.

221. Buhler FR, Bolli P, Kiowski W, et al: Renin profiling to select antihypertensive baseline drugs. Renin inhibitors for high-renin and calcium entry blockers for low-renin patients, Am J Med 77:36–42, 1984.

222. Nishizaka MK, Zaman MA, Calhoun DA: Efficacy of low-dose spironolactone in subjects with resistant hypertension, Am J Hypertens 16:925–930, 2003.

223. Weinberger MH, White WB, Ruilope LM, et al: Effects of eplerenone versus losartan in patients with low-renin hypertension, Am Heart J 150:426–433, 2005.

224. Ganguly A, Weinberger MH: Low renin hypertension: a current review of definitions and controversies, Am Heart J 98:642–652, 1979.

225. Melby SC, Dale SL: Adrenocorticosteroids in experimental and human hypertension, J Endocrinol 81:93P–106P, 1979.

226. Walker BR, Stewart PM, Shackleton CH, et al: Deficient inactivation of cortisol by 11 beta-hydroxysteroid dehydrogenase in essential hypertension, Clin Endocrinol (Oxf) 39:221–227, 1993.

227. Soro A, Ingram MC, Tonolo G, et al: Evidence of coexisting changes in 11 beta-hydroxysteroid dehydrogenase and 5 beta-reductase activity in subjects with untreated essential hypertension, Hypertension 25:67–70, 1995.

228. Agarwal AK, Giacchetti G, Lavery G, et al: CA-Repeat polymorphism in intron 1 of HSD11B2: effects on gene expression and salt sensitivity, Hypertension 36:187–194, 2000.

229. Lovati E, Ferrari P, Dick B, et al: Molecular basis of human salt sensitivity: the role of the 11beta-hydroxysteroid dehydrogenase type 2, J Clin Endocrinol Metab 84:3745–3749, 1999.

230. White PC, Agarwal AK, Li A, et al: Possible association but no linkage of the HSD11B2 gene encoding the kidney isozyme of 11beta-hydroxysteroid dehydrogenase to hypertension in Black people, Clin Endocrinol (Oxf) 55:249–252, 2001.

231. Mantero F, Armanini D, Opocher G, et al: Mineralocorticoid hypertension due to a nasal spray containing 9 alpha-fluoroprednisolone, Am J Med 71:352–357, 1981.

232. Geller DS, Farhi A, Pinkerton N, et al: Activating mineralocorticoid receptor mutation in hypertension exacerbated by pregnancy, Science 289:119–123, 2000.

233. Drucker WD, Hendrikx A, Laragh JH, et al: Effect of administered aldosterone upon electrolyte excretion during and after pregnancy in two women with adrenal cortical insufficiency, J Clin Endocrinol Metab 23:1247–1255, 1963.

234. Sansom S, Muto S, Giebisch G: Na-dependent effects of DOCA on cellular transport properties of CCDs from ADX rabbits, Am J Physiol 253:F753–F759, 1987.

235. Schafer JA, Hawk CT: Regulation of Na$^+$ channels in the cortical collecting duct by AVP and mineralocorticoids, Kidney Int 41:255–268, 1992.

236. Kellenberger S, Gautschi I, Rossier BC, et al: Mutations causing Liddle syndrome reduce sodium-dependent downregulation of the epithelial sodium channel in the Xenopus oocyte expression system, J Clin Invest 101:2741–2750, 1998.

237. Canessa CM, Schild L, Buell G, et al: Amiloride-sensitive epithelial Na+ channel is made of three homologous subunits, Nature 367:463–467, 1994.

238. Furuhashi M, Kitamura K, Adachi M, et al: Liddle's syndrome caused by a novel mutation in the proline-rich PY motif of the epithelial sodium channel beta-subunit, J Clin Endocrinol Metab 90:340–344, 2005.

239. Hansson JH, Schild L, Lu Y, et al: A de novo missense mutation of the beta subunit of the epithelial sodium channel causes hypertension and Liddle syndrome, identifying a proline-rich segment critical for regulation of channel activity, Proc Natl Acad Sci U S A 92:11495–11499, 1995.

240. Rayner BL, Owen EP, King JA, et al: A new mutation, R563Q, of the beta subunit of the epithelial sodium channel associated with low-renin, low-aldosterone hypertension, J Hypertens 21:921–926, 2003.

241. Schild L, Canessa CM, Shimkets RA, et al: A mutation in the epithelial sodium channel causing Liddle disease increases channel activity in the Xenopus laevis oocyte expression system, Proc Natl Acad Sci U S A 92:5699–5703, 1995.

242. Shimkets RA, Warnock DG, Bositis CM, et al: Liddle's syndrome: heritable human hypertension caused by mutations in the beta subunit of the epithelial sodium channel, Cell 79:407–414, 1994.

243. Snyder PM, Price MP, McDonald FJ, et al: Mechanism by which Liddle's syndrome mutations increase activity of a human epithelial Na+ channel, Cell 83:969–978, 1995.

244. Abriel H, Loffing J, Rebhun JF, et al: Defective regulation of the epithelial Na+ channel by Nedd4 in Liddle's syndrome, J Clin Invest 103:667–673, 1999.

245. Goulet CC, Volk KA, Adams CM, et al: Inhibition of the epithelial Na+ channel by interaction of Nedd4 with a PY motif deleted in Liddle's syndrome, J Biol Chem 273:30012–30017, 1998.

246. Botero-Velez M, Curtis JJ, Warnock DG: Brief report: Liddle's syndrome revisited—a disorder of sodium reabsorption in the distal tubule, N Engl J Med 330:178–181, 1994.

247. Palmer BF, Alpern RJ: Liddle's syndrome, Am J Med 104:301–309, 1998.

Chapter 13

MINERALOCORTICOID DEFICIENCY

PAUL M. STEWART and MARCUS QUINKLER

Mineralocorticoid Hormone Action
Biosynthesis
Mineralocorticoid Receptor

Failure of Aldosterone Biosynthesis: Hypoaldosteronism
Combined Glucocorticoid and Mineralocorticoid
   Deficiencies: Adrenal Failure
Isolated Hypoaldosteronism
Syndrome of Hyporeninemic Hypoaldosteronism
Postadrenalectomy Hypoaldosteronism
Pharmacologic Inhibition of Aldosterone

Failure of Aldosterone Action: Mineralocorticoid Resistance
Pseudohypoaldosteronism

Mineralocorticoid Hormone Action

BIOSYNTHESIS

Aldosterone is the principal mineralocorticoid secreted from the outer zona glomerulosa of the adrenal cortex. The daily production rate is approximately 100 to 150 μg/day, compared to the production of cortisol, the principal glucocorticoid, which is 10 to 15 mg/day. Aldosterone biosynthesis is facilitated through the functional zonation of the adrenal cortex, that is, the zonal-specific expression of key steroidogenic enzymes, principally the expression of the product of the *CYP11B2* gene, aldosterone synthase, in the zona glomerulosa. Conversely, the absence of CYP17 in the zona glomerulosa explains why glucocorticoids are not synthesized in this layer. Synthesis is regulated by three principal secretagogues, adrenocorticotropic hormone (ACTH), potassium, and angiotensin II, but of these, angiotensin II plays a dominant role, principally by stimulating aldosterone synthase expression and activity via second messenger pathways that include increased intracellular calcium and induction of calcium/calmodulin-dependent protein kinase.[1]

The renin-angiotensin-aldosterone axis represents a tightly controlled feedback mechanism regulating salt and water homeostasis and blood pressure control. Renin secreted by the juxta-glomerular apparatus of the macula densa in the nephron in response to hypotension, low perfusion pressure, or low sodium concentration cleaves angiotensinogen to angiotensin I. This in turn is acted upon by angiotensin-converting enzyme to yield angiotensin II, which directly stimulates aldosterone secretion. The combined action of angiotensin II and aldosterone to raise blood pressure and increase epithelial sodium reabsorption switches off renin secretion, thereby completing the feedback loop. In addition, hyperkalemia stimulates aldosterone secretion, whereas hypokalemia suppresses it.

MINERALOCORTICOID RECEPTOR

The mineralocorticoid receptor (MR) is a ligand-activated transcription factor of the steroid/thyroid/retinoid superfamily of intracellular receptors. The *MR* gene contains 10 exons, spans over 400 kb, encodes a protein of 984 amino acids and is located on chromosome 4q31.1-4q31.2.[2] Exon 2 contains the translation start site. Alternative transcription of two 5′-untranslated exons (exons 1α and 1β) produces two mRNA isoforms, MRα and MRβ, which are coexpressed in aldosterone target tissues. The MR is expressed mainly in epithelial cells of the distal tubules and collecting duct of the kidney, the distal colon, and the ducts of salivary and sweat glands, as well as in nonepithelial tissues such as the heart, the vasculature, and certain regions of the central nervous system, particularly the hippocampus. The MR is composed of an amino-terminal region that harbors a ligand-independent transactivation function, a centrally located, highly conserved DNA-binding domain, and a complex C-terminal domain responsible for ligand binding and ligand-dependent transactivation. In the absence of ligand, the MR is located mainly in the cytoplasm, associated with chaperone proteins. Upon hormone binding, the MR dissociates from chaperone proteins such as heat shock protein hsp90, hsp70, p23, and p48 proteins, undergoes nuclear translocation in response to localization signals (NLS0, NSL1, and NSL2) and interacts with coactivators (e.g., steroid receptor coactivator 1 [SRC-1]) or corepressors (e.g., SMRT and PIAS1) at the mineralocorticoid response elements. Several MR target genes have been identified so far, such as the amiloride-sensitive epithelial sodium channel in the apical membrane, basolateral Na$^+$,K$^+$-ATPase pump, serum and glucocorticoid–regulated kinase 1 (sgk1), K-ras2-gene, elongation factor ELL, ERK cascade inhibitor GILZ (glucocorticoid-induced leucine zipper protein), plasminogen activator inhibitor

1 (PAI-1), endothelin 1 (ET-1), ubiquitin-specific protease 2-45 (Usp2-45), and channel-inducing factor (CHIF).[3,4] Several down-regulated genes have also been identified.

One paradox was that the cloned MR had a similar affinity for aldosterone and cortisol. At a pre-receptor level, the autocrine expression of the type 2 isozyme of 11β-hydroxysteroid dehydrogenase ensures the inactivation of the higher concentrations of cortisol, thereby permitting aldosterone to bind to the MR in vivo.[5,6]

The classical action of aldosterone is to stimulate epithelial sodium transport. This involves early and late pathways, both of which are mediated via the MR. The principal effector pathway in mediating this sodium transport is the epithelial sodium channel (ENaC), a highly selective sodium channel found at the apical surface of tight epithelia of salt-reabsorbing tissues, including the distal nephron, the distal colon, salivary and sweat glands, lung, and taste buds.[7] It plays a critical role in the control of sodium balance, extracellular fluid volume, and blood pressure, since the ENaC-mediated entry of sodium into the cell in these epithelial tissues represents the rate-limiting step for the movement of sodium from the mucosal side to the serosal side. These channels allow the transport of sodium into the cell by diffusion without coupling to the flow of other solutes and without the direct input of metabolic energy. ENaCs are often referred to as "amiloride-sensitive" because of their high sensitivity to the potassium-sparing diuretic amiloride and its analogues. These channels are stimulated by aldosterone and inhibited by amiloride.[7]

ENaCs are composed of three subunits: α, β, and γ. These three subunits are 35% homologous at the amino acid level and are conserved throughout evolution.[8] Moreover, the three subunits are similar in structure and share the following characteristics: short intracellular proline-rich C-termini, two transmembrane-spanning domains, and a large extracellular loop.[9] The α subunit has been localized to chromosome 12p13.1-pter, and the β and γ subunits have been localized to 16p12.2-13.11.[10] For optimal sodium conductance, the stoichiometry of the channel is 2α:1β:1γ subunits. It is not clear yet how such a two-α subunit stoichiometry of ENaC can be reconciled with the trimeric nature of the channel as suggested by the ASIC crystal structure.[11] Mutations in the C-terminal domains of the β and γ subunits of ENaC explain an autosomal-dominant form of low renin hypertension, Liddle's syndrome.[12-14] Here the ENaC is constitutively active, subsequently shown to occur because of loss of the C-terminal proline-rich sites that target the ENaC subunits for degradation through a ubiquitin ligase known as Nedd-4.[15]

The late-response actions of aldosterone upon sodium conductance (6 to 24 hours) involve direct induction of transcription of the α subunit. However, the early effects (<6 hours), although still operating through the MR, are not mediated directly through ENaC gene transcription. Instead, two separate groups[16,17] identified the rapid induction of sgk-1, which directly phosphorylates the Nedd4 protein that blocks the interaction with the C-terminal domains of the ENaC subunits and hence ubiquitination and degradation of the ENaC channels. This increases surface expression of ENaC and sodium conductance.

In summary, therefore, recent years have seen considerable advances in our understanding of the molecular mechanisms underpinning aldosterone-regulated epithelial sodium transport. Defining normality has uncovered the basis for clinical disorders causing mineralocorticoid deficiency (Fig. 13-1).

Failure of Aldosterone Biosynthesis: Hypoaldosteronism

COMBINED GLUCOCORTICOID AND MINERALOCORTICOID DEFICIENCIES: ADRENAL FAILURE

The causes of primary adrenal failure and its clinical features are described elsewhere. Aldosterone deficiency occurs in congenital adrenal hyperplasia due to 21-hydroxylase and 3β-hydroxysteroid dehydrogenase deficiencies. Patients with 11β-hydroxylase or 17α-hydroxylase deficiency also have hypoaldosteronism but have mineralocorticoid excess because of excess secretion of the mineralocorticoid deoxycorticosterone (DOC) proximal to the enzymatic block. At presentation, most patients with primary autoimmune adrenal failure have evidence of both glucocorticoid and mineralocorticoid deficiency. However, as adrenal failure evolves, selective aldosterone deficiency can occur in the presence of preserved zona fasciculata function. While glucocorticoid responsiveness to ACTH, metyrapone, or insulin-induced hypoglycemia may be normal, plasma renin activity (PRA) is elevated, and plasma aldosterone levels are low or undetectable. This is accompanied by mild metabolic acidosis and, occasionally, hyponatremia. With time, progression to "panadrenal" insufficiency can occur. A year or more can separate the onset of the mineralocorticoid and glucocorticoid deficiencies.[18-20]

It is important to recognize that mineralocorticoid deficiency is not a feature of secondary adrenal failure, caused by hypothalamic or pituitary disease, because the renin-angiotensin system is not affected.

Primary adrenal hypoplasia often affects the zona glomerulosa, causing mineralocorticoid insufficiency and salt loss, as well as impaired glucocorticoid synthesis and release. Mutations in DAX1 (dosage-sensitive sex reversal adrenal hypoplasia congenita–critical region on the X chromosome gene 1) cause X-linked adrenal hypoplasia congenita (AHC).[21] The patients are characterized by primary adrenal failure (combined glucocorticoid and mineralocorticoid deficiency), testicular dysgenesis, and gonadotropin deficiency. Most DAX1 mutations are deletions, nonsense, or frameshift mutations that markedly impair its transcriptional activity. Mild DAX1 mutations, such as the missense mutation (W105C) in the amino-terminal region of the DAX1 gene, are associated with more variable clinical phenotypes and may be a cause of isolated mineralocorticoid deficiency.[22] Aldosterone deficiency also occurs in 10% to 15% of individuals who have ACTH resistance as part of the triple A (Allgrove) syndrome (AAAS, ALADIN), with isolated adrenal failure, alacrima, or upper-gastrointestinal abnormalities such as achalasia of the esophagus.[23] Severe loss-of-function mutations in the MC2R (ACTH-receptor) gene, which is expressed also in the zona glomerulosa, may be found in a significant proportion of children with primary adrenal insufficiency, e.g., familial glucocorticoid deficiency type 1 (FGD1) and who have been diagnosed as having salt-losing forms of adrenal hypoplasia. These findings may suggest a supportive role for ACTH in mineralocorticoid synthesis and release, especially in times of stress (e.g., infection), salt-restriction, heat, or relative mineralocorticoid insensitivity.[24] Mineralocorticoid requirements often decrease with age, as evidenced by the fall in normal mineralocorticoid secretion rates after infancy.

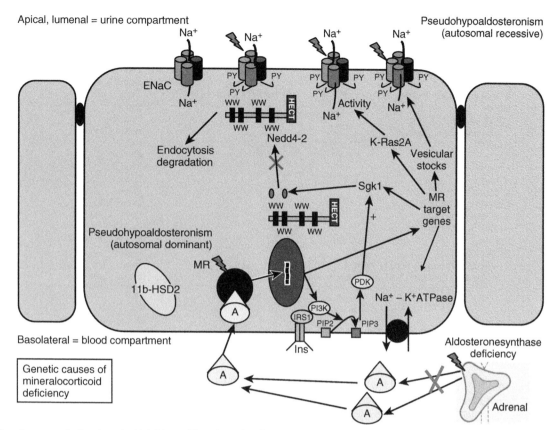

FIGURE 13-1. Genetic causes of mineralocorticoid deficiency. The schematic cell represents a renal cell from the distal tubule/collecting duct segment, which expresses the mineralocorticoid receptor (MR), is aldosterone (A) sensitive, and expresses 11β-hydroxysteroid dehydrogenase type 2 (11β-HSD2), serum and glucocorticoid–regulated kinase 1 (sgk1), and the epithelial sodium channel (ENaC). *CHIF*, Channel-inducing factor; *ERK*, extracellular signal-regulated kinase; *GILZ*, glucocorticoid-induced leucine zipper protein.

ISOLATED HYPOALDOSTERONISM

Selective deficiency of aldosterone secretion without alteration in cortisol production can result from inborn errors in aldosterone biosynthesis, failure of the zona-glomerulosa function of the adrenal gland secondary to drugs, surgery, or the syndrome of hyporeninemic hypoaldosteronism.

Primary Isolated Hypoaldosteronism

Prior to the characterization of the *CYP11B2* gene, which is located on chromosome 8q24,[25,26] the disease was termed *corticosterone methyl oxidase type I (CMO I) deficiency* and *corticosterone methyl oxidase type II (CMO II) deficiency*. Subsequently, both variants were shown to be secondary to mutations in aldosterone synthase and are now termed *type 1 and type 2 aldosterone synthase deficiency*. Aldosterone synthase catalyses the three terminal steps of aldosterone biosynthesis, 11β-hydroxylation of deoxycorticosterone to corticosterone, 18-hydroxylation to 18-hydroxycorticosterone, and 18-oxidation to aldosterone. Patients with type 1 aldosterone synthase deficiency have low to normal levels of 18-hydroxycorticosterone but undetectable levels of aldosterone (or urinary tetrahydroaldosterone), whereas patients with the type 2 variant have high levels of 18-hydroxycorticosterone and only subnormal or even normal levels of aldosterone. This suggests blockade of only the terminal 18-oxidation step, with some residual aldosterone synthase activity. The explanation for the variable biochemical phenotype is unknown, particularly now that the same mutation in the *CYP11B2* gene has been

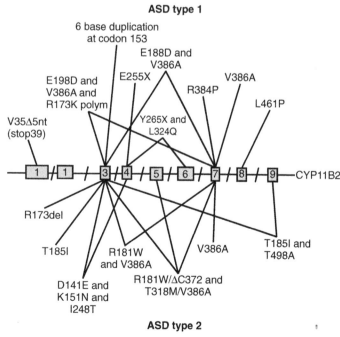

FIGURE 13-2. Schematic representation of identified mutations in the *CYP11B2* gene. The *CYP11B2* gene is represented with its intron/exon structure. Mutations found for aldosterone synthase deficiency (ASD) type 1 are shown *above* the gene structure; those responsible for ASD type 2 are presented *below* the gene structure.

Table 13-1. Aldosterone Synthase Deficiency Type 1 and Type 2

Type	Mutation	Location	Author
1	V35Δ5nt→stop 39	Exon 1	28
1	6 base duplication at codon 153	Exon 3	29
1	E188D and V386A	Exons 3 and 7	30
1	E198D and V386A and polymorphism R173K	Exons 3 and 7	31
1	E255X	Exon 4	32, 33
1	E255X and Q272X stop	Exon 4	34
1	Y265X and L324Q CH	Exons 4 and 6	30
1	R384P	Exon 7	35
1	L451F	Exon 8	36
1	L461P	Exon 8	37
1 or 2	V386A (heterozygous)	Exon 7	33, 38
2	R173del	Exon 3	39
2	R181W and V386A	Exons 3 and 7	28, 40, 41
2	R181W and A319V	Exons 3 and 6	41
2	T185I	Exon 3	42
2	R181W / ΔC372 and T318M / V386A CH	Exons 3, 5, and 7	43
2	GC(435Gly)	Exon 8	44
2	T185I (C554T) and A1492G (T498A) CH	Exons 3 and 9	45
2	D141E and K151N and I248T (gene conversion with *CYP11B1*)	Exons 3 and 4	46

CH, Compound heterozygous.

uncovered in both variants (Fig. 13-2, Table 13-1). It is possible that this may reflect polymorphic variants in the residual and normal product of the *CYP11B1* gene, 11β-hydroxylase.

At variance with the MR knockout mouse model, the aldosterone synthase knockout mouse model is not lethal. As expected, ionic homeostasis is altered in the absence of aldosterone, but high levels of corticosterone and angiotensin II seem to partially rescue sodium balance,[27] underscoring the importance of the MR over its ligand, aldosterone.

Both variants of aldosterone synthase deficiency are rare and inherited as autosomal-recessive traits (see Table 13-1). The type 2 deficiency is found most frequently among Jews of Iranian origin.

The severity of the clinical manifestations is inversely related to the age at diagnosis in both variants. In most infants, the disorders become less severe as the child ages. Aldosterone synthase type 2 deficiency becomes clinically apparent between 1 week and 3 months of age, with severe dehydration, vomiting, and failure to grow and thrive. Hyponatremia, hyperkalemia, and metabolic acidosis are uniformly present. The plasma renin activity is elevated, and plasma aldosterone levels are low. Plasma 18-hydroxycorticosterone levels are markedly elevated, and the ratio of 18-hydroxycorticosterone to aldosterone in plasma exceeds 5. The ratio of the urinary metabolite of 18-hydroxycorticosterone, 18-OH-THA, to the urinary metabolite of aldosterone, TH-Aldo, is also greater than 5. In older children, adolescents, and adults, the abnormal steroid pattern described may be present and may persist throughout life without clinical manifestations. Recently, type 1 aldosterone synthase deficiency has been reported with onset in middle age. Mineralocorticoids are given (9α-fludrocortisone) during infancy and early childhood, but this therapy can be discontinued in the majority of adults. Spontaneous "normalization" of growth can occur in untreated patients. It is not understood why aldosterone deficiency is so much more threatening in infancy than in adult life. It is particularly puzzling that isolated hypoaldosteronism due to low renin secretion in aging patients has clinical significance, while patients with asymptomatic inherited hypoaldosteronism due to aldosterone synthase deficiency exhibit none of the manifestations of hyporeninemic hypoaldosteronism.

Secondary Isolated Hypoaldosteronism

Hyperreninemic hypoaldosteronism can occur in critically ill patients with disorders such as sepsis, cardiogenic shock, or liver cirrhosis.[47,48] Cortisol levels in these patients are elevated and commensurate with the level of stress. In normal subjects, aldosterone, corticosterone, and 18-hydroxycorticosterone levels can be suppressed in 48 to 96 hours with continuous ACTH stimulation.[49-51] Prolonged ACTH secretion is thought to impair aldosterone synthase activity and explain the underlying mechanism of this syndrome. These patients have an increased ratio of plasma 18-hydroxycorticosterone to aldosterone, and the aldosterone response to angiotensin II infusion is impaired. Hypoxia and proinflammatory cytokines may be additional mechanisms that inhibit aldosterone synthesis from the zona glomerulosa, as may elevated circulating levels of atrial natriuretic peptide (ANP).[52] Additionally, many critically ill patients are taking medications that can interfere with aldosterone production (see later). Hyperreninemic hypoaldosteronism is also reported in patients with tumors that have metastasized to the adrenals.

Since no major clinical complications are reported with this form of hypoaldosteronism, it seldom requires treatment. Avoidance of drugs and factors that can exacerbate the condition, however, is essential.

SYNDROME OF HYPORENINEMIC HYPOALDOSTERONISM

The syndrome of hyporeninemic hypoaldosteronism (SHH), also referred to as *type 4 distal renal tubular acidosis* (RTA), is not uncommon and usually occurs in late middle age (median age 68 years) in males more than females. Underlying diabetes mellitus is present in 50% of cases and chronic renal insufficiency in 80% of cases. It is frequent in patients with tubulointerstitial forms of renal disease but has been described in virtually every type of renal abnormality.[53-56] SHH accounts for 50% to 70% of patients with unexplained hyperkalemia and renal disease in patients with relatively preserved glomerular filtration rate (GFR).[53,55,56]

Patients have low PRA and aldosterone levels that cannot be stimulated by provocative tests. Hyperchloremic metabolic acidosis occurs in about 70%, and mild to moderate hyponatremia is seen in about 50% of affected patients. Hyperkalemia that is out of proportion to the degree of renal insufficiency is observed in all patients.[55,56] The pathogenesis is unknown, but proposed mechanisms include hyporeninemia due to damaged juxtaglomerular apparatus, sympathetic insufficiency, altered renal prostaglandin production, and impaired conversion of prorenin to renin.[57,58] Low renin production does not appear to be the sole factor, since PRA can be normal in some patients. It is possible that some cases can be explained by sodium retention leading to volume expansion, with secondary suppression of renin and aldosterone.

The leading causes of interstitial nephritis, in which hyperkalemia occurs early and before chronic renal failure, are anatomic genitourinary abnormalities, analgesic abuse with aspirin or phenacetin, hyperuricemia, nephrocalcinosis, nephrolithiasis, and sickle cell disease. Diabetic patients are predisposed to hyperkalemia because of insulin deficiency and hyperglycemia, and this may be exacerbated by autonomic neuropathy. IgM monoclonal gammopathy has been associated with nodular glomerulosclerosis, a concentrating defect, and hyporeninemic hypoaldosteronism.[59] Patients with acquired immunodeficiency syndrome (AIDS) can have persistent hyperkalemia secondary to adrenal insufficiency or, less frequently, hyporeninemic hypoaldosteronism.

There is no ideal medical therapy for SHH. The majority of patients with mild selective hypoaldosteronism require no therapy. Treatment may be indicated in patients with severe hyperkalemia. Reducing the extracellular potassium load is the single most effective measure in controlling hyperkalemia. Reducing dietary intake of potassium is helpful. The long-term control of glucose homeostasis in diabetes mellitus may reduce the risk of developing SHH, and autonomic insufficiency is probably avoidable in well-controlled diabetes. Since many medications can interfere with the renin-aldosterone axis, avoidance of these drugs is of major importance. β-Adrenergic receptor blockers, prostaglandin synthetase inhibitors, and potassium-sparing diuretics should be avoided in patients with SHH and in diabetic patients with latent hypoaldosteronism. Calcium channel blockers, antidopaminergic agents, and drugs that impair adrenal function must be used with caution. Patients taking angiotensin-converting enzyme (ACE) inhibitors must be monitored carefully for hyperkalemia. The prolonged administration of heparin can worsen hypoaldosteronism[60] and has been associated with lethal hyperkalemia. Fludrocortisone 0.2 mg/day for 2 weeks usually normalizes potassium levels in patients with SHH,[61,62] but there is a risk of salt retention and hypertension. In severe SHH, fludrocortisone acetate, in doses of 0.1 to 1.0 mg/day (equivalent to 200 to 2000 μg aldosterone daily), can be required. Diuretics may be the optimal therapy for patients with SHH and coexisting diseases associated with sodium retention. Older patients with hypertension, mild renal impairment, and congestive heart failure respond better to diuretic therapy than to mineralocorticoid replacement. Since kaliuresis is the goal of diuretic therapy, the diuretic employed should have a potent kaliuretic activity; thiazide diuretics are more effective than loop diuretics and induce less natriuresis.

POSTADRENALECTOMY HYPOALDOSTERONISM

In a patient with a unilateral aldosteronoma (Conn's syndrome), the contralateral zona glomerulosa is frequently suppressed. Without reversal of the chronic volume expansion preoperatively, postadrenalectomy patients may develop severe hyperkalemia and hypotension lasting several days to several weeks after surgery. This may be exacerbated by the use of spironolactone preoperatively. This drug has a long half-life and should be discontinued 2 to 3 days before surgery to minimize the risk of mineralocorticoid deficiency postoperatively.

PHARMACOLOGIC INHIBITION OF ALDOSTERONE

Cyclosporin, heparin sodium, and calcium channel blockers specifically inhibit aldosterone production from the zona glomerulosa. Cyclosporin blocks angiotensin II–induced aldosterone production and inhibits "growth" and steroidogenic capacity of adrenocortical cells.[63] The latter effect may be caused by an impairment of protein synthesis. Additionally, cyclosporin and tacrolimus (FK506) inhibit MR transcription activity without affecting aldosterone binding.[64] Polysulfated glycosaminoglycans, such as heparin sodium, impair aldosterone biosynthesis. With prolonged administration, heparin sodium can produce significant hypoaldosteronism with severe hyperkalemia[65] because of a direct toxic effect on the zona glomerulosa, evidenced by a hyperreninemic hypoaldosteronism and zona glomerulosa atrophy. The least toxic dose of heparin sodium is unknown, but doses as small as 20,000 units/day for 5 days can reduce aldosterone secretion. This is an uncommon cause of hypoaldosteronism but is important to recognize because it is reversible and can be lethal. The offending agent seems to be chlorobutanol, used as a preservative for heparin, rather than the heparin molecule itself. Calcium channel blockers inhibit aldosterone production and under certain clinical conditions can impair aldosterone secretion by inhibiting calcium influx. β-Blockers and prostaglandin synthase inhibitors are frequent causes of hyporeninemic hypoaldosteronism. β-Blockers inhibit renin secretion from the juxtaglomerular apparatus, and prostaglandin synthetase inhibitors, which specifically inhibit cyclooxygenase, block renin release. ACE inhibitors and potassium-sparing diuretics can contribute to hypoaldosteronism and resultant hyperkalemia. ACE inhibitors "inhibit" ACE, thus interrupting the renin-aldosterone axis and leading to iatrogenic hypoaldosteronism. Spironolactone has two effects: it is a mineralocorticoid-receptor antagonist, and it inhibits aldosterone biosynthesis. Triamterene causes potassium retention by a direct action on non-aldosterone-mediated, distal-tubular exchange sites. Amiloride acts on the luminal surfaces of epithelial membranes to block sodium channels, resulting in less sodium resorption and potassium secretion. Drugs that impair adrenal function are increasingly used for the hormonal treatment of breast cancer and medical management of Cushing's syndrome. Most can cause hypoaldosteronism. Aminoglutethimide, metyrapone, and trilostane block various enzymatic steps in the synthesis of mineralocorticoids, glucocorticoids, and adrenal sex steroids. Lower doses of these drugs may not be associated with hyperkalemia, since aldosterone precursors such as deoxycorticosterone may supply the necessary mineralocorticoid activity. Finally, drugs affecting the dopaminergic system can produce significant alterations in aldosterone secretion. It is believed that aldosterone is under tonic dopamine inhibition. Thus, dopaminergic agonists such as bromocriptine may impair aldosterone secretion in certain physiologic situations.

Failure of Aldosterone Action: Mineralocorticoid Resistance

Mineralocorticoid resistance implies a lack of response to aldosterone despite normal or even increased concentrations. The classification of this entity has been confusing, but the elucidation of the molecular basis of many of these conditions has clarified the field. Two main types of so-called pseudohypoaldosteronism fulfill the criteria for mineralocorticoid resistance.

PSEUDOHYPOALDOSTERONISM

Pseudohypoaldosteronism (PHA) is a rare, inherited salt-wasting disorder first described by Cheek and Perry in 1958 as a defective renal tubular response to mineralocorticoid in infancy. Patients present in the neonatal period with dehydration, hyponatremia, hyperkalemia, metabolic acidosis, and failure to thrive despite normal glomerular filtration and normal renal and adrenal function.[66] Renin levels and plasma aldosterone are grossly elevated. When patients fail to respond to mineralocorticoid therapy, PHA is suspected as the underlying disorder.

PHA type 1 can be divided into two distinct disorders based on unique physiologic and genetic characteristics: the renal form of PHA, inherited as an autosomal dominant (AD) trait, and a generalized autosomal recessive (AR) form of PHA. Some de novo cases are described as sporadic. The AD form is usually less severe, with the patient's condition often improving spontaneously within the first several years of life, thus allowing discontinuation of therapy and treatment. Adult patients with the AD form are clinically indistinguishable from their wild-type relatives except for presumably lifelong elevation of renin, angiotensin II, and aldosterone levels. However, it has been suggested that the seemingly benign AD form may have been a fatal neonatal disorder in previous eras, preventing propagation of disease alleles.[67] By contrast, the AR form has a multiorgan disorder, with mineralocorticoid resistance seen in the kidney, sweat and salivary glands, and the colonic mucosa.[68] The latter condition does not spontaneously improve with age.[69] As a result, this form is considered to be more severe because it usually persists into adulthood. Since sodium reabsorption is coupled to potassium and hydrogen ion secretion, patients often show decreased potassium and hydrogen ion secretion with decreased sodium reabsorption. Hence, potassium and hydrogen ions accumulate in the body, and this ultimately leads to hyperkalemia and metabolic acidosis. Moreover, a decrease in vascular volume leads to activation of the renin-angiotensin-aldosterone axis.

The underlying basis for the AD form of PHA is explained on the basis of different heterozygous inactivating mutations in the mineralocorticoid receptor (MR) (Table 13-2). One mutated allele of the *MR* gene is sufficient to lead to the renal phenotype in men. In contrast, MR knockout mice showed hyponatremia, hyperkalemia, a strongly activated renin-angiotensin-aldosterone system (RAAS), significantly reduced ENaC activity in kidney and colon, and the mice died between day 8 and day 13 after birth when they were not treated with isotonic NaCl solutions.[70] By contrast, heterozygous MR knockout mice grow and breed normally and show no salt wasting. This difference between humans and mice might be due to differences in neonatal kidney maturation. However, only heterozygous mutations have been reported in humans, suggesting that the homozygous state may be embryologically lethal. The loss of one allele results in haploinsufficiency sufficient to generate the AD form of PHA symptoms, thus underlining the importance of

Table 13-2. Mineralocorticoid Receptor Mutations in Patients With the Autosomal-Dominant Form of Pseudohypoaldosteronism

Mutation	Location	Author
c.215G>C (−2 in Kozak seq. of translation initiation site) *and*	Intron 1	72
c.754A>G (Ile180Val) *and*	Exon 2	
c.938C>T (Ala241Val)	Exon 2	
c.402T>A (Y134X stop) nonsense	Exon 2	75
c.488C>G (S163stop) nonsense	Exon 2	76
del8bp537; frameshift	Exon 2	77
c.981delC (pSer328 frameshift)	Exon 2	74
c.1029C>A (Tyr343stop); nonsense	Exon 2	74, 78
c.1131dupT (E378X stop)	Exon 2	79
ΔG1226; frameshift leads to premature stop codon	Exon 2	7
c.1308T>A (C436stop); nonsense	Exon 2	80
InsT1354; frameshift	Exon 2	77
ΔT1597; frameshift leads to premature stop codon	Exon 2	71
InsA1715 (Y503Xstop); heterozygous	Exon 2	67
c.1831C>T (R537stop); nonsense	Exon 2	71
c.1679G>A (pTrp560Xstop)	Exon 2	74
c.1757+1G>A; splice donor site	Intron B	78
c.1984C>T (Arg590Xstop); heterozygous	Exon 3	67
c.1768C>T (pArg590Xstop)	Exon 3	74
c.1811delT (pLeu604 frameshift)	Exon 3	74
c.2119G>A (G633R); missense	Exon 3	77
c.2157C>A (Cys645stop); nonsense	Exon 4	77
c.1934G>C (pCys645Ser)	Exon 4	74
c.1954C>T (Arg652stop); nonsense	Exon 4	74, 78
c.1977A>C (pArg659Ser)	Exon 4	74
c.2017C>T (R673Xstop)	Exon 5	79
c.2020A>T (pLys674Xstop)	Exon 5	74
c.2024C>g (S675Xstop)	Exon 5	79
c.2125delA, frameshift T709 leads to L772Xstop	Exon 5	75
c.2275C>T (pPro759Ser)	Exon 5	74
c.2306_2307inv (pLeu769Pro)	Exon 5	74
c.2310C>A (p.Asn770Lys); missense	Exon 5	74, 78
c.2549A>G (Q776R); missense	Exon 5	77
c.2581G>A; splice alteration − nonsense, heterozygous	Exon 5	79
ΔA; aberrant splicing	Intron 5	71
c.2413T>C (pSer805Pro)	Exon 6	74
c.2445C>A (pSer815Arg)	Exon 6	74
c.2669C>T or c2453C>T (S818L); missense, heterozygous	Exon 6	67, 79
InsA2681 (fsH821); frameshift, heterozygous	Exon 6	67
c.2771T>C (L924P); nonsense	Exon 8	81
c.2779+1G>A; abnormal splicing	Exon 8	74
c.2839C>T or c.3055C>T (R947Xstop)	Exon 9	73, 82
InsC2871; frameshift from codon 958	Exon 9	79, 83
c.3115C>T (Q967stop); heterozygous	Exon 9	67
c.2915A>G (E972G)	Exon 9	79
c.3158T>C (L979P); missense	Exon 9	77

a substantial MR protein level, most notably during the neonatal period.[67]

To date, more than 40 mutations in the *MR* gene have been described in patients with the AD form of PHA (see Table 13-2; Fig. 13-3). They include missense, nonsense, frameshift, and splice-site mutations, as well as deletions spread throughout the gene. These mutations are responsible for either an early termination of translation with MR truncation or a defect in MR activity (loss of LBD or DBD), disruption of nucleocytoplasmic shuttling, or alteration in some transcriptional coregulator recruitment. The clinical improvement after infancy cannot yet be explained on the molecular level. The hypothesis that polymorphisms within the three ENaC gene subunits are responsible could not be shown, but today potential candidates might be the ubiquitin protein ligase Nedd4 and the serine-threonine kinases WNK1 and WNK4.

In 1998, Geller et al.[71] described the first four PHA mutations in the *MR* gene: two single base-pair mutations in exon 2 (ΔG1226 and ΔT1597), which result in a frameshift and premature stop codons; one nonsense mutation in exon 2 (C1831T,

R537stop) leading to a premature stop codon; and an intron-5 single base-pair deletion (ΔA) resulting in a splice donor-site deletion. Recently a patient was described[72] with three mutations in the *MR* gene: one mutation (G215C) at position −2 preceding the start codon in exon 2, which may result in an altered translation efficiency of the MR; and two mutations in exon 2 (A754G and C938T), which may affect transactivation function of the MR. Although none of those three mutations alone causes severe disruptions, the combination of the three polymorphisms seems to effectively diminish MR translation and function to result in a clinical picture of PHA. An R947X mutation in exon 9 of the *MR* gene, causing a reduction of the ligand-binding capacity, was found in three unrelated families with the autosomal-dominant form of PHA1.[73] The authors demonstrated the absence of a founder effect for the R947X mutation in these three families and suggested that this mutation might be a hot spot for loss-of-function mutations in PHA1.[73] In a recent large cohort of PHA1 patients, 68% of the mutations were dominantly transmitted, while 18% were de novo mutations.[74]

By contrast, homozygous inactivating mutations in the α and to a lesser extent the β and γ subunits of the *ENaC* gene account for the generalized AR form of PAH. This is therefore the opposite phenotype of Liddle's syndrome, with the small difference that mutations of Liddle's syndrome are found only in the β and γ subunit of the *ENaC* gene, whereas the AR form of PHA has been shown to be explained by mutations in any of the three ENaC subunits. In addition, mutations are not located in the carboxyterminus of the ENaC in PHA (Table 13-3). Generalized loss of ENaC activity leads to renal salt wasting, as seen in the renal form, but in addition, recurrent respiratory infections and neonatal respiratory distress, cholelithiasis, and polyhydramnios. Surprisingly, no colonic phenotype has been described in these patients, despite the presence of ENaC activity in this tissue.

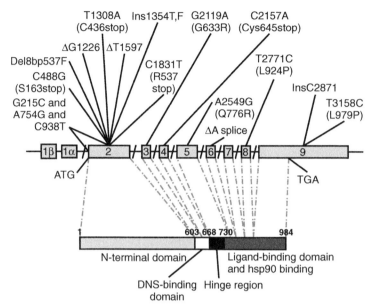

FIGURE 13-3. Schematic representation of identified mutations in the mineralocorticoid receptor (*MR*) gene. The *MR* gene is represented with its intron/exon structure. Eight exons (2 to 9) code for the functional domains, which are shown *below* in the amino acid sequence. The translation initiation site (ATG) and the translation stop codon (TGA) are shown.

Table 13-3. ENaC Mutations in Patients With the Autosomal-Recessive Form of Pseudohypoaldosteronism

ENaC Subunit	Mutation	Location	Author
α	302delTC (Ile68 frameshift)	Exon 2	69
α	C133Y; missense mutation	Exon 2	84, 85
α	R56 stop and R139 deletion CH	Exons 2 and 3	86
α	c.604delAC (T168; frameshift) *and* c.1404delC (F435; frameshift) CH	Exons 3 and 8	86
α	828delA (S243 frameshift) *and* S483 frameshift CH	Exons 4 and 10	91
α	c.1078G>T (Gly327Cys); missense mutation	Exon 5	92
α	c.1439insT (T447; frameshift)	Exon 8	93
α	1449delC (His450; frameshift)	Exon 8	91, 92
α	1455delC (Ser452; frameshift)	Exon 8	92
α	S483; frameshift	Exon 10	91
α	R492 stop; nonsense mutation	Exon 10	94
α	c.1621C>T/p; nonsense mutation and Arg508stop	Exon 11	69, 78, 86, 93
α	S562L missense mutation *and* S483 frameshift CH	Exons 10 and 13	91
α	c.1684T>C (S562P)	Exon 13	95
β	deletion in promoter region	5′-UTR	87
β	c.236G>A (Gly37Ser)	Exon 2	96
β	T216 frameshift *and* D305 frameshift CH	Exons 3 and 5	86
β	C647insA (Leu174; frameshift)	Exon 3	86
β	c.637C>T/p; nonsense mutation and Gln213stop		78
β	915del (Ser263; frameshift)	Exon 5	86
β	1669 + 1G>A; splice-site mutation	Intron 12	92, 93
γ	c.318-1G>A (KYS106-108→N and 134 stop)	Intron 2	88
γ	c.1318C>T/p; nonsense mutation and Arg440stop		78
γ	1570-1G>A substitution at 5′ acceptor splice site of intron 11 CH	Exon 12 and Intron 11	89
γ	1627delG (Val543; frameshift)	Exon 13	89

CH, Compound heterozygous.

Chang et al.[69] found the first two mutations involving the α subunit of ENaC resulting in PHA. A 2-bp deletion at codon 68 introduces a frameshift mutation and thus disrupts the protein before the first transmembrane domain. The other mutation of the α subunit is a single base substitution at codon R508 which truncates the α subunit before the second transmembrane domain by introducing a premature termination codon in the extracellular domain. In the following years, several missense and frameshift mutations, several compound heterozygous, have been described (see Table 13-3). Some mutations are located in the first or second cysteine-rich boxes of the extracellular loop,[84,85] which are involved in disulfide-bond formation and trafficking of the channel to the cell surface.

In the β subunit, Chang et al.[69] reported a point mutation (G37S) which lies within the gating segment preceding the first transmembrane-spanning region that is homologous among all members of the *ENaC* gene family. This mutation on the β subunit has been shown to diminish ENaC activity but does not lead to a complete loss of activity. Recently mutations have been described that lead to deletion of the extracellular loop and the C-terminus of the protein[86] or that delete parts of the promoter region of the β subunit.[87]

Strautnieks et al.[88] identified mutations in the γ subunit of ENaC and further elucidated the cause of the autosomal recessive form of PHA1. The mutation in intron 2 involves the 3′ acceptor splice-site preceding exon 3 and results in two different mRNA products. One mRNA product shows a replacement of a highly conserved amino acid triplet, Lys-Tyr-Ser, by asparagine in the extracellular loop immediately adjacent to the transmembrane domain. The other mRNA product is truncated at amino acid 134, resulting in deletion of the extracellular loop. Adachi et al.[89] reported a compound-heterozygous mutation in the γ subunit consisting of a frameshift mutation in exon 12, resulting in a premature stop codon at position 597, and a mutation in intron 11, resulting in aberrant splicing and inhibition of normal mRNA transcription.

Knockout mice lacking the α-ENaC subunit show poor mobility and appetite after birth, and death ensues within the first 2 days due to lung edema and electrolyte disturbances.[90] Interestingly, β- and γ-ENaC knockout mice show a delayed lung liquid clearance at birth but no respiratory distress syndrome, suggesting that α-ENaC is essential for lung liquid clearance and maturation after birth in mice. The cause of death in this case is hyperkalemia and metabolic acidosis. In humans with the AR form of PHA, neonatal respiratory distress syndrome is reported in only two cases to date, but the lung symptoms occur a few months after birth. In addition, no phenotypic difference between the different ENaC subunit mutations has been reported in men. These species-specific differences in ENaC functions cannot be explained to date.

PHA1 patients are resistant to mineralocorticoid therapy, and thus standard treatment involves supplementation with sodium chloride (2 to 8 g/day) and cation-exchange resins. This usually corrects the patient's biochemical imbalance. However, if a patient shows signs of severe hyperkalemia, peritoneal dialysis

may be necessary. Hypercalciuria has been reported in some cases involving PHA1. In such cases, the recommended course of treatment usually involves either treatment with indomethacin or with hydrochlorothiazide. Indomethacin is thought to act by causing a reduction in the glomerular filtration rate or an inhibition of the effect of prostaglandin E_2 on renal tubules.[97] Indomethacin has been shown to reduce polyuria, sodium loss, and hypercalciuria.

Hydrochlorothiazide, a potassium-losing diuretic, is sometimes also administered to diminish hyperkalemia. In addition, it has been shown to reduce hypercalciuria in PHA1 patients.[97]

In patients with the autosomal-dominant or renal form of PHA1, the signs and symptoms of PHA decrease with age, thus allowing discontinuation of therapy when the patient is a few years old. Nevertheless, these patients usually require salt supplementation for the first 2 to 3 years of life. In patients with the autosomal-recessive or multiorgan type of PHA1, however, resistance to therapy with sodium chloride or drugs that decrease serum potassium concentrations often occurs and may even lead to death in infancy from hyperkalemia. Multiorgan PHA1 patients often require very high amounts of salt in their diet (as high as 45 g NaCl per day).[98]

Carbenoxolone (CBX), a derivative of glycyrrhetinic acid in licorice, has been used with moderate success in helping to reduce the high-salt diets for renal PHA1 patients. CBX acts by inhibiting 11β-hydroxysteroid dehydrogenase type 2 (11β-HSD2) activity. By inhibiting this enzyme, CBX allows unmetabolized cortisol to bind to and activate mineralocorticoid receptors in a manner similar to that of aldosterone.[6,99] However, since PHA involves either a receptor or postreceptor defect, it is not clear why inhibition of 11β-HSD2 should be effective in this condition. In a 1997 study by Hanukoglu et al.[99] (and personal observations in an unrelated case), administration of CBX did not show any improvement in multiorgan PHA1 patients.

Two other variants of PHA have been described: types 2 and 3. Type 2 PHA, or Gordon's syndrome, is in retrospect a misnomer. Patients with Gordon's syndrome[100] share some of the features of patients with PHA type 1, notably hyperkalemia and metabolic acidosis, but exhibit salt retention with mild hypertension and suppressed plasma renin activity rather than salt wasting. The condition is explained by mutations in proteins of the serine-threonine kinase family, WNK1 and WNK4, resulting in an enhanced activity of the thiazide-sensitive Na/Cl cotransporter (NCCT) in the cortical and medullary collecting ducts. Whereas WNK4 is a negative regulator of the NCCT, WNK1 blunts WNK4's inhibitory effect on the NCCT.[101] The condition represents the exact opposite of Gitelman's syndrome but is not a true form of PHA.

Type 3 PHA is an acquired and usually transient form of mineralocorticoid resistance seen in patients with underlying renal pathologies, including obstruction, infection, and in patients with excessive loss of salt through the gut or skin. Reduced GFR is a hallmark of the condition. The cause is unknown, though increased TGF-β-mediated aldosterone resistance has been suggested to be an underlying factor.

REFERENCES

1. Condon JC, Pezzi V, Drummond BM, et al: Calmodulin-dependent kinase Calmodulin-dependent kinase I regulates adrenal cell expression of aldosterone synthase, Endocrinology 143(9):3651–3657, 2002.

2. Arriza JL, Weinberger C, Cerelli G, et al: Cloning of human mineralocorticoid receptor complementary

DNA: structural and functional kinship with the glucocorticoid receptor, Science 237(4812):268–275, 1987.

3. Pearce D, Bhargava A, Cole TJ: Aldosterone: its receptor, target genes, and actions, Vitam Horm 66:29–76, 2003.

4. Rogerson FM, Brennan FE, Fuller PJ: Dissecting mineralocorticoid receptor structure and function, J Steroid Biochem Mol Biol 85(2-5):389–396, 2003.

5. Edwards CR, Stewart PM, Burt D, et al: Localisation of 11 beta-hydroxysteroid dehydrogenase—tissue-

specific protector of the mineralocorticoid receptor, Lancet 2(8618):986–989, 1988.

6. Funder JW, Pearce PT, Smith R, et al: Mineralocorticoid action: target tissue specificity is enzyme, not receptor, mediated, Science 242(4878):583–585, 1988.

7. Garty H, Palmer LG: Epithelial sodium channels: function, structure, and regulation, Physiol Rev 77(2):359–396, 1997.

8. Snyder PM: The epithelial Na$^+$ channel: cell surface insertion and retrieval in Na$^+$ homeostasis and hypertension, Endocr Rev 23(2):258–275, 2002.

9. Rossier BC, PRadervand S, Schild L, et al: Epithelial sodium channel and the control of sodium balance: interaction between genetic and environmental factors, Annu Rev Physiol 64:877–897, 2002.

10. Voilley N, Bassilana F, Mignon C, et al: Cloning, chromosomal localization, and physical linkage of the beta and gamma subunits (SCNN1B and SCNN1G) of the human epithelial amiloride-sensitive sodium channel, Genomics 28(3):560–565, 1995.

11. Jasti J, Furukawa H, Gonzales EB, et al: Structure of acid-sensing ion channel 1 at 1.9 A resolution and low pH, Nature 449(7160):316–323, 2007.

12. Lifton RP: Molecular genetics of human blood pressure variation, Science 272(5262):676–680, 1996.

13. Shimkets RA, Warnock DG, Bositis CM, et al: Liddle's syndrome: heritable human hypertension caused by mutations in the beta subunit of the epithelial sodium channel, Cell 79(3):407–414, 1994.

14. Hansson JH, Nelson-Williams C, Suzuki H, et al: Hypertension caused by a truncated epithelial sodium channel gamma subunit: genetic heterogeneity of Liddle syndrome, Nat Genet 11(1):76–82, 1995.

15. Goulet CC, Volk KA, Adams CM, et al: Inhibition of the epithelial Na$^+$ channel by interaction of Nedd4 with a PY motif deleted in Liddle's syndrome, J Biol Chem 273(45):30012–30017, 1998.

16. Chen SY, Bhargava A, Mastroberardino L, et al: Epithelial sodium channel regulated by aldosterone-induced protein SGK, Proc Natl Acad Sci U S A 96(5):2514–2519, 1999.

17. Naray-Fejes-Toth A, Canessa C, Cleaveland ES, et al: SGK is an aldosterone-induced kinase in the renal collecting duct. Effects on epithelial Na$^+$ channels, J Biol Chem 274(24):16973–16978, 1999.

18. Kokko JP: Primary acquired hypoaldosteronism, Kidney Int 27(4):690–702, 1985.

19. Saenger P, Levine LS, Irvine WJ, et al: Progressive adrenal failure in polyglandular autoimmune disease, J Clin Endocrinol Metab 54(4):863–867, 1982.

20. Williams FA Jr, Schambelan M, Biglieri EG, et al: Acquired primary hypoaldosteronism due to an isolated zona glomerulosa defect, N Engl J Med 309(26):1623–1627, 1983.

21. Muscatelli F, Strom TM, Walker AP, et al: Mutations in the DAX1 gene give rise to both X-linked adrenal hypoplasia congenita and hypogonadotropic hypogonadism, Nature 372:672–676, 1994.

22. Verrijn Stuart AA, Ozisik G, De Vroede MA, et al: An amino-terminal DAX1 (NROB1) missense mutation associated with isolated mineralocorticoid deficiency, J Clin Endocrinol Metab 92(3):755–761, 2007.

23. Metherell LA, Chapple JP, Cooray S, et al: Mutations in MRAP, encoding a new interacting partner of the ACTH receptor, cause familial glucocorticoid deficiency type 2, Nat Genet 37(2):166–170, 2005.

24. Lin L, Hindmarsh PC, Metherell LA, et al: Severe loss-of-function mutations in the adrenocorticotropin receptor (ACTHR, MC2R) can be found in patients diagnosed with salt-losing adrenal hypoplasia, Clin Endocrinol (Oxf) 66(2):205–210, 2007.

25. Mornet E, Dupont J, Vitek A, et al: Characterization of two genes encoding human steroid 11 beta-hydroxylase (P-450[11] beta), J Biol Chem 264(35):20961–20967, 1989.

26. Taymans SE, Pack S, Pak E, et al: Human CYP11B2 (aldosterone synthase) maps to chromosome 8q24.3, J Clin Endocrinol Metab 83(3):1033–1036, 1998.

27. Makhanova N, Sequeira-Lopez ML, Gomez RA, et al: Disturbed homeostasis in sodium-restricted mice heterozygous and homozygous for aldosterone synthase gene disruption, Hypertension 48(6):1151–1159, 2006.

28. Mitsuuchi Y, Kawamoto T, Miyahara K, et al: Congenitally defective aldosterone biosynthesis in humans: inactivation of the P-450C18 gene (CYP11B2) due to

nucleotide deletion in CMO I deficient patients, Biochem Biophys Res Commun 190:864–869, 1993.

29. Kayes-Wandover KM, Schindler RE, Taylor HC, et al: Type 1 aldosterone synthase deficiency presenting in a middle-aged man, J Clin Endocrinol Metab 86(3):1008–1012, 2001.

30. Lopez-Siguero JP, Garcia-Garcia E, Peter M, et al: Aldosterone synthase deficiency type I: hormonal and genetic analyses of two cases, Horm Res 52(6):298–300, 1999.

31. Portrat-Doyen S, Tourniaire J, Richard O, et al: Isolated aldosterone synthase deficiency caused by simultaneous E198D and V386A mutations in the CYP11B2 gene, J Clin Endocrinol Metab 83(11):4156–4161, 1998.

32. Peter M, Fawaz L, Drop SL, et al: Hereditary defect in biosynthesis of aldosterone: aldosterone synthase deficiency 1964–1997, J Clin Endocrinol Metab 82(11):3525–3528, 1997.

33. Peter M, Bünger K, Drop SLS, et al: Molecular genetic study in two patients with congenital hypoaldosteronism (types I and II) in relation to previously published hormonal studies, Eur J Endocrinol 139:96–100, 1998.

34. Williams TA, Mulatero P, Bosio M, et al: A particular phenotype in a girl with aldosterone synthase deficiency, J Clin Endocrinol Metab 89(7):3168–3172, 2004.

35. Geley S, Johrer K, Peter M, et al: Amino acid substitution R384P in aldosterone synthase causes corticosterone methyloxidase type I deficiency, J Clin Endocrinol Metab 80(2):424–429, 1995.

36. Nguyen HH, Hannemann F, Hartmann MF, et al: Aldosterone synthase deficiency caused by a homozygous L451F mutation in the CYP11B2 gene, Mol Genet Metab 93(4):458–467, 2008.

37. Nomoto S, Massa G, Mitani F, et al: CMO I deficiency caused by a point mutation in exon 8 of the human CYP11B2 gene encoding steroid 18-hydroxylase (P450$_{C18}$), Biochem Biophys Res Commun 234:382–385, 1997.

38. Wasniewska M, De Luca F, Valenzise M, et al: Aldosterone synthase deficiency type I with no documented homozygous mutations in the CYP11B2 gene, Eur J Endocrinol 144(1):59–62, 2001.

39. Peter M, Nikischin W, Heinz-Erian P, et al: Homozygous deletion of arginine-173 in the CYP11B2 gene in a girl with congenital hypoaldosteronism: corticosterone methyloxidase deficiency type II, Horm Res 50:222–225, 1998.

40. Pascoe L, Curnow KM, Slutsker L, et al: Mutations in the human CYP11B2 (aldosterone synthase) gene causing corticosterone methyloxidase II deficiency, Proc Natl Acad Sci U S A 89(11):4996–5000, 1992.

41. Leshinsky-Silver E, Landau Z, Unlubay S, et al: Congenital hyperreninemic hypoaldosteronism in Israel: sequence analysis of CYP11B2 gene, Horm Res 66(2):73–78, 2006.

42. Peter M, Bunger K, Solyom J, et al: Mutation THR-185 ILE is associated with corticosterone methyl oxidase deficiency type II, Eur J Pediatr 157(5):378–381, 1998.

43. Zhang G, Rodriguez H, Fardella CE, et al: Mutation T318M in the CYP11B2 gene encoding P450c11AS (aldosterone synthase) causes corticosterone methyl oxidase II deficiency, Am J Hum Genet 57(5):1037–1043, 1995.

44. Kuribayashi I, Kuge H, Santa RJ, et al: A missense mutation (GGC[435Gly]→AGC[Ser]) in exon 8 of the CYP11B2 gene inherited in Japanese patients with congenital hypoaldosteronism, Horm Res 60(5):255–260, 2003.

45. Dunlop FM, Crock PA, Montalto J, et al: A compound heterozygote case of type II aldosterone synthase deficiency, J Clin Endocrinol Metab 88(6):2518–2526, 2003.

46. Fardella CE, Hum DW, Rodriguez H, et al: Gene conversion in the CYP11B2 gene encoding P450c11AS is associated with, but does not cause, the syndrome of corticosterone methyloxidase II deficiency, J Clin Endocrinol Metab 81(1):321–326, 1996.

47. Davenport MW, Zipser RD: Association of hypotension with hyperreninemic hypoaldosteronism in the critically ill patient, Arch Intern Med 143(4):735–737, 1983.

48. Du CD, Bouchet B, Cauquelin B, et al: Hyperreninemic hypoaldosteronism syndrome, plasma concentrations of interleukin 6 and outcome in critically ill patients

with liver cirrhosis, Intensive Care Med 34(1):116–124, 2008.

49. Bartter FC, Duncan LE, Liddle GW: Dual mechanism regulating adrenocortical function in man, Am J Med 21(3):380–386, 1956.

50. Biglieri EG, Chang B, Hirai J, et al: Adrenocorticotropin inhibition of mineralocorticoid hormone production, Clin Sci 57(Suppl 5):307s–311s, 1979.

51. Aguilera G, Fujita K, Catt KJ. Mechanisms of inhibition of aldosterone secretion by adrenocorticotropin, Endocrinology 108:522–528, 1981.

52. Tuchelt H, Eschenhagen G, Bahr V, et al: Role of atrial natriuretic factor in changes in the responsiveness of aldosterone to angiotensin II secondary to sodium loading and depletion in man, Clin Sci (Lond) 79(1):57–65, 1990.

53. DeFronzo RA: Hyperkalemia and hyporeninemic hypoaldosteronism, Kidney Int 17(1):118–134, 1980.

54. Schambelan M, Stockigt JR, Biglieri EG: Isolated hypoaldosteronism in adults. A renin-deficiency syndrome, N Engl J Med 287(12):573–578, 1972.

55. Schambelan M, Sebastian A, Biglieri EG: Prevalence, pathogenesis, and functional significance of aldosterone deficiency in hyperkalemic patients with chronic renal insufficiency, Kidney Int 17(1):89–101, 1980.

56. Weidmann P, Reinhart R, Maxwell MH, et al: Syndrome of hyporeninemic hypoaldosteronism and hyperkalemia in renal disease, J Clin Endocrinol Metab 36(5):965–977, 1973.

57. Tan SY, Shapiro R, Franco R, et al: Indomethacin-induced prostaglandin inhibition with hyperkalemia. A reversible cause of hyporeninemic hypoaldosteronism, Ann Intern Med 90(5):783–785, 1979.

58. Schambelan M, Sebastian A: Hyporeninemic hypoaldosteronism, Adv Intern Med 24:385–405, 1979.

59. Nakamoto Y, Imai H, Hamanaka S, et al: IgM monoclonal gammopathy accompanied by nodular glomerulosclerosis, urine-concentrating defect, and hyporeninemic hypoaldosteronism, Am J Nephrol 5(1):53–58, 1985.

60. Leehey D, Gantt C, Lim V: Heparin-induced hypoaldosteronism. Report of a case, JAMA 246(19):2189–2190, 1981.

61. Tan SY, Burton M: Hyporeninemic hypoaldosteronism. An overlooked cause of hyperkalemia, Arch Intern Med 141(1):30–33, 1981.

62. Sebastian A, Schambelan M, Lindenfeld S, et al: Amelioration of metabolic acidosis with fludrocortisone therapy in hyporeninemic hypoaldosteronism, N Engl J Med 297(11):576–583, 1977.

63. Rebuffat P, Kasprzak A, Andreis PG, et al: Effects of prolonged cyclosporine-A treatment on the morphology and function of rat adrenal cortex, Endocrinology 125(3):1407–1413, 1989.

64. Deppe CE, Heering PJ, Viengchareun S, et al: Cyclosporine a and FK506 inhibit transcriptional activity of the human mineralocorticoid receptor: a cell-based model to investigate partial aldosterone resistance in kidney transplantation, Endocrinology 143(5):1932–1941, 2002.

65. Ponce SP, Jennings AE, Madias NE, et al: Drug-induced hyperkalemia, Medicine (Baltimore) 64(6):357–370, 1985.

66. Zennaro MC, Borensztein P, Soubrier F, et al: The enigma of pseudohypoaldosteronism, Steroids 59(2):96–99, 1994.

67. Geller DS, Zhang J, Zennaro MC, et al: Autosomal dominant pseudohypoaldosteronism type 1: mechanisms, evidence for neonatal lethality, and phenotypic expression in adults, J Am Soc Nephrol 17(5):1429–1436, 2006.

68. Ulick S, Wang JZ, Morton DH: The biochemical phenotypes of two inborn errors in the biosynthesis of aldosterone, J Clin Endocrinol Metab 74(6):1415–1420, 1992.

69. Chang SS, Grunder S, Hanukoglu A, et al: Mutations in subunits of the epithelial sodium channel cause salt wasting with hyperkalaemic acidosis, pseudohypoaldosteronism type 1, Nat Genet 12(3):248–253, 1996.

70. Berger S, Bleich M, Schmid W, et al: Mineralocorticoid receptor knockout mice: pathophysiology of Na$^+$ metabolism, Proc Natl Acad Sci U S A 95(16):9424–9429, 1998.

71. Geller DS, Rodriguez-Soriano J, Vallo BA, et al: Mutations in the mineralocorticoid receptor gene cause

autosomal dominant pseudohypoaldosteronism type I, Nat Genet 19(3):279–281, 1998.

72. Arai K, Nakagomi Y, Iketani M, et al: Functional polymorphisms in the mineralocorticoid receptor and amiloride-sensitive sodium channel genes in a patient with sporadic pseudohypoaldosteronism, Hum Genet 112(1):91–97, 2003.

73. Fernandes-Rosa FL, de Castro M, Latronico AC, et al: Recurrence of the R947X mutation in unrelated families with autosomal dominant pseudohypoaldosteronism type 1: evidence for a mutational hot spot in the mineralocorticoid receptor gene, J Clin Endocrinol Metab 91(9):3671–3675, 2006.

74. Pujo L, Fagart J, Gary F, et al: Mineralocorticoid receptor mutations are the principal cause of renal type 1 pseudohypoaldosteronism, Hum Mutat 28(1):33–40, 2007.

75. Balsamo A, Cicognani A, Gennari M, et al: Functional characterization of naturally occurring NR3C2 gene mutations in Italian patients suffering from pseudohypoaldosteronism type 1, Eur J Endocrinol 156(2):249–256, 2007.

76. Riepe FG, Krone N, Morlot M, et al: Identification of a novel mutation in the human mineralocorticoid receptor gene in a German family with autosomal-dominant pseudohypoaldosteronism type 1: further evidence for marked interindividual clinical heterogeneity, J Clin Endocrinol Metab 88(4):1683–1686, 2003.

77. Sartorato P, Lapeyraque AL, Armanini D, et al: Different inactivating mutations of the mineralocorticoid receptor in fourteen families affected by type I pseudohypoaldosteronism, J Clin Endocrinol Metab 88(6):2508–2517, 2003.

78. Belot A, Ranchin B, Fichtner C, et al: Pseudohypoaldosteronisms, report on a 10-patient series, Nephrol Dial Transplant 23(5):1636–1641, 2008.

79. Riepe FG, Finkeldei J, de Sanctis L, et al: Elucidating the underlying molecular pathogenesis of NR3C2 mutants causing autosomal dominant pseudohypoaldosteronism type 1, J Clin Endocrinol Metab 91(11):4552–4561, 2006.

80. Nystrom AM, Bondeson ML, Skanke N, et al: A novel nonsense mutation of the mineralocorticoid receptor gene in a Swedish family with pseudohypoaldosteronism type I (PHA1), J Clin Endocrinol Metab 89(1):227–231, 2004.

81. Tajima T, Kitagawa H, Yokoya S, et al: A novel missense mutation of mineralocorticoid receptor gene in one Japanese family with a renal form of pseudohypoaldosteronism Type 1, J Clin Endocrinol Metab 85(12):4690–4694, 2000.

82. Riepe FG, Krone N, Morlot M, et al: Autosomal-dominant pseudohypoaldosteronism type 1 in a Turkish family is associated with a novel nonsense mutation in the human mineralocorticoid receptor gene, J Clin Endocrinol Metab 89(5):2150–2152, 2004.

83. Viemann M, Peter M, Lopez-Siguero JP, et al: Evidence for genetic heterogeneity of pseudohypoaldosteronism type 1: identification of a novel mutation in the human mineralocorticoid receptor in one sporadic case and no mutations in two autosomal dominant kindreds, J Clin Endocrinol Metab 86(5):2056–2059, 2001.

84. Grunder S, Chang SS, Lifton R, et al: A novel thermosensitive mutation in the ectodomain of alpha ENaC, J Am Soc Nephrol 9, 1998.

85. Firsov D, Robert-Nicoud M, Gruender S, et al: Mutational analysis of cysteine-rich domains of the epithelium sodium channel (ENaC). Identification of cysteines essential for channel expression at the cell surface, J Biol Chem 274(5):2743–2749, 1999.

86. Kerem E, Bistritzer T, Hanukoglu A, et al: Pulmonary epithelial sodium-channel dysfunction and excess airway liquid in pseudohypoaldosteronism, N Engl J Med 341(3):156–162, 1999.

87. Thomas CP, Zhou J, Liu KZ, et al: Systemic pseudohypoaldosteronism from deletion of the promoter region of the human beta epithelial Na⁺ channel subunit, Am J Respir Cell Mol Biol 27(3):314–319, 2002.

88. Strautnieks SS, Thompson RJ, Gardiner RM, et al: A novel splice-site mutation in the gamma subunit of the epithelial sodium channel gene in three pseudohypoaldosteronism type 1 families, Nat Genet 13(2):248–250, 1996.

89. Adachi M, Tachibana K, Asakura Y, et al: Compound heterozygous mutations in the gamma subunit gene of ENaC (1627delG and 1570-1G→A) in one sporadic Japanese patient with a systemic form of pseudohypoaldosteronism type 1, J Clin Endocrinol Metab 86(1):9–12, 2001.

90. Hummler E, Barker P, Gatzy J, et al: Early death due to defective neonatal lung liquid clearance in alpha-ENaC-deficient mice, Nat Genet 12(3):325–328, 1996.

91. Schaedel C, Marthinsen L, Kristoffersson AC, et al: Lung symptoms in pseudohypoaldosteronism type 1 are associated with deficiency of the alpha subunit of the epithelial sodium channel, J Pediatr 135(6):739–745, 1999.

92. Edelheit O, Hanukoglu I, Gizewska M, et al: Novel mutations in epithelial sodium channel (ENaC) subunit genes and phenotypic expression of multisystem pseudohypoaldosteronism, Clin Endocrinol (Oxf) 62(5):547–553, 2005.

93. Saxena A, Hanukoglu I, Saxena D, et al: Novel mutations responsible for autosomal recessive multisystem pseudohypoaldosteronism and sequence variants in epithelial sodium channel alpha-, beta-, and gamma-subunit genes, J Clin Endocrinol Metab 87(7):3344–3350, 2002.

94. Bonny O, Knoers N, Monnens L, et al: A novel mutation of the epithelial Na⁺ channel causes type 1 pseudohypoaldosteronism, Pediatr Nephrol 17(10):804–808, 2002.

95. Riepe FG, van Bemmelen MX, Cachat F, et al: Revealing a subclinical salt-losing phenotype in heterozygous carriers of the novel S562P mutation in the alpha subunit of the epithelial sodium channel, Clin Endocrinol (Oxf) 2008.

96. Grunder S, Firsov D, Chang SS, et al: A mutation causing pseudohypoaldosteronism type 1 identifies a conserved glycine that is involved in the gating of the epithelial sodium channel, EMBO J 16(5):899–907, 1997.

97. Stone RC, Vale P, Rosa FC: Effect of hydrochlorothiazide in pseudohypoaldosteronism with hypercalciuria and severe hyperkalemia, Pediatr Nephrol 10(4):501–503, 1996.

98. White PC: Disorders of aldosterone biosynthesis and action, N Engl J Med 331(4):250–258, 1994.

99. Hanukoglu A, Joy O, Steinitz M, et al: Pseudohypoaldosteronism due to renal and multisystem resistance to mineralocorticoids respond differently to carbenoxolone, J Steroid Biochem Mol Biol 60(1–2):105–112, 1997.

100. Wilson FH, Disse-Nicodeme S, Choate KA, et al: Human hypertension caused by mutations in WNK kinases, Science 293(5532):1107–1112, 2001.

101. Faure S, Delaloy C, Leprivey V, et al: WNK kinases, distal tubular ion handling and hypertension, Nephrol Dial Transplant 18(12):2463–2467, 2003.

Chapter 14

PHEOCHROMOCYTOMA

KAREL PACAK, HENRI J.L.M. TIMMERS, and GRAEME EISENHOFER

Pheochromocytomas are rare but treacherous catecholamine-secreting tumors that, if missed or not properly treated, almost invariably prove fatal.[1-3] Prompt diagnosis therefore is essential for effective treatment, usually by surgical resection, which is curative in most cases. Thus, it is crucially important for the clinician to first think of the tumor based on knowledge of its manifestations and clinical settings. The manifestations are diverse, and the tumor can mimic a variety of conditions, often resulting in erroneous diagnoses.[1] Autopsy studies have shown that significant numbers of pheochromocytomas remain undiagnosed until death, and that up to 50% of these unrecognized tumors may have contributed to patient mortality.[4] Recent advances in biochemical diagnosis, tumor localization, and surgical approaches, as well as improved understanding of the pathophysiology and genetics of pheochromocytoma, are leading to earlier diagnosis and changes in management strategies and therapeutic options.[1,2,5-11]

Pheochromocytomas typically arise in about 85% of cases from adrenal medullary chromaffin tissue (also designated adrenal paragangliomas) and in about 15% of cases from extra-adrenal chromaffin tissues. Those arising from extra-adrenal tissue are commonly known as paragangliomas. Paragangliomas are divided into two groups: those that arise from parasympathetic-associated tissues (most commonly along the cranial nerves and vagus; e.g., glomus tumors, chemodectoma, carotid body tumor) and those that arise from sympathetic-associated chromaffin tissue (often designated extra-adrenal pheochromocytomas). Extra-adrenal pheochromocytomas arise mainly from chromaffin tissue adjacent to sympathetic ganglia; they arise less commonly from the pelvis, and they arise rarely from the mediastinum (2%) and the neck (less than 1%) (Fig. 14-1). Extra-adrenal pheochromocytomas in the abdomen most commonly arise from a collection of chromaffin tissue around the origin of the inferior mesenteric artery or aortic bifurcation called the organ of Zuckerkandl.[1] Adrenal and extra-adrenal paragangliomas display similar histopathologic characteristics.

Most pheochromocytomas arise sporadically, but based on recent reports, up to 24% are familial.[12] In contrast to sporadic pheochromocytomas that usually are unicentric and unilateral, familial pheochromocytomas are often multifocal and bilateral.[1,5,13]

History

The name pheochromocytoma, proposed by Pick in 1912,[14] comes from the Greek words *phaios* ("dusky") and *chroma* ("color"); it refers to the staining that occurs when the tumors are treated with chromium salts. The first diagnosis of pheochromocytoma was made in 1886 by Frankel,[15] who found bilateral tumors of the adrenal gland at autopsy in an 18-year-old girl who had died suddenly. Extra-adrenal pheochromocytoma was

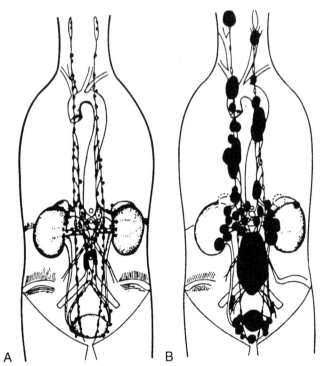

FIGURE 14-1. **A,** Anatomic distribution of extra-adrenal chromaffin tissue in the newborn. **B,** Locations of extra-adrenal pheochromocytomas reported in the literature up to 1965. (From Coupland R: The Natural History of the Chromaffin Cell, Essex, UK, Longsman Green, 1965.)

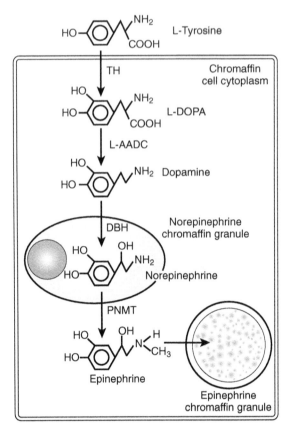

FIGURE 14-2. Diagram illustrating the catecholamine biosynthetic pathway in an adrenal chromaffin cell. *DBH,* Dopamine β-hydroxylase; *L-AADC,* L-aromatic amino acid decarboxylase; *PNMT,* phenylethanolamine N-methyltransferase; *TH,* tyrosine hydroxylase.

first reported by Alezais and Peyron in 1908.[16] The important association of paroxysmal hypertension with pheochromocytoma was first described by L'Abbe and colleagues in 1922.[17] The first successful surgical removals of pheochromocytomas were performed by Roux in France in 1926 and by C. H. Mayo in the United States in 1927.[18,19] In 1929, Rabin[20] reported that a pheochromocytoma contained an excess amount of the normal pressor agent present in the adrenal gland, and suggested that this might account for the main clinical manifestations (i.e., hypertension and tachycardia). In 1936, epinephrine (also known as adrenaline) was isolated from a pheochromocytoma by Kelly and colleagues,[21] but it was not until 1946 that von Euler and his coworkers, and 1947 that Holtz and his coworkers, reported independently the occurrence of norepinephrine (noradrenaline) in the body.[22-24] In 1949, Holton[25] first demonstrated the presence of norepinephrine in a pheochromocytoma. The first large series of successful surgical removals with pharmacologic blockade was reported by Kvale and colleagues in 1956.[26]

According to different reviews and statistics, pheochromocytomas account for approximately 0.05% to 0.1% of patients with any degree of sustained hypertension[1,5,18]; however, this probably includes only 50% of persons harboring the tumor, when it is considered that about half the patients with pheochromocytoma have only paroxysmal hypertension or are normotensive. Also, despite the low incidence of pheochromocytoma in patients with sustained hypertension, it must be considered that the current prevalence of sustained hypertension in the adult population of Western countries is up to 30%.[27-29] In Western countries, the prevalence of pheochromocytoma can be estimated at between 1 : 4500 and 1 : 1700, with an annual incidence of 3 to 8 cases per 1 million per year in the general population.[30] Pheochromocytoma occurs at any age, but most often in the fourth and fifth decades, and it occurs equally in men and women.

Catecholamine Synthesis, Release, and Metabolism

Pheochromocytomas are often described as tumors that synthesize, store, and secrete catecholamines. It is rarely appreciated that pheochromocytomas also metabolize catecholamines, and that this is a more consistent process than that of catecholamine secretion.[31] Failure to recognize this key feature is probably caused by several misconceptions about the storage and metabolism of catecholamines, perhaps the most pervasive being that metabolism occurs mainly after catecholamine release. In fact, substantial amounts of catecholamines are metabolized in the same cells where the amines are synthesized, and much of this is independent of catecholamine release. The nature of the metabolites produced depends on the neuronal or chromaffin cell phenotype and the types of catecholamines synthesized within the tumor cells.

BIOSYNTHESIS

Catecholamine synthesis begins with the amino acid tyrosine, which comes from the diet or via hydroxylation of phenylalanine in the liver. L-Tyrosine is converted to dihydroxyphenylalanine (dopa) by tyrosine hydroxylase (TH) (Fig. 14-2). This reaction requires molecular oxygen and the cofactor tetrahydrobiopterin and represents the rate-limiting step in catecholamine biosynthesis (Fig. 14-3).[32] Tissue sources of catecholamines therefore are principally dependent on the presence of this enzyme, which is largely confined to dopaminergic and noradrenergic neurons of

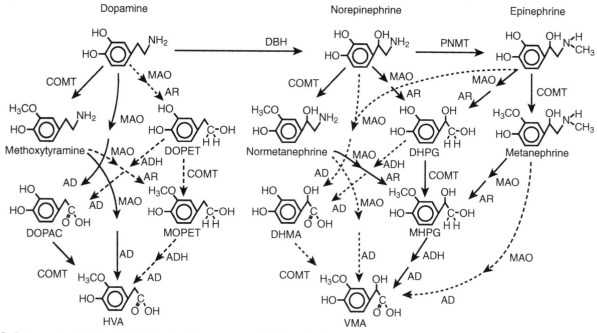

FIGURE 14-3. Pathways of metabolism of catecholamines. Enzymes responsible for each pathway are shown at the heads of arrows. *Solid arrows* indicate the major pathways, whereas *dotted arrows* indicate pathways of negligible importance. Pathways of sulfate conjugation are not shown. *AD*, Aldehyde dehydrogenase; *ADH*, alcohol dehydrogenase; *AR*, aldose or aldehyde reductase; *COMT*, catechol *O*-methyltransferase; *DBH*, dopamine β-hydroxylase; *DHMA*, 3,4-dihydroxymandelic acid; *DHPG*, 3,4-dihydroxyphenyl-glycol; *DOPAC*, 3,4-dihydroxyphenylacetic acid; *DOPET*, 3,4 dihydroxyphenylethanol; *HVA*, homovanillic acid; *MAO*, monoamine oxidase; *MHPG*, 3-methoxy-4 hydroxyphenyl-glycol; *MOPET*, 3-methoxy-4 hydroxyphenyletanol; *PNMT*, phenolethanolamine *N*-methyltransferase; *VMA*, vanillylmandelic acid.

the central nervous system, and to sympathetic nerves and chromaffin cells of the adrenal medulla and extramedullary paraganglia in the periphery.

Dopa is decarboxylated by aromatic L-amino acid decarboxylase to produce dopamine. The dopamine formed in neurons and chromaffin cells is translocated from the cytoplasm into vesicular storage granules. In dopaminergic neurons of the central nervous system, dopamine serves as the end product neurotransmitter. Large amounts of dopamine are produced as an end product of catecholamine synthesis in peripheral non-neuronal cells of the gastrointestinal tract and kidneys.[33] The dopamine present in urine is derived mainly from decarboxylation of dopa taken up from the circulation by the kidneys.

The dopamine formed in noradrenergic neurons and chromaffin cells is converted to norepinephrine by dopamine β-hydroxylase (DBH), an enzyme that is found only in the vesicles of cells that synthesize norepinephrine and epinephrine.

In adrenal medullary chromaffin cells, norepinephrine is metabolized by the cytosolic enzyme phenylethanolamine *N*-methyltransferase (PNMT) to form epinephrine.[34] Epinephrine then is translocated into chromaffin granules, where the amine is stored while awaiting release.[35] PNMT activity is induced by high levels of glucocorticoid production in the adrenal cortex.

Presumably because expression of PNMT is dependent on high local concentrations of glucocorticoids, pheochromocytomas that produce large amounts of epinephrine typically have an adrenal location, whereas those in extra-adrenal locations usually produce only norepinephrine.[36] Pheochromocytomas that lack both PNMT and DBH and that predominantly produce dopamine are extremely rare. Dopamine production is a more common finding in individuals with parasympathetic-associated paragangliomas.

Conversion of tyrosine to dopa by TH represents the pivotal step in regulating synthesis and in maintaining stores of catechol-

amines in response to changes in catecholamine turnover associated with variations in exocytotic release. Rapid activation of TH is achieved by phosphorylation of serine residues at the regulatory domain, under the control of multiple Ca^{2+} and cyclic adenosine monophosphate (cAMP)-dependent pathways influenced by changes in nerve activity and actions of peptides and other coactivators.[37] Long-term regulation involves induction of synthesis of the enzyme at the transcriptional level. Feedback inhibition by catecholamines provides a further mechanism for the short-term regulation of enzyme activity.

α-Methyl-L-tyrosine or metyrosine (Demser) is an analogue of tyrosine that inhibits TH, thereby decreasing catecholamine stores. The drug is used occasionally in patients with pheochromocytoma (particularly those with extensive metastatic disease) or preoperatively.

STORAGE AND RELEASE

Translocation of catecholamines into vesicular granules for storage is facilitated by two vesicular monoamine transporters.[38] Both transporters have wide specificity for different monoamine substrates. It is important to note that vesicular stores of catecholamines do not exist in a static state, simply waiting for a signal for exocytotic release. Rather, vesicular stores of catecholamines exist in a highly dynamic equilibrium with the surrounding cytoplasm, with passive outward leakage of catecholamines into the cytoplasm counterbalanced by inward active transport under control of the vesicular monoamine transporters.[31]

Catecholamines share the acidic environment of the storage granule matrix with adenosine triphosphate (ATP), peptides, and proteins, the most well known of which are the chromogranins.[39] The chromogranins are ubiquitous components of secretory vesicles, and their widespread presence among endocrine tissues has led to their measurement in plasma as useful, albeit relatively nonspecific, markers of neuroendocrine tumors, including pheochromocytomas.

Catecholamines are stored in several types of vesicular granules that differ in size and type of protein and peptide components, the specific functions of which are incompletely understood. Two populations of chromaffin cells have been described with morphologically distinct vesicles, which preferentially store norepinephrine or epinephrine, and which release the two catecholamines differentially in response to different stimuli. Most adrenal pheochromocytomas secrete both norepinephrine and epinephrine; about a third exclusively produce norepinephrine, and a much smaller proportion exclusively produce and secrete epinephrine.

The process of exocytosis occurs at specialized locations on sympathetic varicosities dictated by the cell-surface expression of specialized docking proteins that interact with other proteins on the surfaces of secretory vesicles. The process is stimulated by an influx of Ca^{2+}, which in neurons is controlled primarily by nerve impulse–mediated membrane depolarization, and in adrenal medullary cells by acetylcholine release from innervating splanchnic nerves. The wide range of voltage-, receptor-, G protein–, and second messenger–operated Ca^{2+} channels provide numerous points for regulation of Ca^{2+}-triggered exocytosis. In this way, a variety of peptides, neurotransmitters, and humoral factors provide additional mechanisms for stimulation of exocytosis or may act to modulate nerve impulse–stimulated release of catecholamines. Norepinephrine also inhibits its own release through occupation of presynaptic α_2-adrenoceptors. The mechanisms regulating catecholamine release are closely coordinated so as to regulate the enzymes responsible for synthesis, thereby ensuring appropriate replenishment of the catecholamines lost through exocytosis.[40]

UPTAKE AND METABOLISM

Because the enzymes responsible for the metabolism of catecholamines have intracellular locations, the primary mechanism limiting the life span of catecholamines in the extracellular space is uptake by active transport, not metabolism by enzymes.[41] Uptake is facilitated by transporters that belong to two families with mainly neuronal and extraneuronal locations. The neuronal norepinephrine transporter provides the principal mechanism for rapid termination of the signal in sympathoneuronal transmission, whereas transporters at extraneuronal locations are more important for limiting the spread of the signal and for clearing catecholamines from the bloodstream. For norepinephrine released by sympathetic nerves, about 90% is removed back into nerves by neuronal uptake, 5% is removed by extraneuronal uptake, and 5% escapes these processes to enter the bloodstream. In contrast, for epinephrine released directly into the bloodstream from the adrenals, about 90% is removed by extraneuronal monoamine transport processes, the liver being particularly important. The presence of these highly active transport processes means that catecholamines are rapidly cleared from the bloodstream with a circulatory half-life of less than 2 minutes.

Irreversible inactivation of released catecholamines occurs in a series arrangement, with uptake followed by metabolism. Metabolism occurs through a multiplicity of pathways catalyzed by an array of enzymes and resulting in a variety of metabolites (see Figs. 14-3 and 14-4).[42] Deamination of catecholamines by monoamine oxidase (MAO) yields reactive aldehyde intermediate metabolites that are metabolized further to deaminated acids (by aldehyde dehydrogenase) or to deaminated alcohols (by alde-

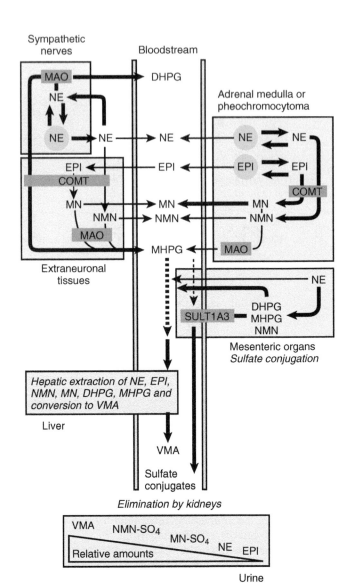

FIGURE 14-4. Model showing contributions of the adrenal medulla or a pheochromocytoma, in relation to sympathetic nerves and other tissues, to production of circulating catecholamines and catecholamine metabolites. Most metabolism occurs in the same cells where catecholamines are synthesized, mainly from catecholamines leaking from storage granules. In sympathetic nerves, where normally most catecholamine metabolism occurs, norepinephrine (NE) is deaminated by monoamine oxidase (MAO) to 3,4-dihydroxyphenylglycol (DHPG). The additional presence of catechol O-methyltransferase (COMT) in adrenal medullary cells leads to conversion of NE to normetanephrine (NMN) and of epinephrine (EPI) to metanephrine (MN). Normally, O-methylation is a minor pathway of catecholamine metabolism, but when a pheochromocytoma is present, O-methylation can represent a major pathway of metabolism. NMN and MN are converted to the sulfate-conjugated metabolites by sulfotransferase type 1A3 (SULT1A3), an enzyme present in high concentrations in digestive tissues. Vanillylmandelic acid (VMA), the main catecholamine metabolite excreted in urine, is formed in the liver largely from methoxyhydroxyphenylglycol (MHPG). MHPG is normally largely derived from extraneuronal O-methylation of DHPG produced in sympathetic nerves.

hyde or aldose reductase). The aldehyde intermediate formed from dopamine is a good substrate for aldehyde dehydrogenase but not for aldehyde or aldose reductase. In contrast, the aldehyde intermediates formed from the β-hydroxylated catecholamines (i.e., norepinephrine and epinephrine) are good substrates for aldehyde or aldose reductase but are poor substrates for aldehyde dehydrogenase. Therefore, norepinephrine and epinephrine are preferentially deaminated to 3,4-dihydroxyphenylglycol (DHPG), the alcohol metabolite. Deamination to the deaminated acid metabolite, 3,4-dihydroxymandelic acid (DHMA), is not a favored pathway.

Catechol-*O*-methyltransferase (COMT) is responsible for the second major pathway of catecholamine metabolism: catalyzing *O*-methylation of dopamine to methoxytyramine, norepinephrine to normetanephrine, and epinephrine to metanephrine. COMT is not present in catecholamine-producing neurons, which contain exclusively MAO, but it is present along with MAO in most extraneuronal tissues. The membrane-bound isoform of COMT, which has high affinity for catecholamines, is especially abundant in adrenal chromaffin and pheochromocytoma tumor cells.[43] As a result of differences in expression of metabolizing enzymes, catecholamines produced in neurons and adrenal medullary or pheochromocytoma tumor cells follow different neuronal and extraneuronal pathways of metabolism (see Figs. 14-3 and 14-4).

Neuronal pathways are quantitatively far more important than are extraneuronal pathways for the metabolism of norepinephrine produced in sympathetic nerves (see Fig. 14-4). The reasons for this are twofold. First, much more norepinephrine released by sympathetic nerves is removed by neuronal uptake than by extraneuronal uptake. Second, under resting conditions, much more of the norepinephrine metabolized intraneuronally is derived from transmitter leaking from storage vesicles than from transmitter recaptured after exocytotic release. Thus, most of the norepinephrine produced in the body is metabolized initially to DHPG, mainly from transmitter deaminated intraneuronally after leakage from storage vesicles or after release and reuptake.

DHPG is further *O*-methylated by COMT in non-neuronal tissues to 3-methoxy-4-hydroxyphenylglycol (MHPG), a metabolite that is also produced to a limited extent by deamination of normetanephrine and metanephrine. Compared with DHPG, normetanephrine and metanephrine are produced in small amounts and only at extraneuronal locations, with the single largest source representing adrenal chromaffin cells, which account for more than 90% of circulating metanephrine and 24% to 40% of circulating normetanephrine.[44] Within the adrenals, normetanephrine and metanephrine are produced similarly to DHPG in sympathetic nerves, from norepinephrine and epinephrine leaking from storage granules into the chromaffin cell cytoplasm.

The MHPG produced from DHPG and metanephrines is conjugated or metabolized to vanillylmandelic acid (VMA) by the sequential actions of alcohol dehydrogenase and aldehyde dehydrogenase. The former enzyme is localized largely to the liver. Thus, at least 90% of the VMA formed in the body is produced in the liver, mainly from hepatic uptake and metabolism of circulating DHPG and MHPG.[45]

With the exception of VMA, all the catecholamines and their metabolites are metabolized to sulfate conjugates by a specific sulfotransferase isoenzyme type 1A3 (SULT1A3). In humans, a single amino acid substitution confers the enzyme with particularly high affinity for dopamine and the *O*-methylated metabolites of catecholamines, including normetanephrine, metanephrine, and methoxytyramine. The SULT1A3 isoenzyme is found in high concentrations in gastrointestinal tissues, which therefore represent a major source of sulfate conjugates.

In humans, VMA and the sulfate and glucuronide conjugates of MHPG represent the main end products of norepinephrine and epinephrine metabolism. HVA and the conjugates of HVA are the main metabolic end products of dopamine metabolism. These end products and the other conjugates are eliminated mainly by urinary excretion. As a result, their circulatory clearance is slow and their plasma concentrations are high relative to those of the precursor amines.

Clinical Presentation

SIGNS AND SYMPTOMS

The presence of pheochromocytoma usually is characterized by clinical signs and symptoms (Table 14-1) that result from hemodynamic and metabolic actions of circulating catecholamines or, less commonly, of other amines and co-secreted neuropeptides.[18] Clinical findings such as hypertension, headache, unusual sweating, frequent arrhythmias, and the presence of pallor during hypertensive episodes are highly suggestive of pheochromocytoma. Although headache, palpitations, and sweating are nonspecific symptoms, their presence in patients with hypertension should arouse immediate suspicion for a pheochromocytoma because this triad constitutes the most commonly encountered symptoms in patients with a pheochromocytoma.

Sustained or paroxysmal hypertension (equally present) is the most common clinical sign (85% to 90%). Up to 13% of patients typically present with persistently normal blood pressure,[5,18] but this proportion can be much higher in patients with adrenal incidentalomas or in those who undergo periodic screening for familial pheochromocytoma.[12,46,47] In the latter group, tumors now are being found at an earlier stage, usually are quite small, and secrete low amounts of catecholamines. Other factors that may affect pheochromocytoma-associated elevations in blood pressure include the nature of catecholamine secretion, that is, receptor downregulation caused by consistently high levels of catecholamines, hypovolemia, and associated changes in sympathetic nerve function.[48] Pheochromocytoma also may present with hypotension, particularly with postural hypotension or with alternating episodes of high and low blood pressure.[5,49] This is commonly seen in patients who harbor tumors that are

Table 14-1. Signs and Symptoms of Pheochromocytoma*

Symptoms		Signs	
Headaches	++++	Hypertension	++++
Palpitations	+++	Tachycardia or reflex bradycardia	+++
Sweating	+++		
Anxiety/nervousness	++	Postural hypotension	+++
Tremulousness	++	Hypertension, paroxysmal	++
Nausea/emesis	++		
Pain in chest/abdomen	++	Weight loss	++
		Pallor	++
Weakness/fatigue	++	Hypermetabolism	++
Dizziness	+	Fasting hyperglycemia	++
Heat intolerance	+	Tremor	++
Paresthesias	+	Increased respiratory rate	++
Constipation	+		
Dyspnea	+	Decreased gastrointestinal motility	++
Visual disturbances	+	Psychosis (rare)	+
Seizures, grand mal	+	Flushing, paroxysmal (rare)	+

From Plouin PE et al.[53]
*Incidence: ++++, 76% to 100%; +++, 51% to 75%; ++, 26% to 50%; +, 1% to 25%.

secreting epinephrine or compounds causing vasodilatation, or after higher doses of antihypertensive therapy. Hypotension also may occur secondary to hypovolemia, abnormal autonomic reflexes, or differential stimulation of α- and β-adrenergic receptors, or as a result of the type of neuropeptide that is co-secreted.

Headache, which occurs in up to 90% of patients with pheochromocytoma,[1,18] may be mild or severe, short or long in duration, and may last for up to several days. In some patients, catecholamine-induced headache may be similar to tension headache.

Excessive generalized sweating occurs in approximately 60% to 70% of patients presenting with pheochromocytoma.[1,18] Other complaints are palpitations and dyspnea, weight loss despite normal appetite (caused by catecholamine-induced glycogenolysis and lipolysis), and generalized weakness.[49,50]

Some patients present with new and commonly more severe episodes of anxiety or panic attacks.[49] Palpitations, anxiety, and nervousness are more common in patients with pheochromocytomas that produce epinephrine.[49] Less common clinical manifestations include fever of unknown origin (hypermetabolic state) and constipation secondary to catecholamine-induced decrease in intestinal motility, or possibly enkephalins.[51] Some patients say that they feel flushed[18,52]; however, in our experience, the observation of an actual flush during a paroxysmal hypertensive episode in a patient with pheochromocytoma is an exceedingly rare event. Occasionally, Raynaud's phenomenon is noted. Patients also may present with tremor, seizures, hyperglycemia, hypermetabolism, weight loss (usually noted only in patients with malignant pheochromocytoma), fever, and even mental changes.[18,52]

Pheochromocytoma-induced metabolic or hemodynamic attacks may last from a few seconds to several hours, with intervals between attacks varying widely; some occur only once every few months. A typical paroxysm is characterized by a sudden major increase in blood pressure; a severe, often pounding headache; profuse sweating over most of the body, especially the trunk; palpitations with or without tachycardia; prominent anxiety or a sense of doom; skin pallor; nausea, with or without emesis; and pain in the abdomen, the chest, or both.[18,52,53] After an episode, patients usually feel drained and exhausted, and some may urinate more frequently. Initially, the episodes may be mild, of short duration, and infrequent.

Unusual symptoms related to paroxysmal blood pressure elevations during diagnostic procedures such as endoscopy, administration of anesthesia (caused by a sudden fall in blood pressure or any activation of the sympathetic nervous system, such as occurs during the induction phase of general anesthesia), or ingestion of food or beverages containing tyramine (e.g., certain cheeses, beers, wines, bananas, and chocolate) should arouse immediate suspicion of pheochromocytoma. The use of certain drugs such as histamine, metoclopramide, adrenocorticotropic hormone (ACTH), phenothiazine, methyldopa, monoamine oxidase inhibitors, tricyclic antidepressants, opiates (e.g., morphine, fentanyl), naloxone, droperidol, metoclopramide, glucagon, and chemotherapy may precipitate a hypertensive episode.[18,52,54-60] Moreover, micturition or bladder distention in the case of a pheochromocytoma of the urinary bladder (more than half of these individuals have painless hematuria) should promptly arouse suspicion of the presence of this tumor. Causes that account for episodic catecholamine secretion often remain unestablished, but in some situations, it may be caused by intentional or accidental tumor manipulation coupled with an increase

in intra-abdominal pressure from palpation, defecation, a fall, an automobile accident, or pregnancy.[18,52,61] Psychological stress does not usually precipitate a hypertensive crisis.[18,52,61] Timing of attacks may be unpredictable, and attacks may also occur at rest. However, about 8% to 10% of patients may be completely asymptomatic, usually because of a very small (less than 1 cm) tumor associated with nonsignificant catecholamine secretion or tumor dedifferentiation characterized by the absence of catecholamine-synthesizing enzymes and resulting in no production of catecholamines.[5] Normal plasma and urine catecholamines and metanephrines due to absence of catecholamine production have been observed in patients with metastatic pheochromocytoma, often due to an underlying mutation of the succinate dehydrogenase subunit B gene.[62] The defect was identified as an absence of tyrosine hydroxylase, the enzyme that catalyzes the initial and rate-limiting step in catecholamine biosynthesis (personal communication). These patients with so-called biochemically silent pheochromocytoma usually present at an advanced stage of the disease with symptoms and signs related to tumor mass effects rather than with symptoms and signs of catecholamine excess.

The hyperglycemia is usually mild, occurs with the hypertensive episodes, is accompanied by a subnormal level of plasma insulin (because of α-adrenergic inhibition of insulin release),[63] and usually does not require treatment; however, it can be sustained and severe enough to require insulin and even to present as diabetic ketoacidosis.[64] Hypoglycemia has also been reported.

Hypercalcemia has been reported in some patients with pheochromocytoma, sometimes as part of multiple endocrine neoplasia type 2 (MEN2)[54] but at other times without evidence of parathyroid disease[65] because the hypercalcemia disappears after the tumor is resected. Likewise, high levels of serum calcitonin, suggestive of medullary thyroid carcinoma, have been reported; these return to normal after the tumor is removed.[66] In addition, pheochromocytoma has presented as Cushing's syndrome with the tumor as the ectopic source of ACTH.[67] Because catecholamines suppress intestinal motility, constipation is common, and occasionally even adynamic ileus occurs. Rarely, pheochromocytoma has produced vasoactive intestinal peptide with resultant watery diarrhea, hypokalemia, and achlorhydria (Verner-Morrison syndrome).[68] Lactic acidosis without shock or sepsis has been reported.[69] Interleukin-6 (IL-6) may have caused fever and multiorgan failure in one patient with pheochromocytoma with increased serum IL-6 and in another with pheochromocytoma and Castleman's disease (IL-6–mediated B cell proliferation) because these conditions were reversed in each patient when the tumor was removed.[70,71] Many patients with pheochromocytoma are asymptomatic or have only minor signs and symptoms; therefore, the diagnosis is easily missed, often with tragic consequences. Several studies of routine autopsies have indicated that most pheochromocytomas are first discovered after death.[4] This pattern has continued into more recent studies, which show that the diagnosis is missed much more often in elderly patients.[72] This may result from the fact that elderly patients often have other, more common diseases (e.g., coronary or cerebral atherosclerosis) that could easily explain the minor symptoms that patients report.[72] A list of emergency situations characteristic for the presence of pheochromocytoma are described in Table 14-2.

Estrogen, growth hormone, vitamin D, and retinol A (Accutane) have been shown to induce pheochromocytoma in experimental animals.[73] Whether these hormones contribute to the higher incidence of clinical pheochromocytoma or to an increase

Table 14-2. Emergency Situations Related to Catecholamine Excess Released from Pheochromocytoma

Clinical Setting	Symptoms
Pheochromocytoma multisystem crisis (PMC)	Hypertension and/or hypotension, multiple organ failure, temperature of 40° C, encephalopathy
Cardiovascular	Collapse
	Hypertensive crisis
	Upon induction of anesthesia
	Medication-induced or other mechanisms
	Shock or profound hypotension
	Acute heart failure
	Myocardial infarction
	Arrhythmia
	Cardiomyopathy
	Myocarditis
	Dissecting aortic aneurysm
	Limb ischemia, digital necrosis or gangrene
Pulmonary	Acute pulmonary edema
	Adult respiratory distress syndrome
Abdominal	Abdominal bleeding
	Paralytic ileus
	Acute intestinal obstruction
	Severe enterocolitis and peritonitis
	Colon perforation
	Bowel ischemia plus generalized peritonitis
	Mesenteric vascular occlusion
	Acute pancreatitis
	Cholecystitis
	Megacolon
Neurologic	Hemiplegia
	Limb weakness
Renal	Acute renal failure
	Acute pyelonephritis
	Severe hematuria
Metabolic	Diabetic ketoacidosis
	Lactic acidosis

Adapted from Brouwers FM, Lenders JW, Eisenhofer G, Pacak K: Pheochromocytoma as an endocrine emergency, Rev Endocr Metab Disord 4:121-128, 2003.

Table 14-3. Differential Diagnosis for Pheochromocytoma

Neuroblastoma, ganglioneuroblastoma, ganglioneuroma
Adrenal medullary hyperplasia
Hyperadrenergic essential hypertension
Baroreflex failure
Thyrotoxicosis
Anxiety, panic attacks
Migraine or cluster headaches
Autonomic epilepsy
Abrupt clonidine withdrawal
Amphetamines
Cocaine
Alcoholism
Ingestion of tyramine-containing foods or proprietary cold preparations while taking monoamine oxidase inhibitors
Hypoglycemia, insulin reaction
Paroxysmal tachycardias including postural tachycardia syndrome
Angina pectoris or myocardial infarction
Mitral valve prolapse
Abdominal catastrophe/aortic dissection
Cardiovascular deconditioning
Renal parenchymal or renal artery diseases
Intracranial lesions, cerebral vasculitis, and hemorrhage
Menopausal syndrome
Lead poisoning
Toxemia of pregnancy
Unexplained shock
Acute intermittent porphyria

in malignant potential is unknown; however, recently at least two patients chronically receiving Accutane treatment were found to have pheochromocytoma (personal communications).

In summary, the following patients should be evaluated for a pheochromocytoma: (1) anyone with the triad of headaches, sweating, and tachycardia, whether or not the subject has hypertension; (2) anyone with a known mutation of one of the susceptibility genes and/or a family history of pheochromocytoma; (3) anyone with an incidental adrenal mass; (4) anyone whose hypertension is associated with borderline increases in catecholamine production reflected by elevated plasma catecholamine or metanephrine levels; (5) anyone whose blood pressure is poorly responsive to standard therapy; and (6) anyone who has had hypertension, tachycardia, or an arrhythmia in response to anesthesia, surgery, or medications known to precipitate symptoms in patients with pheochromocytoma.[48]

DIFFERENTIAL DIAGNOSIS

The differential diagnosis of pheochromocytoma includes a long list of conditions that may suggest the presence of the tumor (Table 14-3).[18,52,61] Many of these conditions can be excluded readily on the basis of a good history and physical examination. The most common mimic is hyperadrenergic hypertension, which is characterized by tachycardia, sweating, anxiety, and increased cardiac output.[74,75] These patients often have increased levels of catecholamines in blood and urine and may be excluded by use of the clonidine suppression test, which shows that the

excess catecholamines are caused by excess central sympathetic nervous activity and are not caused by a tumor (see the following).[48] Another common problem involves differentiating patients with pheochromocytoma from those with anxiety or panic attacks. This generally requires close observation of the patient during an episode.

Differentiation from an acute myocardial infarction may be difficult because angina pectoris and myocardial damage may occur in the absence of coronary artery disease in a patient with a pheochromocytoma. Many nonspecific electrocardiographic (ECG) changes have been reported, as well as various supraventricular and ventricular tachycardias, in patients with pheochromocytoma.

In the very rare situation in which a strong discordance is noted between symptoms and laboratory findings, one must consider the possibility of factitious administration of catecholamines. In this rare situation, as in other cases of factitious illness, an association of the individual with someone in the medical profession appears to be one of the common elements and should raise appropriate suspicion.

Patterns of biochemical test results that are more suggestive of sympathoadrenomedullary activation than of a tumor (e.g., as occurs in hypernoradrenergic hypertension, renovascular hypertension, congestive heart failure, panic disorder, and dumping syndrome) include proportionally larger elevations above the normal limits of plasma norepinephrine or epinephrine than of plasma normetanephrine or metanephrine.

Although severe paroxysmal hypertension should always raise suspicion of pheochromocytoma, it can also reflect a clinical entity called *pseudopheochromocytoma*. Pseudopheochromocytoma refers to the large majority of individuals (often women) with severe paroxysmal hypertension, whether normotensive or hypertensive between episodes, in whom pheochromocytoma has been ruled out.[76,77] Recent evidence indicates that pseudopheochromocytoma is a heterogeneous clinical condition subdivided into a primary and a secondary form. In contrast to a primary form, a secondary form is associated with various pathologies (e.g., hypoglycemia, autonomic epilepsy, baroreceptor failure) and medications, or with drug abuse.

The most common clinical characteristics of this syndrome might be attributable in many cases to short-term activation of the sympathetic nervous system. Paroxysmal hypertension usually is associated with tachycardia, palpitations, nervousness, tremor, weakness, excessive sweating, pounding headache, feeling hot, and facial paleness or (rarely) redness. In contrast to pheochromocytoma, patients with pseudopheochromocytoma more often present with panic attacks or anxiety, flushing, nausea, and polyuria.[76-78] All these symptoms well resemble a syndrome described by Page.[79] Equally interesting were his observations that "an attack is brought on by excitement" and that the syndrome has a clear predominance in women. Among the important features distinctive from pheochromocytoma are the circumstances under which episodes occur. In pseudopheochromocytoma, symptoms may be provoked rarely by some identifiable event. It is important, therefore, in questioning these patients, to search for specific provocative factors that may have precipitated these episodes. Similar to pheochromocytoma, episodes may last from a few minutes to several hours and may occur daily or once every few months. Between episodes, blood pressure is normal or may be mildly elevated. Pseudopheochromocytoma is sometimes treatable by antihypertensive drugs or psychotherapy.

Pathology

Sporadic pheochromocytomas are generally solitary, well-circumscribed, encapsulated tumors (Fig. 14-5A).[80] They usually are located in the adrenal gland or in its immediate vicinity. However, the adrenal gland may not be in its expected place atop the kidney, but actually may be located anywhere superior, inferior, medial, lateral, dorsal, or ventral to the kidney. Thus, pheochromocytoma may still be considered intra-adrenal in origin if the cortex of the adrenal is found in close relationship to the pheochromocytoma. Malignant tumors appear to be larger, to contain more necrotic tissue, and to be composed of smaller cells than are benign adrenal pheochromocytomas.[18,81] However, it is difficult, if not impossible, to distinguish malignant from benign pheochromocytomas on the basis of histopathologic features. Capsular invasion, vascular penetration, coarse nodularity, the presence of atypical nuclei, higher mitotic count, absence of intracytoplasmic hyaline granules, and mitosis exist in both types of pheochromocytoma.[80] Only tumor invasion of tissues and the presence of metastatic lesions (most commonly in the liver, lungs, lymphatic nodes, and bones) are consistent with the diagnosis of malignant pheochromocytoma.[18,82] As described by Linnoila and colleagues, fewer neuropeptides are expressed in malignant than in benign pheochromocytoma cells.[83] No differences have been noted in immunohistochemical expression of cathepsins, basic fibroblastic growth factor, c-met, or collagenase between benign and malignant pheochromocytomas.[84] Clarke and colleagues recently reported that MIB-1 appears to be a good indicator of the potential of metastatic pheochromocytoma, with a specificity of 100% and a sensitivity of 50%.[84]

Most pheochromocytomas range in size from 3 to 5 cm.[18,52,80] The largest tumor reported was 20 cm in diameter.[85] Tumors often show areas of hemorrhage, as well as areas of necrosis with cystic degeneration. These areas of hemorrhage and necrosis are the cause of the inhomogeneity seen in the images of pheochromocytoma on computed tomography (CT) scans.

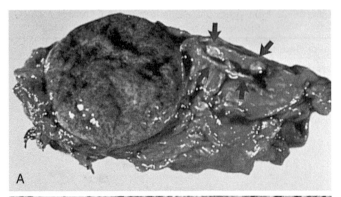
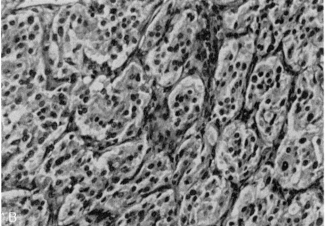
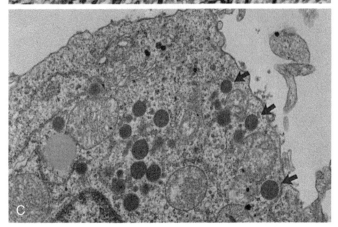

FIGURE 14-5. **A,** Cross section of a well-demarcated intra-adrenal pheochromocytoma with stippled areas of congestion. The normal adrenal cortex, which was a characteristic yellow-orange when fresh, is marked with arrows. **B,** The typical histology of an adrenal pheochromocytoma is shown with cells in nests and trabeculae separated by a thin vascular stroma (hematoxylin-eosin, ×400). **C,** Electron microscopy view of an adrenal pheochromocytoma with many large core catecholamine-containing granules, some marked with arrows. These granules, with a thin uniform halo between the core and the investing membrane, are the epinephrine-containing type. Granules with a prominent eccentric lucent space between the core and the limiting membrane are the norepinephrine-containing type (×13,500).

The chromaffin reaction, originally described by Henle in 1865, is a deep brown color of the adrenal medulla that occurs at least 12 hours after the tissue is placed in a dichromate solution.[86] The reaction is caused by the oxidation of the catecholamines epinephrine and norepinephrine into adrenochrome pigments. When this pattern is well developed, it mimics tumor cell nests or "zellballen," seen also in parasympathetic paragangliomas in the head and neck. Another pattern consists of anas-

Table 14-4. Pathologic Conditions Associated With Pheochromocytoma

Syndrome	Genetic Abnormality	Phenotypic Abnormalities
Multiple Endocrine Neoplasia Syndromes		
Multiple endocrine neoplasia type 2A (Sipple's syndrome)	Chromosome 10 (10q11.2)	Medullary carcinoma of the thyroid
	RET proto-oncogene mutations affect tyrosine kinase ligand-binding domain	Hyperparathyroidism
Multiple endocrine neoplasia type 2B	Chromosome 10 (10q11.2)	Medullary carcinoma of the thyroid
	RET proto-oncogene mutations affect tyrosine kinase catalytic site	Mucosal neuromas
		Intestinal ganglioneuroma
		Megacolon
		Marfanoid habitus
Neuroectodermal Syndromes		
Neurofibromatosis (von Recklinghausen's disease) type 1 (NF-1)	Chromosome 17 (17q11) mutations affect NF-1, tumor suppressor gene	Peripheral neurofibromas
Cerebelloretinal hemangioblastomatosis (von Hippel-Lindau syndrome, VHL) type 2	Chromosome 3 (3p25-26) missense mutations affect VHL, tumor suppressor gene	Retinal angiomas
		Cerebellar and spinal cord hemangioblastomas
		Renal cell cancer
		Pancreatic, renal, epididymal, and endolymphatic cysts/tumors
Succinate Dehydrogenase Gene Family Syndromes		
SDHB: paraganglioma (PGL) type 4	Chromosome 1 (1p36) missense, nonsense, and frameshift mutations	(Malignant) pheochromocytoma, parasympathetic paraganglioma
SDHC: PGL type 3	Chromosome 1 (1q21)	Parasympathetic paraganglioma, pheochromocytoma (rare)
SDHD: PGL type 1	Chromosome 11 (11q23) missense, nonsense, and frameshift mutations maternal imprinting	Parasympathetic paraganglioma, pheochromocytoma

tomosing cords of cells (trabecular). The third and most common pattern is a mixture of anastomosing cell cords and nests of cells (see Fig. 14-5B).[80] The tumor cells are usually polygonal with an intermediate amount of lightly colored eosinophilic granular cytoplasm. Cells may vary in size from small to large. Nuclei are well demarcated and generally eccentric in location. Nuclear pleomorphism with enlargement and hyperchromatism may be seen[80]; this is not diagnostic of malignancy. Occasionally, tumor cells resemble ganglion cells with rounded, eccentric nuclei and prominent nucleoli.

Touch preparations of the freshly cut surface of the tumor can be dried for several days over sodium hydroxide or another drying agent and then exposed to formaldehyde vapor. Examination under ultraviolet light reveals brightly colored catecholamine-containing granules within the cells of a pheochromocytoma.

Electron microscopy reveals the presence of membrane-bound, dense-core, neurosecretory granules 150 to 250 nm in diameter (see Fig. 14-5C).[80] In most tumors, the predominant granule is the one associated with norepinephrine, whereas in the normal gland, the predominant granule is the one associated with epinephrine.[87]

Chromaffin cells have the ability to synthesize and secrete various amines and certain peptide hormones (i.e., ACTH, chromogranins, neuropeptide Y, calcitonin, angiotensin-converting enzyme, renin, vasoactive intestinal polypeptide, adrenomedullin, enkephalins, and atrial natriuretic factor), and this accounts for some of the different presentations of pheochromocytoma (e.g., Cushing's syndrome, watery diarrhea). Antigens,[88] protein gene product 9.5,[89] galanin,[90] renin,[91] angiotensin-converting enzyme,[92] and synaptophysin[93] have been found in neuroendocrine neoplasms, including pheochromocytoma.

Genetics of Pheochromocytoma

Up to 24% of pheochromocytomas are inherited.[12,18,46,52,61] Hereditary pheochromocytoma is associated with multiple endocrine neoplasia type 2 (MEN2A or MEN2B), von Recklinghausen's neurofibromatosis type 1 (NF-1), von Hippel-Lindau (VHL) syndrome, and familial paraganglioma caused by germline mutations of genes encoding succinate dehydrogenase subunits B, C, and D (Table 14-4). In general, the traits are inherited in an autosomal dominant pattern.

MULTIPLE ENDOCRINE NEOPLASIA SYNDROMES

MEN2 is an autosomal dominantly inherited syndrome (Sipple's syndrome) that consists of pheochromocytoma, medullary carcinoma of the thyroid, and hyperparathyroidism.[94-96] It affects about 1 in 40,000 individuals and is characterized by medullary thyroid carcinoma, pheochromocytoma, and parathyroid hyperplasia/adenoma.[97]

The gene responsible for MEN2 is a proto-oncogene called RET.[98] In contrast to MEN1, RET is specifically expressed in neural crest–derived cells such as calcitonin-producing C cells in the thyroid gland and catecholamine-producing chromaffin cells in the adrenal gland. Whether it is also expressed in the parathyroid glands remains to be ascertained, especially when the low rate of hyperparathyroidism in patients with MEN2A and the lack of hyperparathyroidism in those with MEN2B are considered, although both conditions are caused by mutations in the RET gene. RET plays a role in normal gastrointestinal neuronal and kidney development, as exemplified by the RET knockout mouse, which has a Hirschsprung-like phenotype and renal cyst or agenesis.[99] RET is located on chromosome 10q11.2 and encodes a receptor tyrosine kinase, RET protein. As an oncogene, activation of RET leads to hyperplasia of target cells in vivo. Subsequent secondary events then lead to tumor formation.[100] RET consists of 21 exons with 6 so-called "hot spot exons" (exons 10, 11, 13, 14, 15, and 16) in which mutations are identified in 97% of patients with MEN2. Recently, it has been proposed that in addition to other events, RET protein accumulation, secondary to absent or reduced VHL protein, may then cause transformation of selected chromaffin cells to pheochromocytoma.[100] Additional studies are needed to clarify whether such somatic VHL gene alterations in MEN2-associated tumors play a role in early or late tumorigenesis or rather in tumor progression. RET germline mutation screening is commercially available (in the US, http://endocrine.mdacc.tmc.edu; Mayo Clinic, Rochester, MN) and has widely replaced the cumbersome provocative testing of calcitonin stimulation (with calcium and/or pentagastrin), which has been unreliable.

Pheochromocytomas (at least 70% of which are bilateral) develop on a background of adrenomedullary hyperplasia and become manifest (e.g., biochemically or on imaging) in about 50% of patients. MEN2-associated pheochromocytomas are almost exclusively benign (with <5% reported to be malignant) and localized to the adrenals. The peak age is around 40 years, but children as young as 10 years can be affected.[101,102]

Patients with MEN2-related pheochromocytoma often lack sustained hypertension or other symptoms (they occur only in about 50%). Because MEN-related pheochromocytomas secrete epinephrine, stimulation of β-adrenergic receptors causes palpitations and tachycardia. Therefore, their detection is based mainly on elevated plasma metanephrine and epinephrine levels. In patients with pheochromocytomas that exclusively produce normetanephrine, MEN2 can be excluded. MEN2-related pheochromocytomas are almost always intra-adrenal, are often bilateral (≈30% at diagnosis), and are rarely malignant (<5%).[46,103] In addition, as with most epinephrine-secreting pheochromocytomas, the hypertension is more likely to be paroxysmal than sustained. For these reasons, the diagnosis is easy to miss.

Medullary thyroid carcinoma is found in most patients with MEN2A, pheochromocytoma in a somewhat lesser percentage, and hyperparathyroidism in only about 25% of affected patients. Pheochromocytomas in MEN 2A most often are diagnosed at between 30 and 40 years of age. The syndrome results from germline mutations in the RET proto-oncogene on chromosome 10 (10q11.2).[98]

Patients with MEN2B have pheochromocytoma, medullary carcinoma of the thyroid, ganglioneuromatosis, multiple mucosal neuromas of eyelids, lips, and tongue, and some connective tissue disorders that include marfanoid habitus, scoliosis, kyphosis, pectus excavatum, slipped femoral epiphysis, and pes cavus.[104] This syndrome also appears to be caused by germline mutations in the RET proto-oncogene on chromosome 10, but these mutations affect the tyrosine kinase catalytic site of the protein.[105] In children with MEN2B-associated pheochromocytomas, a higher risk of malignancy compared with MEN2A or sporadic disease is found.[106]

MEN1 (Wermer's syndrome) consists of hyperparathyroidism, pituitary adenomas, and pancreatic islet cell tumors. Pheochromocytoma is not usually part of this complex; however, the occurrence of pheochromocytoma and pancreatic islet cell tumors has been reported in some families.[107] Often, the islet cell tumors are nonfunctional. Various "crossover" syndromes have been reported in which pheochromocytoma has been associated with characteristics of MEN1, MEN2A, MEN2B, von Recklinghausen's neurofibromatosis (NF), VHL, and the Zollinger-Ellison syndrome.[108] It has been proposed that the combination of neurofibromatosis, duodenal carcinoid, and pheochromocytoma constitutes a neuroendocrine syndrome that is separate from the combination of VHL, islet cell tumor, and pheochromocytoma.[109]

VON HIPPEL-LINDAU SYNDROME

Another neuroectodermal syndrome commonly associated with pheochromocytoma is VHL syndrome, which is caused by mutations in chromosome 3 (3p25-26), which encodes the VHL tumor suppressor gene.[110] Pheochromocytomas in VHL disease typically develop according to Knudson's two-hit model, including an inherited germline mutation of VHL and loss of function of the wild-type allele of the VHL gene. The disease has been divided into two types based on the significant genotype-phenotype correlations observed. Type 1 includes mainly large deletions or mutations and expresses the full phenotype of vascular lesions of the retina, cysts or solid tumors in the brain or spinal cord, pancreatic cysts, renal cell carcinoma, epididymal cystadenoma, and endolymphatic sac tumors, but no pheochromocytoma. Type 2 has missense mutations, pheochromocytoma, and the full phenotype.[111] Patients often are asymptomatic when they present with other aspects of this disease. This syndrome is variable in terms of the different organ systems involved and the extent of involvement from patient to patient and from family to family. Overall, less than 30% of patients with a VHL germline mutation develop a pheochromocytoma. Pheochromocytomas as part of the VHL syndrome have an exclusively noradrenergic phenotype, reflecting the production of norepinephrine only.[112] These tumors are located mainly intra-adrenally and are bilateral in about 50% of patients, with a less than 7% incidence of metastases. Because they do not express glucagon receptors, the glucagon test should not be used for detection of these tumors. These tumors are commonly found on the basis of periodic annual screening, or during searches for other tumors that are part of this syndrome. Therefore, when detected, these tumors are commonly small; they often fail to be detected by nuclear imaging methods. Furthermore, about 80% of pheochromocytomas found in patients with VHL during screening are asymptomatic and are not associated with hypertension.

NEUROFIBROMATOSIS TYPE 1

Von Recklinghausen's NF is now divided into two types: NF-1 has neurofibromas of peripheral nerves, whereas NF-2 has central neurofibromas. NF-1 is inherited in an autosomal dominant pattern. The association with pheochromocytoma is one between a relatively common disease and a rare disease. Thus, although less than 1% to 2% of patients with NF have pheochromocytoma, about 5% of patients with pheochromocytoma have NF.[113] Pheochromocytoma associated with NF-1 is caused by germline mutations in chromosome 17 (17q11), where the NF-1 gene encodes for the protein neurofibromin. These mutations lead to inactivation of this tumor suppressor gene and its protein.[114] Similar mutations introduced into the NF-1 gene in mice lead to pheochromocytoma, which is otherwise rare in these animals.[115] Pheochromocytoma in patients with NF-1 is rarely seen in children, because it usually occurs at a later age (around 50 years). Only 12% of patients with NF-1 are diagnosed with bilateral and multifocal pheochromocytomas, and less than 6% of patients have metastatic pheochromocytoma.[116]

The incidence of pheochromocytoma in NF-1 is relatively low (about 1%) compared with other hereditary syndromes, and routine screening of such patients generally is not recommended. However, if a patient with NF-1 has hypertension, then a pheochromocytoma should be considered and excluded.[113]

SUCCINATE DEHYDROGENASE GENE FAMILY

Recently, pheochromocytoma susceptibility has been associated with germline mutations of the *succinate dehydrogenase (SDH)* gene family.[117,118] The *SDH* genes (*SDHA, SDHB, SDHC,* and *SDHD*) encode the four subunits of complex II of the mitochondrial electron transport chain,[119] which is essential for the generation of ATP (oxidative phosphorylation). *SDHB* and *SDHD* mutations can lead to complete loss of SDH enzymatic activity, a phenomenon that has been linked to tumorigenesis through upregulation of hypoxic-angiogenetic responsive genes.[120] Unlike the *SDHA* gene, mutations of *SDHB, SDHC,* and *SDHD* genes are associated with the presence of familial and nonfamilial pheochromocytoma and parasympathetic paraganglioma. Frameshift, missense, and nonsense mutations were identified for the *SDH* gene family. In recent studies, it has been found that about 4% to 12% of sporadic pheochromocytomas[12,121] and up to 50% of familial pheochromocytomas[121] have *SDHD* or *SDHB* mutations. The *SDHB, SDHC,* and *SDHD* traits are inherited in an autosomal dominant fashion and give rise to familial paraganglioma (PGL) syndromes 4, 3, and 1, respectively (see Table 14-4). The penetrance of these traits is incomplete, however. Furthermore, *SDHD*-related disease is characterized by maternal genomic imprinting. Because of silencing of the maternal allele by methylation, individuals who inherit a mutation from their mother remain free of paraganglioma but still may pass on the mutation to their offspring. *SDHB* mutations predispose to mainly extra-adrenal pheochromocytomas with a high malignant potential, and less frequently to benign parasympathetic head and neck paragangliomas.[62,122-124] *SDHD* mutations typically are associated with multifocal parasympathetic head and neck paragangliomas and usually with benign extra-adrenal and adrenal pheochromocytomas.[122,124] Metastastic pheochromocytoma is rare in *SDHD* mutation carriers, but it can occur.[123,125] *SDHC* mutations are rare and are almost exclusively associated with parasympathetic head and neck paraganglioma,[126] although rare cases of *SDHC*-associated extra-adrenal pheochromocytoma have been reported.[127,128] Most *SDHB*-related paragangliomas secrete norepinephrine or both norepinephrine and dopamine,[62] a profile that is consistent with mainly extra-adrenal tumors. Some *SDHB*-related PGLs exclusively overproduce dopamine, but not other catecholamines.[62,129-131] Therefore, measurement of plasma levels of dopamine or its *O*-methylated metabolite methoxytyramine should be considered in *SDHB*-related pheochromocytoma. As mentioned, ≈10% of *SDHB*-related sympathetic paragangliomas are "biochemically silent." The biochemical phenotype of *SDHD*-associated pheochromocytoma has not been studied consistently.

We recommend to offer genetic testing, preceded by careful genetic counseling, to all first-degree family members of patients with *SDH*-related pheochromocytoma and paraganglioma,[132] and to subsequently carry out a periodic clinical, biochemical, and radiologic tumor screening among mutation carriers, especially those with an *SDHB* mutation. No evidence-based protocol has been used for tumor screening among children with a known *SDHB*, or any other mutation. We recommend periodic biochemical and total body magnetic resonance imaging (MRI) screening from as early as age 7.

SPORADIC AND OTHER PHEOCHROMOCYTOMAS

Genetic analyses of DNA from sporadic pheochromocytoma have yielded variable results, with up to 20% *RET* mutations (half MEN2A and half MEN2B) in some series, and up to 20% VHL mutations in others.[46,133,134] In another study, 45% of sporadic adrenal pheochromocytomas had loss of heterozygosity at the VHL gene locus, but no genetic abnormalities were found in sporadic extra-adrenal pheochromocytomas.[135] Genetic analysis provides positive identification of carriers in familial syndromes and thus identifies who should be screened and who need not be screened for the various traits of the phenotype.

Pheochromocytoma also may occur as part of Carney's triad (i.e., gastric leiomyosarcoma, pulmonary chondroma, and extra-adrenal pheochromocytoma).[136] The syndrome is very rare; fewer than 30 cases have been reported, and only 25% of patients manifest all three parts of the triad. It occurs sporadically and is clearly nonfamilial.[137] Recently, a new syndrome called the Stratakis-Carney syndrome, or the "dyad of gastrointestinal stromal tumor and paraganglioma" associated with *SDHB, SDHC,* and *SDHD* mutations, was identified.[138]

For the genetic diagnosis of pheochromocytoma, a panel of experts at the International Symposium on Pheochromocytoma 2005 held in Bethesda, Maryland, agreed that, although there is now a reasonable argument for more widespread genetic testing, it is neither appropriate nor currently cost-effective to test for every disease-causing gene in every patient with a pheochromocytoma or paraganglioma. Rather, it was stressed that the decision to test, and which genes to test, requires judicious consideration of numerous factors, several of which are noted in Fig. 14-6.

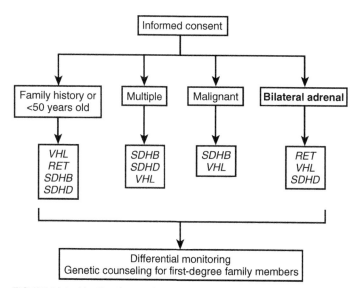

FIGURE 14-6. Algorithm for genetic testing for genes associated with pheochromocytoma. The algorithm should be applied if there is a family history of pheochromocytoma, the patient is <50 years old, or multiple malignant or bilateral tumors are present. The biochemical phenotype of a tumor should also be considered in selection of the most appropriate genes to test. The term *multiple* in the figure indicates tumors in separate anatomic locations. Patients with multiple endocrine neoplasia type 2 might have multiple tumors in a single adrenal gland. It should be considered that multiple or bilateral tumors often do not occur simultaneously. *RET*, Rearranged during transfection; *SDHB*, *succinate dehydrogenase subunit B gene*; *SDHD*, succinate dehydrogenase subunit D gene; *VHL*, von Hippel-Lindau gene. (Adapted from Pacak et al.[154,155])

Biochemical Diagnosis of Pheochromocytoma

INITIAL BIOCHEMICAL TESTING

Missing a pheochromocytoma can have deadly consequences. Therefore, one of the most important considerations in the choice of an initial biochemical test is a high level of reliability that the test will provide a positive result in that rare patient with the tumor. Such a test also provides confidence that a negative result reliably excludes the tumor, thereby avoiding the need for multiple or repeat biochemical tests or even costly and unnecessary imaging studies to rule out the tumor. Therefore, the initial workup of a patient with suspected pheochromocytoma should include a suitably sensitive biochemical test.

Catecholamine secretion by pheochromocytomas can be episodic or, in patients who are asymptomatic, negligible in nature. Thus, measurements of urinary or plasma catecholamines do not provide reliable biochemical tests for detection of the tumor. This is particularly problematic during screening for pheochromocytoma in patients with a predisposing hereditary condition, where 26% to 29% of tumors can be expected to be associated with normal urinary excretion or plasma concentrations of catecholamines.[139] Because of the intermittent nature of catecholamine secretion, it has been recommended that urine or blood samples are best collected when the patient is hypertensive. Hypertension, however, can be present in some patients independently of catecholamine release by a tumor. Thus, normal catecholamines in a patient with hypertension do not exclude pheochromocytoma.

Because metanephrines are produced continuously within pheochromocytoma tumor cells, and independently of catecholamine release, these measurements obviate any need for collection of blood or urine samples during hypertensive episodes. This understanding has provided a rationale for subsequent studies examining the utility of measurements of plasma free metanephrines for diagnosis of pheochromocytoma.[8,9,139-144] At the National Institutes of Health (NIH), the superiority of plasma free metanephrines over other tests was established in a series of three published reports,[9,139,143] culminating in a study involving more than 850 patients, including 214 with pheochromocytoma.[9] Plasma free metanephrines showed superior combined diagnostic sensitivity and specificity over all other tests examined, including urinary and plasma catecholamines, urinary vanillylmandelic acid, and urinary total and fractionated metanephrines. Analysis of receiver-operating characteristic curves showed that at equivalent levels of sensitivity, the specificity of plasma free metanephrines was higher than that of all other tests, and that, at equivalent levels of specificity, the sensitivity of plasma free metanephrines was also higher than that of all other tests, even when the latter were combined.

The high diagnostic sensitivity of measurements of plasma free metanephrines has now been independently confirmed by four other groups of investigators.[8,140,142] All together, the five independent studies—with 336 patients with pheochromocytoma and close to 2500 patients in whom the tumor was excluded—have indicated an overall diagnostic sensitivity of 98% and specificity of 92% for measurement of plasma free metanephrines.

Metanephrines in urine usually are measured after a deconjugation step that liberates free metanephrines from sulfate- or glucuronide-conjugated metanephrines,[145,146] whereas plasma metanephrines are measured most often in the free form, but they can also be measured after a deconjugation step (Fig. 14-7). Conjugated metanephrines are present in urine and plasma at much higher concentrations than are free metanephrines. Adding to the confusion in terminology is the fact that historically metanephrines were measured in urine by spectrophotometric methods as "total" metanephrines, representing the combined sum of deconjugated normetanephrine (the O-methylated metabolite of norepinephrine) and deconjugated metanephrine (the O-methylated metabolite of epinephrine).

Spectrophotometric measurements of total metanephrines have been largely phased out in favor of newer chromatographic methods that allow fractionated measurements of normetanephrine and metanephrine (hence the term *fractionated metanephrines*). Reports of "fractionated" metanephrines still often include a value for "total" metanephrines as a holdover from earlier spectrophotometic measurements, but this vestigial line in the report offers little value to the clinician. Because many pheochromocytomas produce mainly (or solely) only one of the two metabolites, separate measurements of normetanephrine and metanephrine ensure that small or mild increases in one metabolite are not diluted by normal levels of the other. Separate measurements also allow distinction of norepinephrine from epinephrine-producing pheochromocytomas, which as discussed later can provide additional useful information about a possible pheochromocytoma.

SAMPLING PROCEDURES AND INTERFERENCES

The conditions under which blood or urine samples are collected can be crucial to the reliability and interpretation of test results. Blood for measurements of plasma-free metanephrines or catecholamines ideally should be collected with patients supine for at least 20 minutes before sampling.[147] To avoid any stress associated with the needlestick, samples ideally should be collected through a previously inserted IV. Alternatively, the sample may be taken by needlestick from a seated patient, provided that upper reference limits obtained after supine rest using an indwelling IV are used.[148] False positives in this situation are more prevalent. Thus, if the seated test returns a positive result, sampling should be repeated after rest in the supine position to rule out a false-positive initial test. Patients should have refrained from nicotine and alcohol for at least 12 hours and, to minimize analytic interference, should have fasted overnight before blood sampling.

A 24-hour collection of urine is often favored over blood sampling, because this avoids the rigid sampling conditions associated with blood collection and is more convenient for clinical staff to implement. However, 24-hour collections of urine are not always easily, conveniently, or reliably collected by patients, particularly pediatric patients. Also, the influences of diet and of sympathoneuronal and adrenal medullary systems activation (associated with physical activity or changes in posture) are not controlled as easily as they are for blood collections. Thus, some investigators advocate spot or overnight urine collections with output of catecholamines or metanephrines normalized against urinary creatinine excretion.[149] Additional considerations for urine collected under these conditions include dietary protein, muscle mass, level of physical activity, and time of day, all of which influence creatinine excretion and confound interpretation of results.

Dietary constituents or medications can cause direct analytic interference in measurements of catecholamines and metabolite levels or may influence the physiologic processes that determine

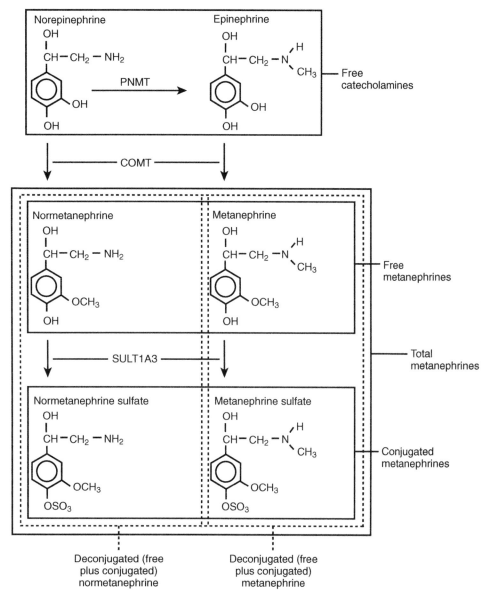

FIGURE 14-7. Pathway of production of free and sulfate-conjugated metanephrines, illustrating differences in free metanephrines measured in plasma and deconjugated metanephrines (free plus conjugated metanephrines) measured in urine. Deconjugated metanephrines in urine may be measured as fractionated metanephrines (i.e., separate measurements of deconjugated normetanephrine and metanephrine) or as total metanephrines (i.e., the combined sum of deconjugated normetanephrine and metanephrine). *COMT,* Catechol *O*-methyltransferase; *PNMT,* phenylethanolamine *N*-methyltransferase; *SULT1A3,* monoamine-preferring phenol sulfotransferase.

these levels. Analytic interference can be highly variable, depending on the particular measurement method used, whereas physiologic interference is usually of a more general nature and is independent of the measurement method used (Table 14-5). Tricyclic antidepressants, in particular, are a major source of physiologic interference.[150] The high incidence of false-positive results for plasma or urinary norepinephrine and normetanephrine in patients taking tricyclics is presumably caused by the primary inhibitory actions of these agents on monoamine reuptake. The result is an increased escape of norepinephrine from sympathetic nerve terminals into the bloodstream.

The development of new drugs, variations in assay techniques, and continuing improvements in analytic procedures make it difficult to identify which directly interfering medications should be avoided for a given analytic test. Labetalol and its metabolites, which were common sources of analytic interference with spectrometric and fluorometric measurements of cat-

echolamines and metanephrines, now represent only a variable source of interference for high-pressure liquid chromatographic (HPLC) measurements of catecholamines, with interference mainly affecting epinephrine determinations.[151] The anxiolytic agent buspirone (Buspar) is another drug that can cause falsely elevated levels of urinary metanephrine in some but not all HPLC assays of urinary fractionated metanephrines.[150] Similarly, acetaminophen can directly interfere with measurements of normetanephrine in some HPLC assays, but not in others.[152,153]

BIOCHEMICAL ALGORITHM

Expert recommendations for initial biochemical testing from the International Symposium on Pheochromocytoma include measurements of fractionated metanephrines in urine or plasma, or both, as available.[154,156] No consensus was reached on whether plasma or urine measurement should be the preferred test. Both tests offer similarly high diagnostic sensitivity (provided appro-

Table 14-5. Medications That May Cause Physiologically Mediated False-Positive Elevations of Plasma and Urinary Catecholamines or Metanephrines

	Catecholamines		Metanephrines	
	NE	E	NMN	MN
Tricyclic antidepressants				
Amitriptyline (Elavil), imipramine (Topfranil), nortriptyline (Aventyl)	+++	−	+++	−
α-Blockers (nonselective)				
Phenoxybenzamine (Dibenzyline)	+++	−	+++	−
α-Blockers (α₁-selective)				
Doxazosin (Cardura), terazosin (Hytrin), prazosin (Minipress)	+	−	−	−
β-Blockers				
Atenolol (Tenormin), metoprolol (Lopressor), propranolol (Inderal), labetalol (Normadyne)*	+	+	+	+
Calcium channel antagonists				
Nifedipine (Procardia), amlodipine (Norvasc), diltiazem (Cardizem), verapamil (Calan)	+	+	−	−
Vasodilators				
Hydralazine (Apresoline), isosorbide (Isordil, Dilatrate), minoxidil (Loniten)	+	−	Unknown	
Monoamine oxidase inhibitors				
Phenelzine (Nardil), tranylcypromine (Parnate), selegiline (Eldepryl)	−	−	+++	+++
Sympathomimetics				
Ephedrine, pseudoephedrine (Sudafed), amphetamines, albuterol (Proventil)	++	++	++	++
Stimulants				
Caffeine (coffee*, tea), nicotine (tobacco), theophylline	++	++	Unknown	
Miscellaneous				
Levodopa, carbidopa (Sinemet)*	++	−	Unknown	
Cocaine	++	++	Unknown	

E, Epinephrine; MN, metanephrine; NE, norepinephrine; NMN, normetanephrine; +++, substantial increase; ++, moderate increase; +, mild increase if any; −, little or no increase.

*Indicates a drug that can also cause direct analytic interference with some methods.

priate reference ranges are used), so that a negative result for either test appears equally effective for excluding pheochromocytoma. However, because of differences in specificity, tests of plasma free metanephrines exclude pheochromocytoma in more patients without the tumor than do tests of urinary fractionated metanephrines. Additional measurements of urinary or plasma catecholamines may be carried out, but in our experience are unlikely to lead to detection of additional tumors not indicated by elevated levels of normetanephrine or metanephrine. Exceptions include rare tumors that produce exclusively dopamine.[8] With a mind to the above exception, the decision to rule out pheochromocytoma should be based primarily on findings of negative test results for measurements of normetanephrine and metanephrine. An algorithm for the biochemical diagnosis of pheochromocytoma is given in Fig. 14-8.

FOLLOW-UP BIOCHEMICAL TESTING

Follow-up biochemical testing usually should be necessary only in patients with positive results of initial tests of plasma free or urinary fractionated metanephrines. Exceptions include patients at high risk for pheochromocytoma because of a hereditary syndrome or a prior history of the tumor, all of whom should undergo periodic screening. In these patients, and occasionally in others with adrenal incidentalomas, the tumors may be too small to produce signs and symptoms or a positive result by any available biochemical test. In these patients, positive results likely will follow enlargement of tumors.

Because of the large numbers of patients tested for pheochromocytoma and the rarity of the tumor, false-positive results can be expected to outnumber true-positive results, even for tests with reasonably high specificity. Thus, the likelihood of pheochromocytoma in a patient with a positive result is usually low. Follow-up tests are invariably required to unequivocally confirm or exclude the tumor, the extent and nature of this requiring informed and sound clinical decision making. Thus, the clinician who judges the likelihood of a pheochromocytoma from a single positive test result should first take into account the degree of initial clinical suspicion or pretest probability of the tumor, which affects the posttest probability of a tumor.

The extent of the increase in a positive test result is crucially important for judging the likelihood of a pheochromocytoma. Most patients with the tumor have increases in plasma or urinary metanephrines well in excess of those more commonly encountered as false-positive results in patients without the tumor. Increases in plasma concentrations of normetanephrine to above 400 ng/L (2.2 nmol/L) or of metanephrine to above 236 ng/L (1.2 nmol/L) are extremely rare in patients without pheochromocytoma, but occur in about 80% of patients with the tumor.[9] Similarly, increases in urinary output of normetanephrine to above 1500 μg/day (8.2 μmol/day) or of metanephrine to above 600 μg/day (3.0 μmol/day) are rare in patients without pheochromocytoma, but occur in about 70% of patients with the tumor. Provided that biochemical test results are accurate, the likelihood of pheochromocytoma in such a patient is so high that the immediate task is to locate the tumor.

When concern is expressed about the analytic accuracy of a positive plasma test result, this can be checked by a follow-up urinary test, and vice versa concern arises about an initial urinary test result. Such follow-up testing may be particularly prudent in patients with milder increases in plasma free or urinary fractionated metanephrines, where the posttest probability of pheochromocytoma remains low, and where subtle analytic interferences can be difficult for the testing laboratory to recognize. A similar pattern of increases in urinary and plasma normetanephrine or metanephrine not only helps confirm the accuracy of results but increases the likelihood of a pheochromocytoma.

Before follow-up testing is implemented, some consideration should be given to sources of false-positive results, including accompanying medical conditions, inappropriate sampling conditions, dietary influences, and medications likely to directly interfere with analytic results or to increase levels of normeta-

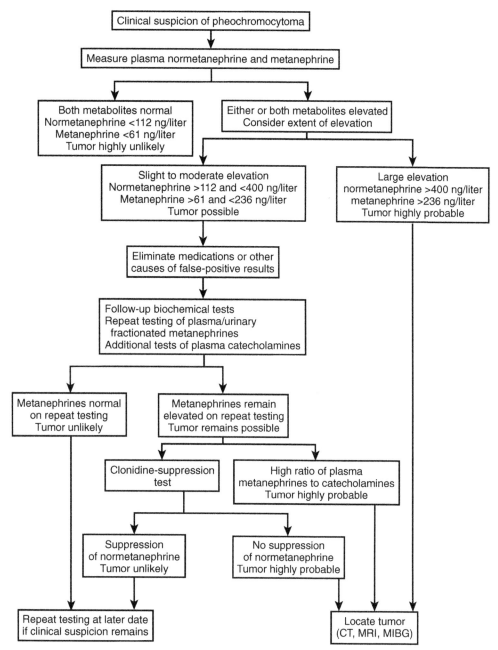

FIGURE 14-8. Algorithm for biochemical diagnosis of pheochromocytoma.

nephrine or metanephrine (see Table 14-5). Among the latter, tricyclic antidepressants and phenoxybenzamine (Dibenzyline) can be common sources of false-positive results.[150] Tricyclic antidepressants elevate plasma and urinary norepinephrine and normetanephrine through blockade of norepinephrine reuptake at sympathetic nerve endings, and these are contraindicated in patients with pheochromocytoma. Phenoxybenzamine also increases plasma and urinary norepinephrine and normetanephrine, presumably by blocking presynaptic α_2-adrenoceptors and releasing sympathetic nerves from the inhibitory effects of occupation of these receptors on norepinephrine release. Therefore, phenoxybenzamine should not be used for treatment until biochemical testing is complete and confirms the presence of tumor.

Additional sampling for plasma catecholamines, in combination with plasma free metanephrines or urinary catecholamines,

in combination with urinary fractionated metanephrines, can provide further useful information to help distinguish true-positive from false-positive results.[150] Because free metanephrines are produced continuously within pheochromocytoma tumor cells by a process that is independent of catecholamine release, patients with true-positive results usually have larger percent increases in plasma metanephrines to above the upper reference limits than percent increases in the parent catecholamines. Conversely, because substantial amounts of metanephrine (greater than 90%) and normetanephrine (26% to 40%) are normally produced within adrenal medullary cells, independently of catecholamine release, increases in metanephrines during activation of sympathoneuronal and adrenal medullary systems are smaller than increases in catecholamines. Thus, patients with false-positive results caused by sympathoneuronal and adrenal medullary systems activation usually have larger percent increases in plasma norepinephrine than in plasma normetanephrine or plasma epinephrine than in metanephrine.

Because of relatively poor diagnostic sensitivity, measurements of urinary VMA or of urinary "total" metanephrines are of limited value for detecting or excluding pheochromocytoma. Such tests rarely provide useful diagnostic information beyond that attained by measurement of plasma or urinary fractionated metanephrines, where normetanephrine and metanephrine are measured separately. Exceptions include metastases confined to the liver or to mesenteric organs where the vascular drainage from tumors enters the liver, the main site in the body for formation of VMA from catecholamines and catecholamine metabolites.

PHARMACOLOGIC TESTS

Various pharmacologic tests have been used over the years in an attempt to improve diagnostic accuracy for pheochromocytoma. This was especially true years ago, when the assays for catecholamines and their metabolites were new, crude, and often undependable. However, provocative tests are inherently dangerous, as indicated by the several deaths that have been reported during histamine testing.[157] In light of the much improved quality of present assays, the use of these pharmacologic procedures has been greatly reduced. On the other hand, suppression tests may be useful and bear lower risk.

Clonidine (Catapres) is now the drug used most often in suppression tests to identify a pheochromocytoma.[48,158] It is a centrally acting α_2-adrenergic agonist that suppresses central sympathetic nervous outflow; this normally results in lower levels of plasma catecholamines. Blood is drawn for plasma catecholamines before and 3 hours after the oral administration of clonidine 0.3 mg/70 kg body weight. Tricyclic antidepressants and diuretics are reported to compromise reliability of the test[159]; therefore, these medications should be withdrawn before testing is begun. Profound hypotensive responses to clonidine can be troublesome in some patients taking antihypertensive medications; therefore, these should be stopped on the day of the test. Plasma catecholamine levels will decrease if they are under normal physiologic control, whereas in patients with pheochromocytoma, plasma catecholamines will not decrease.

The clonidine suppression test is unreliable in patients with normal or only mildly increased plasma catecholamine levels.[160] In such patients, normal suppression of plasma norepinephrine may occur after administration of clonidine despite the presence of a pheochromocytoma. Presumably, normal suppression occurs because much of the norepinephrine is derived from sympathetic nerves and remains responsive to clonidine. The clonidine suppression test therefore is recommended for patients with plasma catecholamine levels over 5.9 nmol/L (1000 pg/mL), with a normal response defined as a fall to within the normal range.[158] This recommendation makes it problematic to use the test in patients with normal or only mildly elevated plasma catecholamine levels, which is particularly troublesome because such patients represent those in whom it is most difficult to conclusively diagnose pheochromocytoma.

Additional measurements of plasma normetanephrine before and after clonidine provide a method for overcoming the above limitation in patients with elevated plasma concentrations of normetanephrine, but normal or mildly elevated plasma concentrations of norepinephrine.[150] A decrease in plasma levels of normetanephrine of more than 40% or to below the upper reference limit (0.61 nmol/L = 112 pg/mL) was present in all patients without pheochromocytoma, indicating a diagnostic specificity of 100%. This was similar to that for norepinephrine (specificity = 98%), where pheochromocytoma could be excluded by a decrease in norepinephrine of more than 50% or a level of norepinephrine after clonidine below 2.94 nmol/L (498 pg/mL). Among patients with pheochromocytoma, only 2 of 48 had plasma levels of normetanephrine that fell by more than 40% or to below 0.61 nmol/L (112 pg/mL) after clonidine. This indicated a diagnostic sensitivity for normetanephrine responses to clonidine of 98%, which represents a substantial improvement over the sensitivity of only 67% for norepinephrine responses. Thus, the clonidine suppression test, combined with measurements of plasma normetanephrine, provides an efficient and reasonably reliable method for distinguishing false-positive from true-positive elevations in plasma normetanephrine.

As was noted previously, provocative tests are inherently dangerous and are rarely called for. Glucagon is the drug that is usually used.[75,161] A positive test result is usually defined as an increase in plasma norepinephrine of greater than threefold or to more than 2000 pg/mL, 2 minutes after an IV bolus of 1.0 mg.[162] The test has high diagnostic specificity but limited sensitivity. Phentolamine must always be at hand for the treatment of any episodes of severe hypertension.

ADDITIONAL INTERPRETATIVE CONSIDERATIONS

Pheochromocytomas differ considerably in rates of catecholamine synthesis, turnover, and release, and in the types of catecholamines and metabolites produced. These differences may explain variations in presenting signs and symptoms; they also can provide useful information about the tumor, including the adrenal or extra-adrenal location, the underlying mutation, tumor size, and the presence of metastatic disease.

Adrenal pheochromocytomas may produce near exclusively norepinephrine, or both norepinephrine and epinephrine. In contrast, extra-adrenal pheochromocytomas almost invariably produce exclusively norepinephrine.[36] Differences in plasma concentrations or urinary outputs of normetanephrine and metanephrine reflect underlying differences in tumor catecholamine phenotype better than do differences in plasma or urinary norepinephrine and epinephrine. Thus, patients with increases in only normetanephrine may have tumors with an adrenal or extra-adrenal location, whereas those with additional or exclusive increases in metanephrine are likely to have a tumor with an adrenal location. Exceptions to the above rule have been described in patients with recurrence or spread from a primary epinephrine-producing tumor with an adrenal location.[163]

Pheochromocytomas that produce mainly epinephrine (and hence also produce large amounts of metanephrine) tend to present more often with alternating hypertension and hypotension and to be more paroxysmal in nature than do those that produce exclusively norepinephrine.[164,165] Patients with tumors that secrete large amounts of epinephrine may present with signs and symptoms that reflect the potent actions of epinephrine on glucose metabolism and pulmonary physiology (e.g., hyperglycemia, dyspnea, pulmonary edema).[59,166] Among patients with hereditary pheochromocytoma, differences in metanephrine production distinguish MEN2 from VHL, and can provide a supplementary guide to clinical presentation for deciding which gene to test to unambiguously identify the underlying germline mutation.[167]

Mutation-dependent differences in expression of genes may explain the progression from benign to malignant pheochromocytoma, which often is characterized by a dedifferentiated state.

Norepinephrine is usually the predominant catecholamine produced.[168,169] Metastatic pheochromocytomas sometimes can be characterized by high tissue, plasma, and urinary levels of dopa and dopamine, the immediate precursors of norepinephrine.[169-171] Elevations in plasma or urinary dopa and dopamine are not in themselves particularly sensitive or specific markers of benign or metastatic pheochromocytoma. However, when accompanied by elevations in plasma norepinephrine or other clinical evidence of pheochromocytoma, such elevations should arouse immediate suspicion of metastatic disease.

A consequence of the considerable variation in catecholamine release noted among patients with pheochromocytoma is that plasma concentrations or urinary excretion of catecholamines is poorly correlated with tumor size.[44] In contrast, because of metabolism of catecholamines within tumors and the independence of this process on catecholamine release, urinary excretion or plasma concentrations of metanephrines show strong positive correlation with tumor size and can be useful for judging the extent and progression of disease.[139,172]

Localization of Pheochromocytoma

According to expert recommendations from the International Symposium on Pheochromocytoma,[154] localization of pheochromocytoma should be initiated only if clinical evidence for the presence of tumor is reasonably compelling. If suspicion is derived from signs and symptoms of catecholamine excess, biochemical test results should be strongly positive. If the pretest probability of a tumor is higher, as in patients with a hereditary predisposition or previous history of the tumor, less compelling biochemical evidence might justify imaging studies. The finding of a mass in an adrenal gland does not prove that the mass is a pheochromocytoma: it proves only that there is a mass in the adrenal. Similarly, failure to find a mass in either adrenal gland does not prove that the patient does not have a pheochromocytoma. A detailed history and careful physical examination may yield vital clues as to the location of a pheochromocytoma, as in the case of postmicturition hypertension secondary to a pheochromocytoma of the urinary bladder.

Overall, pheochromocytomas located in the adrenal gland are identified more easily than are those in extra-adrenal tissues, because clinicians usually focus on the adrenal gland as the main source of catecholamine production. Although appropriate imaging techniques are usually chosen to locate tumors in the adrenal gland, clinicians are often uncertain as to which algorithm to follow and what technique to choose for the detection of extra-adrenal pheochromocytoma.[173] Furthermore, often it is not considered that up to 24% of patients with apparent sporadic pheochromocytoma in fact may be carriers of germline mutations, some of which involve a predisposition to extra-adrenal pheochromocytoma[12]; that malignant pheochromocytoma accounts for up to 35% of cases, depending on the type of tumor; and that about 10% of patients with pheochromocytoma present with metastatic disease at the time of their initial workup.[174] After initial failed surgery, patients with metastatic pheochromocytoma are commonly reevaluated through the use of meta-iodobenzylguanidine (MIBG) scintigraphy, a modality that actually should be performed before surgery to confirm that a tumor was indeed a pheochromocytoma, or to rule out metastatic disease.[176] Therefore, ruling out metastatic pheochromocytoma before initial surgery would be useful, because the detection of other lesions may affect treatment plan and follow-up.

According to expert recommendations,[154] the localization and confirmation of pheochromocytoma should involve at least two imaging modalities. Anatomic imaging studies (CT and MRI) should be combined with functional (nuclear medicine) imaging studies for optimal results in locating primary, recurrent, or metastatic pheochromocytoma. The exception to this rule could be a small adrenal pheochromocytoma with a clearly positive picture on T_2 MRI image and a predominantly adrenergic (epinephrine-producing) phenotype, as is typically seen in many patients with MEN2.[177]

ANATOMIC IMAGING

In most institutions, computed tomography (CT) of the abdomen, with or without contrast, provides the initial method of localizing pheochromocytoma because this imaging technique is easy, widely available, and relatively inexpensive. CT can be used to localize adrenal tumors 1 cm or larger and extra-adrenal tumors 2 cm or larger (sensitivity is about 95%, but specificity is only about 70%).[178] Administration of intravenous contrast media for CT scanning is preferred, but these agents have been suggested to evoke catecholamine release from tumors. However, a study in which the nonionic contrast medium iohexol was used did not find any support for this notion.[179] In our experience, intravenous contrast does not elicit increases in plasma catecholamines, blood pressure, or heart rate.

A homogeneous mass with a density measurement of less than 10 HU on unenhanced CT is most probably a nonfunctioning benign adenoma, as opposed to most pheochromocytomas, which usually exhibit a density of more than 10 HU and an inhomogeneous appearance. The disadvantage of CT is that it may fail to localize recurrent pheochromocytomas because of postoperative anatomic changes and the presence of surgical clips. Because extra-adrenal pheochromocytomas are located most commonly in the abdomen, we suggest that CT of the abdomen, including the pelvis, be done first. This should be followed by chest and neck imaging if abdominal CT is negative.

MRI with or without gadolinium enhancement is also a very reliable method of detection and may identify more than 95% of tumors; it is superior to CT in detecting extra-adrenal tumors.[180] On MRI T1 sequences, pheochromocytoma has a signal similar to that of liver, kidney, and muscle, and can be differentiated with ease from adipose tissue. Chemical shift MRI characterizes adrenal masses on the basis of the presence of fat in benign adenomas and the absence of fat in pheochromocytoma, metastases, hemorrhagic pseudocysts, or malignant tumors. The hypervascularity of pheochromocytoma makes them appear characteristically bright, with a high signal on T2 sequence and no signal loss on opposed-phase images. More particularly, almost all pheochromocytomas have a more intense signal than that of the liver or muscle and often more intense than fat on T2-weighted images. However, such intense signals can be elicited by hemorrhage or hematomas, adenomas, and carcinomas, so an overlap with pheochromocytoma must be considered, and specific additional imaging is needed to confirm that the tumor is pheochromocytoma.[181] Atypical pheochromocytomas may show medium signal quality on T2-weighted images and an inhomogeneous appearance, especially if they are cystic.

Among the advantages of MRI imaging of pheochromocytoma are its high sensitivity in detecting adrenal disease (93% to 100%) and the lack of exposure to ionizing radiation.[182] MRI is a good imaging modality for the detection of intracardiac, juxtacardiac, and juxtavascular pheochromocytomas because it reduces cardiac and respiratory motion-induced artifacts, whereas the use of T2 sequences enables better differentiation from surrounding tissues. MRI offers the possibility of multi-planar imaging and of superior assessment of the relationship between a tumor and its surrounding vessels (the great vessels in particular) compared with CT, rendering this modality of utmost importance in the evaluation of patients with pheochromocytoma in these areas, and especially to rule out vessel invasion. However, its overall sensitivity for detection of extra-adrenal, metastatic, or recurrent pheochromocytoma is lower compared with that of adrenal disease (90%). Overall, the specificity of MRI is about 70%.[178] MRI should be used as the initial imaging procedure when there is pregnancy or allergy to the contrast materials used for CT scans. However, MRI is more expensive than CT. Currently, no consensus indicates whether CT or MRI is preferred for initial localization of a tumor. Anatomic imaging should focus initially on the abdomen and pelvis.[154] We do not recommend ultrasound to localize pheochromocytoma: exceptions to this rule include children and pregnant women when MRI is not available.

FUNCTIONAL IMAGING

Functional imaging studies (enabled by the presence of the cell membrane and vesicular catecholamine transport systems in pheochromocytoma cells) include ^{123}I- or ^{131}I-MIBG scintigraphy, 6-^{18}F-fluorodopamine, ^{18}F-dihydroxyphenylalanine (^{18}F-dopa), ^{11}C-hydroxyephedrine, and ^{11}C-epinephrine positron emission tomography (PET).[6,7,163,183-185] These modalities can be used to confirm that a tumor is a pheochromocytoma and can detect most cases of metastatic disease.

However, it should be noted that malignant pheochromocytoma may undergo tumor dedifferentiation with loss of specific neurotransmitter transporters, leading to an inability to accumulate these isotopes and consequent lack of localization. ^{18}F-fluoro-deoxyglucose (FDG)-PET scanning or somatostatin receptor scintigraphy may be required as the only next step of the imaging algorithm. FDG is a nonspecific imaging agent whose accumulation is based on the higher metabolic rate of tumors compared with surrounding normal tissue. Another characteristic of dedifferentiated tumors involves the loss or the gain of specific receptors. More particularly, malignant pheochromocytomas often express somatostatin receptors,[186] thus enabling somatostatin receptor scintigraphy with the somatostatin analogue octreotide (Octreoscan).

METAIODOBENZYLGUANIDINE SCINTIGRAPHY

In rare cases, pheochromocytoma cannot be localized by CT or MRI studies. This may be caused by very small tumor size or by unusual location of a tumor (e.g., in the heart or neck). In such cases, whole body scanning using MIBG labeled with radioiodine (^{123}I or ^{131}I) should be considered. It is capable of showing multiple lesions simultaneously, as well as showing those in unusual locations. Other tumors arising from neuroendocrine cells may also take up ^{123}I- or ^{131}I-MIBG, and this has been reported for chemodectomas, nonsecreting paragangliomas, and carcinoids, and in both sporadic and familial medullary carcinomas of the thyroid.[187] MIBG yields nearly 100% specificity in detection of this tumor.[188]

MIBG labeled with ^{131}I provides negative results in up to 15% of patients with proven pheochromocytomas. However, much better sensitivity is available with MIBG labeled with ^{123}I.[183,189] Another advantage of ^{123}I over ^{131}I-labeled MIBG is its additional utility for imaging by single-photon emission computed tomog-

raphy (SPECT). The agent also has a shorter half-life compared with ^{131}I-MIBG (13 hours vs. 8.2 days), so that higher doses can be used.[183] The sensitivity of ^{123}I-MIBG scintigraphy is 92% to 98% for nonmetastatic pheochromocytoma,[190] but only 57% to 79% for metastases.[190-192] The accumulation of MIBG can be decreased by several types of drugs: (1) agents that deplete catecholamine stores, such as sympathomimetics, reserpine, and labetalol; (2) agents that inhibit cell catecholamine transporters, including cocaine and tricyclic antidepressants; and (3) other drugs such as calcium channel blockers and certain α- and β-adrenergic receptor blockers.[193] It is suggested that most of these drugs be withheld for about 2 weeks before undergoing MIBG scintigraphy. Both ^{123}I-MIBG and ^{131}I-MIBG require saturated solution of potassium iodine (SSKI, 100 mg twice a day for 4 or 7 days, respectively) to be used to block thyroid gland accumulation of free $^{123/131}$I. It should be noted that $^{123/131}$I-MIBG is normally accumulated in the myocardium, spleen, liver, urinary bladder, lungs, salivary glands, large intestine, and cerebellum. Moreover, the normal adrenal gland may show MIBG uptake in as many as 75% of patients.[194,195] Some of the MIBG is taken up by platelets, and thrombocytopenia may occur.

The study is relatively expensive, and the patient usually must be scanned at 24 hours and again at 48 or 72 hours after injection of the radioisotope to determine whether images that appear on the early scan are physiologic and will fade, or are tumors and will persist or increase in intensity on the later scan.

In summary, we recommend the use of ^{123}I-MIBG rather than ^{131}I-MIBG. ^{123}I-MIBG scintigraphy has a limited sensitivity for pheochromocytoma metastases but can be useful if ^{131}I-MIBG therapy is anticipated. Positron emission tomography, if available, is preferred for comprehensive localization of metastatic disease.

POSITRON EMISSION TOMOGRAPHY

PET imaging is done within minutes or hours after injection of short-lived positron-emitting agents. Low radiation exposure and superior spatial resolution are among the advantages of PET, whereas cost and limited availability of radiopharmaceuticals and PET equipment (including cyclotron) still prohibit more widespread use.

Most PET radiopharmaceuticals used for the detection of pheochromocytoma enter the pheochromocytoma cell using the cell membrane norepinephrine transporter. Dopamine is a better substrate for the norepinephrine transporter than are most other amines, including norepinephrine. Thus, a labeled analogue of dopamine should be useful as a scintigraphic imaging agent. 6-^{18}F-fluorodopamine, a sympathoneuronal imaging agent developed at the NIH, is a positron-emitting analogue of dopamine and was found to be a good substrate for the plasma membrane and for intracellular vesicular transporters in catecholamine-synthesizing cells.[196]

We recently published a series of 28 patients with known pheochromocytoma in whom 6-^{18}F-fluorodopamine-PET scans were positive and localized pheochromocytoma tumors in all.[6] In another study,[197] it was shown that in patients with metastatic pheochromocytoma, 6-^{18}F-fluorodopamine-PET localized pheochromocytomas in all patients and showed a large number of foci that were not imaged with ^{131}I-MIBG scintigraphy (Fig. 14-9). Thus, 6-^{18}F-fluorodopamine-PET was found to be a superior imaging method in patients with metastatic pheochromocytoma. More recently, however, we have identified several pheochromocytomas that were negative on 6-^{18}F-fluorodopamine-PET scans

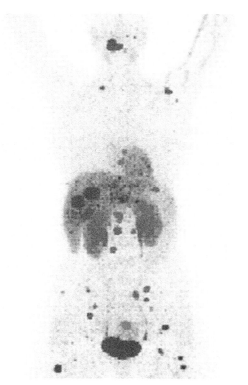

FIGURE 14-9. Reprojected coronal 6-(18F)-fluorodopamine positron emission tomographic scan in a patient with metastatic pheochromocytoma.

(unpublished observations). All these pheochromocytomas also had negative [131]I- or ^{123}I-MIBG scintigraphy.

[11]C-hydroxyephedrine and ^{11}C-epinephrine[198] are other PET imaging agents that have been shown to have a limited diagnostic yield because of their less than perfect sensitivity and/or specificity. This could be caused in part by their limited affinity for cell membrane and vesicular norepinephrine transporter systems, as well as the short half-life of ^{11}C radiopharmaceuticals (20 minutes), which renders the implementation of whole-body scans difficult. ^{18}F-fluorodopa PET has shown promising results in initial studies in a limited number of patients with pheochromocytoma.[184,199] The sensitivity of ^{18}F-fluorodopa appears to be limited for metastases, however (unpublished observations).

Increased glucose metabolism characterizes various malignant tumors; thus the uptake of glucose labeled with ^{18}F-fluoride can be useful in imaging these tumors. In one study of 17 patients, FDG-PET was used with some success in imaging of metastatic pheochromocytoma and revealed more metastases than [123]I- or ^{131}I-MIBG scintigraphy.[185] Malignant pheochromocytomas may accumulate FDG more avidly than benign pheochromocytomas; nevertheless, FDG cannot distinguish malignant from benign disease. It should be noted that the use of FDG is not recommended in the initial diagnostic localization of pheochromocytoma. This radiopharmaceutical is nonspecific for this tumor. However, it can be useful in those patients in whom other imaging modalities are negative, and in rapidly growing metastatic pheochromocytoma that is becoming undifferentiated and thus losing the property to accumulate more specific agents.[173] Moreover, ^{18}F-FDG PET is the preferred technique for localization of *SDHB*-associated metastatic pheochromocytoma, as previously described.[191] Impairment of mitochondrial function due to loss of SDHB function may cause tumor cells to shift from oxidative phosphorylation to aerobic glycolysis, a phenomenon known

as the "Warburg effect."[200] Higher glucose requirements due to a switch to less efficient pathways for cellular energy production may explain increased ^{18}F-FDG uptake by malignant *SDHB*-related pheochromocytoma. This possible bioenergenetic signature on imaging awaits confirmation at a molecular level.

Overall, the advantages of PET are that it can be done within minutes or hours after injection of short-lived positron-emitting agents, radiation exposure is low, and spatial resolution is superior. Cost and limited availability of the radiopharmaceuticals and PET equipment prohibit more widespread use of this imaging modality.

OCTREOSCAN

Somatostatin receptor scintigraphy using octreotide has been used in patients with pheochromocytoma[201]; however, the sensitivity of this imaging modality is low, especially in the detection of solitary tumors, and this modality is inferior to MIBG scintigraphy.[201] However, in patients with metastatic pheochromocytoma, Octreoscan can be useful, especially in those tumors that express somatostatin receptors and are negative on MIBG scintigraphy and 6-^{18}F-fluorodopamine-PET.[173]

Vena caval sampling for catecholamines and metanephrines is rarely called for except when extra-adrenal tumors have escaped removal during previous surgery and cannot be located with [123/131]I-MIBG scanning or other localizing techniques.[163]

In summary, the strategies outlined above provide the basis for diagnostic localization of pheochromocytoma as described in Fig. 14-10. Although CT and MRI have excellent sensitivity, these anatomic imaging approaches lack the specificity required to unequivocally identify a mass as a pheochromocytoma. The higher specificity of functional imaging—the test of choice is currently ^{123}I-MIBG scintigraphy—offers an approach by which the limitations of anatomic imaging can be overcome.[154]

Treatment for Pheochromocytoma

The optimal therapy for a pheochromocytoma is prompt surgical removal of the tumor, because an unresected tumor represents a time bomb waiting to explode with a potentially lethal hypertensive crisis.[18,52] Safe surgical removal requires the efforts of a team made up of an internist, an anesthesiologist, and a surgeon, preferably all with previous experience with pheochromocytoma.

MEDICAL THERAPY AND PREPARATION FOR SURGERY

Preoperative medical treatment is directed at controlling hypertension (including hypertensive crises during the removal of pheochromocytoma), maintaining stable blood pressure during surgery, and minimizing adverse effects during anesthesia and other clinical signs and symptoms caused by high plasma catecholamine levels.[202,204]

Maintenance of adequate blood pressure control for 2 weeks before the operation is an important aspect of management once a tumor is diagnosed. Phenoxybenzamine (Dibenzyline; irreversible noncompetitive α-adrenoceptor blocker) is used most commonly for preoperative blockade. Phenoxybenzamine has a long-lasting effect that diminishes only after de novo α-adrenoceptor synthesis. The initial dose of long-acting phenoxybenzamine is usually 10 mg twice a day; this is increased until clinical manifestations are controlled or side effects appear. For most patients, a total daily dose of 1 mg/kg is sufficient. Some

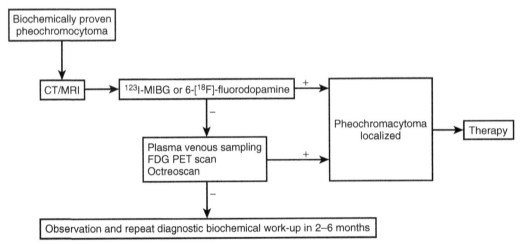

FIGURE 14-10. Algorithm for localization of pheochromocytoma. In patients with biochemically proven pheochromocytoma, we suggest the use of anatomic imaging methods (either computed tomography [CT] or magnetic resonance imaging [MRI]) for initial imaging of the adrenals. In children or pregnancy, MRI is preferable, but ultrasound may also be considered. A lesion on unenhanced CT with attenuation values lower than 10 Hounsfield units excludes the presence of pheochromocytoma, whereas values higher than 10 Hounsfield units may be followed by contrast-enhanced and delayed-enhanced CT examination. If MRI is done, T2 sequences should be obtained (pheochromocytomas is bright on T2 image). Negative imaging of the adrenals should be followed by abdominal, chest, and neck CT or MRI scans. Except in a few situations, as previously described, the presence of pheochromocytoma should always be ruled out or confirmed with functional imaging. The functional imaging test of choice at present is (^{123}I)-meta-iodobenzylguanidine (MIBG), or, if this is not possible, (^{131}I)-MIBG. If the MIBG scan is negative, positron emission tomography (PET) studies should be performed with specific ligands, preferably 6-(18F)-fluorodopamine. If these are also negative, pheochromocytoma is most likely dedifferentiated (commonly seen in malignant tumors). In such a situation, (18F)-fluorodeoxyglucose (FDG)-PET or Octreoscan should be carried out. Venous sampling with measurement of catecholamines or (preferably) metanephrines to localize tumor is an ultimate modality to be used with caution in only selected cases in which all imaging methods have failed. Sometimes, repeated noninvasive localization workup after 2 to 6 months is a preferable choice.

patients may require much larger doses, and the dosage may be increased in increments of 10 to 20 mg every 2 to 3 days. If the drug is given in too high an initial dosage, the patient will have significant postural hypotension. As the correct dose is approached, paroxysmal hypertensive episodes will be brought under control, and when the right dose is achieved, the patient will become normotensive.

Other α-blocking agents of use are prazosin (Minipress), terazosin (Hytrin), and doxazosin (Cardura).[205] All three are specific, competitive, and therefore short-acting α$_1$-adrenergic antagonists, and all three have the potential for severe postural hypotension immediately after the first dose, which therefore should be given just as the patient is ready to go to bed. Thereafter, the dosage can be increased as needed. Prazosin is administered in doses of 2 to 5 mg two or three times a day, whereas terazosin is given in doses of 2 to 5 mg once daily, and doxazosin in doses of 2 to 8 mg once daily. Labetalol (Normodyne or Trandate), a drug with both α- and β-antagonistic activity, may also be used at a dosage of 200 to 600 mg twice daily.[206] Advantages of labetalol are that an α-blocker and a β-blocker are given simultaneously, and both oral and IV formulations of the drug are readily available. However, with labetalol, one is forced to use a fixed ratio of α- to β-antagonistic activity (i.e., 1:4 or 1:6). This often means that more slowing of the heart occurs, rather than control of hypertension, when what usually is needed is a drug with an α/β ratio of 4:1 or greater. It usually is better to use the amounts needed of individual α- and β-blockers. Large doses of any of these drugs may be necessary to control blood pressure. If blood pressure is controlled, and the patient is given a normal or high-salt diet, the patient's diminished blood volume will be restored to normal. As normal blood volume is restored, the degree of postural hypotension decreases. β-Adrenergic blocking agents are needed only when significant tachycardia or a catecholamine-induced arrhythmia occurs. A β-blocker should never be used

in the absence of an α-blocker because the former will exacerbate epinephrine-induced vasoconstriction by blocking its vasodilator component. This will make hypertensive episodes worse in subjects on a β-blocker alone.

In our experience, metyrosine (Demser) is a valuable drug in the treatment of patients with pheochromocytoma. The drug competitively inhibits tyrosine hydroxylase, the rate-limiting step in catecholamine biosynthesis.[207] It significantly but not completely depletes catecholamine stores with maximum effect after about 3 days of treatment. Thus, it facilitates blood pressure control both before and during surgery, especially during the induction of anesthesia and surgical manipulation of the tumor—times when extensive sympathetic activation or catecholamine release may occur. Treatment is started at a dosage of 250 mg given orally every 6 to 8 hours; thereafter, the dose is increased by 250 to 500 mg every 2 to 3 days or as necessary up to a total dose of 1.5 to 4.0 g/day. The drug is a substituted amino acid (i.e., α-methyl-L-tyrosine), and therefore it readily crosses the blood-brain barrier. Thus, it inhibits catecholamine synthesis in the brain as well as in the periphery, and often causes sedation, depression, anxiety, and galactorrhea; it rarely causes extrapyramidal signs (e.g., Parkinsonism) in older patients. These symptoms are reversed rapidly when the dosage is lowered or the drug is discontinued. If dreaming abnormalities are reported by the patient, then the dosage should be reduced to the previous lower dose for 1 or 2 days, or until the abnormality disappears. Then the dosage should be increased more slowly until the desired effects are reached. Metyrosine is not generally available in all countries and institutions.

Various calcium channel blockers have been used to control blood pressure both before and during surgery.[208] In our experience, if both metyrosine and α-antagonists are used, the blood pressure of the patient is much less labile during anesthesia and surgery, intraoperative blood loss is reduced, and less volume

Table 14-6. Main Classes of Drugs With Contraindications in Patients With Pheochromocytoma

Drug Class	Relevant Clinical Uses
β-Adrenergic blockers*	May be used to treat conditions that result from catecholamine excess (e.g., hypertension, cardiac dysrhythmias), cardiomyopathy, heart failure, panic attacks, migraine, tachycardia
Dopamine D2 receptor antagonists	Control of nausea, vomiting, psychosis, and hot flashes and for tranquilizing effect
Tricyclic antidepressants	Treatment for insomnia, neuropathic pain, nocturnal enuresis in children, headaches, depression (rarely)
Other antidepressants (serotonin and NE reuptake inhibitors)	Depression, anxiety, panic attacks, antiobesity agents
Monoamine oxidase inhibitors	Nonselective agents rarely used as antidepressants (due to cheese effect)
Sympathomimetics*	Control of low blood pressure during surgical anesthesia; decongestants; antiobesity agents
Chemotherapeutic agents*	Antineoplastic actions; treatment for malignant pheochromocytoma
Opiate analgesics*	Induction of surgical anesthesia
Neuromuscular blocking agents*	Induction of surgical anesthesia
Peptide and steroid hormones*	Diagnostic testing

Adapted from Pacak.[202,203]

NE, Norepinephrine.

*These drugs have therapeutic or diagnostic use in pheochromocytoma, but usually only after pretreatment with appropriate antihypertensives (e.g., α-adrenoceptor blockers).

replacement is required during surgery than if only α-antagonists are used.[209] It is our custom to administer 1 mg/kg of phenoxybenzamine and 0.5 to 0.75 g of metyrosine orally at midnight on the evening before surgery.

Hypertensive crises that can manifest as severe headache, visual disturbances, acute myocardial infarction, congestive heart failure, or cerebrovascular accident are appropriately treated with an intravenous bolus of 5 mg phentolamine (Regitine). Phentolamine has a very short half-life; therefore, if necessary, the same dose can be repeated every 2 minutes until hypertension is adequately controlled, or phentolamine can be given as a continuous infusion (100 mg of phentolamine in 500 mL of 5% dextrose in water). A continuous intravenous infusion of sodium nitroprusside (preparation similar to phentolamine) or, in some cases, nifedipine (10 mg orally or sublingually) can be used to control hypertension. Due attention should also be given to the possibility that some drugs (e.g., tricyclic antidepressants, metoclopramide, naloxone) can cause hypertensive crisis in patients with pheochromocytoma (Table 14-6).

In patients with clinical manifestations caused by β-adrenoceptor stimulation (e.g., tachycardia or arrhythmias, angina, nervousness), β-adrenergic receptor blockers such as propranolol, atenolol, or metoprolol are indicated. β-Adrenoceptor blockers, however, should never be employed before α-adrenoceptor blockers are administered, because unopposed stimulation of α-adrenoceptors and loss of β-adrenoceptor–mediated vasodilatation may cause a serious and life-threatening elevation of blood pressure. Labetalol, a combined α- and β-adrenoceptor blocker, is not preferred because in some patients it may cause hypertension (perhaps through its greater effect on β- than α-adrenoceptors).[210] It should be noted that both α- and β-adrenoceptor blockers may elevate plasma free normetanephrine levels.[150] In contrast, calcium channel blockers, also used to control hypertension and tachycardia in patients with pheochromocytoma, does not affect plasma metanephrine levels. A proposed algorithm for preoperative treatment is given in Fig. 14-11.[202]

For most abdominal pheochromocytomas smaller than 6 cm, laparoscopy has replaced laparotomy as the procedure of choice because of significant postoperative benefits.[211,212]

POSTOPERATIVE MANAGEMENT

Volume replacement is the treatment of choice if hypotension should occur during surgery (i.e., after the tumor is removed) or in the postoperative period. The use of pressor agents is ill advised, especially if long-acting α-blockers have been used, because of the high doses of drug that must be used and the difficulty with which patients are weaned from these agents. Control of postoperative hypotension is even more imperative if both metyrosine and phenoxybenzamine are used preoperatively, because the former inhibits catecholamine synthesis by both the tumor and the sympathetic nervous system, whereas the latter blocks the action of any catecholamines that are synthesized. In this situation, the vascular bed is effectively paralyzed in a dilated state. Therefore, the best way to control blood pressure is via adequate volume replacement.

The volume of fluid required is often large (0.5 to 1.5 times the patient's total blood volume) during the first 24 to 48 hours after removal of the tumor. This is because the half-lives of both metyrosine and phenoxybenzamine are approximately 12 hours, and thus it takes nearly three half-lives or 36 hours for the sympathetic nervous system to resume autoregulation. When this occurs, renal output begins to increase, and blood pressure and heart rate remain stable. It is at this time that normal replacement volumes (i.e., 125 mL/hr) can be used. If the last dose of medication was administered on the midnight before surgery, autoregulation usually occurs at about noon on the first postoperative day. Both the type and the amount of fluid replacement needed are readily determined by observation of the blood pressure, heart rate, central venous pressure, and urinary output. It is not unusual for patients to show a 10% to 12% increase in body weight by the time diuresis is begun.

Postoperative hypertension may mean that some tumor tissue was not resected. However, during the first 24 hours after surgery, hypertension is most likely attributed to pain, volume overload, or autonomic instability; these are all readily treated symptomatically. If hypertension persists in a patient even after he or she has returned to dry weight, the coexistence of essential hypertension is still the most likely diagnosis. However, any attempt to collect specimens for biochemical evidence of a residual tumor should be delayed at least 5 to 7 days post surgery to ensure that the large increases in both plasma and urinary catecholamines produced by surgery have dissipated. We normally repeat the postoperative urine collection just before the patient is to be discharged from the hospital, or when the patient is last seen by the surgeons 4 to 6 weeks post operation. Repeat measurements should be made if symptoms reappear, or approximately yearly, for a total of 5 years, if the patient remains asymptomatic. Operative mortality at the Mayo Clinic from 1980 to 1986 was 1.3%, or 1 in 77 patients.[213] The long-term survival of patients after successful removal of a benign pheochromocytoma is essentially the same as that of age-adjusted normal individuals.[214] At least 25% of patients remain hypertensive, but this is usually easily controlled with medication.[61,215]

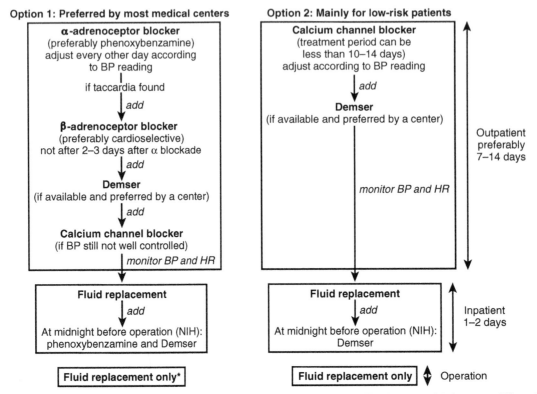

FIGURE 14-11. Proposed algorithm for the preoperative treatment of patients with pheochromocytoma. *BP,* Blood pressure; *HR,* heart rate. (*If α₁-adrenoceptor blockers are used, then give one dose in the morning before surgery.) (Adapted from Pacak.[202])

Special Presentations and Therapeutic Problems

MALIGNANT PHEOCHROMOCYTOMA

Malignant pheochromocytoma is established by the presence of metastases at the sites where chromaffin cells are normally absent.[83] Pheochromocytoma metastasizes via hematogenous or lymphatic pathways, and the most common metastatic sites are lymph nodes, bone, lung, and liver.[159,168,216-218] Among all pheochromocytomas, the frequency of malignant pheochromocytomas ranges from 13% to 34%, with a slight male predominance.[218] It is recognized that one half of malignant tumors present are found at the initial presentation, whereas the second half develop at a median interval of 5.6 years.[219] The prevalence of an underlying *SDHB* mutation among patients with malignant pheochromocytoma is 30%, and even higher (48%) if the tumor originates from an extra-adrenal location.[220] Two groups of patients can be distinguished on the basis of location of metastatic lesions. The first group represents short-term survivors with the presence of metastatic lesions, especially in liver and lungs. Their survival is usually less than 2 years. The second group represents long-term survivors with the presence of bone metastatic lesions. Patients in this group can survive longer than 20 years after the initial diagnosis. The overall 5-year survival rate varies between 34% and 60%.[171,221] The survival of patients with metastatic disease due to an underlying *SDHB* mutation is lower than in non-*SDHB* patients.[222] Recent advances in biochemical testing and nuclear imaging techniques, as discussed previously, have greatly improved our ability to diagnose and localize malignant pheochromocytoma at much earlier stages.

Clinical manifestations of malignant pheochromocytoma are similar to those of its benign counterpart, and no characteristic symptoms or group of symptoms would suggest a tentative diagnosis of malignancy.[159,168,216-219] The most common manifestations are hypertension, headache, sweating, palpitations, and other symptoms. It should be noted that some patients have minimal symptoms despite markedly elevated catecholamine levels, most likely because of desensitization of adrenergic receptors by constant exposure to high concentrations of catecholamines. Furthermore, patients can present with symptoms caused by local invasion of tumors into various organs, especially in cases of *SDHB*-related disease.[62]

Similar to benign pheochromocytomas, malignant pheochromocytomas predominantly secrete norepinephrine.[42,165,223] However, patients with malignant disease tend to have higher levels of plasma and urinary metanephrines, reflecting a larger tumor size.[216,221] In addition, increased excretion of dopamine and its metabolites, VMA and 3-methoxytyramine, is often associated with malignant pheochromocytoma because of an intraneuronal loss of dopamine-β-hydroxylase as a consequence of cell dedifferentiation.[42,168,171,219] The presence of normal epinephrine concentrations, together with that of excessive norepinephrine levels, also reflects tissue immaturity due to the tumor's inability to N-methylate.[223]

Various attempts have been made to develop ancillary criteria to distinguish malignant from benign pheochromocytomas before they develop metastases. Young age, extra-adrenal tumor location, large tumor size, and adrenal pheochromocytomas that fail to take up MIBG all have been associated with an increased likelihood of malignancy.[168,171,216,218,219,223] Persistent postoperative arterial hypertension is reported to be more common in malignant pheochromocytoma.[171]

Conventional pathologic features such as tumor necrosis, vascular or capsular invasion, nuclear atypia, and mitotic index do not consistently predict the malignant behavior of pheochromocytomas.[168,171,216-219,223] In two different studies from the Mayo Clinic, pheochromocytomas that exhibited a diploid DNA pattern were associated with benign behavior, whereas a nondiploid DNA pattern seemed requisite for recurrence or metastasis.[224] However, several studies thereafter did not confirm any correlation between DNA ploidy and malignant behavior in pheochromocytomas.[225,226] Several molecular markers for distinguishing benign from malignant pheochromocytomas have been investigated, but none appear to reliably indicate malignant behavior in an individual patient.[227-229] Therefore, long-term follow-up of patients with pheochromocytoma is mandatory.

As described previously, it is recognized that various peptides are produced and stored in the chromaffin granules in the adrenal medulla. In pheochromocytomas, these substances are secreted excessively, along with catecholamines. They may cause a systemic effect and may modify the clinical features of pheochromocytomas. In addition, they can be helpful (e.g., chromogranin A) in the diagnosis and follow-up of pheochromocytomas.[227]

Localization of malignant pheochromocytoma follows the same steps and algorithm as for benign pheochromocytoma. The exception (as described previously) is that malignant pheochromocytoma often may be dedifferentiated, thus losing the expression of cell membrane and vesicular transporter systems. In such a situation, FDG-PET can be more helpful than the use of a specific positron-emitting agent or MIBG scintigraphy, especially in *SDHB*-associated pheochromocytoma.[191]

Successful management of malignant pheochromocytoma requires a multidisciplinary approach.[174] Treatment is performed with the intention of attaining possible cure for limited disease and the goal of palliation for advanced disease. The treatment regimen should be individualized to meet the goal of controlling endocrine activity, decreasing tumor burden, and alleviating local symptoms.

Pharmacologic treatment for malignant pheochromocytoma does not differ from that provided for benign disease. For patients with limited disease, surgery may be the only curative modality of therapy. However, for patients with multiple metastatic lesions, radical surgical resection is often impossible, and other surgical procedures may be associated with complications such as those related to significant catecholamine release during tumor manipulation. Furthermore, at present it is not clear whether such an approach can prolong survival of patients; additional detailed, large, and prospective studies are needed. However, debulking often results in smaller tumor burden that may respond much better to radiotherapy and chemotherapy and a significant decrease in catecholamine levels, reflecting improvement of many symptoms and signs.

The first-line systemic treatment for malignant pheochromocytoma is targeted radiotherapy with the use of ^{131}I-MIBG. ^{131}I-MIBG therapy is used in MIBG-positive tumors, especially those that are unresectable. Doses vary from as low as 50 mCi up to 900 mCi as a single dose (such high doses require bone marrow rescue). However, more often, multiple doses of around 200 mCi are given at intervals of 3 to 6 months. The procedure is well tolerated, with minimal toxicity (if lower doses are used) that includes nausea; mild bone marrow suppression, especially thrombocytopenia; mildly elevated liver enzymes; and some renal toxicity. Thrombocytopenia usually is seen a few weeks after MIBG is administered. Patients take SSKI (100 mg three times a day) or potassium perchlorate (200 mg twice a day, if the patient is allergic to iodides), to block thyroid accumulation of radioiodine generated via deiodination of ^{131}I-MIBG. Blocking medication is initiated 1 day before the patient receives ^{131}I-MIBG and is continued for 30 days. Even with the blockade, some risk of decreased thyroid function is present. Overall, only one third of patients show partial response (less than 50% reduction of tumor mass) and improvement in symptoms and signs.[230] Disease progression is common after 2 years. Use of higher doses of around 700 mCi may result in better response, but additional studies are needed.[231] Radiotherapy with the use of radiolabeled somatostatin analogues such as [^{111}In]-pentetreotide appears to be largely ineffective in metastatic pheochromocytoma.[232] In this context, [^{90}Y-DOTA]-D-Phe[1]-Tyr[3]-octreotide requires further investigation.[233]

In rapidly progressive metastatic pheochromocytoma, chemotherapy rather than MIBG therapy is recommended. A combination of cyclophosphamide 750 mg/m[2] body surface area on day 1; vincristine 1.4 mg/m[2] on day 1; and dacarbazine 600 mg/m[2] on days 1 and 2 (CVD), administered IV in 21 day cycles, was used.[234] Fifty-seven percent of patients had a complete or partial tumor response (i.e., at least a 50% reduction in the size of all measurable tumor). In addition, 79% of patients had a complete or partial biochemical response (i.e., at least a 50% reduction in urinary excretion of catecholamines and catecholamine metabolites). All responding patients showed objective improvement in performance status and in blood pressure, and the duration of response lasted from 6 months to over 2 years. Chemotherapy stops when the patient shows the development of new lesions or a 25% increase in the size of old lesions in spite of continued treatment. A major reason for the development of resistance of malignant pheochromocytoma to treatment with the CVD regimen is induction of *MDR-1* gene activity. So far, attempts to block the activity of this gene have been unsuccessful. Data on alternative chemotherapy protocols remain limited. Very recently, a radiologic response was reported in one of three cases of metastatic pheochromocytoma among 29 patients with neuroendocrine tumors treated with an oral regimen of temozolomide (median dose, 150 mg/day) and thalidomide (median dose, 100 mg/day).[235] Notable toxic effects in the whole study population included lymphocytopenia (69%), thrombocytopenia (14%), and neuropathy (38%).

Patients with large tumor burdens may present with massive release of catecholamines within the first few hours after administration of the first course of chemotherapy.[236] A similar massive release of catecholamines was reported after chemotherapy with cyclophosphamide, vincristine, and prednisone in a patient with pheochromocytoma and lymphocytic lymphoma.[237] These instances of "catecholamine storm" are manifested by the sudden onset of extreme tachycardia, severe hypertension, or both. Because these events are not predictable, we generally advise that the first course of chemotherapy, in any patient, be administered in hospital. It is important to intervene immediately with β-blockers if severe tachycardia occurs, or with α-blockers if extreme hypertension develops, or a combination of α- and β-blockers if both occur. Unless this is done rapidly, we have seen patients go into severe congestive heart failure with resultant decreases in cardiac ejection fraction to as low as 6% to 10%.[236] These patients must not be abandoned at this point but must be given appropriate support. The catecholamine-stunned heart can respond, and we have seen recovery within 7 to 10 days.

In summary, no generally effective systemic treatment with antineoplastic potential is available for malignant pheochromocytoma. A considerable proportion of patients respond to MIBG radiotherapy or to cytotoxic chemotherapy. However, because

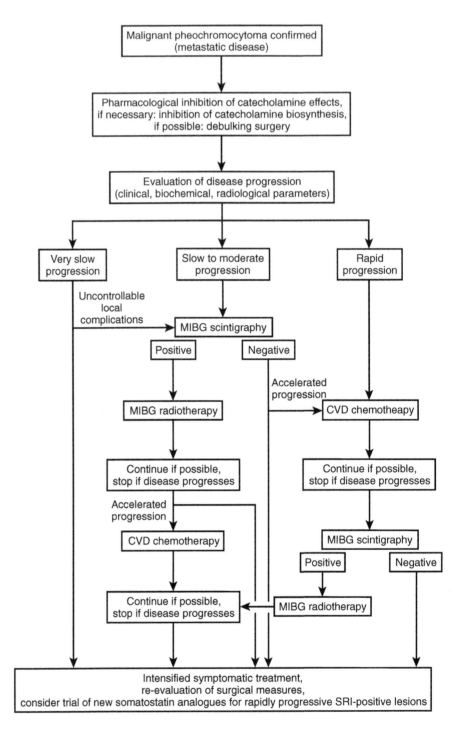

FIGURE 14-12. Proposed algorithm for the treatment of metastatic pheochromocytoma. (Adapted from Scholz et al.[174])

there are no published randomized controlled studies, it remains unclear whether these responses have an overall impact on survival or quality of life. Fig. 14-12 shows a proposed algorithm for the treatment of metastatic pheochromocytoma.

External beam radiation is used for palliation of chronic pain and symptoms of local compression arising from these tumors.[238,239] However, no systemic effects on tumor burden or hormone levels were observed. Successful infarction of pheochromocytoma by embolization has been demonstrated in individual case reports.[240] Recently, radiofrequency ablation, cryotherapy, and percutaneous microwave coagulation have been used for treatment of malignant pheochromocytoma.[11,241,242]

PHEOCHROMOCYTOMA IN CHILDREN

Although pheochromocytomas are the most common endocrine tumors in children, they account for only 5% to 10% of all pheochromocytomas, with an incidence of 2 per million per year.[243-245] In children, pheochromocytomas are commonly familial (40%), extra-adrenal (8% to 43%), bilateral adrenal (7% to 53%), and multifocal.[106,246-249] Childhood pheochromocytomas peak at 10 to 13 years, with a male predominance (male vs. female, 2:1) before puberty.[106,246,250] Less than 10% of pediatric pheochromocytomas are malignant,[106,246,251,252] with reported mean survival rates of 73% at 3 years and 40% to 50% at 5 years after diagnosis.[230,250,253] In 1960, Hume[250] reported that 24% of pheochromocytomas in children are bilateral—a much higher incidence than is found in adults. Children also have a higher incidence of extra-adrenal pheochromocytomas, especially in the organ of Zuckerkandl and the urinary bladder. Recurrent pheochromocytomas are rare in children, but recurrent tumors may appear years after initial diagnosis, emphasizing the importance of close long-term follow-up.[252]

In contrast to adult patients, in whom sustained hypertension is found in only 50% of cases, more than 70% to 90% of children present with sustained hypertension.[243,246,252] Pheochromocytoma is the underlying cause in 1% to 2% of cases of pediatric hypertension and should be considered after exclusion of more common causes such as renal disease and renal artery stenosis.[106] Pheochromocytomas secreting epinephrine may present with hypotension, particularly postural hypotension.[49] Sweating, visual problems, weight loss, and nausea and vomiting are more common in children than in adults,[254] as are polyuria and polydipsia. In addition, children commonly present with palpitations, anxiety, and hyperglycemia.[18] Other signs of catecholamine excess are pallor and flushing.[18] As summarized by Manger and Gifford,[18] some children occasionally present with a reddish blue mottling of the skin and a puffy red and cyanotic appearance of the hands. Less common clinical manifestations include fever and constipation. Similar to adult patients, the presence of the triad of headache, palpitations, and sweating in children, in combination with hypertension, should arouse immediate suspicion of a pheochromocytoma.

Because neuroblastomas (the most common solid tumors in childhood), ganglioneuroblastomas, and ganglioneuromas can synthesize and excrete catecholamines and their metabolites, the differential diagnosis of a pheochromocytoma is somewhat difficult or, at times, impossible.

Measurement of plasma free metanephrines under standardized conditions, with the use of age- and gender-specific reference ranges, appears to be the biochemical test of choice for detecting childhood pheochromocytoma.[255]

In children, more than 90% of pheochromocytomas are localized in the abdomen; therefore imaging studies should be directed to this part of the body. Although CT localizes about 95% of pheochromocytomas, MRI is the preferred imaging modality in children to avoid radiation exposure. MIBG scintigraphy is used to confirm that the tumor is indeed a pheochromocytoma and to rule out metastatic disease. We suggest genetic counseling and testing for underlying mutations in all children with pheochromocytoma.

Treatment of childhood pheochromocytoma is similar to that for pheochromocytomas that occur in adult patients.

PHEOCHROMOCYTOMA IN PREGNANCY

Pheochromocytoma in pregnancy demands special attention because it carries a high morbidity and mortality if pheochromocytoma is unsuspected (≈38% maternal mortality and ≈33% fetal mortality among published cases). Both maternal and fetal mortality can be greatly reduced if the diagnosis is made antenatally.[256,257] Nevertheless, in two series it was found that pheochromocytoma remained unrecognized antepartum in 47% to 65% of patients.[256,257]

Hypertensive crisis caused by pheochromocytoma in pregnancy is highly unpredictable. Direct tumor stimulation leading to marked catecholamine release can occur as the result of examination, postural changes, pressure from the uterus, labor contractions, fetal movements, and tumor hemorrhage. It is seen most commonly during the period surrounding delivery. Acute hypertensive crisis may manifest itself as severely elevated blood pressure, arrhythmia, or pulmonary edema.

The clinical picture of hypertensive crisis can be easily mistaken for acute toxemia of pregnancy. In contrast to acute toxemia, hypertension or hypertensive crisis can occur early in pregnancy (before the third trimester) and can be paroxysmal, or it may be accompanied by postural hypotension, in which proteinuria or edema is often absent.[258] Biochemical diagnosis can be hindered if a patient is on methyldopa, which can result in a false-positive test. Therefore, if pheochromocytoma is suspected, treatment with methyldopa should be suspended or delayed for the measurement of metanephrines. The sensitivity of plasma metanephrines in the detection of pheochromocytoma appears to be maintained during pregnancy.

Localization of a suspected pheochromocytoma is vital and is best accomplished by MRI and/or ultrasonography. It is important to administer α-adrenergic blocking agents as soon as the diagnosis is confirmed. The agent of choice is phenoxybenzamine. With the exception of mild perinatal depression and transient hypotension in the newborn, no reports have described adverse fetal effects during treatment.[259] β-Blockers have been used to control tachycardia, but they may be associated with intrauterine growth retardation.[256]

Approximately 25% of published cases presented with a cardiovascular emergency (e.g., myocardial ischemia, cardiac shock, pulmonary edema, cerebral hemorrhage). Maternal hypertensive crisis is always very dangerous for the fetus; it commonly results in uteroplacental insufficiency, early separation of the placenta, or fetal death.[260] In situations of hypertensive crisis, IV phentolamine, given as a bolus of 1 to 5 mg or as a continuous infusion of 1 mg/min, can be used to control blood pressure. As a final resort, sodium nitroprusside may be used, but this has to be infused at a rate of less than 1 μg/kg/min to avoid fetal cyanide toxicity.[261]

If the patient is in the first two trimesters, then the tumor should be removed as soon as the patient has been adequately prepared with α-blockers. Recently, this has been accomplished laparoscopically.[262] In most instances, the fetus will remain undisturbed, but a spontaneous abortion is possible. In the third trimester, it is appropriate for the patient to be treated with α-blockers and carefully monitored until the fetus reaches sufficient maturity to be viable. At that point, a cesarean section should be performed, because vaginal delivery can be extremely hazardous.[18,52,263] The tumor can be removed during the same operation. Anesthetic management is critical during the cesarean section and removal of the tumor, whether these procedures are done at the same time or in sequence.[264] However, if uncontrolled hypertension, hemorrhage, or other emergency occurs, the tumor should be removed at once.[18,52] Magnesium sulfate has been used to control hypertensive emergencies during labor and during resection of the tumor in pregnant patients with pheochromocytoma.[265] The efficacy of the drug was severely limited if an adequate blood level of magnesium could not be achieved because of preexisting hypomagnesemia. Labor and vaginal delivery should be avoided because these may cause tumor stimulation and increase catecholamine secretion with severe hypertensive crisis despite adrenergic blockade.

Acknowledgment

The authors acknowledge with gratitude the assistance of Ms. Kathryn S. King in preparing this chapter.

REFERENCES

1. Manger WM, Gifford RW: Pheochromocytoma, J Clin Hypertens 4(1):62–72, 2002.
2. Pacak K, Linehan WM, Eisenhofer G, et al: Recent advances in genetics, diagnosis, localization, and treatment of pheochromocytoma, Ann Intern Med 134(4):315–329, 2001.
3. Brouwers FM, Lenders JW, Eisenhofer G, et al: Pheochromocytoma as an endocrine emergency, Rev Endocr Metab Disord 4(2):121–128, 2003.
4. Sutton MG, Sheps SG, Lie JT: Prevalence of clinically unsuspected pheochromocytoma, review of a 50-year autopsy series, Mayo Clin Proc 56(6):354–360, 1981.
5. Bravo EL, Tagle R: Pheochromocytoma: state-of-the-art and future prospects, Endocr Rev 24(4):539–553, 2003.
6. Pacak K, Eisenhofer G, Carrasquillo JA, et al: 6-[18F]fluorodopamine positron emission tomographic (PET) scanning for diagnostic localization of pheochromocytoma, Hypertension 38(1):6–8, 2001.
7. Pacak K, Eisenhofer G, Carrasquillo JA, et al: Diagnostic localization of pheochromocytoma: the coming of age of positron emission tomography, Ann N Y Acad Sci 970:170–176, 2002.
8. Sawka AM, Jaeschke R, Singh RJ, et al: A comparison of biochemical tests for pheochromocytoma: measurement of fractionated plasma metanephrines compared with the combination of 24-hour urinary metanephrines and catecholamines, J Clin Endocrinol Metab 88(2):553–558, 2003.
9. Lenders JW, Pacak K, Walther MM, et al: Biochemical diagnosis of pheochromocytoma: which test is best? JAMA 287(11):1427–1434, 2002.
10. Kaouk JH, Matin S, Bravo EL, et al: Laparoscopic bilateral partial adrenalectomy for pheochromocytoma, Urology 60(6):1100–1103, 2002.
11. Munver R, Del Pizzo JJ, Sosa RE: Adrenal-preserving minimally invasive surgery: the role of laparoscopic partial adrenalectomy, cryosurgery, and radiofrequency ablation of the adrenal gland, Curr Urol Rep 4(1):87–92, 2003.
12. Neumann HP, Bausch B, McWhinney SR, et al: Germline mutations in nonsyndromic pheochromocytoma, N Engl J Med 346(19):1459–1466, 2002.
13. Kuchel O: Pheochromocytoma. In Genest J, Kuchel O, Hamet P, et al, editors: Hypertension: Physiopathology and Treatment, ed 2, New York, 1983, McGraw-Hill, pp 947–963.
14. Pick L: Das Ganglioma embryonale sympathicum (Sympathoma embryonale), eine typisch bosartige Geschwulstform des sympathischen Nervensystems, Klin Wochenschr 49:16–22, 1912.
15. Frankel F: Ein fall von doppelseitigem, vollig latent verlaufenden Nebennieren tumor und gleichzeitiger Nephritis mit Veranderungen am Circulationsapparat und Retinitis, Virchows Arch 103:244–263, 1886.
16. Alezais H, Peyron A: Un groupe nouveau de tumeurs epitheliales: les paraganglions, Compte Rend Soc Biol (Paris) 65:745–747, 1908.
17. L'Abbe M, Tinel J, Doumer A: Crises solaires et hypertension paroxystique en rapport avec une tumeur surrenale, Bull Mem Soc Med Hop (Paris) 46:982–990, 1922.
18. Manger WM, Gifford RW: Clinical and Experimental Pheochromocytoma, ed 2, Cambridge, MA, 1996, Blackwell Science.
19. Mayo CH: Paroxysmal hypertension with tumor of retroperitoneal nerve. Report of case, JAMA 89:1047–1050, 1927.
20. Rabin CB: Chromaffin cell tumor of the suprarenal medulla (pheochromocytoma), Arch Pathol 7:228–243, 1929.
21. Kelly HM, Piper MC, Wilder RE: Case of paroxysmal hypertension with paraganglioma of the right suprarenal gland, Mayo Clin Proc 11:65–70, 1936.
22. von Euler US: Presence of a substance with sympathin E properties in spleen extracts, Acta Physiol Scand 11:168–186, 1946.
23. von Euler US: The presence of a sympathomimetic substance in extracts of mammalian heart, J Physiol 105:38–44, 1946.
24. Holtz P, Credner K, Kroneberg G: Uber das sympathicomimetische pressorische Prinizip des Harns ("Urosympathin"), Arch Exp Pathol Pharmakol 204:228–243, 1947.
25. Holton P: Noradrenaline in tumors of the adrenal medulla, J Physiol 108:525–529, 1949.
26. Kvale WF, Roth GM, Manger WM, et al: Pheochromocytoma, Circulation 14:622–630, 1956.
27. Epstein FH, Eckhoff RD: The epidemiology of high blood pressure—geographic distributions and etiologic factors. In Stamler J, Stamler R, Pullman TN, editors: The epidemiology of hypertension, New York, 1967, Grune and Stratton, pp 155–166.
28. Page LB: Epidemiologic evidence on the etiology of human hypertension and its possible prevention, Am Heart J 91(4):527–534, 1976.
29. McBride W, Ferrario C, Lyle PA: Hypertension and medical informatics, J Natl Med Assoc 95(11):1048–1056, 2003.
30. Pacak K, Chrousos GP, Koch CA, et al: Pheochromocytoma: progress in diagnosis, therapy, and genetics. In: Margioris A, Chrousos GP, editors: Adrenal Disorders, ed 1, Totowa, 2001, Humana Press, pp 479–523.
31. Eisenhofer G, Goldstein DS, Kopin IJ, et al: Pheochromocytoma: rediscovery as a catecholamine-metabolizing tumor, Endocr Pathol 14(3):193–212, 2003.
32. Udenfriend S: Tyrosine hydroxylase, Pharmacol Rev 18(1):43–51, 1966.
33. Eisenhofer G, Goldstein DS: Peripheral dopamine systems. In Robertson D, Low P, Burnstock G, et al, editors: Primer on the Autonomic Nervous System, San Diego, 2004, Elsevier, in press.
34. Axelrod J: Methylation reactions in the formation and metabolism of catecholamines and other biogenic amines, Pharmacol Rev 18(1):95–113, 1966.
35. Johnson RG Jr: Accumulation of biological amines into chromaffin granules: a model for hormone and neurotransmitter transport, Physiol Rev 68(1):232–307, 1988.
36. Brown WJ, Barajas L, Waisman J, et al: Ultrastructural and biochemical correlates of adrenal and extra-adrenal pheochromocytoma, Cancer 29(3):744–759, 1972.
37. Nagatsu T: Tyrosine hydroxylase: human isoforms, structure and regulation in physiology and pathology, Essays Biochem 30:15–35, 1995.
38. Henry JP, Sagne C, Bedet C, et al: The vesicular monoamine transporter: from chromaffin granule to brain, Neurochem Int 32(3):227–246, 1998.
39. O'Connor DT, Wu H, Gill BM, et al: Hormone storage vesicle proteins, transcriptional basis of the widespread neuroendocrine expression of chromogranin A, and evidence of its diverse biological actions, intracellular and extracellular, Ann N Y Acad Sci 733:36–45, 1994.
40. Nagatsu T, Stjarne L: Catecholamine synthesis and release. Overview, Adv Pharmacol 42:1–14, 1998.
41. Eisenhofer G: The role of neuronal and extraneuronal plasma membrane transporters in the inactivation of peripheral catecholamines, Pharmacol Ther 91(1):35–62, 2001.
42. Eisenhofer G, Huynh TT, Hiroi M, et al: Understanding catecholamine metabolism as a guide to the biochemical diagnosis of pheochromocytoma, Rev Endocr Metab Disord 2(3):297–311, 2001.
43. Eisenhofer G, Keiser H, Friberg P, et al: Plasma metanephrines are markers of pheochromocytoma produced by catechol-O-methyltransferase within tumors, J Clin Endocrinol Metab 83(6):2175–2185, 1998.
44. Eisenhofer G, Rundqvist B, Aneman A, et al: Regional release and removal of catecholamines and extraneuronal metabolism to metanephrines, J Clin Endocrinol Metab 80:3009–3017, 1995.
45. Eisenhofer G, Aneman A, Hooper D, et al: Mesenteric organ production, hepatic metabolism, and renal elimination of norepinephrine and its metabolites in humans, J Neurochem 66:1565–1573, 1996.
46. Neumann HP, Berger DP, Sigmund G, et al: Pheochromocytomas, multiple endocrine neoplasia type 2, and von Hippel-Lindau disease, N Engl J Med 329(21):1531–1538, 1993.
47. Neumann HP, Bender BU, Januszewicz A, et al: Inherited pheochromocytoma, Adv Nephrol Necker Hosp 27:361–376, 1997.
48. Bravo EL, Tarazi RC, Fouad FM, et al: Clonidine-suppression test: a useful aid in the diagnosis of pheochromocytoma, N Engl J Med 305(11):623–626, 1981.
49. Bravo EL, Gifford RW Jr: Pheochromocytoma, Endocrinol Metab Clin North Am 22(2):329–341, 1993.
50. Gifford RW Jr, Bravo EL, Manger WM: Diagnosis and management of pheochromocytoma, Cardiology 72(Suppl 1):126–130, 1985.
51. Bouloux PG, Fakeeh M: Investigation of phaeochromocytoma, Clin Endocrinol (Oxf) 43(6):657–664, 1995.
52. Manger WM Jr, GRW: Pheochromocytoma, New York, Springer-Verlag, 1977.
53. Plouin PF, Degoulet P, Tugaye A, et al: [Screening for phaeochromocytoma: in which hypertensive patients? A semilogical study of 2585 patients, including 11 with phaeochromocytoma (author's transl)], Nouv Presse Med 10(11):869–872, 1981.
54. Steiner AL, Goodman AD, Powers SR: Study of a kindred with pheochromocytoma, medullary thyroid carcinoma, hyperparathyroidism and Cushing's disease: multiple endocrine neoplasia, type 2, Medicine (Baltimore) 47(5):371–409, 1968.
55. Bittar DA: Innovar-induced hypertensive crises in patients with pheochromocytoma, Anesthesiology 50(4):366–369, 1979.
56. Barancik M: Inadvertent diagnosis of pheochromocytoma after endoscopic premedication, Dig Dis Sci 34(1):136–138, 1989.
57. Schorr RT, Rogers SN: Intraoperative cardiovascular crisis caused by glucagon, Arch Surg 122(7):833–834, 1987.
58. Jan T, Metzger BE, Baumann G: Epinephrine-producing pheochromocytoma with hypertensive crisis after corticotropin injection, Am J Med 89(6):824–825, 1990.
59. Page LB, Raker JW, Berberich FR: Pheochromocytoma with predominant epinephrine secretion, Am J Med 47(4):648–652, 1969.
60. Cook RF, Katritsis D: Hypertensive crisis precipitated by a monoamine oxidase inhibitor in a patient with phaeochromocytoma, BMJ 300(6724):614, 1990.
61. Young JB, Landsberg L: Catecholamines and the Adrenal Medulla. In Wilson JD, Foster DW, editors: William's Textbook of Endocrinology 9:665–728, 1998.
62. Timmers HJ, Kozupa A, Eisenhofer G, et al: Clinical presentations, biochemical phenotypes, and genotype-phenotype correlations in patients with succinate dehydrogenase subunit B-associated pheochromocytomas and paragangliomas, J Clin Endocrinol Metab 92(3):779–786, 2007.
63. Colwell JA: Inhibition of insulin secretion by catecholamines in pheochromocytoma, Ann Intern Med 71(2):251–256, 1969.
64. Edelman ER, Stuenkel CA, Rutherford JD, et al: Diabetic ketoacidosis associated with pheochromocytoma, Cleve Clin J Med 59(4):423–427, 1992.
65. Stewart AF, Hoecker JL, Mallette LE, et al: Hypercalcemia in pheochromocytoma. Evidence for a novel mechanism, Ann Intern Med 102(6):776–779, 1985.
66. Heath H 3rd, Edis AJ: Pheochromocytoma associated with hypercalcemia and ectopic secretion of calcitonin, Ann Intern Med 91(2):208–210, 1979.
67. Spark RF, Connolly PB, Gluckin DS, et al: ACTH secretion from a functioning pheochromocytoma, N Engl J Med 301(8):416–418, 1979.
68. Viale G, Dell'Orto P, Moro E, et al: Vasoactive intestinal polypeptide-, somatostatin-, and calcitonin- producing adrenal pheochromocytoma associated with the watery diarrhea (WDHH) syndrome. First case report with immunohistochemical findings, Cancer 55(5):1099–1106, 1985.
69. Bornemann M, Hill SC, Kidd GS 2nd: Lactic acidosis in pheochromocytoma, Ann Intern Med 105(6):880–882, 1986.
70. Salahuddin A, Rohr-Kirchgraber T, Shekar R, et al: Interleukin-6 in the fever and multiorgan crisis of pheochromocytoma, Scand J Infect Dis 29(6):640–642, 1997.
71. Stelfox HT, Stewart AK, Bailey D, et al: Castleman's disease in a 44-year-old male with neurofibromatosis and pheochromocytoma, Leuk Lymphoma 27(5–6):551–556, 1997.
72. Stenstrom G, Svardsudd K: Pheochromocytoma in Sweden 1958–1981. An analysis of the National

Cancer Registry Data, Acta Med Scand 220(3):225–232, 1986.

73. Moon HD, Koneff AA, Li CC, et al: Pheochromocytomas of adrenals in male rats chronically injected with pituitary growth hormone, Proc Soc Exp Biol Med 93:74–77, 1956.

74. Esler M, Julius S, Zweifler A, et al: Mild high-renin essential hypertension, neurogenic human hypertension? N Engl J Med 296(8):405–411, 1977.

75. Bravo EL, Tarazi RC, Gifford RW, et al: Circulating and urinary catecholamines in pheochromocytoma. Diagnostic and pathophysiologic implications, N Engl J Med 301(13):682–686, 1979.

76. Kuchel O: Pseudopheochromocytoma, Hypertension 7(1):151–158, 1985.

77. Kuchel O: New Insights Into Pseudopheochromocytoma and Emotionally Provoked Hypertension. In Mansoor GA, editor: Secondary Hypertension, Totowa, 2004, Humana Press.

78. White WB, Baker LH: Episodic hypertension secondary to panic disorder, Arch Intern Med 146(6):1129–1130, 1986.

79. Page IH: A syndrome simulating diencephalic stimulation occurring in patients with essential hypertension, Am J Med Sci 190:9–14, 1935.

80. Lack EE: Pathology of the Adrenal Glands. In Roth LM, editor: Contemporary Issues in Surgical Pathology, New York, 1990, Churchill Livingstone, pp 14.

81. Raikhlin NT, Baronin AA, Smirnova EA, et al: Ultrastructural criteria of malignancy of adrenal medullary tumor, Bull Exp Biol Med 134(1):64–68, 2002.

82. Yu J, Pacak K: Management of malignant pheochromocytoma, Endocrinologist 12:291–299, 2002.

83. Linnoila RI, Keiser HR, Steinberg SM, et al: Histopathology of benign versus malignant sympathoadrenal paragangliomas: clinicopathologic study of 120 cases including unusual histologic features [see comments], Hum Pathol 21(11):1168–1180, 1990.

84. Clarke MR, Weyant RJ, Watson CG, et al: Prognostic markers in pheochromocytoma, Hum Pathol 29(5):522–526, 1998.

85. Modlin I, Farndon J, Shepherd A, et al: Pheochromocytomas in 72 patients: clinical and diagnostic features, treatment and long term results, Br J Surg 66(7):456–465, 1979.

86. Henle J, cited by Lack EE: Pathology of the adrenal glands. In Roth LM, editor: Contemporary Issues in Surgical Pathology, New York, 1990, Churchill Livingstone, pp 14.

87. Pearse AG: Common cytochemical and ultrastructural characteristics of cells producing polypeptide hormones (the APUD series) and their relevance to thyroid and ultimobranchial C cells and calcitonin, Proc R Soc Lond B Biol Sci 170(18):71–80, 1968.

88. Trojanowski JQ, Lee VM: Expression of neurofilament antigens by normal and neoplastic human adrenal chromaffin cells, N Engl J Med 313(2):101–104, 1985.

89. Thompson RJ, Doran JF, Jackson P, et al: PGP 9.5—a new marker for vertebrate neurons and neuroendocrine cells, Brain Res 278(1–2):224–228, 1983.

90. Bauer FE, Hacker GW, Terenghi G, et al: Localization and molecular forms of galanin in human adrenals: elevated levels in pheochromocytomas, J Clin Endocrinol Metab 63(6):1372–1378, 1986.

91. Mizuno K, Ojima M, Hashimoto S, et al: Biochemical identification of renin in human pheochromocytoma, Res Commun Chem Pathol Pharmacol 50(3):419–433, 1985.

92. Gonzalez-Garcia C, Keiser HR: Angiotensin II and angiotensin converting enzyme binding in human adrenal gland and pheochromocytomas, J Hypertens 8(5):433–441, 1990.

93. Miettinen M: Synaptophysin and neurofilament proteins as markers for neuroendocrine tumors, Arch Pathol Lab Med 111(9):813–818, 1987.

94. Sipple JH: The association of pheochromocytoma with carcinoma of the thyroid gland, Am J Med 31:163–166, 1961.

95. Sarosi G, Doe RP: Familial occurrence of parathyroid adenomas, pheochromocytoma, and medullary carcinoma of the thyroid with amyloid stroma (Sipple's syndrome), Ann Intern Med 68(6):1305–1309, 1968.

96. Pacak K, Ilias I, Adams KT, et al: Biochemical diagnosis, localization and management of pheochromocytoma: focus on multiple endocrine neoplasia type 2 in relation to other hereditary syndromes and sporadic forms of the tumour, J Intern Med 257(1):60–68, 2005.

97. Brandi ML, Gagel RF, Angeli A, et al: Guidelines for diagnosis and therapy of MEN type 1 and type 2, J Clin Endocrinol Metab 86(12):5658–5671, 2001.

98. Mulligan LM, Kwok JB, Healey CS, et al: Germ-line mutations of the RET proto-oncogene in multiple endocrine neoplasia type 2A, Nature 363(6428):458–460, 1993.

99. Lore F, Talidis F, Di Cairano G, et al: Multiple endocrine neoplasia type 2 syndromes may be associated with renal malformations, J Intern Med 250(1):37–42, 2001.

100. Koch CA, Pacak K, Chrousos GP: The molecular pathogenesis of hereditary and sporadic adrenocortical and adrenomedullary tumors, J Clin Endocrinol Metab 87(12):5367–5384, 2002.

101. Gagel RF, Tashjian AH Jr, Cummings T, et al: The clinical outcome of prospective screening for multiple endocrine neoplasia type 2a. An 18-year experience, N Engl J Med 318(8):478–484, 1988.

102. Jadoul M, Leo JR, Berends MJ, et al: Pheochromocytoma-induced hypertensive encephalopathy revealing MEN-IIa syndrome in a 13-year old boy. Implications for screening procedures and surgery, Horm Metab Res Suppl 21:46–49, 1989.

103. Casanova S, Rosenberg-Bourgin M, Farkas D, et al: Phaeochromocytoma in multiple endocrine neoplasia type 2A: survey of 100 cases, Clin Endocrinol 38:531–537, 1993.

104. Khairi MR, Dexter RN, Burzynski NJ, et al: Mucosal neuroma, pheochromocytoma and medullary thyroid carcinoma: multiple endocrine neoplasia type 3, Medicine (Baltimore) 54(2):89–112, 1975.

105. Eng C, Smith DP, Mulligan LM, et al: Point mutation within the tyrosine kinase domain of the RET proto-oncogene in multiple endocrine neoplasia type 2B and related sporadic tumours, Hum Mol Genet 3(2):237–241, 1994.

106. Ross JH: Pheochromocytoma. Special considerations in children, Urol Clin North Am 27(3):393–402, 2000.

107. Carney JA, Go VL, Gordon H, et al: Familial pheochromocytoma and islet cell tumor of the pancreas, Am J Med 68(4):515–521, 1980.

108. Cameron D, Spiro HM, Landsberg L: Zollinger-Ellison syndrome with multiple endocrine adenomatosis type II: N Engl J Med 299(3):152–153, 1978.

109. Griffiths DF, Williams GT, Williams ED: Duodenal carcinoid tumours, phaeochromocytoma and neurofibromatosis: islet cell tumour, phaeochromocytoma and the von Hippel-Lindau complex: two distinctive neuroendocrine syndromes, Q J Med 64(245):769–782, 1987.

110. Latif F, Tory K, Gnarra J, et al: Identification of the von Hippel-Lindau disease tumor suppressor gene, Science 260(5112):1317–1320, 1993.

111. Chen F, Kishida T, Yao M, et al: Germline mutations in the von Hippel-Lindau disease tumor suppressor gene: correlation with phenotype, Hum Mutat 5:66–75, 1995.

112. Eisenhofer G, Walther MM, Huynh TT, et al: Pheochromocytomas in von Hippel-Lindau syndrome and multiple endocrine neoplasia type 2 display distinct biochemical and clinical phenotypes, J Clin Endocrinol Metab 86(5):1999–2008, 2001.

113. Kalff V, Shapiro B, Lloyd R, et al: The spectrum of pheochromocytoma in hypertensive patients with neurofibromatosis, Arch Intern Med 142(12):2092–2098, 1982.

114. Colman SD, Wallace MR: Neurofibromatosis type 1, Eur J Cancer 30A(13):1974–1981, 1994.

115. Jacks T, Shih TS, Schmitt EM, et al: Tumour predisposition in mice heterozygous for a targeted mutation in Nf1, Nat Genet 7(3):353–361, 1994.

116. Walther MM, Herring J, Enquist E, et al: von Recklinghausen's disease and pheochromocytomas, J Urol 162(5):1582–1586, 1999.

117. Astuti D, Douglas F, Lennard TW, et al: Germline SDHD mutation in familial phaeochromocytoma, Lancet 357(9263):1181–1182, 2001.

118. Baysal BE, Ferrell RE, Willett-Brozick JE, et al: Mutations in SDHD, a mitochondrial complex II gene, in hereditary paraganglioma, Science 287(5454):848–851, 2000.

119. Astrom K, Cohen JE, Willett-Brozick JE, et al: Altitude is a phenotypic modifier in hereditary paraganglioma type 1: evidence for an oxygen-sensing defect, Hum Genet 113(3):228–237, 2003.

120. Gimenez-Roqueplo AP, Favier J, Rustin P, et al: Functional consequences of a SDHB gene mutation in an apparently sporadic pheochromocytoma, J Clin Endocrinol Metab 87(10):4771–4774, 2002.

121. Astuti D, Latif F, Dallol A, et al: Gene mutations in the succinate dehydrogenase subunit SDHB cause susceptibility to familial pheochromocytoma and to familial paraganglioma, Am J Hum Genet 69(1):49–54, 2001.

122. Benn DE, Gimenez-Roqueplo AP, Reilly JR, et al: Clinical presentation and penetrance of pheochromocytoma/paraganglioma syndromes, J Clin Endocrinol Metab 91(3):827–836, 2006.

123. Havekes B, Corssmit EP, Jansen JC, et al: Malignant paragangliomas associated with mutations in the succinate dehydrogenase D gene, J Clin Endocrinol Metab 92(4):1245–1248, 2007.

124. Neumann HP, Pawlu C, Peczkowska M, et al: Distinct clinical features of paraganglioma syndromes associated with SDHB and SDHD gene mutations, JAMA 292(8):943–951, 2004.

125. Timmers HJ, Pacak K, Bertherat J, et al: Mutations associated with succinate dehydrogenase d-related malignant paragangliomas, Clin Endocrinol (Oxf) 4(68):561–566, 2008.

126. Schiavi F, Boedeker CC, Bausch B, et al: Predictors and prevalence of paraganglioma syndrome associated with mutations of the SDHC gene, JAMA 294(16):2057–2063, 2005.

127. Mannelli M, Ercolino T, Giache V, et al: Genetic screening for pheochromocytoma: should SDHC gene analysis be included? J Med Genet 44(9):586–587, 2007.

128. Peczkowska M, Cascon A, Prejbisz A, et al: Extra-adrenal and adrenal pheochromocytomas associated with a germline SDHC mutation, Nat Clin Pract Endocrinol Metab 4(2):111–115, 2008.

129. Eisenhofer G, Goldstein DS, Sullivan P, et al: Biochemical and clinical manifestations of dopamine-producing paragangliomas: utility of plasma methoxytyramine, J Clin Endocrinol Metab 90:2068–2075, 2005.

130. Eisenhofer G, Goldstein DS, Sullivan P, et al: Biochemical and clinical manifestations of dopamine-producing paragangliomas: utility of plasma methoxytyramine, J Clin Endocrinol Metab 90(4):2068–2075, 2005.

131. Timmers HJ, Kozupa A, Eisenhofer G, et al: Clinical presentations, biochemical phenotypes, and genotype-phenotype correlations in patients with succinate dehydrogenase subunit B-associated pheochromocytomas and paragangliomas, J Clin Endocrinol Metab 92(3):779–786, 2007.

132. Young WF Jr, Abboud AL: Editorial: paraganglioma—all in the family, J Clin Endocrinol Metab 91(3):790–792, 2006.

133. Beldjord C, Desclaux-Arramond F, Raffin-Sanson M, et al: The RET protooncogene in sporadic pheochromocytomas: frequent MEN 2-like mutations and new molecular defects, J Clin Endocrinol Metab 80(7):2063–2068, 1995.

134. Eng C, Crossey PA, Mulligan LM, et al: Mutations in the RET proto-oncogene and the von Hippel-Lindau disease tumour suppressor gene in sporadic and syndromic phaeochromocytomas, J Med Genet 32(12):934–937, 1995.

135. Vargas MP, Zhuang Z, Wang C, et al: Loss of heterozygosity on the short arm of chromosomes 1 and 3 in sporadic pheochromocytoma and extra-adrenal paraganglioma, Hum Pathol 28(4):411–415, 1997.

136. Carney JA: The triad of gastric epithelioid leiomyosarcoma, pulmonary chondroma, and functioning extra-adrenal paraganglioma: a five-year review, Medicine (Baltimore) 62(3):159–169, 1983.

137. Margulies KB, Sheps SG: Carney's triad: guidelines for management, Mayo Clin Proc 63(5):496–502, 1988.

138. Pasini B, McWhinney SR, Bei T, et al: Clinical and molecular genetics of patients with the Carney-Stratakis syndrome and germline mutations of the genes coding for the succinate dehydrogenase subunits SDHB, SDHC, and SDHD, Eur J Hum Genet 16(1):79–88, 2008.

139. Eisenhofer G, Lenders J, Linehan W, et al: Plasma normetanephrine and metanephrine for detecting pheochromocytoma in von Hippel-Lindau disease and multiple endocrine neoplasia type 2, N Engl J Med 340:1872–1879, 1999.

140. Raber W, Raffesberg W, Bischof M, et al: Diagnostic efficacy of unconjugated plasma metanephrines for the detection of pheochromocytoma, Arch Intern Med 160(19):2957–2963, 2000.

141. Unger N, Pitt C, Schmidt IL, et al: Diagnostic value of various biochemical parameters for the diagnosis of pheochromocytoma in patients with adrenal mass, Eur J Endocrinol 154(3):409–417, 2006.

142. Vaclavik J, Stejskal D, Lacnak B, et al: Free plasma metanephrines as a screening test for pheochromocytoma in low-risk patients, J Hypertens 25(7):1427–1431, 2007.

143. Lenders J, Keiser H, Goldstein D, et al: Plasma metanephrines in the diagnosis of pheochromocytoma, Ann Intern Med 123(2):101–109, 1995.

144. de Jong WH, Graham KS, van der Molen JC, et al: Plasma free metanephrine measurement using automated online solid-phase extraction HPLC tandem mass spectrometry, Clin Chem 53(9):1684–1693, 2007.

145. Boyle JG, Davidson DF, Perry CG, et al: Comparison of diagnostic accuracy of urinary free metanephrines, vanillyl mandelic acid, and catecholamines and plasma catecholamines for diagnosis of pheochromocytoma, J Clin Endocrinol Metab 92(12):4602–4608, 2007.

146. Perry CG, Sawka AM, Singh R, et al: The diagnostic efficacy of urinary fractionated metanephrines measured by tandem mass spectrometry in detection of pheochromocytoma, Clin Endocrinol (Oxf) 66(5):703–708, 2007.

147. Eisenhofer G: Editorial: biochemical diagnosis of pheochromocytoma—is it time to switch to plasma-free metanephrines? J Clin Endocrinol Metab 88(2):550–552, 2003.

148. Lenders JW, Willemsen JJ, Eisenhofer G, et al: Is supine rest necessary before blood sampling for plasma metanephrines? Clin Chem 53(2):352–354, 2007.

149. Peaston R, Lennard T, Lai L: Overnight excretion of urinary catecholamines and metabolites in the detection of pheochromocytoma, J Clin Endocrinol Metab 81:1378–1384, 1996.

150. Eisenhofer G, Goldstein DS, Walther MM, et al: Biochemical diagnosis of pheochromocytoma: how to distinguish true- from false-positive test results, J Clin Endocrinol Metab 88(6):2656–2666, 2003.

151. Bouloux PM, Perrett D: Interference of labetalol metabolites in the determination of plasma catecholamines by HPLC with electrochemical detection, Clin Chim Acta 150(2):111–117, 1985.

152. Lenders JW, Eisenhofer G, Armando I, et al: Determination of metanephrines in plasma by liquid chromatography with electrochemical detection, Clin Chem 39(1):97–103, 1993.

153. Roden M, Raffesberg W, Raber W, et al: Quantification of unconjugated metanephrines in human plasma without interference by acetaminophen, Clin Chem 47(6):1061–1067, 2001.

154. Pacak K, Eisenhofer G, Ahlman H, et al: Pheochromocytoma: recommendations for clinical practice from the First International Symposium, Nat Clin Pract Endocrinol Metab 3(2):92–102, 2007.

155. Pacak K, Eisenhofer G, Ahlman H, et al: Pheochromocytoma: recommendations for clinical practice from the First International Symposium, October 2005, Nat Clin Pract Endocrinol Metab 3(2):92–102, 2007.

156. Grossman A, Pacak K, Sawka A, et al: Biochemical diagnosis and localization of pheochromocytoma: can we reach a consensus? Ann N Y Acad Sci 1073:332–347, 2006.

157. Sheps SG, Maher FT: Comparison of the histamine and tyramine hydrochloride tests in the diagnosis of pheochromocytoma, JAMA 195(4):265–267, 1966.

158. Bravo EL, Gifford RW Jr: Current concepts. Pheochromocytoma: diagnosis, localization and management, N Engl J Med 311(20):1298–1303, 1984.

159. Bravo E: Evolving concepts in the pathophysiology, diagnosis, and treatment of pheochromocytoma, Endocr Rev 15(3):356–368, 1994.

160. Sjoberg RJ, Simcic KJ, Kidd GS: The clonidine suppression test for pheochromocytoma. A review of its utility and pitfalls, Arch Intern Med 152(6):1193–1197, 1992.

161. Lawrence AM: Glucagon provocative test for pheochromocytoma, Ann Intern Med 66(6):1091–1096, 1967.

162. Grossman E, Goldstein D, Hoffman A, et al: Glucagon and clonidine testing in the diagnosis of pheochromocytoma, Hypertension 17:733–741, 1991.

163. Pacak K, Goldstein DS, Doppman JL, et al: A "pheo" lurks: novel approaches for locating occult pheochromocytoma, J Clin Endocrinol Metab 86(8):3641–3646, 2001.

164. Lance JW, Hinterberger H: Symptoms of pheochromocytoma, with particular reference to headache, correlated with catecholamine production, Arch Neurol 33(4):281–288, 1976.

165. Ito Y, Fujimoto Y, Obara T: The role of epinephrine, norepinephrine, and dopamine in blood pressure disturbances in patients with pheochromocytoma, World J Surg 16(4):759–763, 1992.

166. Aronoff SL, Passamani E, Borowsky BA, et al: Norepinephrine and epinephrine secretion from a clinically epinephrine-secreting pheochromocytoma, Am J Med 69(2):321–324, 1980.

167. Bryant J, Farmer J, Kessler LJ, et al: Pheochromocytoma: the expanding genetic differential diagnosis, J Natl Cancer Inst 95(16):1196–1204, 2003.

168. Schlumberger M, Gicquel C, Lumbroso J, et al: Malignant pheochromocytoma: clinical, biological, histologic and therapeutic data in a series of 20 patients with distant metastases, J Endocrinol Invest 15:631–642, 1992.

169. van der Harst E, de Herder WW, de Krijger RR, et al: The value of plasma markers for the clinical behaviour of phaeochromocytomas, Eur J Endocrinol 147(1):85–94, 2002.

170. Goldstein DS, Stull R, Eisenhofer G, et al: Plasma 3,4-dihydroxyphenylalanine (dopa) and catecholamines in neuroblastoma or pheochromocytoma, Ann Intern Med 105(6):887–888, 1986.

171. John H, Ziegler WH, Hauri D, et al: Pheochromocytomas: can malignant potential be predicted? Urology 53(4):679–683, 1999.

172. Stenstrom G, Waldenstrom J: Positive correlation between urinary excretion of catecholamine metabolites and tumour mass in pheochromocytoma. Results in patients with sustained and paroxysmal hypertension and multiple endocrine neoplasia, Acta Med Scand 217(1):73–77, 1985.

173. Ilias I, Pacak K: Current approaches and recommended algorithm for the diagnostic localization of pheochromocytoma, J Clin Endocrinol Metab 89(2):479–491, 2004.

174. Scholz T, Eisenhofer G, Pacak K, et al: Clinical review: current treatment of malignant pheochromocytoma, J Clin Endocrinol Metab 92(4):1217–1225, 2007.

175. Deleted in pages.

176. Grumbach MM, Biller BM, Braunstein GD, et al: Management of the clinically inapparent adrenal mass ("incidentaloma"), Ann Intern Med 138(5):424–429, 2003.

177. Miskulin J, Shulkin BL, Doherty GM, et al: Is preoperative iodine 123 meta-iodobenzylguanidine scintigraphy routinely necessary before initial adrenalectomy for pheochromocytoma? Surgery 134(6):918–922, 2003, discussion 22–23.

178. Maurea S, Cuocolo A, Reynolds JC, et al: Diagnostic imaging in patients with paragangliomas. Computed tomography, magnetic resonance and MIBG scintigraphy comparison, Q J Nucl Med 40(4):365–371, 1996.

179. Mukherjee JJ, Peppercorn PD, Reznek RH, et al: Pheochromocytoma: effect of nonionic contrast medium in CT on circulating catecholamine levels, Radiology 202(1):227–231, 1997.

180. Schmedtje JFJ, Sax S, Pool JL, et al: Localization of ectopic pheochromocytomas by magnetic resonance imaging, Am J Med 83:770–772, 1987.

181. Prager G, Heinz-Peer G, Passler C, et al: Can dynamic gadolinium-enhanced magnetic resonance imaging with chemical shift studies predict the status of adrenal masses? World J Surg 26(8):958–964, 2002.

182. Honigschnabl S, Gallo S, Niederle B, et al: How accurate is MR imaging in characterisation of adrenal masses: update of a long-term study, Eur J Radiol 41(2):113–122, 2002.

183. Shapiro B, Gross MD, Shulkin B: Radioisotope diagnosis and therapy of malignant pheochromocytoma, Trends Endocrinol Metab 12(10):469–475, 2001.

184. Hoegerle S, Nitzsche E, Altehoefer C, et al: Pheochromocytomas: detection with 18F DOPA whole body PET—initial results, Radiology 222(2):507–512, 2002.

185. Shulkin BL, Thompson NW, Shapiro B, et al: Pheochromocytomas: imaging with 2-[fluorine-18]fluoro-2-deoxy-D-glucose PET, Nucl Med 212:35–41, 1999.

186. Epelbaum J, Bertherat J, Prevost G, et al: Molecular and pharmacological characterization of somatostatin receptor subtypes in adrenal, extraadrenal, and malignant pheochromocytomas, J Clin Endocrinol Metab 80(6):1837–1844, 1995.

187. Von Moll L, McEwan AJ, Shapiro B, et al: Iodine-131 MIBG scintigraphy of neuroendocrine tumors other than pheochromocytoma and neuroblastoma, J Nucl Med 28(6):979–988, 1987.

188. Shapiro B, Copp JE, Sisson JC, et al: Iodine-131 metaiodobenzylguanidine for the locating of suspected pheochromocytoma: experience in 400 cases, J Nucl Med 26(6):576–585, 1985.

189. Nakatani T, Hayama T, Uchida J, et al: Diagnostic localization of extra-adrenal pheochromocytoma: comparison of (123)I-MIBG imaging and (131)I-MIBG imaging, Oncol Rep 9(6):1225–1227, 2002.

190. Van Der Horst-Schrivers AN, Jager PL, Boezen HM, et al: Iodine-123 metaiodobenzylguanidine scintigraphy in localising phaeochromocytomas—experience and meta-analysis, Anticancer Res 26(2B):1599–1604, 2006.

191. Timmers HJ, Kozupa A, Chen CC, et al: Superiority of fluorodeoxyglucose positron emission tomography to other functional imaging techniques in the evaluation of metastatic SDHB-associated pheochromocytoma and paraganglioma, J Clin Oncol 25(16):2262–2269, 2007.

192. van der Harst E, de Herder WW, Bruining HA, et al: [(123)I]metaiodobenzylguanidine and [(111) In]octreotide uptake in benign and malignant pheochromocytomas, J Clin Endocrinol Metab 86(2):685–693, 2001.

193. Solanki KK, Bomanji J, Moyes J, et al: A pharmacological guide to medicines which interfere with the biodistribution of radiolabelled meta-iodobenzylguanidine (MIBG), Nucl Med Commun 13(7):513–521, 1992.

194. Lynn MD, Shapiro B, Sisson JC, et al: Portrayal of pheochromocytoma and normal human adrenal medulla by m-[123I]iodobenzylguanidine: concise communication, J Nucl Med 25(4):436–440, 1984.

195. Elgazzar A, Gelfand M, Washburn L, et al: I-123 MIBG scintigraphy in adults, Clin Nucl Med 20(2):147–152, 1993.

196. Goldstein DS, Eisenhofer G, Dunn BB, et al: Positron emission tomographic imaging of cardiac sympathetic innervation using 6-[18F]fluorodopamine: initial findings in humans, J Am Coll Cardiol 22(7):1961–1971, 1993.

197. Ilias I, Yu J, Carrasquillo JA, et al: Superiority of 6-[18F]-fluorodopamine positron emission tomography versus [131I]-metaiodobenzylguanidine scintigraphy in the localization of metastatic pheochromocytoma, J Clin Endocrinol Metab 88(9):4083–4087, 2003.

198. Shulkin BL, Wieland DM, Schwaiger M, et al: PET scanning with hydroxyephedrine: an approach to the localization of pheochromocytoma, J Nucl Med 33(6):1125–1131, 1992.

199. Timmers HJ, Hadi M, Carrasquillo JA, et al: The effects of carbidopa on uptake of 6–18F-Fluoro-L-DOPA in PET of pheochromocytoma and extraadrenal abdominal paraganglioma, J Nucl Med 48(10):1599–1606, 2007.

200. Warburg O: On the origin of cancer cells, Science 123(3191):309–314, 1956.

201. Kaltsas G, Korbonits M, Heintz E, et al: Comparison of somatostatin analog and meta-iodobenzylguanidine radionuclides in the diagnosis and localization of advanced neuroendocrine tumors, J Clin Endocrinol Metab 86(2):895–902, 2001.

202. Pacak K: Preoperative management of the pheochromocytoma patient, J Clin Endocrinol Metab 92(11):4069–4079, 2007.

203. Pacak K: Preoperative management of the pheochromocytoma patient, J Clin Endocrinol Metab 92(11):4069–4079, 2007.

204. Mannelli M: Management and treatment of pheochromocytomas and paragangliomas, Ann N Y Acad Sci 1073:405–416, 2006.

205. Nicholson JP Jr, Vaughn ED Jr, Pickering TG, et al: Pheochromocytoma and prazosin, Ann Intern Med 99(4):477–479, 1983.

206. Van Stratum M, Levarlet M, Lambilliotte JP, et al: Use of labetalol during anesthesia for pheochromocytoma removal, Acta Anaesthesiol Belg 34(4):233–240, 1983.
207. Sjoerdsma A, Engelman K, Spector S, et al: Inhibition of catecholamine synthesis in man with alpha-methyltyrosine, an inhibitor of tyrosine hydroxylase, Lancet 2(7422):1092–1094, 1965.
208. Colson P, Ribstein J: [Simplified strategy for anesthesia of pheochromocytoma]. Ann Fr Anesth Reanim 10(5):456–462, 1991.
209. Perry R, Keiser H, Norton J, et al: Surgical management of pheochromocytoma with the use of metyrosine, Ann Surg 212:621–628, 1990.
210. Briggs RS, Birtwell AJ, Pohl JE: Hypertensive response to labetalol in phaeochromocytoma, Lancet 1(8072):1045–1046, 1978.
211. Vargas H, Kavoussi L, Bartlett D, et al: Laparoscopic adrenalectomy: a new standard of care, Urology 49:673–678, 1997.
212. Winfield HN, Hamilton BD, Bravo EL, et al: Laparoscopic adrenalectomy: the preferred choice? A comparison to open adrenalectomy, J Urol 160(2):325–329, 1998.
213. Sheps SG, Jiang NS, Klee GG, et al: Recent developments in the diagnosis and treatment of pheochromocytoma, Mayo Clin Proc 65(1):88–95, 1990.
214. Stenstrom G, Ernest I, Tisell LE: Long-term results in 64 patients operated upon for pheochromocytoma, Acta Med Scand 223(4):345–352, 1988.
215. Amar L, Servais A, Gimenez-Roquepla AP, et al: Year of diagnosis, features at presentation, and risk of recurrence in patients with pheochromocytoma or secreting paraganglioma, J Clin Endocrinol Metab 90(4):2110–2116, 2005.
216. Goldstein RE, O'Neill JA Jr, Holcomb GW 3rd, et al: Clinical experience over 48 years with pheochromocytoma, Ann Surg 229(6):755–764, 1999.
217. Kopf D, Goretzki PE, Lehnert H: Clinical management of malignant adrenal tumors, J Cancer Res Clin Oncol 127(3):143–155, 2001.
218. Glodny B, Winde G, Herwig R, et al: Clinical differences between benign and malignant pheochromocytomas, Endocr J 48(2):151–159, 2001.
219. Mornex R, Badet C, Peyrin L: Malignant pheochromocytoma: a series of 14 cases observed between 1966 and 1990, J Endocrinol Invest 15(9):643–649, 1992.
220. Brouwers FM, Eisenhofer G, Tao JJ, et al: High frequency of SDHB germline mutations in patients with malignant catecholamine-producing paragangliomas: implications for genetic testing, J Clin Endocrinol Metab 91(11):4505–4509, 2006.
221. Mundschenk J, Lehnert H: Malignant pheochromocytoma, Exp Clin Endocrinol Diabetes 106(5):373–376, 1998.
222. Amar L, Baudin E, Burnichon N, et al: Succinate dehydrogenase B gene mutations predict survival in patients with malignant pheochromocytomas or paragangliomas, J Clin Endocrinol Metab 92(10):3822–3828, 2007.
223. Stumvoll M, Fritsche A, Pickert A, et al: Features of malignancy in a benign pheochromocytoma, Horm Res 48(3):135–136, 1997.
224. Hosaka Y, Rainwater LM, Grant CS, et al: Pheochromocytoma: nuclear deoxyribonucleic acid patterns studied by flow cytometry, Surgery 100(6):1003–1010, 1986.
225. Brown HM, Komorowski RA, Wilson SD, et al: Predicting metastasis of pheochromocytomas using DNA flow cytometry and immunohistochemical markers of cell proliferation: A positive correlation between MIB-1 staining and malignant tumor behavior, Cancer 86(8):1583–1589, 1999.
226. Tormey WP, Fitzgerald RJ, Thomas G, et al: Catecholamine secretion and ploidy in phaeochromocytoma, Int J Clin Pract 54(8):520–523, 2000.
227. Rao F, Keiser HR, O'Connor DT: Malignant pheochromocytoma. Chromaffin granule transmitters and response to treatment, Hypertension 36(6):1045–1052, 2000.
228. Yon L, Guillemot J, Montero-Hadjadje M, et al: Identification of the secretogranin II-derived peptide EM66 in pheochromocytomas as a potential marker for discriminating benign versus malignant tumors, J Clin Endocrinol Metab 88(6):2579–2585, 2003.
229. Elder EE, Xu D, Hoog A, et al: KI-67 AND hTERT expression can aid in the distinction between malignant and benign pheochromocytoma and paraganglioma, Mod Pathol 16(3):246–255, 2003.
230. Loh KC, Fitzgerald PA, Matthay KK, et al: The treatment of malignant pheochromocytoma with iodine-131 metaiodobenzylguanidine (131I-MIBG): a comprehensive review of 116 reported patients, J Endocrinol Invest 20(11):648–658, 1997.
231. Rose B, Matthay KK, Price D, et al: High-dose 131I-metaiodobenzylguanidine therapy for 12 patients with malignant pheochromocytoma, Cancer 98(2):239–248, 2003.
232. Lamarre-Cliche M, Gimenez-Roquepla AP, Billaud E, et al: Effects of slow-release octreotide on urinary metanephrine excretion and plasma chromogranin A and catecholamine levels in patients with malignant or recurrent phaeochromocytoma, Clin Endocrinol (Oxf) 57(5):629–634, 2002.
233. Forster GJ, Engelbach MJ, Brockmann JJ, et al: Preliminary data on biodistribution and dosimetry for therapy planning of somatostatin receptor positive tumours: comparison of (86)Y-DOTATOC and (111)In-DTPA-octreotide, Eur J Nucl Med 28(12):1743–1750, 2001.
234. Averbuch SD, Steakley CS, Young RC, et al: Malignant pheochromocytoma: effective treatment with a combination of cyclophosphamide, vincristine, and dacarbazine, Ann Intern Med 109(4):267–273, 1988.
235. Kulke MH, Stuart K, Enzinger PC, et al: Phase II study of temozolomide and thalidomide in patients with metastatic neuroendocrine tumors, J Clin Oncol 24(3):401–406, 2006.
236. Quezado ZN, Keiser HR, Parker MM: Reversible myocardial depression after massive catecholamine release from a pheochromocytoma, Crit Care Med 20(4):549–551, 1992.
237. Taub MA, Osburne RC, Georges LP, et al: Malignant pheochromocytoma. Severe clinical exacerbation and release of stored catecholamines during lymphoma chemotherapy, Cancer 50(9):1739–1741, 1982.
238. Siddiqui MZ, Von Eyben FE, Spanos G: High-voltage irradiation and combination chemotherapy for malignant pheochromocytoma, Cancer 62(4):686–690, 1988.
239. Yu L, Fleckman AM, Chadha M, et al: Radiation therapy of metastatic pheochromocytoma: case report and review of the literature, Am J Clin Oncol 19(4):389–393, 1996.
240. Takahashi K, Ashizawa N, Minami T, et al: Malignant pheochromocytoma with multiple hepatic metastases treated by chemotherapy and transcatheter arterial embolization, Intern Med 38(4):349–354, 1999.
241. Pacak K, Fojo T, Goldstein DS, et al: Radiofrequency ablation: a novel approach for treatment of metastatic pheochromocytoma, J Natl Cancer Inst 93(8):648–649, 2001.
242. Ohkawa S, Hirokawa S, Masaki T, et al: [Examination of percutaneous microwave coagulation and radiofrequency ablation therapy for metastatic liver cancer], Gan To Kagaku Ryoho 29(12):2149–2151, 2002.
243. Fonkalsrud EW: Pheochromocytoma in childhood, Prog Pediatr Surg 26:103–111, 1991.
244. Havekes B, Romijn JA, Eisenhofer G, et al: Update on pediatric pheochromocytoma, Pediatr Nephrol 24(5):943–950, 2009.
245. Bloom DA, Fonkalsrud EW: Surgical management of pheochromocytoma in children, J Pediatr Surg 9(2):179–184, 1974.
246. Caty MG, Coran AG, Geagen M, et al: Current diagnosis and treatment of pheochromocytoma in children. Experience with 22 consecutive tumors in 14 patients, Arch Surg 125(8):978–981, 1990.
247. Barontini M, Levin G, Sanso G: Characteristics of pheochromocytoma in a 4- to 20-year-old population, Ann N Y Acad Sci 1073:30–37, 2006.
248. De Krijger RR, Van Nederveen FH, Korpershoek E, et al: Frequent genetic changes in childhood pheochromocytomas, Ann N Y Acad Sci 1073:166–176, 2006.
249. Ludwig AD, Feig DI, Brandt ML, et al: Recent advances in the diagnosis and treatment of pheochromocytoma in children, Am J Surg 194(6):792–796, 2007, discussion 6–7.
250. Hume DM: Pheochromocytoma in the adult and in the child, Am J Surg 99:458–496, 1960.
251. Kaufman BH, Telander RL, van Heerden JA, et al: Pheochromocytoma in the pediatric age group: current status, J Pediatr Surg 18(6):879–884, 1983.
252. Reddy VS, O'Neill JA Jr, Holcomb GW 3rd, et al: Twenty-five-year surgical experience with pheochromocytoma in children, Am Surg 66(12):1085–1091, 2000, discussion 92.
253. Coutant R, Pein F, Adamsbaum C, et al: Prognosis of children with malignant pheochromocytoma. Report of 2 cases and review of the literature, Horm Res 52(3):145–149, 1999.
254. Fonseca V, Bouloux PM: Phaeochromocytoma and paraganglioma, Baillieres Clin Endocrinol Metab 7(2):509–544, 1993.
255. Weise M, Merke D, Pacak K, et al: Utility of plasma free metanephrines for detecting childhood pheochromocytoma, J Clin Endocrinol Metab 87(5):1955–1960, 2002.
256. Harper MA, Murnaghan GA, Kennedy L, et al: Phaeochromocytoma in pregnancy. Five cases and a review of the literature, Br J Obstet Gynaecol 96(5):594–606, 1989.
257. Oishi S, Sato T: Pheochromocytoma in pregnancy: a review of the Japanese literature, Endocr J 41(3):219–225, 1994.
258. Schenker JG, Chowers I: Pheochromocytoma and pregnancy. Review of 89 cases, Obstet Gynecol Surv 26(11):739–747, 1971.
259. Ahlawat SK, Jain S, Kumari S, et al: Pheochromocytoma associated with pregnancy: case report and review of the literature, Obstet Gynecol Surv 54(11):728–737, 1999.
260. Brunt LM: Phaeochromocytoma in pregnancy, Br J Surg 88(4):481–483, 2001.
261. Molitch ME: Endocrine emergencies in pregnancy, Baillieres Clin Endocrinol Metab 6(1):167–191, 1992.
262. Demeure MJ, Carlsen B, Traul D, et al: Laparoscopic removal of a right adrenal pheochromocytoma in a pregnant woman, J Laparoendosc Adv Surg Tech A 8(5):315–319, 1998.
263. Ein SH, Shandling B, Wesson D, et al: Recurrent pheochromocytomas in children, J Pediatr Surg 25(10):1063–1065, 1990.
264. Mitchell SZ, Freilich JD, Brant D, et al: Anesthetic management of pheochromocytoma resection during pregnancy, Anesth Analg 66(5):478–480, 1987.
265. James MF, Huddle KR, Owen AD, et al: Use of magnesium sulphate in the anaesthetic management of phaeochromocytoma in pregnancy, Can J Anaesth 35(2):178–182, 1988.

Chapter 15

ADRENAL SURGERY

PHILIP W. SMITH and JOHN B. HANKS

The first known surgical extirpation of the adrenal gland is thought to have occurred in 1889 during the performance of a radical nephrectomy; the first planned adrenalectomy was performed in 1914. Surgical excision is now the standard of care for many adrenal pathologies, and the field continues to evolve and advance. The enhanced sophistication of image-guided surgery and the increasing use of laparoscopic procedures have had great impacts on abdominal surgery and particularly on adrenal surgery.

Prior to 1992, adrenalectomies were performed exclusively by open techniques. These were mainly performed through an open anterior approach via midline or subcostal incision, or through a posterior approach through the 11th or 12th ribs. In 1992, the laparoscopic technique was described by Gagner in Canada and by Higashihara in Japan.[1,2] Initially, laparoscopic approaches to adrenalectomy were limited to small benign lesions, but indications continue to expand. Currently, laparoscopy is the gold standard for excision of the majority of benign adrenal lesions.[3-5] The use of laparoscopy for lesions greater than 10 cm or in

clearly malignant lesions remains under debate. Recently, robotic surgery has been applied to adrenalectomy, although the role of this technology remains unclear.

In parallel to advances in surgical techniques, imaging technology has become increasingly sophisticated, allowing a greater understanding of endocrinologic disorders. CT and MRI have allowed excellent visualization of the retroperitoneal space and both adrenal glands. Enhanced CT and MRI virtually eliminated the necessity of retroperitoneal exploration in situations such as familial pheochromocytoma, allowing the use of a unilateral approach and subsequent periodic imaging to evaluate possible recurrence.[6]

Indications and Contraindications

Adrenal masses are common and are frequently found incidentally on imaging obtained for other reasons.[7] The workup of an adrenal mass is straightforward and is focused on determining if a mass is functional or may represent malignancy, both indications for adrenalectomy (Table 15-1). The specifics of this workup are discussed in detail elsewhere in this text. Although the majority of adrenal masses are benign, the finding of malignant adrenal masses is not uncommon, and as many as 15% of incidentally found adrenal masses are functionally active.[8] Benign adrenal masses include the nonfunctioning ("incidentaloma") and the functioning adrenal mass (Conn's Syndrome, Cushing's tumor, pheochromocytoma, or an androgen-secreting tumor). Primary malignancies of the adrenal may have their own characteristic imaging finding; however, this is often difficult to determine with certainty preoperatively, and size of the mass is used as an important predictor. A final class of adrenal masses includes metastatic lesions.

Much of the workup and diagnostic decision making depends on biochemical studies and image review (e.g., CT, MIBG, MRI, CT, arteriogram, PET, or other specialized studies). Fine-needle aspiration biopsy has very limited application in the evaluation of adrenal lesions, unlike its utility in thyroid nodules. The primary use of fine-needle aspiration is for suspicion of an extraadrenal malignancy metastatic to the adrenal. Fine-needle aspiration of an adrenal mass should never be considered until

Table 15-1. Indications for Adrenalectomy

Mass

Functioning
  Pheochromocytoma
  Aldosteronoma
  Cushing's syndrome
  Androgen-secreting
Nonfunctioning
  Larger than 4 cm
  Recent growth of >1 cm over last 12 months
  Solitary metastasis

Hyperplasia (Bilateral)

Macronodular (unresponsive to medical therapy)
Ectopic adrenocorticotropic hormone (ACTH)
Failed pituitary resection for Cushing's disease with persistent ACTH

completing a workup for pheochromocytoma, because inadvertent fine-needle aspiration of such a lesion may lead to catastrophic, uncontrolled hypertension.

Of the benign lesions mentioned, pheochromocytoma has an increased chance of being bilateral or ectopic. Careful evaluation should be made prior to the initial operation, documenting the location of ectopic tissue. Previously, MEN2 patients underwent bilateral adrenalectomy and retroperitoneal exploration. In 1993, Wells and colleagues advocated that if a unilateral lesion is found, it may be reasonable to resect it, followed by surveillance of the remaining adrenal.[6] Only 50% of patients with unilateral pheochromocytoma in the MEN2 population will require contralateral adrenalectomy within 5 years, thereby decreasing their exposure to exogenous corticosteroid replacement for that time. This allows for less invasive, more direct approaches, including flank incision (and later, laparoscopy), with greatly reduced morbidity and mortality.

Contraindications to adrenal surgery after appropriate selection are relatively few. It has been emphasized that prior to considering resection, several factors must be taken into account. For example, a 2-cm, nonfunctioning incidentaloma should not (in general) be surgically removed, whereas a 6-cm lesion should.[9] A 2-cm functioning tumor should be removed, whereas a 2-cm metastasis to the adrenal should be carefully considered with regard to prognosis. An asymptomatic angiomyelolipoma of almost any size need not be resected if the diagnosis is certain. Therefore, although the surgical capability to perform adrenalectomy is usually available, it must be tempered by presurgical judgment. If the laparoscopic approach is to be considered, it is clear that experience is needed both in endocrine surgery and in laparoscopy. Caution should be used in the appropriate choice of technique for adrenal or retroperitoneal procedures.

Laparoscopy has emerged as the standard for surgical removal of most lesions of the adrenal gland.[3-5] Although no prospective randomized trial has been reported comparing laparoscopic adrenalectomy to open adrenalectomy, in multiple reviews, laparoscopy has proven to be as safe and effective as the open approach and offers less pain, shorter hospital stay, and more rapid convalescence.[5] Gagner et al. had suggested that increased intraoperative catecholamine secretion occurs during laparoscopic surgery, possibly related to CO_2 insufflation.[10] Other studies have not shown that CO_2 had any different effect than helium insufflation, and most recent studies have confirmed the intraoperative safety of the technique.[11]

Metastatic or regionally advanced carcinoma of the adrenal, or the presence of regionally metastatic pheochromocytoma,

makes the laparoscopic approach less appropriate.[12] Such a clinical situation might require en bloc resection, possibly involving kidney or other organs as well as regional lymph nodes. Despite advances in minimally invasive techniques, it still is believed that adrenal masses that demonstrate evidence of local invasion should be approached with an open resection, and reported series of laparoscopic adrenalectomy have excluded these patients.

The size of the adrenal lesion may affect the choice of operative approach. There are two primary concerns regarding resecting large adrenal lesions through minimally invasive techniques. The first is the technical difficulty of safely dissecting and removing bulky lesions. The second major concern is the possibility of laparoscopically resecting a known or unknown adrenocortical carcinoma, which remains a debated practice. The likelihood of an undiagnosed lesion harboring malignancy increases dramatically with the size of the lesion. According to the NIH consensus statement for the management of undiagnosed adrenal masses, the incidence of adrenocortical carcinomas increases from 2% in lesions ≤40 mm, to 6% in lesions 41 to 60 mm, to 25% in lesions >60 mm.[13]

Adrenocortical carcinomas are rare and have poor prognoses, with 12% to 38% 5-year survival.[14] Complete resection offers the only hope of cure (see Chapter 11). Therefore, patients with carcinomas often require more extensive resection, which may include local lymph nodes, kidney, spleen, and/or partial resection of the pancreas or liver. The standard approach for documented adrenal malignancy has been an open laparotomy. Early, limited reports of laparoscopic resections of primary adrenal malignancies were associated with very high rates of early recurrence, including in laparoscopic port sites as well as peritoneal carcinomatosis.[15] It was believed that insufflation, which is necessary for laparoscopy, contributed to disease spread. This belief now has been replaced by an understanding that the operation must follow basic oncologic principles regardless of the technique employed for resection. As additional experience has accumulated, improved outcomes are now reported with laparoscopy for primary adrenal malignancy.[15] Table 15-2 summarizes 15 publications that included laparoscopic resections for primary adrenal malignancies, all published between 2002 and 2008 (adapted from McCauley[15]). This aggregate includes 60 primary adrenal malignancies; the low number is reflective of the rarity of these tumors. In this analysis, six of the reported tumor recurrences and all five instances of port-site recurrence and carcinomatosis occurred in a single series.[16] Of note, those five patients represent a highly selected group, all of whom presented with recurrent disease prior to the resection reported in this series, identifying them as high risk for aggressive tumor behavior. Even including these five patients, oncologic results in the overall group compare favorably to open series; 35% had recurrence during approximately 3 years of mean follow-up. This compares well with results reported in open series which report similar or higher recurrence rates.[15,16]

Although the question is not settled, there is a growing consensus in the literature that minimally invasive techniques may be employed for excision of primary adrenal malignancy in appropriately selected cases. It also is now becoming evident that laparoscopy provides similar long-term results to open adrenalectomy when employed for solitary metastases to the adrenal.[15] Appropriate planning and patient selection are imperative. If preoperative imaging suggests invasion into surrounding structures or vena caval thrombus, one should proceed with open resection. Principles of resection that apply in open surgery must

Table 15-2. Summary of Series Reporting Laparoscopic Adrenalectomy for Primary Adrenal Malignancies from 2002 to 2008

Author	# LA	# Primary Malignant Adrenal Neoplasms	Median or Mean Tumor Size	Median or Mean Follow-Up (Months)	Recurrence	Port-Site/Peritoneal Metastasis	Survival
Corcione[45]	100	2 ACC	8.5 cm	13.6	1 local	0	1 alive, DF 1 alive w/dis
Eto[46]	150	1 ACC	4.5 cm	106	Local	0	1 alive w/dis
Gill[47]	250	6 ACC, 1 malignant pheo	5 cm*	26	2 local 1 distant	0	3 alive, DF 1 alive w/dis 2 dead of dis
Gonzalez[16]	6	6 ACC	5.3 cm	28	6 local and distant	5	2 alive w/dis 4 dead of dis
Henry[48]	233	6 ACC	7.4 cm	47	1 distant	0	5 alive, DF 1 dead of dis
Kirshtein[49]	14	5 ACC	4 cm*	Unknown	0	0	Unknown
Liao[18]	210	4 ACC	6.2 cm	39	1 local and distant 2 distant	0	1 alive, DF 1 alive w/dis 2 dead of dis
Lombardi[50]	79	4 ACC, 3 malignant pheo	5.9 cm*	23	1 local 1 distant	0	4 alive, DF 2 alive w/dis 1 dead, unrelated
Nocca[51]	131	4 ACC	8.5 cm	34	1 distant	0	3 alive, DF 1 dead of dis
Palazzo[52]	391	3 ACC	6.8 cm	34	1 distant	0	2 alive, DF 1 dead of dis
Parnaby[21]	101	3 ACC	Unknown	48	0	0	3 alive, DF
Porpiglia[53]	205	5 ACC 1 myxoid ACC	6.9 cm	30	0	0	5 alive, DF 1 dead, unrelated
Ramacciato[19]	107	2 ACC	8.5 cm	45	0	0	2 alive, DF
Schlamp[54]	1	1 ACC	7.5 cm	4	Local	0	1 alive w/dis
Soon[20]	16	3 ACC	3.1 cm*	18	0	0	3 alive, DF
Totals	1994	55 ACC 1 myxoid 4 malignant pheo	6.3 cm	35	21	5	33 alive, DF 8 alive w/dis 11 dead of dis 2 dead, unrelated

Data from McCauley and Nguyen.[15]

ACC, Adrenocortical carcinoma; DF, disease free; LA, laparoscopic adrenalectomy; pheo, pheochromocytoma.
*Indicates that size includes all tumor types for these series.

be maintained in laparoscopy, including preservation and dissection of tissue planes and avoidance of fracture or rupture of the lesion. The specimen should be removed from the body in an impermeable retrieval bag to avoid exposure of the port site. It is obvious that the surgeon must be experienced in both laparoscopy and endocrine surgery. Because malignancy may be undiagnosed prior to resection, all of these principles should be applied to laparoscopic and open adrenalectomy in general, with particular attention in large or suspicious lesions.

There remains debate in the literature regarding how large of a lesion should be approached laparoscopically, both for oncologic and technical reasons. A large lesion makes the operation more challenging. Most series reporting resection of large masses, including those in Table 15-1, emphasize the lateral transperitoneal technique, which allows the greatest visualization and operative space. Even with this approach, however, visualization can be a challenge in large lesions. Large lesions also may have aberrant vascular supply, thus leading to potential for operative bleeding. While lesions as large as 15 cm have been resected laparoscopically,[17] the appropriate size restrictions for laparoscopic adrenalectomy has not been universally agreed upon. Multiple series have now been published of laparoscopic adrenalectomy for lesions over 6 cm.[15,18-21] Hospital length of stay, operative blood loss, and overall morbidity are not necessarily worsened following laparoscopic resections of large lesions. Rosoff's review concludes that tumor size alone should not preclude laparoscopic approaches, but that larger lesions should be managed by experienced laparoscopic surgeons who also are

adept at the open procedure, should conversion be required. The review also emphasizes the importance of adhering to the oncologic principles discussed earlier.[22] Previous upper-abdominal surgery such as nephrectomy, splenectomy, or hepatic resection is not an absolute contraindication to laparoscopy but does make the procedure more difficult. This could necessitate conversion to an open procedure, potentially in an urgent fashion if difficult dissection leads to operative bleeding. Retroperitoneal laparoscopic approach has been reported to circumvent these problems, but this procedure is technically challenging and not widely practiced.

Robotic surgery is a fairly recent development in adrenal surgery. Robotic computer-assisted telemanipulation systems were developed to overcome some of the limitations of standard laparoendoscopic techniques and to facilitate surgeon hand motions in limited operating spaces. The surgeon operates from a remote console, and hand motions are reproduced in scaled proportion through robotically controlled microwrist instruments inserted through the body wall. Purported advantages of robotic-assisted laparoscopic surgery over conventional laparoscopy include hand motions intuitive even to the nonlaparoscopic surgeon,[23] seven degrees of freedom of motion (compared to four with standard laparoscopy), three-dimensional image projection, tremor suppression, motion scaling, and the potential to perform remote "telesurgery."

Robotic approaches have been applied in a wide variety of urologic, cardiothoracic, gynecologic, and general surgical procedures. The first report of robotic adrenalectomy was by Piazza et al. in 1999.[24] Hanly and colleagues reported 30 robotic adrenalectomies without any conversions to open procedures.[25] They felt that the robotic system permitted improved identification and control of the multiple adrenal arteries. Although all other reports of robotic adrenalectomy have been for benign lesions, a robotic resection of an 8-cm adrenal lesion that proved to be adrenocortical carcinoma with clean margins has now been reported, with good early results.[26]

Several reports have compared robotic to laparoscopic adrenalectomy. No difference was found in perioperative quality of life measures between laparoscopic and robotic adrenalectomy.[27] An earlier randomized series compared one hospital's first 10 robotic adrenalectomies to 10 laparoscopic adrenalectomies[28] and reported that laparoscopy was superior to robotics in terms of morbidity and cost. More recently, a retrospective review of prospectively collected data compared 50 patients undergoing robotic unilateral adrenalectomy to 59 patients undergoing laparoscopic unilateral transperitoneal adrenalectomy.[29] They found that the robotic approach was associated with lower blood loss but longer operative times early in their series. Interestingly, they reported a learning curve of 20 robotic adrenalectomies, after which the difference in operative time was absent. Furthermore, operative times were not affected by obesity or large tumors in the robotic group, while these factors led to significantly longer operative times in the laparoscopic group. Conversion rate, morbidity, and hospital stay were similar between groups.

Limitations of robotics and robotic adrenalectomy include the high cost of the permanent equipment and the semi-reusable instruments, the absence of good data for benefit compared to standard laparoscopy, the learning curve, and the lack of tactile feedback to the surgeon. While the role and future of this technology remain to be determined, one expects that the lessons and advances from robotics will allow further advances in adrenal surgery.

Preoperative History and Evaluation

Patients with functional adrenal tumors may present with characteristic metabolic disorders. Patients with nonfunctional masses or malignancies should undergo routine evaluation for general anesthesia, which is required for either minimally invasive or open adrenalectomy. In the patient with a functioning adrenal mass, specific attention may be needed to correct any metabolic abnormality. The patient with an aldosterone-secreting tumor, hypertension, and significant hypokalemia will require medical correction. Potassium replacement with oral supplementation is usually sufficient. Hypertension treatment can be undertaken with a variety of medications, including calcium channel blockers and angiotensin-converting enzyme (ACE) inhibitors. Hyperglycemia occurs in as many as 15% of these patients, and they may require insulin treatment. The patient presenting with Cushing's syndrome and a unilateral adrenal mass may have suppression of the contralateral adrenal. Therefore, preoperative preparation with stress-dose steroids (e.g., 100 mg of hydrocortisone) is generally indicated. This dose is also adequate for patients undergoing bilateral adrenalectomy for persistent ACTH-secreting syndromes. The former group of patients will require postsurgical steroid tapering, whereas the latter group will require lifelong exogenous steroid replacement.

The patient with pheochromocytoma deserves particular attention (see Chapter 14). Once this diagnosis is made, medical management must address hypertension, decreased intravascular volume, and possible cardiac arrhythmias. The use of phenoxybenzamine, a long-acting α-adrenoceptor blocker, is usually suggested for 1 to 3 weeks prior to surgery (see also Chapter 14). More recently, some groups have reported the use of preoperative blockade with selective postsynaptic α₁-adrenergic receptor antagonists such as prazosin hydrochloride or doxazosin. Such selective agents are thought not to produce reflex tachycardia and have a shorter half-life. These agents may avoid postoperative hypotension that are associated with the longer-acting drugs. These are important considerations, yet phenoxybenzamine remains a standard and time-tested preoperative blockade. The use of calcium channel blockers or ACE inhibitors has also gained acceptance. Because these medications are given in the preoperative period, attention should be given to oral salt and fluid intake to address expansion of intravascular volume prior to surgery. This preoperative regimen must be closely watched. During this time, patients will retain fluid and demonstrate side effects of the medication, possibly including sinus discomfort and orthostatic hypotension. Additionally, a small subset of patients may have arrhythmias which may require β-adrenoceptor blockade. Effective β-blockers include propranolol and nadolol.[30] Our group has had excellent experience with metyrosine, 1 to 4 g/day for 10 to 14 days prior to surgery, in addition to phenoxybenzamine. Metyrosine is a tyrosine hydroxylase inhibitor and is very effective in reducing blood pressure; it is associated with fatigue and sinus discomfort. Patients need to be instructed carefully about its side effects.

Preoperative imaging must be evaluated by expert interpretation and also should be studied by the operating surgeon. CT and MRI form the cornerstones of workup and preoperative diagnosis. These films must be of adequate technique and quality to allow investigation of the retroperitoneum and the contralateral adrenal, as well as any other anatomy relevant to the diagnostic workup (e.g., the lung fields, in the case of metastasis). In the case of aldosterone excess, the diagnosis of a solitary adrenal mass must be made to secure the diagnosis of Conn's syndrome. If both adrenals are not investigated, occasional macronodular bilateral hyperplasia might present with a unilateral nodule that, although appearing to be dominant, might draw attention away from less discrete nodularity in the contralateral gland (Figs. 15-1, 15-2). This situation might require bilateral adrenal vein

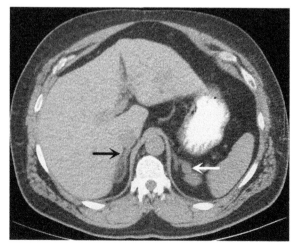

FIGURE 15-1. CT scan of 36-year-old female with hypertension and hypokalemia. Initial workup demonstrated a 1.2-cm left adrenal mass *(white arrow)*. However, subsequent targeted imaging suggests a mass in the right adrenal *(black arrow)*, raising the question of bilateral macromodular hyperplasia.

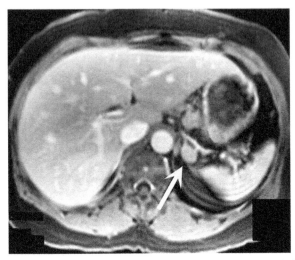

FIGURE 15-2. MRI scan shows an enlarged left adrenal mass in a patient with Conn's syndrome *(arrow)*. Right adrenal is seen behind the vena cava and is normal size.

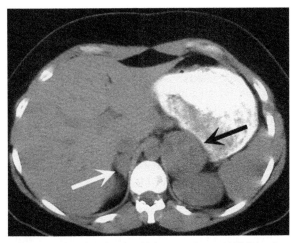

FIGURE 15-3. A 42-year-old female with hypertension and MEN2 syndrome. CT scan reveals bilateral adrenal masses, which were pheochromocytomas.

sampling for aldosterone levels (see Chapter 12). In the case of the pheochromocytoma, multicentric tumors in the retroperitoneum and the contralateral adrenal must be excluded. Any suspicious masses may require MIBG radionuclide study or T1- and T2-weighted MRI scanning (Fig. 15-3).

The experienced endocrine surgeon should personally investigate any or all preoperative laboratory and imaging studies, using local or regional expertise in imaging. Repeat studies are warranted if there is any doubt as to the diagnosis, since operative and perioperative management vary with different pathologies.

Surgical Anatomy, Approaches, and Techniques

The surgical approach to the adrenal requires a complete understanding of the surgical anatomy and the available preoperative and intraoperative options. One of several approaches can be chosen. The open technique allows access to both adrenals and

the retroperitoneum (transabdominal). The lateral techniques (open, laparoscopic, or robotic) allow a more focused approach to unilateral adrenal masses and to retroperitoneal areas and kidney. The posterior approach (open or laparoscopic) allows fairly limited access to the adrenal gland on either side but is thought to be associated with fewer postoperative complications.

SURGICAL ANATOMY

The adrenal glands are retroperitoneal organs. They are slightly nodular with a firm texture, and they are surrounded by a layer of loose connective tissue. The arterial supply of both sides consists of multiple small branches that enter the superior, medial, and inferior surfaces of the gland. Venous drainage is much more constant and usually is via a single adrenal vein, with different drainage for the right and left gland.

The right adrenal gland is situated adjacent and medial to the superior pole of the right kidney. It is immediately anterior to the posterior reflection of the diaphragm and adjacent to the right and posterior border of the inferior vena cava. The right adrenal is inferior to segment VII of the liver. The arterial supply is from the inferior phrenic artery and from branches of the renal artery, lumbar arteries, and aorta. The right adrenal vein is approximately 3 mm in size; it courses medially and empties directly into the inferior vena cava. In very rare cases, the adrenal vein can course superiorly to empty into the right hepatic vein.

The left adrenal gland is also superior and medial to the superior pole of the left kidney. This position is posterior to the stomach and pancreas in the retroperitoneal area, behind the lesser sac. The medial aspect of the left adrenal gland lies along the left crus of the diaphragm and aorta. Dissection in this area will usually expose the esophagus. Like the right adrenal, the arterial supply is from the renal artery, inferior phrenic artery, lumbar arteries, and aorta. The left adrenal vein often courses inferiorly, emptying into the left renal vein. Occasionally, the left adrenal vein can course medially, joining with a phrenic vein before emptying into the renal vein. Approaching either adrenal, the surgeon must be aware that the vessels of the renal hilum are near the inferior aspect of the dissection, and that extreme care must be taken not to stray into vessels supplying the renal parenchyma.

SURGICAL APPROACHES

General endotracheal anesthetic is used in all cases. Foley catheter and gastric decompression are instituted. Depending on the approach, appropriate padding and support must be used to protect weight-bearing areas and prevent compression or stretch neurapraxic injury to areas such as the brachial plexus and peroneal nerve. Antibiotics are administered 30 minutes prior to skin incision. Compression boots or stockings are instituted for mechanical thromboprophylaxis prior to anesthetic induction.

Open Transabdominal (Anterior) Approach

Until 20 years ago, this was the classic surgical approach, particularly in the case of familial pheochromocytoma. It allows access to both adrenals and full exploration of intraabdominal and retroperitoneal extraadrenal deposits of tumor. The midline or bilateral subcostal incision is employed, allowing access to the peritoneal cavity with the patient positioned supine. The right adrenal gland is approached by mobilizing the hepatic flexure of the colon and right lobe of the liver. A generous Kocher maneuver is performed, mobilizing the duodenum medially (Fig. 15-4). In this manner, a full view is gained of the vena cava from

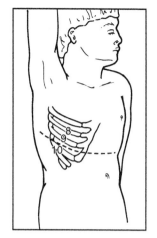

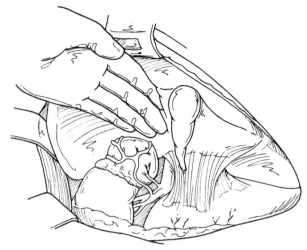

FIGURE 15-4. Approach to a right adrenal mass via open transabdominal technique. The incision can be extended laterally to a thoracoabdominal incision via the 9th-10th interspace. (From Scott HW Jr, Oates JA, Nies AS et al: Pheochromocytoma: present diagnosis and management, Ann Surg 183:587, 1976.)

the level of the right renal vein to the diaphragm. The adrenal gland is usually dissected from a lateral position, mobilizing it off of the kidney and from the retroperitoneal tissues; the gland is mobilized medially until the right adrenal vein is seen and securely ligated.

The left adrenal gland is approached by entering the lesser sac and taking down the short gastric vessels along the greater curve of the stomach. The spleen and tail of the pancreas are mobilized medially by dividing the splenocolic ligament and mobilizing the spleen and tail of the pancreas medially, thereby allowing a full view of the left retroperitoneal space. The left adrenal gland is then approached, either by (1) isolating the hilum of the left kidney and identifying the left adrenal vein or (2) superiorly, by tracing the inferior phrenic vein to the top of the adrenal. Medial dissection usually allows release of the adrenal from the aorta. Care must be used in the most inferior aspect of this dissection while identifying the adrenal vein. Additional care must be used in the space between the adrenal and kidney to avoid damage to any arterial branches coursing superiorly to the superior pole of the left kidney.

Open Lateral Approach

This approach has been used more commonly since the 1980s and before the advances in laparoscopic procedures. After inducing general anesthesia, the patient is placed in the lateral decubitus position, with the table flexed just above the anterior superior iliac spine; this accentuates the area between the costal margin and the iliac crest on the side of the lesion. The patient is rolled forward slightly, which has the added advantage of allowing the abdominal pannus to fall out of the surgical field, allowing excellent exposure of the costoiliac area. In patients with Cushing's syndrome, this maneuver is particularly helpful. The tip of the 11th or 12th rib can be palpated fairly easily in this position even if the patient is somewhat obese. A curvilinear incision is employed on the 11th rib. The periosteum is stripped off of the rib, which is then resected at the base. Care must be used to preserve the intercostal neurovascular bundle. By incising through the medial aspect of this incision, the abdominal musculature can be divided, and the peritoneum can be pushed anteriorly and not entered. The pleura can be usually demonstrated and pushed superiorly. If the pleura is entered, it can be repaired under positive-pressure ventilation, which usually does not require a chest tube. Immediately inferior to the edge of the diaphragm is the area of perinephric fat at the superior aspect of

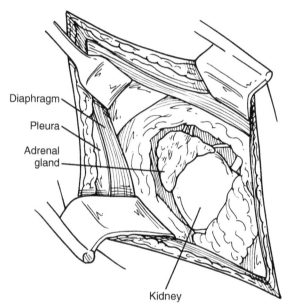

FIGURE 15-5. Lateral open approach to an adrenal mass on the right through an 11th-rib resection. Diaphragm and pleura are retracted superiorly, and Gerota's fascia is incised, allowing exposure of the mass. (From Scott HW, Liddle GW, Mulherin JL et al: Surgical experience with Cushing's disease, Ann Surg 185:524, 1977.)

the kidney; Gerota's fascia is encountered here and incised. This area is entered, and by proceeding medially, the surgeon can identify either the adrenal tumor or normal-appearing cortex of the adrenal, which stands out in contrast to the surrounding fat (Fig. 15-5). These procedures can be performed through an 8- to 10-cm incision, employing self-retaining retractors to gain optimal exposure. On the left, the surgeon must be careful about vigorous retraction on the spleen; on the right, similar care must be used on the liver. The dissection of each adrenal gland proceeds as described for the anterior open approach.

After completion of the adrenalectomy, the patient is taken out of the flex position on the table, and the incision is closed in layers. The intercostal bed is closed. This should be done with full view of the intercostal neurovascular bundle, so as not to injure them and cause bothersome postoperative pain. Often the intercostal nerve can be injected at this time with 0.25% Marcaine. The latissimus dorsi and abdominal muscles can then also be closed using a running suture. A chest tube is not usually required unless parenchymal damage to the lung has occurred. Every effort should be made to close any small holes in the pleura, which can occur if an 11th rib or higher approach is used.

Open Posterior Approach

Perhaps the most direct anatomic route to the adrenal glands is through a posterior approach. This is particularly true for smaller tumors. There is general agreement that this is not a preferred approach for lesions larger than 5 cm. Prior to the advent of laparoscopy, it was felt that the posterior approach allowed for the shortest hospitalization and lowest morbidity.

The patient is placed in a prone position, with the operating table in a flex position. Hyperflexion of the lower back area is achieved by positioning the table and by the use of pillows under the abdomen. In this fashion, the area between the posterior iliac crest and the posterior costal margin is accentuated. The advantage of this position is that it allows access to both adrenals. The disadvantage is very limited exposure; therefore, the incision and consequent dissection must be carefully planned. A curvilinear incision starting parallel to and about 3 inches lateral to the spine and turning sharply out over the 12th rib is preferred. This allows exposure to the latissimus dorsi muscle and the sacrospinal fascia. The latissimus dorsi and the lateral aspect of the sacrospinal are divided, and the 12th rib is identified. The periosteum is stripped along the entire length of the rib, taking care to preserve the intercostal neurovascular bundle. The rib is removed, and the bed of the rib is incised. This allows access to the retroperitoneum, exposing the perinephric fat. Superior retraction identifies the parietal pleura and the lateral arcuate ligament of the diaphragm. The pleura should be reflected upward, allowing reasonable exposure to the perinephric fat. Dissection through the fat exposes the upper pole of the kidney, which is retracted inferiorly. It is at this time that distinct limitations in visibility can be appreciated if the appropriate dissection has not been done (Fig. 15-6). The gland on either the right or

left side should be identified in the perinephric fat. Superior dissection usually allows enough mobilization to gain access to the adrenal vein, coursing into the vena cava (on the right side) or coursing inferiorly into the left adrenal vein (on the left side).

Closure is as described for the lateral approach, reapproximating the rib bed and musculature. Any holes in the pleura should be searched for and closed. It is usually not necessary to place a chest tube unless the parenchyma of the lung has been damaged.

Lateral Laparoscopic Transperitoneal Approach

This is the most commonly employed approach to laparoscopic adrenalectomy.[5] The patient is placed in the lateral decubitus position, as previously described. Again, the appropriate side should be hyperextended, maximizing the space between the costal margin and the iliac crest. The operating surgeon and camera driver should be on the patient's abdominal side. The initial skin incision, approximately 1 cm in length, is made 2 cm below and parallel to the costal margin, medial to the anterior axillary line. The port is placed, and the abdomen is insufflated with CO_2, either by a Veress needle or by placing a 10-mm Hassan trocar under direct vision. Through this initial incision, a 30-degree, 10-mm laparoscope is placed into the peritoneal cavity, and the peritoneal cavity is then visualized. On the left side, two additional 5- or 10-mm trocars are inserted under direct laparoscopic visualization (Fig. 15-7A). The first is placed inferiorly and slightly medial to the tip of the 11th rib; the other is inserted slightly anterior and medial to the initial trocar. The two most lateral ports are used for the dissecting instruments, and the visualizing laparoscope is placed at the most medial of these. On the left side, this allows good mobilization of the splenic flexure, and dissection then proceeds as described for the left adrenalectomy. After the spleen is fully mobilized it will fall medially, and the retroperitoneum can be almost completely visualized (see Fig. 15-7B, C, and D). Occasionally, a fourth trocar can be inserted 3 to 5 cm posterior to the previous lateral port. This trocar could be used to retract the spleen and kidney or surrounding fat for better exposure. Laparoscopic ultrasound can be used if there is difficulty in finding the gland or the lesion within the gland. Careful dissection is then needed in the space between the aorta and the superior pole of the adrenal. Our preferred method is to isolate the left adrenal vein at its junction into the renal vein and divide it securely between clips (see Fig. 15-7E). Dissection can then be continued superiorly, mobilizing the adrenal from the surrounding perinephric fat. After ligation of the adrenal vein, almost all the other left adrenal vasculature can be coagulated using cautery or the harmonic scalpel.

Once the adrenal gland is freed from its attachments, it can be removed through the 10-mm port by placing it in a sterile nylon or Silastic bag. This bag can then be removed via the original trocar site. For larger tumors, this might require spreading the abdominal-wall musculature. All incisions are then closed with absorbable suture.

For a laparoscopic transperitoneal right adrenalectomy, the patient is placed in the right lateral decubitus position, with the surgeon and his assistant on the patient's abdominal side. The peritoneum is insufflated in the same fashion as previously described; the laparoscope is placed, and the abdomen is inspected. Three additional 5- or 10-mm trocars are placed under the ribs in the same position as previously described (Fig. 15-8A). The dissecting instruments are used through the most lateral trocar sites. Under laparoscopic visualization, the hepatic flexure of the colon is taken down, and the right lobe of the liver is retracted medially. A fan-type liver retractor can be inserted

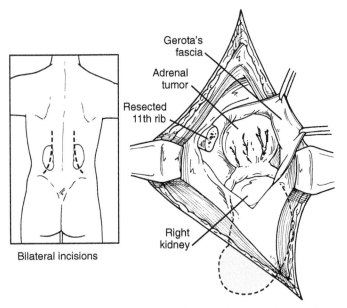

FIGURE 15-6. Posterior, transdiaphragmatic approach to adrenal mass. Bilateral incisions may be used for bilateral tumors. (From Scott HW Jr, Foster JH, Liddle G, Davidson ET: Cushing's syndrome due to adrenocortical tumor, Ann Surg 162:505, 1965.)

Bilateral incisions

Gerota's fascia

Adrenal tumor

Resected 11th rib

Right kidney

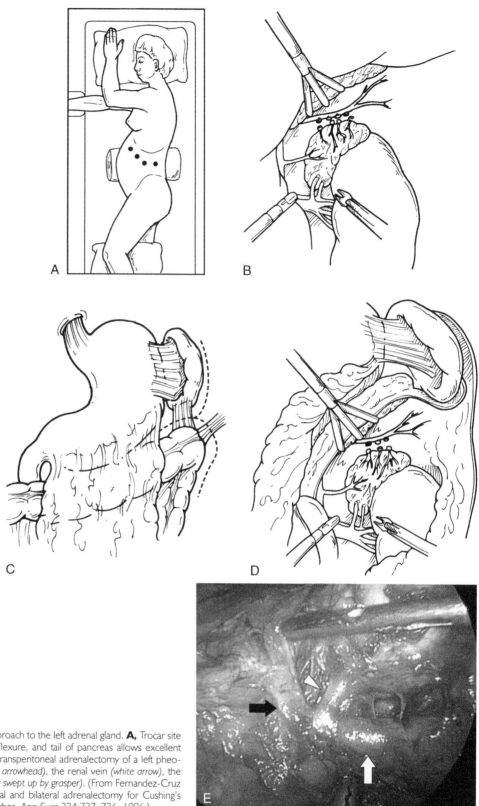

FIGURE 15-7. Lateral laparoscopic transperitoneal approach to the left adrenal gland. **A,** Trocar site placement. **B, C, D,** Mobilization of spleen, splenic flexure, and tail of pancreas allows excellent exposure. **E,** Intraoperative view during laparoscopic transperitoneal adrenalectomy of a left pheochromocytoma, demonstrating the adrenal vein *(white arrowhead)*, the renal vein *(white arrow)*, the phrenic vein *(black arrow)*, and the adrenal lesion *(being swept up by grasper)*. (From Fernandez-Cruz L, Sachz A, Benarroch G et al: Laparoscopic unilateral and bilateral adrenalectomy for Cushing's syndrome: transperitoneal and retroperitoneal approaches, Ann Surg 224:727–736, 1996.)

through a medial port to reflect the right hepatic lobe medially. This necessitates taking down the right lateral hepatic attachments and the triangular ligament, using laparoscopic scissors or the harmonic scalpel. This dissection is usually carried up to the level of the diaphragm, allowing full visualization of the area

behind the liver and in the retroperitoneum (see Fig. 15-8B, C, and D). The perinephric fat appears in the area between the diaphragm and the superior pole of the kidney. The inferior portion of the adrenal can be immobilized using electrocautery and the grasper dissector. If this dissection is carried medially

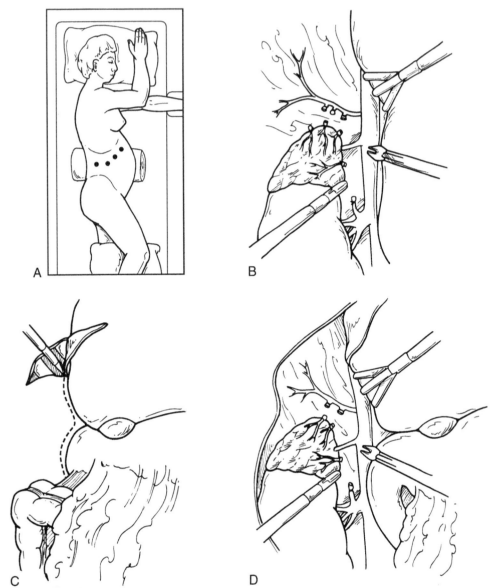

FIGURE 15-8. Lateral laparoscopic transperitoneal approach to the right adrenal gland. **A,** Trocar site placement. **B-D,** Exposure of the right adrenal by mobilization of the right lobe of liver and visualization of the vena cava. (From Fernandez-Cruz L, Sachz A, Benarroch G et al: Laparoscopic unilateral and bilateral adrenalectomy for Cushing's syndrome: transperitoneal and retroperitoneal approaches, Ann Surg 224:727–736, 1996.)

and superiorly, the lateral edge of the vena cava is identified. Ultrasound can be used to identify adrenal tissue or masses. The right adrenal vein is almost always in the midportion of the body of the adrenal, coursing transversely. As one carefully dissects in this area, the right adrenal vein will almost always be encountered, and it can be clipped at this time. At least two clips should remain on the vena cava side. If the vein is not found in this position, careful search for a superior route into the hepatic vein must be considered. Once the adrenal vein is divided, the adrenal gland can be mobilized more easily, and dissection should be carried superiorly. Smaller branches from the inferior phrenic vessels will be encountered, and these should be divided. Occasionally, particularly in larger adrenal masses, there will be increased vascularity and attachments encountered on the posterior surface of the liver. These must be carefully dissected, particularly in the case of hypercortisolism, in an effort to remove all cortical tissue. After complete mobilization, the adrenal gland can be placed within a sterile nylon bag and removed through

one of the 10-mm laparoscopic ports. Closure of the individual trocar sites is performed as previously described.

We have had recent satisfactory experience using 5-cm trocar sites in the more lateral positions. All trocar sites should be injected with 0.25% Marcaine to alleviate postoperative pain.

Endoscopic Retroperitoneal Adrenalectomy

The patient is placed under general anesthesia, and then is placed in lateral decubitus position, with the affected side exposed. As described previously, the OR table is then flexed until the space between the costal margin and iliac crest is maximized (Fig. 15-9). A 2-cm, muscle-splitting incision is made in the midaxillary line just beneath the tip of the 11th rib. The surgeon's finger is placed through this incision and into the retroperitoneal space, palpating the lower pole of the kidney. A transparent, disposable dissecting balloon is introduced and insufflated under visual control to create a retroperitoneal working space. The balloon must be directly visualized and placed posteriorly to prevent

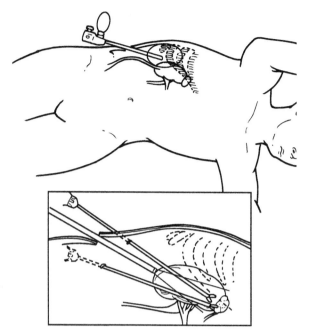

FIGURE 15-9. Patient position and trocar placement for endoscopic retroperitoneal right adrenalectomy. (From Bonjer HJ: Endoscopic retroperitoneal adrenalectomy: lessons learned from 111 consecutive cases, Ann Surg 232:796, 2000.)

penetration of the peritoneal sac. After this insufflation technique is completed, the balloon is deflated and replaced by a Hasson trocar. The CO_2 is then insufflated to a pressure of 12 to 15 mm Hg, and a 10-mm laparoscope is introduced. A second 5-mm trocar is inserted immediately adjacent to the 12th rib, through which a dissecting instrument can be inserted. Continued dissection of the retroperitoneal space allows the introduction of third and fourth trocar sites to the medial side of the first trocar site. Again, every effort must be made not to perforate the peritoneal sac. At this time, the lateral conal fascia appears as a thin, avascular, white-gray membrane that connects the peritoneum to the quadratus lumborum muscle; this is opened. This allows the identification of the upper renal pole. On the left, the inferior rim of the adrenal gland, as well as the ventral and lateral aspects of the adrenal gland, are exposed through this view. As previously described, dissection must now proceed carefully, without damaging the surface of the gland, and gaining access to the left adrenal vein before complete removal can be accomplished. After this dissection is complete, the adrenal gland can be removed in a Silastic bag. All trocar sites are closed in a method described previously.

For the endoscopic retroperitoneal right adrenalectomy, exposure is done in exactly the same fashion. Working in the space created by the insufflating bag dissection, the lateral conal fascia is likewise divided. This gains access to the superior pole of the right kidney. Occasionally, an inferior adrenal artery can be found in this dissection, arising from an upper renal artery along the inferior rim of the adrenal. Care should be taken to dissect this arterial supply and to ligate the artery close to the adrenal to avoid disrupting renal arterial branches. The short right adrenal vein on this side should be carefully exposed after dissection of the vena cava along the medial side of the adrenal. Mobilization, dissection, and removal of the gland is performed using a Silastic laparoscopic bag as described previously, and closure is likewise performed as previously described. These procedures require extensive laparoscopic expertise. Often, peri-

toneal anatomy is not straightforward when visualized through this approach. Laparoscopic ultrasound is very useful to help direct the surgeon and to locate the lesion.

Robotic Adrenalectomy

The Da Vinci Robotic Surgical System (Intuitive Surgical, Sunny Valley, CA) is the primary robotic surgery system currently in use and consists of a robotic manipulator and a remote console where the first operator is seated during the procedure. Once pneumoperitoneum is created by either Veress needle or Hasson technique, trocars are placed and the robot arms are connected. Next, the operating surgeon controls the robot at the console, while the first assistant handles the laparoscopic instruments inserted through one or two accessory trocars.

Right adrenalectomy is performed with the patient in the left lateral decubitus position. The first port, a 12-mm camera port, is placed midway between the umbilicus and the right costal margin. Two robotic instrument ports, both 8 mm, are then placed along a line two fingerbreadths from the costal margin. A 10-mm liver retraction port is placed in the midline in the epigastrium. A 10-mm accessory port (fifth trocar) is placed in the right abdomen, through which the assistant can use a clip applier. Left adrenalectomy is performed with the patient in the right lateral decubitus position. Positioning is the mirror image of that for the right adrenalectomy described earlier. The role of the assistant at the operating table is to change the robotic instruments as necessary, to use the clip applier for division of the adrenal vein, and to manipulate the suction. Otherwise, the sequential steps for dissection and excision of the gland are the same as those for a lateral transperitoneal adrenalectomy by traditional laparoscopic techniques described previously.[29]

Partial Adrenalectomy

Classically, the finding of an adrenal mass on one side has resulted in the complete removal of that adrenal gland. More recently, there has been some interest in preserving adrenal function in the case of benign tumors. For patients requiring bilateral adrenalectomy, adrenal-sparing procedures may avoid the need for lifelong steroid replacement and avoid the significant risk of Addisonian crisis. Even in patients undergoing unilateral adrenalectomy, there may be inadequate hormonal reserve to respond to stress.[31] Therefore, it may be in the patient's best interest to preserve adrenal tissue when possible. This technique is generally applied to those patients with Conn's syndrome, a cortisol-producing adenoma, and hereditary pheochromocytoma. Partial adrenalectomy is not appropriate when there is significant concern for malignancy.

Partial adrenalectomy may be performed through any of the surgical approaches described. A large series of posterior endoscopic adrenalectomies reported by Walz et al. in 2006 included 149 partial adrenalectomies in 139 patients.[32] This group has reported 100% biochemical cure which persisted through follow-up. Other groups have also reported excellent cure rates, with very low rates of recurrence and negative surgical margins.

Familial pheochromocytoma has usually been associated with bilateral adrenalectomy and exogenous steroid dependency. Recent experience has documented the use of partial adrenalectomy, preserving a portion of normal adrenal tissue and its blood supply. This can be done through either an open or a laparoscopic approach. However, long-term follow-up is mandatory because recurrence is a distinct possibility. Lee described partial adrenalectomy, sparing cortical tissue, in 14 patients with MEN2 and von Hippel-Lindau syndrome.[33] Thirteen of these patients (93%) had normal cortisol levels after surgery and were free of exogenous steroids. Nine patients showed no recurrent tumor at 90 months after surgery. In 1999, Neumann et al.[34] and Walther et al.[35] reported series of 39 and 13 patients, respectively, with excellent results and little increased morbidity. More recently, Diner et al. reported the National Cancer Institute's experience with 33 patients with hereditary pheochromocytoma treated with partial adrenalectomy.[36] Although 15% of these patients required steroid replacement in the early postoperative period, by 3 months only 3% continued to be dependent on exogenous steroid, and all patients experienced normalization of catecholamine levels. One issue particular to partial adrenalectomy for pheochromocytoma is that there is a greater degree of gland manipulation than during total adrenalectomy, which may increase the risk of hypertensive crisis, although this has not been observed in reported series.

Recurrence is an obvious potential risk in partial adrenalectomy. In the National Cancer Institute experience with hereditary pheochromocytoma, 6% of patients had recurrence, requiring completion adrenalectomy.[36] Reviews of other series have shown that recurrent tumors developed in 15% to 20% of patients with von Hippel-Lindau at a median of 18 to 40 months of follow-up, and in 33% of patients with MEN2 at 58 to 84 months follow-up.[37] In patients with aldosterone-producing adenomas, aldosterone may be produced by other, nondominant, nodules within the gland. Although excellent results generally are reported, there is a definite incidence of persistent hyperaldosteronism, in one series occurring in 7% of partial adrenalectomies.[38]

Although the body of literature employing this approach has grown, partial adrenalectomy remains controversial. Issues remaining to be resolved include patient selection, the amount of tissue to excise, which technical method to use to divide the gland, and whether or not to divide the adrenal vein.[37] Some groups performing partial adrenalectomy have reported that it is not necessary to preserve the adrenal vein so long as at least a third of the gland volume is preserved,[32] but others have found that adrenal vein preservation is essential.[39]

Special Circumstances

MANIPULATION OF THE ADRENAL

The adrenal parenchyma fractures easily with overzealous manipulation. This can result in bleeding which, although rarely life threatening, is a particular nuisance during laparoscopy. The operative field becomes less distinct, and the visual field is less optimal. Additionally, such fracture can result in tumor spillage and possible tumor seeding of the area. This has particular relevance for adrenal malignancy but can also affect the long-term outcome for resection of functioning tumors, such as pheochromocytoma, and ACTH-dependent Cushing's syndrome. Therefore, gentle handling of all tissue in periadrenal planes is important. For open procedures, finger traction and dissection is very effective. For laparoscopic procedures, avoidance of grasping the adrenal directly is also important. There is increased manipulation of the adrenal in partial adrenalectomy, which is of at least theoretic concern (see prior discussion). Use of the harmonic scalpel has greatly helped hemostasis and dissection in these techniques. For all operative approaches, good visualization, gentle dissection, and knowledge of landmarks is essential.

INTRAOPERATIVE BLEEDING

Troublesome bleeding can be encountered if there is failure to identify and adequately dissect the adrenal vein. On the left side, a longer adrenal vein runs inferiorly into the left renal vein. Bleeding in the hilum of the kidney or in the adrenal vein itself may result in significant blood loss. On the right, the adrenal vein courses into the inferior vena cava and is much shorter. During laparoscopic adrenalectomy, lack of image clarity, uncertainty as to the anatomy, or overwhelming bleeding may well require rapid conversion to an open adrenalectomy. Additionally, vena caval lacerations during a right laparoscopic adrenalectomy can result in CO_2 embolus caused by the pneumoperitoneum.

It is our experience that one should dissect the hilar vessels of the kidney on the left side and be certain as to the course of the adrenal vein prior to ligating it. On the right side, lateral mobilization of the gland and careful dissection on the lateral border of the inferior vena cava will allow access to the short right adrenal vein. There is usually enough space to place at least three clips (leaving two on the vena cava side) with security.

INTRAOPERATIVE MANAGEMENT OF HYPERTENSION

Pheochromocytoma deserves special comment in this regard. In the usual circumstance, the patient has received pharmacologic blockade prior to surgery. It is important that adequate peripheral and central venous access be available and also that a radial artery catheter be placed preoperatively for continuous hemodynamic monitoring. Additionally, a Swan-Ganz catheter may be placed, as required, because of cardiac disease or other cardiopulmonary indications. Intraoperatively, manipulation of a pheochromocytoma can result in acute hypertension. To control hypertension, sodium nitroprusside is an excellent choice by the anesthesiologist (Fig. 15-10): it has a direct-acting vasodilator effect and a rapid half-life. Therefore, within seconds of discontinuing the infusion, its effect ends, allowing for precision in dealing with possible rapid fluctuations of hypertension and hypotension. Other potent vasodilators, such as nitroglycerin, can be used with or instead of nitroprusside. Dysrhythmias may occur before or after tumor removal and can be treated with propranolol, esmolol, or lidocaine. Esmolol has the shortest half-life, and is gaining popularity as the preferred β-adrenoceptor blocker intraoperatively.[40]

Hypotension can occur immediately after the removal of pheochromocytoma, particularly if pharmacologic agents are still being infused. This can be treated with crystalloid or, if necessary, pressor support. Therefore, careful communication between the surgeon and the anesthesiologist is extremely important. Post-removal hypotension can be treated with volume and/or dopamine infusion, in addition to discontinuing vasodilators.

Postoperative Care

The patient who has undergone adrenalectomy through a transabdominal open approach requires the same considerations for postoperative care as for any laparotomy. Nasogastric suction may be employed until return of bowel function is demonstrated. Wound care, either for a midline or a subcostal incision, is relatively standard.

For patients undergoing laparoscopic procedures, there is little doubt that there are decreased analgesic requirements, and

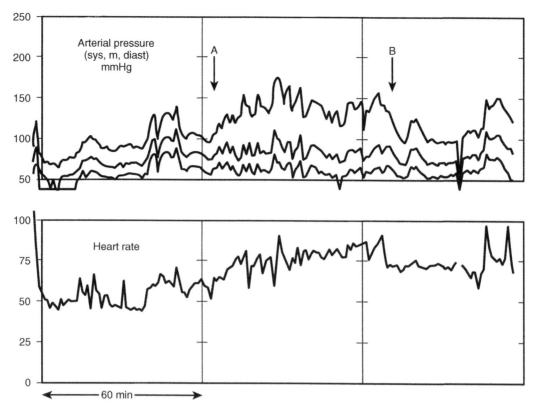

FIGURE 15-10. On-line arterial pressure measurements during pheochromocytoma resection. *A,* The intraperitoneal dissection and tumor manipulation begins, with systolic and diastolic blood pressure peaks. These are rapidly and effectively treated with esmolol and nitroprusside infusions. *B,* The adrenal vein is ligated and the tumor removed. No further infusions are necessary or administered.

earlier ambulation can be expected. Most likely this will result in a decreased incidence of postoperative complications such as pulmonary embolus. Recent reports of experience with transperitoneal or retroperitoneal laparoscopic procedures report patient discharge in 1 or 2 days.

Postoperative considerations are also determined by the initial diagnosis. Adjustments of medication and patient education are important aspects of posthospital care, depending on the preoperative diagnosis.

CONN'S SYNDROME

Patients with Conn's syndrome (Fig. 15-11) most likely have been on significant antihypertensive medication as well as potassium supplementation. After successful adrenal surgery, the patient will be able to decrease this potassium medication relatively rapidly; however, blood pressure evaluation needs to continue. Lo's group reported on 46 consecutive patients undergoing removal of an aldosterone-secreting tumor between 1983 and 1994[41]; there was no operative mortality. In patients undergoing long-term follow-up, 10 of 44 patients (23%) remained on medical therapy for hypertension. Interestingly, younger patients (aged 44 versus 52 years) and patients who responded to preoperative spironolactone antihypertensive therapy were statistically likely to have a better blood pressure response to surgery. Hypokalemia was corrected in all patients.

PHEOCHROMOCYTOMA

Patients with pheochromocytoma (Fig. 15-12) also have been on significant antihypertensive medication as well as preoperative blockade. The preoperative α- and β-adrenoceptor blockade can be immediately discontinued; in fact, it may be dangerous if

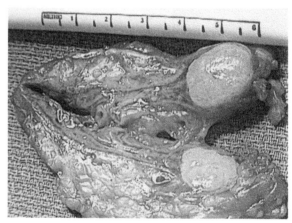

FIGURE 15-11. This 1.5-cm cortical tumor of the right adrenal was removed laparoscopically (Conn's syndrome).

taken after surgery. The hypertension of a pheochromocytoma quickly resolves after resection. The patient needs to be educated in terms of blood pressure monitoring during convalescence. These patients may have significant fluid shifts postoperatively, and they require careful monitoring, especially those with a preoperative cardiac history. Brunt's group has reported results using the laparoscopic approach for familial pheochromocytoma[42]; from 1993 to 2001, 21 such patients had surgery. Operative times averaged 216 ± 57 minutes, and average blood loss was 168 mL. No blood transfusion was necessary in any patient. Fifteen patients (71%) had intraoperative hypertension and/or tachycardia requiring medication; all responded to nitroprusside

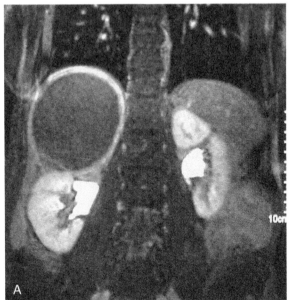

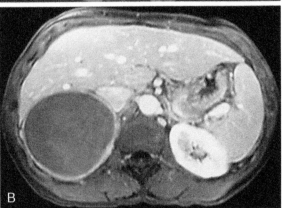

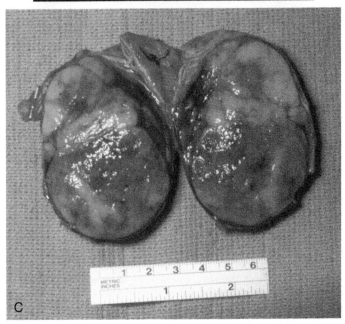

FIGURE 15-12. **A,** Coronal and **B,** transverse MRI of an 11-cm adrenal mass in a 40-year-old female with hypertension. The mass is a pheochromocytoma and was removed via an open lateral retroperitoneal approach. **C,** Sectioned gross specimen of pheochromocytoma demonstrating medullary lesion.

and/or nitroglycerin and labetalol. Only two (10%) had intraoperative systolic hypertension exceeding 200 mm Hg.

CUSHING'S SYNDROME

For the patient undergoing adrenalectomy for an ACTH-independent Cushing's tumor of the adrenal, it should be expected that the contralateral adrenal is probably suppressed. Therefore, the patient should have received preoperative steroids and will need to be educated regarding post-hospitalization steroid requirements and tapering of the dose in the months after surgery. The equivalent of 200 to 300 mg of cortisol daily should be given for the first 2 to 4 days. A maintenance dose equivalent to 7.5 to 10 mg prednisone should then be instituted and tapered gradually. Such a steroid taper may take 3 to 6 months. Endogenous cortisol responses to synthetic ACTH or a more direct physiologic stimulation should be documented prior to terminating exogenous steroids.

Cushing's disease patients who have failed pituitary surgery and for whom bilateral adrenalectomy is being considered (Fig. 15-13) also have special postoperative circumstances. Some of these patients may have panhypopituitary syndromes. Their medications may include pituitary replacement medications such as desmopressin. These patients must be carefully evaluated preoperatively, and the extent of any pituitary deficiency as a result of previous surgery should be completely assessed. Postoperatively, these patients can have significant fluid and electrolyte abnormalities and may require replacement with desmopressin. After successful bilateral adrenalectomy, close monitoring of glucocorticoid and mineralocorticoid replacement must be continued for life. Patients with Cushing's disease are also at increased risk of complications due to obesity, impaired healing, increased susceptibility to infection, and increased risk of thromboembolism, compared to those undergoing adrenalectomy for other indications.[43] In some centers, preoperative treatment with adrenolytic therapy may be instituted for 1 to 3 months before surgery.

PAIN MANAGEMENT

One of the significant advantages to minimally invasive procedures of the adrenal is the anticipated decreased pain requirements. The port sites should be injected with a long-acting

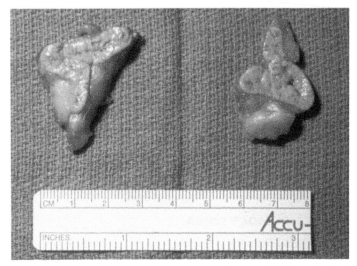

FIGURE 15-13. Bilateral adrenalectomy specimens demonstrating bilateral adrenal cortical hyperplasia due to refractory Cushing's Disease.

anesthetic agent (e.g., Marcaine) to provide postoperative relief. For the patient undergoing an open transperitoneal or flank approach, epidural anesthesia and patient-controlled anesthesia (PCA) have been reported to result in excellent postoperative pain control and enhanced respiratory function. Epidural patient-controlled devices are removed prior to discharge; however, the pain relief they provide is striking. If the patient has chosen not to have epidural catheterization, good postoperative pain relief can be obtained by intercostal nerve blocks at the time of closing flank incisions. Marcaine injections into the neurovascular bundle of the appropriately selected ribs provide excellent postoperative pain relief.

Future Directions

Virtually every part of the medical field has been affected by technologic changes, and surgery has been affected as much as any other. Continued advancements in imaging, miniaturization, and computer enhancement techniques will drive the continued application of minimally invasive surgery. Yet the thought processes, anatomy, and indications for surgical approach will remain the same. For example, with wider application of high-resolution axial imaging, adrenal incidentalomas may be found in as many as 4.4% of all abdominal CT scans, vastly increasing the number of patients being brought to the attention of physicians.[7] However, the workup and the indications for removal remain the same despite the temptation to apply novel surgical techniques. Dr. Sam Wells has warned "… the availability of a technique for easily removing these lesions is not necessarily an indication for doing so."[44]

There is no doubt, however, that technology has allowed huge advances and better results. Twenty years ago, patients with pheochromocytoma might receive bilateral exploration via an anterior transabdominal approach, with an appreciable morbidity and mortality. Currently, after appropriate preoperative imaging, the same patient might receive a laparoscopic procedure and be discharged in less than half the time formerly required. Continued advancements in techniques may only improve on this experience, and robotics may play a role in this advancement.

The future may not be so bright for adrenal malignancy. Little progress has been made over the last 20 years in treatment (see Chapter 11). Continued efforts will be needed if any breakthrough in altering the grim prognosis of this disease is to be expected. Perhaps genetic mapping will allow the discovery of a proto-oncogene, as has been discovered for medullary carcinoma of the thyroid, allowing earlier surgical intervention. In any event, advances in technology, as well as increased understanding of normal and altered adrenal physiology, are sure to continue to have an impact on surgical approaches, as has been seen over the last 20 years.

REFERENCES

1. Gagner M, Lacroix A, Bolte E: Laparoscopic adrenalectomy in Cushing's syndrome and pheochromocytoma, N Engl J Med 327(14):1033, 1992.
2. Higashihara E, Tanaka Y, Horie S, et al: A case report of laparoscopic adrenalectomy, Nippon Hinyokika Gakkai Zasshi 83(7):1130–1133, 1992.
3. Assalia A, Gagner M: Laparoscopic adrenalectomy, Br J Surg 91(10):1259–1274, 2004.
4. Smith CD, Weber CJ, Amerson JR: Laparoscopic adrenalectomy: new gold standard, World J Surg 23(4):389–396, 1999.
5. Gumbs AA, Gagner M: Laparoscopic adrenalectomy, Best Pract Res Clin Endocrinol Metab 20(3):483–499, 2006.
6. Lairmore TC, Ball DW, Baylin SB, et al: Management of pheochromocytomas in patients with multiple endocrine neoplasia type 2 syndromes, Ann Surg 217(6):595–601, 1993.
7. Bovio S, Cataldi A, Reimondo G, et al: Prevalence of adrenal incidentaloma in a contemporary computerized tomography series, J Endocrinol Invest 29(4):298–302, 2006.
8. Mantero F, Terzolo M, Arnaldi G, et al: A survey on adrenal incidentaloma in Italy. Study Group on Adrenal Tumors of the Italian Society of Endocrinology, J Clin Endocrinol Metab 85(2):637–644, 2000.
9. Siren J, Tervahartiala P, Sivula A, et al: Natural course of adrenal incidentalomas: seven-year follow-up study, World J Surg 24(5):579–582, 2000.
10. Gagner M, Breton G, Pharand D, et al: Is laparoscopic adrenalectomy indicated for pheochromocytomas? Surgery 120(6):1076–1079, 1996.
11. Fernandez-Cruz L, Saenz A, Taura P, et al: Helium and carbon dioxide pneumoperitoneum in patients with pheochromocytoma undergoing laparoscopic adrenalectomy, World J Surg 22(12):1250–1255, 1998.
12. Gagner M, Pomp A, Heniford BT, et al: Laparoscopic adrenalectomy: lessons learned from 100 consecutive procedures, Ann Surg 226(3):238–246, 1997.
13. NIH state-of-the-science statement on management of the clinically inapparent adrenal mass ("incidentaloma"), NIH Consens State Sci Statements 19(2):1–25, 2002.
14. Paton BL, Novitsky YW, Zerey M, et al: Outcomes of adrenal cortical carcinoma in the United States, Surgery 140(6):914–920, 2006.
15. McCauley LR, Nguyen MM: Laparoscopic radical adrenalectomy for cancer: long-term outcomes, Curr Opin Urol 18(2):134–138, 2008.
16. Gonzalez RJ, Shapiro S, Sarlis N, et al: Laparoscopic resection of adrenal cortical carcinoma: a cautionary note, Surgery 138(6):1078–1085, 2005.
17. Kebebew E, Siperstein AE, Duh QY: Laparoscopic adrenalectomy: the optimal surgical approach, J Laparoendosc Adv Surg Tech A 11(6):409–413, 2001.
18. Liao CH, Chueh SC, Lai MK, et al: Laparoscopic adrenalectomy for potentially malignant adrenal tumors greater than 5 centimeters, J Clin Endocrinol Metab 91(8):3080–3083, 2006.
19. Ramacciato G, Mercantini P, La Torre M, et al: Is laparoscopic adrenalectomy safe and effective for adrenal masses larger than 7 cm? Surg Endosc 22(2):516–521, 2008.
20. Soon PS, Yeh MW, Delbridge LW, et al: Laparoscopic surgery is safe for large adrenal lesions, Eur J Surg Oncol 34(1):67–70, 2008.
21. Parnaby CN, Chong PS, Chisholm L, et al: The role of laparoscopic adrenalectomy for adrenal tumours of 6 cm or greater, Surg Endosc 22(3):617–621, 2008.
22. Rosoff JS, Raman JD, Del Pizzo JJ: Laparoscopic adrenalectomy for large adrenal masses, Curr Urol Rep 9(1):73–79, 2008.
23. Bentas W, Wolfram M, Brautigam R, et al: Laparoscopic transperitoneal adrenalectomy using a remote-controlled robotic surgical system, J Endourol 16(6):373–376, 2002.
24. Piazza L, Caragliano P, Scardilli M, et al: Laparoscopic robot-assisted right adrenalectomy and left ovariectomy [case reports], Chir Ital 51(6):465–466, 1999.
25. Hanly EJ, Talamini MA: Robotic abdominal surgery, Am J Surg 188(4A Suppl):19S–26S, 2004.
26. Zafar SS, Abaza R: Robot-assisted laparoscopic adrenalectomy for adrenocortical carcinoma: initial report and review of the literature, J Endourol 22:985–989, 2008.
27. Brunaud L, Bresler L, Zarnegar R, et al: Does robotic adrenalectomy improve patient quality of life when compared to laparoscopic adrenalectomy? World J Surg 28(11):1180–1185, 2004.
28. Morino M, Beninca G, Giraudo G, et al: Robot-assisted vs laparoscopic adrenalectomy: a prospective randomized controlled trial, Surg Endosc 18(12):1742–1746, 2004.
29. Brunaud L, Bresler L, Ayav A, et al: Robotic-assisted adrenalectomy: what advantages compared to lateral transperitoneal laparoscopic adrenalectomy? Am J Surg 195(4):433–438, 2008.
30. Grant CS: Pheochromocytomas. In Clark OH, Duh QY, editors: Textbook of Endocrine Surgery, ed 1, Philadelphia, 1997, Saunders, pp 579–582.
31. Nakada T, Kubota Y, Sasagawa I, et al: Therapeutic outcome of primary aldosteronism: adrenalectomy versus enucleation of aldosterone-producing adenoma, J Urol 153(6):1775–1780, 1995.
32. Walz MK, Alesina PF, Wenger FA, et al: Posterior retroperitoneoscopic adrenalectomy—results of 560 procedures in 520 patients, Surgery 140(6):943–948, 2006.
33. Lee JE, Curley SA, Gagel RF, et al: Cortical-sparing adrenalectomy for patients with bilateral pheochromocytoma, Surgery 120(6):1064–1070, 1996.
34. Neumann HP, Bender BU, Reincke M, et al: Adrenal-sparing surgery for phaeochromocytoma, Br J Surg 86(1):94–97, 1999.
35. Walther MM, Keiser HR, Choyke PL, et al: Management of hereditary pheochromocytoma in von Hippel-Lindau kindreds with partial adrenalectomy, J Urol 161(2):395–398, 1999.
36. Diner EK, Franks ME, Behari A, et al: Partial adrenalectomy: the National Cancer Institute experience, Urology 66(1):19–23, 2005.
37. Disick GI, Munver R: Adrenal-preserving minimally invasive surgery: update on the current status of laparoscopic partial adrenalectomy, Curr Urol Rep 9(1):67–72, 2008.
38. Ishidoya S, Ito A, Sakai K, et al: Laparoscopic partial versus total adrenalectomy for aldosterone producing adenoma, J Urol 174(1):40–43, 2005.
39. Jeschke K, Janetschek G, Peschel R, et al: Laparoscopic partial adrenalectomy in patients with aldosterone-producing adenomas: indications, technique, and results, Urology 61(1):69–72, 2003.
40. Ulchaker JC, Goldfarb DA, Bravo EL, et al: Successful outcomes in pheochromocytoma surgery in the modern era, J Urol 161(3):764–767, 1999.
41. Lo CY, Tam PC, Kung AW, et al: Primary aldosteronism. Results of surgical treatment, Ann Surg 224(2):125–130, 1996.

42. Brunt LM, Lairmore TC, Doherty GM, et al: Adrenalectomy for familial pheochromocytoma in the laparoscopic era, Ann Surg 235(5):713–720, 2002.
43. Poulin EC, Schlachta CM, Burpee SE, et al: Laparoscopic adrenalectomy: pathologic features determine outcome, Can J Surg 46(5):340–344, 2003.
44. Wells SA, Merke DP, Cutler GB Jr, et al: Therapeutic controversy: the role of laparoscopic surgery in adrenal disease, J Clin Endocrinol Metab 83(9):3041–3049, 1998.
45. Corcione F, Miranda L, Marzano E, et al: Laparoscopic adrenalectomy for malignant neoplasm: our experience in 15 cases, Surg Endosc 19(6):841–844, 2005.
46. Eto M, Hamaguchi M, Harano M, et al: Laparoscopic adrenalectomy for malignant tumors, Int J Urol 15(4):295–298, 2008.
47. Gill IS: The case for laparoscopic adrenalectomy, J Urol 166(2):429–436, 2001.
48. Henry JF, Sebag F, Iacobone M, et al: Results of laparoscopic adrenalectomy for large and potentially malignant tumors, World J Surg 26(8):1043–1047, 2002.
49. Kirshtein B, Yelle JD, Moloo H, et al: Laparoscopic adrenalectomy for adrenal malignancy: a preliminary report comparing the short-term outcomes with open adrenalectomy, J Laparoendosc Adv Surg Tech A 18(1):42–46, 2008.
50. Lombardi CP, Raffaelli M, De Crea C, et al: Role of laparoscopy in the management of adrenal malignancies, J Surg Oncol 94(2):128–131, 2006.
51. Nocca D, Aggarwal R, Mathieu A, et al: Laparoscopic surgery and corticoadrenalomas, Surg Endosc 21(8):1373–1376, 2007.
52. Palazzo FF, Sebag F, Sierra M, et al: Long-term outcome following laparoscopic adrenalectomy for large solid adrenal cortex tumors, World J Surg 30(5):893–898, 2006.
53. Porpiglia F, Fiori C, Tarabuzzi R, et al: Is laparoscopic adrenalectomy feasible for adrenocortical carcinoma or metastasis? BJU Int 94(7):1026–1029, 2004.
54. Schlamp A, Hallfeldt K, Mueller-Lisse U, et al: Recurrent adrenocortical carcinoma after laparoscopic resection, Nat Clin Pract Endocrinol Metab 3(2):191–195, 2007.

Chapter 16

CUSHING'S SYNDROME

DAMIAN G. MORRIS, ASHLEY GROSSMAN, and LYNNETTE K. NIEMAN

Harvey Cushing[1,2] was the first to codify the symptom complex of obesity, diabetes, hirsutism, and adrenal hyperplasia, and to postulate that the basophilic adenomas found at autopsy in six of eight patients caused the disease that now bears his name. Shortly thereafter, Walters and colleagues[3] identified the etiologic contribution of adrenal tumors and the therapeutic role of adrenalectomy. Over the ensuing century, our understanding of the pathogenesis of Cushing's syndrome has expanded to include ectopic production of adrenocorticotropic hormone (ACTH)[4] and corticotropin-releasing hormone (CRH),[5] and recognition of bilateral adrenal stimulation by factors other than ACTH.[6-9] Because florid Cushing's syndrome is ultimately fatal, early diagnosis and treatment have always been important. A plethora of tests have been developed over the years to improve the diagnostic yield. Similarly, the treatment options for Cushing's syndrome have increased to include medical agents that decrease the secretion or block the activity of circulating cortisol and surgical resection of eutopic and ectopic ACTH-producing tumors. Despite all these advances, Cushing's syndrome continues to tax endocrinologists and is likely to continue to do so. This chapter reviews the manifestations, causes, approaches to diagnosis, and treatments for this complicated and multifaceted syndrome.

DEFINITION

Cushing's syndrome is a symptom complex that reflects chronic excessive tissue exposure to glucocorticoids. The diagnosis cannot be made unless both clinical features and biochemical abnormalities are present.

ETIOLOGY AND PATHOPHYSIOLOGY

Cushing's Syndrome

The causes of Cushing's syndrome can be divided into those that are ACTH dependent and those that are ACTH independent (Table 16-1). The ACTH-dependent forms are characterized by excessive ACTH production from a corticotroph adenoma (known as pituitary-dependent Cushing's syndrome or Cushing's disease), from an ectopic tumoral source (ectopic ACTH syndrome), or (rarely) from normal corticotrophs under the influence of excessive CRH production (ectopic CRH secretion). ACTH stimulates all three layers of the adrenal cortex to grow and secrete steroids. When excessive, this results in histologic hyperplasia and increased adrenal weight. Micronodules and macronodules (>1 cm) may be seen. Circulating glucocorticoids are increased, often in association with some increase in adrenal androgens.

ACTH-independent forms, apart from exogenous administration of glucocorticoids, represent adrenal activation by mechanisms other than trophic ACTH support. This enlarging group includes unilateral disease (adenoma and carcinoma), bilateral disease (primary pigmented nodular adrenal disease, McCune-Albright syndrome, and macronodular adrenal disease related to aberrations of the cyclic AMP signaling pathway, or caused by ectopic expression of G protein–coupled receptors), and hyperfunction of adrenal rest tissue.

Adrenal adenomas, composed of zona fasciculata cells, generally produce only glucocorticoids, in contrast to activation of the entire adrenal cortex as seen in other causes of Cushing's syndrome. ACTH levels are suppressed by hypercortisolism and the nonadenomatous tissue atrophies because of lack of this trophic factor. As a result, androgenic signs, such as pustular acne and hirsutism, are relatively uncommon, and dehydroepiandrosterone sulfate levels are typically low. By contrast, case reports have described patients with macronodular adrenal disease with secretion of mineralocorticoids, estrones, or androgens, in addition to cortisol.

Cushing's Disease

Cushing's disease is almost always caused by a solitary (probably monoclonal) corticotroph adenoma.[10] Although nodular corticotroph hyperplasia without evidence of a CRH-producing neoplasm does occur, it represents 2% or less of large surgical series,[11,12] and some doubt its existence. Most tumors are intrasellar microadenomas (<1 cm in diameter), although macroadenomas account for approximately 5% to 10% of tumors, and extrasellar extension or invasion may occur. The cause of Cushing's disease remains unknown, despite much work on the molecular characterization of these tumors. Traditionally, whether the development of pituitary adenomas is due to abnormal hypothalamic hormonal stimulation or feedback regulation or an intrinsic pituitary defect has been the subject of debate, although most data support a primary pituitary abnormality or a series of abnormalities. More recently, a model has been proposed that encompasses both theories. Here, tumors can arise either as a clonal expansion from a primary intrinsic pituitary defect or as excessive hormonal stimulation/abnormal feedback leading to hyperplasia, which in turn predisposes the cells to mutate, with subsequent clonal expansion.[13] Analysis of the primary corticotroph stimulatory and negative feedback pathways has not revealed a common defect.[14,15] Similarly, the common oncogenes and tumor suppressor genes implicated in other cancers do not seem to be commonly involved in the pathogenesis of corticotropinomas. Studies of knockout mice and analysis of human pituitary tumor samples have implicated

the cyclin-dependent kinase inhibitor p27 (Kip1) in corticotroph tumorigenesis. Overall, reduced p27 protein levels in corticotropinomas and a high phosphorylated p27/p27 ratio suggest increased inactivation of this negative cell-cycle regulator, although the cause of this change remains to be elucidated.[16] Cytogenetic studies have revealed a surprising number of gross chromosomal changes in benign pituitary adenomas, and although the number of corticotroph tumors studied has been small, gain of chromosome 6p and loss of chromosomes 2, 15q, and 22 seem to be the most common abnormalities.[17-19] Perhaps improvement in molecular biologic techniques, particularly microarray analysis, will lead to the implication of new genes in the pathogenesis of these tumors that then will require further study.[20]

Ectopic Adrenocorticotropic Hormone Syndrome

The syndrome of ectopic hormone secretion was first codified by Liddle and colleagues, who defined it as "any hormone produced by a neoplasm which is derived from tissue not normally engaged in the production of the hormone in question."[4] ACTH and other pro-opiomelanocortin (POMC) products were subsequently identified in many noncorticotroph tumors, although not all were associated with increased circulating levels or the development of Cushing's syndrome.[4,21]

Although small cell lung cancer is probably the most common cause of ectopic ACTH syndrome, it is not the most common seen in larger series of generally less obvious tumors investigated at endocrine centers, as discussed later (Table 16-2). An intrathoracic neoplasm (carcinoma of the lung or carcinoid of the bronchus or thymus) accounts for approximately 60% of ectopic ACTH secretion, followed by pancreatic tumors (islet cell or carcinoid), pheochromocytoma (≈5% to 10%), and medullary carcinoma of the thyroid (<5%).

The mechanism whereby the POMC gene becomes derepressed in noncorticotroph tumors is not understood. One hypothesis is that these cells are derived from a common multipotential progenitor cell capable of producing peptide hormones, such that ACTH production is a reversion to a less differentiated state.[22] The speculation that many ACTH-producing tumors are derived from neural crest amine precursor uptake and decarboxylation (APUD) cells may support this view,[23] although this embryological hypothesis is not supported by the most recent data. However, because endodermally derived tumors also produce ACTH, the acquisition of APUD characteristics may be but one manifestation of dedifferentiation and may not represent the cause of ectopic ACTH production.

Although the mechanism of gene derepression is not understood, the regulation of POMC production and processing has

Table 16-1. Causes of Cushing's Syndrome

ACTH-dependent
  Pituitary-dependent Cushing's syndrome (Cushing's disease)
  Ectopic ACTH syndrome
  Ectopic CRH secretion
  Exogenous ACTH administration
ACTH-independent
  Adrenal adenoma
  Adrenal carcinoma
  Primary pigmented nodular adrenal disease (PPNAD), sporadic or
    associated with the Carney complex
AIMAH
AIMAH secondary to abnormal hormone receptor expression/signaling
McCune-Albright syndrome
Exogenous glucocorticoid administration

ACTH, Adrenocorticotropic hormone; *AIMAH*, ACTH-independent bilateral macronodular adrenal hyperplasia; *CRH*, corticotropin-releasing hormone.

Table 16-2. Percentage Incidence of Tumor Types Causing Ectopic Adrenocorticotropic Hormone Syndrome in Four Large Series from 1969 to 2003

Tumor Type	Liddle et al., 1969[4] (N = 104)	Jex et al., 1985[428] (N = 21)	Torpy et al., 2002[429] (N = 58)	Morris and Grossman, 2003[430] (N = 32)
Lung carcinoma	50	20	2	19
Bronchial carcinoid	5	28	40	41
Thymic carcinoid	10	8	10	3
Pancreatic tumor	10	20	7	12
Pheochromocytoma, paraganglioma, neuroblastoma	5	12	5	3
Medullary thyroid carcinoma	2		3	9
Miscellaneous*	17	8	2	12

*Other tumors reported to uncommonly secrete adrenocorticotropic hormone include appendix, breast, cloacogenic carcinoma of the anal canal, colon, esophagus, gallbladder, gastric carcinoid, kidney, melanoma, mesothelioma, myeloblastic leukemia, ovary, prostate, salivary glands, and testes.

been investigated. POMC, corticotropin-like intermediate lobe protein, and larger forms of ACTH ("big" or pro-ACTH) that are not usually secreted may circulate, and the intracellular ratio of the POMC products may be abnormal.[24,25] Investigation of cell lines of small cell carcinoma of the lung that synthesize POMC and pro-ACTH showed that only ACTH precursors were secreted, suggesting that processing to ACTH is defective.[26] The pattern of POMC mRNA species in ACTH-producing tumors has been characterized. A 1200 bp transcript similar to that of a corticotroph adenoma,[27] a shorter than normal 800 bp mRNA lacking a signal sequence for secretion,[27,28] and a larger 1400 to 1500 bp POMC transcript have been identified. The larger species appears to originate upstream of the usual pituitary promoter, with preservation of the normal translation start site.[29,30] It is possible that the promoters that initiate this transcription are not regulated by glucocorticoids, and this may explain in part the lack of responsiveness to glucocorticoid suppression noted clinically in these patients. In vitro investigation of human small cell cancer cell lines and pancreatic islet cell tumors with normal glucocorticoid receptor binding has found, for the most part, no regulation of POMC, tyrosine aminotransferase, or the glucocorticoid receptor mRNA at doses of hydrocortisone that would normally suppress pituitary production.[31-33] However, clinical observation of suppression of ACTH production by some bronchial carcinoids during glucocorticoid administration suggests retention of a functional glucocorticoid response element that regulates POMC production, at least in some ectopic tumors.[34]

Ectopic Corticotropin-Releasing Hormone Secretion

Tumor secretion of CRH with or without ACTH secretion is a rare cause of Cushing's syndrome. Although many tumors immunostain for CRH, its secretion is less common, and most patients do not develop cushingoid features.[35] Thus, the diagnosis primarily rests on the demonstration of elevated plasma CRH levels (requiring an assay that is not readily available). The literature includes fewer than 20 patients who fit this criterion. Tumors may have negative immunostaining for ACTH, but this may be related to reduced storage and rapid secretion. In cases such as these, a CRH and ACTH gradient across the tumor bed can be suggestive that, in fact, the tumor secretes both peptides.[36] Tumors include bronchial and thymic carcinoids, small cell lung cancer, medullary thyroid carcinoma, pheochromocytoma, gangliocytoma, prostate carcinoma, and ganglioneuroblastoma.[37,38] The biochemical responses to diagnostic tests can be similar to those seen in ectopic ACTH secretion or in pituitary ACTH-dependent disease.[38] It is important to note that many, if not all, ectopic secretors of CRH causing Cushing's syndrome are also ectopic ACTH secretors.

Primary Adrenal Disease

The primary adrenal forms of Cushing's syndrome do not share a common cause. Although the cause of adrenocortical neoplasia is not known, some events important in the development of adrenal cancer have been identified. Paternal isodisomy at 11p15.5 with overexpression of insulin-like growth factor-2 (IGF-2) and reduced expression of CDKN1C (a G1 cyclin-dependent kinase inhibitor) and H19 (a putative growth suppressor) seems to be a key event. Mutations of *p53* may be involved in a small subset of carcinomas, and mutations of *β-catenin* may be an early event. Other genes important in pathogenesis remain to be elucidated, although potential loci have been identified at chromosomes 17p, 1p, 2p16, and 11q13 for tumor suppressor genes, and at chromosomes 4, 5, and 12 for

oncogenes.[39] Adenomas and carcinomas tend to be monoclonal, although the nodular hyperplasias are often polyclonal.[40] Adrenal adenomas are encapsulated benign tumors, usually less than 40 g in weight. Adrenal carcinomas usually are encapsulated, generally weigh more than 100 g, and may lack classic histologic features of malignancy, although nuclear pleomorphism, necrosis, mitotic figures, and vascular or lymphatic invasion suggest the diagnosis.[41] The adjacent adrenal tissue is atrophic in both conditions.

Primary pigmented nodular adrenal disease (PPNAD), also known as micronodular adrenal disease, is a rare form of Cushing's syndrome characterized histologically by small to normal-size glands (combined weight <12 g) with cortical micronodules (average 2 to 3 mm) that may be dark or black in color. The intervening cortex is usually atrophic.[42] Most cases of PPNAD occur as part of the Carney complex in association with a variety of other abnormalities, including myxomatous masses of the heart, skin, or breast; blue nevi or lentigines; and other endocrine disorders (sexual precocity; Sertoli cell, Leydig cell, or adrenal rest tumors; acromegaly). The Carney complex is inherited as an autosomal dominant condition, and Cushing's syndrome occurs in approximately 30% of cases. The tumor suppressor gene *PRKAR1A*, coding for the type 1A regulatory subunit of protein kinase A, has been shown to be mutated in approximately one half of patients with Carney complex. Mutations in this gene and also the phosphodiesterase 11A (*PDE11A*) gene have been shown to be associated with an isolated distinct form of PPNAD.[43]

Cushing's syndrome resulting from bilateral nodular adrenal disease is an uncommon feature of the McCune-Albright syndrome,[44] which is characterized by fibrous dysplasia of bone, café-au-lait skin pigmentation, and endocrine dysfunction (usually precocious puberty). In this disease, an activating mutation at codon 201 of the α subunit of the G protein that stimulates cyclic adenosine monophosphate formation occurs in a mosaic pattern in early embryogenesis.[45] If this affects some adrenal cells, constitutive activation of adenylate cyclase and the steroidogenic cascade leads to nodule formation and glucocorticoid excess. The internodular adrenal cortex, where the mutation is not present, becomes atrophic.[46]

A missense mutation of the ACTH receptor, resulting in its constitutive activation and ACTH-independent Cushing's syndrome, also has been reported.[47]

ACTH-independent bilateral macronodular adrenal hyperplasia (AIMAH) is a rare form (<1%) of Cushing's syndrome that involves large or even huge adrenal glands, usually with definite nodules on imaging. Most cases are sporadic, but a few familial cases have been reported.[48] Although the cause remains unclear in most cases, some nodules express increased numbers of receptors normally found on the adrenal gland, or ectopic receptors for circulating ligands that then can stimulate cortisol production. Perhaps the best known example of this phenomenon is food-dependent Cushing's syndrome. The normal postprandial increase in gastric inhibitory peptide (GIP) appeared to cause Cushing's syndrome in two middle-aged women with bilateral multinodular adrenal enlargement, mildly elevated urinary free cortisol (UFC) values, and undetectable plasma ACTH values. Fasting morning serum cortisol values were low or normal. Cortisol values increased dramatically after meals and after in vivo or in vitro exposure to GIP.[7,8] In one patient, curative bilateral adrenalectomy revealed multinodular adrenal glands weighing 20 and 35 g.[8] In the other, treatment with octreotide ameliorated the syndrome.[7] Ectopic expression of GIP receptors was found in these patients. Aberrant expression of vasopressin, β-adrenergic luteinizing hormone/human chorionic gonadotropin, serotonin, angiotensin, leptin, glucagon, interleukin (IL)-1, and thyroid-stimulating hormone (TSH) has been described as functionally linked to cortisol production.[49] However, it is possible that this apparent ectopic induction of receptors on the adrenal is a response to the adrenal hyperplasia rather than its cause.

Adrenal rest tissue in the liver, in the adrenal beds, or in association with the gonads may rarely cause Cushing's syndrome, usually in the setting of ACTH-dependent disease after adrenalectomy.[50-53] Ectopic cortisol production by an ovarian carcinoma has been reported.[54]

PSEUDO-CUSHING'S STATES

A pseudo-Cushing's state may be defined as one in which some or all of the clinical features that resemble true Cushing's syndrome, and some evidence of hypercortisolism, are present but disappear after resolution of the underlying condition.[55] The pathophysiology of these states has not been established. One hypothesis is that these stressful conditions increase the activity of the CRH neuron, resulting in excessive ACTH secretion, adrenal hyperplasia, and increased cortisol production.[56] The model predicts only intermittent and modest hypercortisolism because of appropriate corticotroph reduction in ACTH secretion in response to negative feedback by cortisol (Fig. 16-1). This construct presumes also that hypertrophied adrenal glands produce excessive glucocorticoids in response to normal ACTH levels, an assumption that is supported by the blunted ACTH, but not cortisol, response to exogenous CRH in anorexia nervosa,[57] depression,[58] and obligate athleticism.[59]

EPIDEMIOLOGY

Iatrogenic causes account for most cases of Cushing's syndrome because of the common therapeutic use of high-dose glucocorticoids. Large series have reported the distribution of endogenous cases as follows: Cushing's disease (68%), adrenal adenomas (8% to 19%), adrenal carcinoma (6% to 7%), ectopic ACTH syndrome (6% to 15%), and nodular adrenal hyperplasia (2%).[55,60] However, a paucity of information is available on the true incidence of these causes. Perhaps the best data come from a population-based study covering the whole of Denmark (population of 5.3 million), which used stringent methods of data collection, aided by the small number of centers treating the disorder.[61] The incidences of Cushing's disease, adrenal adenoma, and adrenal carcinoma were 1.2 per million per year, 0.6 per million per year, and 0.2 per million per year, respectively. The reported incidence of ectopic ACTH syndrome was extremely low (0.1 per million per year). This is probably due (as the authors concede) to the fact that many cases were never recognized, but may be explained in part by a group of patients with ACTH-dependent Cushing's syndrome (0.5 per million per year) with presumed but unproven pituitary disease. Some of these may well have had ectopic ACTH syndrome. The incidence of ectopic ACTH syndrome most certainly is underestimated in the endocrine literature because most cases reaching endocrinologists are those caused by occult tumors as opposed to those caused by overt malignancy. However, given that Cushing's syndrome will be present in 3% to 12% of cases of small cell lung cancer,[62,63] and that the recent incidence of small cell lung cancer in Europe is approximately 120 per million per year in men and 40 per million per year in women,[64] this is by far the most common cause. Other epidemiologic studies have looked at just the incidence of Cushing's disease and have found rates between 0.7 per million per year in northern Italy[65] and 2.4 per million per year in northern Spain.[66]

Gender and age distribution varies with the cause of Cushing's syndrome. Adrenal adenomas and Cushing's disease present much more commonly in women than in men, and adrenal carcinoma is approximately 1.5 times as common as in men.[55,60] Nodular adrenal hyperplasia has an approximately equal gender ratio.

Ectopic ACTH syndrome is the only cause of the syndrome that is more common in men (other than Cushing's disease in prepubertal children), although this may change as more women are developing small cell lung cancer. Lung cancer is more common after age 40, and this accounts for the increased mean age of patients with ectopic ACTH syndrome compared with Cushing's disease, which occurs between 25 and 40 years of age.[67] The other major cause of ectopic ACTH secretion, intrathoracic carcinoids, has a peak incidence around 40 years and only a slightly increased male-to-female ratio.[68] The age distribu-

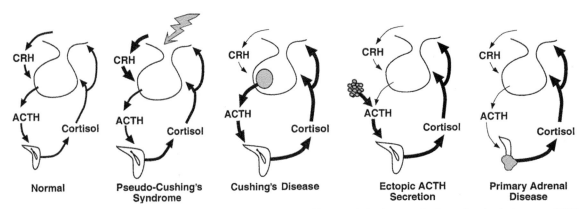

FIGURE 16-1. Physiology of the hypothalamic-pituitary-adrenal axis in normal individuals and hypercortisolemic states. Corticotropin-releasing hormone (CRH) secretion from the hypothalamus normally stimulates adrenocorticotropic hormone (ACTH) secretion from the pituitary gland. This in turn results in increased cortisol production from the adrenal glands. The system is modulated by negative feedback inhibition by cortisol of both CRH and ACTH secretion. In pseudo-Cushing's syndrome, the CRH neuron is activated by central input *(large shaded arrow)*, resulting in increased CRH output that eventuates in hypercortisolism. Increased cortisol production restrains corticotroph activation but does not completely reverse the activation of the CRH neuron, so that mild to moderate hypercortisolism may persist. In Cushing's disease, a corticotroph adenoma secretes ACTH in excess and is inhibited only partially by rising cortisol levels. In this setting and that of ectopic ACTH secretion and primary adrenal disease, the CRH neuron is suppressed by hypercortisolism. In ectopic ACTH secretion, excessive secretion of ACTH from a nonpituitary tumor is not inhibited by glucocorticoid feedback. In this setting and that of autonomous production of cortisol by the adrenal gland, ACTH secretion by normal corticotrophs is suppressed by hypercortisolism.

tion of adrenal cancer is bimodal, with peaks in childhood and adolescence and late in life, although adrenal adenoma occurs most often around 35 years of age.

CLINICAL FEATURES

Excessive cortisol production has widespread systemic effects[67,69-72] (Table 16-3). Although the full-blown cushingoid phenotype is unmistakable, the clinical diagnosis may be equivocal for patients with few of the typical characteristics (Fig. 16-2). Some nonspecific features consistent with the diagnosis of Cushing's syndrome, such as obesity, hypertension, and menstrual irregularity, are common in the general population and may provoke unwarranted and costly screening tests for patients not likely to be affected.

One useful strategy when the diagnosis of Cushing's syndrome is considered, is to look for evidence of progressive physical changes by examination of serial photographs, especially of individuals photographed at annual events such as holidays, birthdays, or school milestones (Fig. 16-3). Another approach relies on identification of signs and symptoms that correctly classify patients suspected of having the disorder. Truncal obesity, ecchymoses, plethora, proximal muscle weakness, and osteopenia are useful discriminant indices for Cushing's syndrome, with osteoporosis, ecchymoses, and muscle weakness being the most reliable.[69,73,74]

Increased deposition of fat, one of the earliest signs, occurs in almost all patients and is reported as increasing weight or difficulty in maintaining weight. The distribution of fat is altered in both men and women, with increased amounts in the visceral compartments[75] and subcutaneous sites on the face and neck. Increased intra-abdominal fat results in the truncal obesity described by Cushing in approximately 50% of patients. Increased fat in the face (moon facies), the supraclavicular or temporal fossae, and the dorsocervical area ("buffalo hump") is uncommon in normal people.

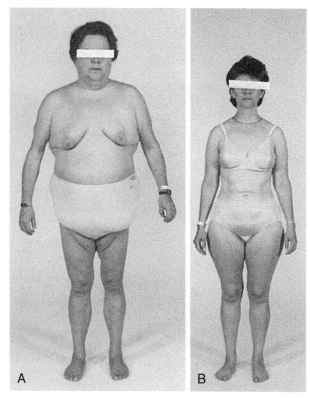

FIGURE 16-2. Body habitus of two patients with proven Cushing's syndrome. Features typical of the syndrome—central obesity, round face, and supraclavicular fat pads—are present in the patient in **A,** but not in the patient in **B,** illustrating that the diagnosis is not always apparent from the initial physical examination.

Table 16-3. Percentage Frequency of Clinical Signs and Symptoms of Cushing's Syndrome as Described in Six Large Studies from 1952 to 2003

Signs and Symptoms (Men/Women)	Plotz et al., 1952[67] (N = 33)	Sprague et al., 1956[72] (N = 100)	Soffer et al., 1961[71] (N = 50)	Urbanic and George, 1981[70] (N = 31)	Ross & Linch, 1982[69] (N = 70)	Giraldi et al., 2003[125] (N = 280)
Obesity or weight gain	97	84	86	79	97	85/86
Hypertension	84	90	88	77	74	68/67
Weakness/muscle atrophy	83		58	90	56	64/46
Plethora	89	81	78		94	89/81
Round face	89	92	92		88	
Striae	60	64	50	51	56	72/51
Thin skin				84		
Ecchymoses	60	62	68	77	62	21/32
Hirsutism	73	74	84	64	81	
Acne	82	64		35	21	19/28
Female balding			51		13	
Dorsocervical fat pad		67	34		54	51/54
Edema	60		66	48	50	
Menstrual changes	86	35	72	69	84	
Decreased libido	86		100/33	55	100/47	
Headache	58					
Backache	83			39	43	
Psychiatric disturbance	67		40	48	62	26/34
Recurrent infection		14		25		
Poor wound healing/severe infection	42					
Abdominal pain					21	
Renal calculi					15	21/6
Osteoporosis/fracture	83		56	48	50	47/32
Abnormal glucose tolerance	94		84	39	50	43/45

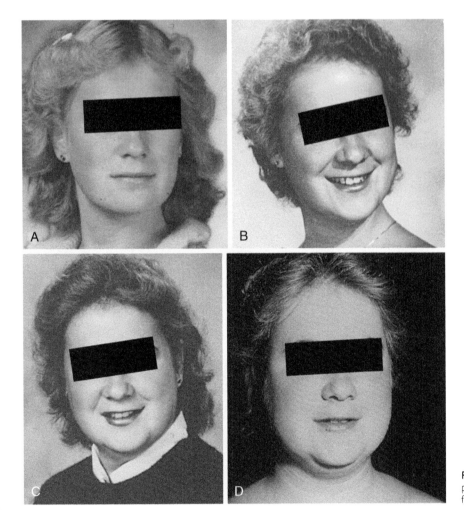

FIGURE 16-3. Progression of cushingoid features as shown in photographs taken at 1-year intervals (**A** through **D,** progress from earliest to latest).

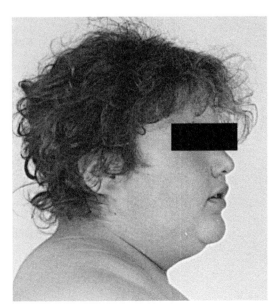

FIGURE 16-4. Fat may fill or, in this case, rise above the supraclavicular fossa of patients with Cushing's syndrome.

When extreme, the supraclavicular fat may present as a "collar" rising above the clavicles (Fig. 16-4); filling of the temporal fossae may prevent eyeglass frames from seating properly. Abnormal fat deposition may occur in the epidural space. Spinal epidural lipomatosis causing neurologic deficit, a rare complication of long-term exogenous steroid use, has been reported in a few patients with endogenous Cushing's syndrome.[76,77] Lumbosacral findings were seen in both men and women, whereas thoracic obstruction was restricted to men. The condition can be diagnosed by magnetic resonance imaging (MRI).[78]

Loss of subcutaneous tissue results in a variety of skin abnormalities that are unusual in the general population and suggest hypercortisolism. Ecchymoses, often after minimal trauma, and cutaneous atrophy, seen as a fine "cigarette paper" wrinkling or tenting over the dorsum of the hand and elbows, are typical. Cutaneous atrophy is influenced by gender and age, with men and the young having greater skin thickness. Two maxims follow: First, it is useful to compare the patient's skin with that of a near age- and gender-matched healthy person; and second, skin thickness is relatively preserved in cushingoid women with increased androgen production or preservation of ovarian function (Fig. 16-5).

Facial plethora, especially over the cheeks, also reflects loss of subcutaneous tissue. Although plethora is more obvious in pale Caucasian individuals, it may be present and should be sought in darker-skinned persons. Because erythema may be induced in normal persons by ultraviolet radiation from lamps or sunlight, wind, or medications (including topical drying agents, glucocorticoids, and antipsoriatic treatments), exposure to these agents should be ascertained before plethora is ascribed to endogenous hypercortisolism. A demarcation line, representing collar, sleeve, or shoulder straps, may differentiate exogenous from endogenous causes. Flushing caused by other conditions (e.g., mastocytosis, thyrotoxicosis, vasomotor instability or estrogen insufficiency in women, carcinoid syndrome) also should be considered.

Purple striae more than 1 cm in diameter are virtually pathognomonic for Cushing's syndrome (Fig. 16-6). Although the silvery, healed striae that are typical postpartum are not caused by active Cushing's syndrome, other pink, less pigmented, and thinner striae may be seen. Although most common over the abdomen, striae occur also over the hips, buttocks, thighs, breasts, and upper arms. The tear in the subcutaneous tissue may be best appreciated by indirect (side) lighting, which throws the striae into relief, or by light stroking of the skin. The violaceous hue is not dependent on ACTH-dependent pigmentation and may be seen in Cushing's syndrome in association with primary adrenal causes.

Proximal muscle weakness with preservation of distal strength is a hallmark of Cushing's syndrome. Histologically, this is reflected in profound atrophy of fibers without necrosis.[79-81] Weakness is best assessed historically by questions related to the use of these muscles: Is there difficulty or weakness in climbing

stairs, getting up from a chair or bed without using hand propulsion, or performing activities using the shoulders (e.g., brushing hair, reaching objects in overhead cabinets, changing ceiling light bulbs)? Formal muscle testing is useful. Assess the strength of the hip flexors by asking the patient to get out of a chair without using his or her arms. If this can be done, the patient is asked to rise from a squat. Inability to perform either task, in the absence of hip or lower extremity arthropathy or other myopathic processes, is suggestive of Cushing's syndrome. Leg extension while seated is a quantifiable test of proximal muscle strength. The number of seconds for which this position is held can be used to judge deterioration or progress after treatment.

Osteopenia is common. A history of fractures, typically of the feet, ribs, or vertebrae, may be one of the only signs of Cushing's syndrome, especially in men.[70,71,82] Avascular necrosis of bone, a rare complication of endogenous hypercortisolism, is more common in iatrogenic hypercortisolism.[83,84] It usually occurs in the hips, but we have also seen it in the knees.

Vellous hypertrichosis of the forehead or upper cheeks distinguishes Cushing's syndrome from the more common causes of hirsutism and may be appreciated only by careful visual and tactile inspection (Fig. 16-7). Excessive terminal hair on the face and body, and acne—pustular, reflecting increased androgens, or papular, reflecting pure glucocorticoid excess—may be present.[85] Severe hirsutism and virilization are uncommon and suggest adrenal carcinoma.

Most patients experience emotional and cognitive changes (including increased fatigue, irritability, crying, and restlessness, depressed mood, decreased libido, insomnia, anxiety, impaired memory, concentration, and verbal communication) and changes in appetite. These changes correlate with the degree of hypercortisolism.[86] Irritability, characterized as a decreased threshold for uncontrollable verbal outbursts, may be one of the earliest symptoms. Global impairment in neuropsychological function correlates well with the performance of seven serial subtractions and recall of the names of three cities—bedside tests that can be used by the clinician to quantify this symptom complex.[87]

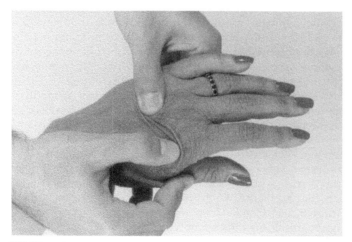

FIGURE 16-5. Thinning of the skin may be demonstrated by twisting the skin on the dorsum of the hand.

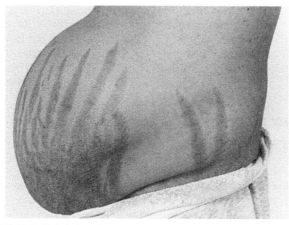

FIGURE 16-6. Typical abdominal striae of a patient with hypercortisolism. These are greater than 1 cm in width and are violaceous.

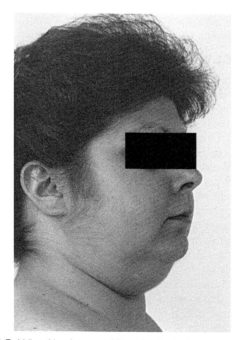

FIGURE 16-7. Vellous hirsutism, especially on the cheeks, is often present in women with Cushing's syndrome.

Approximately 80% of patients meet strict criteria for a major affective disorder—50% with unipolar depression and 30% with bipolar illness.[88,89] Although the quality of the depressed mood ranges from suicide attempts to sadness, the time course is characteristically intermittent, rarely lasting longer than 3 days, in contrast to the constant dysphoria reported by depressed patients without Cushing's syndrome.[86] A minority of patients are manic. The improvement in neuropsychiatric findings after treatment of Cushing's syndrome, coupled with similar features in patients treated with exogenous steroids, and the association of hypercortisolism with poor cognitive performance in depressed patients suggest glucocorticoid excess as a cause.[90,91]

Hypertension is present in approximately 80% of patients, and although hypertension is also common in the general population, its presence in patients younger than 40 years of age, especially if difficult to control, may alert one to the syndrome. Hypertension usually resolves with treatment of the Cushing's syndrome but may persist, possibly as the result of microvessel remodeling and/or underlying essential hypertension.[92]

The association of hypercortisolism and fungal infections of the skin, such as mucocutaneous candidiasis and pityriasis versicolor, with poor wound healing is a common feature. Wound dehiscence occurs less often but is an important consideration in patients who are treated surgically without medical pretreatment.

Patients with marked hypercortisolism (plasma cortisol >43 μg/dL [1200 nmol/L], UFC >2000 μg/day [5520 nmol/day]) are at risk for two potentially catastrophic events: perforation of the viscera and severe infection, either bacterial or opportunistic, such as *Pneumocystis carinii*, aspergillosis, nocardiosis, cryptococcosis, histoplasmosis, and *Candida*.[93-95] Classic clinical signs, such as loss of bowel sounds and fever, may be absent in peritonitis, and the typical leukocytosis of hypercortisolism may not increase further. Thus, the threshold of suspicion for opportunistic infection and a surgical abdomen must be low in patients with severe hypercortisolism.

Libido is decreased uniformly in men and to a lesser extent (44%) in women,[70] in whom *increased* libido may indicate excess androgen production by an adrenocortical carcinoma. Menstrual irregularities, amenorrhea, and infertility are common and may be the presenting complaints.[96] Impotence is common.

PATHOLOGY

The cardinal laboratory findings in endogenous Cushing's syndrome reflect overproduction of glucocorticoids. Although morning plasma cortisol values may be normal, an increased nighttime nadir blunts or obliterates the normal diurnal rhythm.[97-99] This increase in mean 24-hour plasma values is reflected in increased levels of free, or unbound, cortisol in urine[100] and saliva.[101] The capacity of corticosteroid-binding globulin for cortisol is exceeded at a serum cortisol value of approximately 20 μg/dL (≈600 nmol/L). At this point, the excretion of free cortisol increases dramatically in direct proportion to the increased unbound circulating cortisol values.

Hypokalemic metabolic alkalosis usually is observed when daily urine cortisol excretion is greater than 1500 μg (4100 nmol), and thus mainly in cases of ectopic ACTH syndrome.[102] This probably represents a mineralocorticoid action of cortisol at the renal tubule due to saturation of the enzyme 11β-hydroxysteroid dehydrogenase type 2, which inactivates cortisol to cortisone.[103] However, although a common feature of ectopic ACTH secretion, it also may occur in approximately 10% of patients with Cushing's disease. Serum albumin is inversely correlated with

cortisol levels, but this is of clinical significance only at very high cortisol levels, and it reverses with treatment for Cushing's syndrome.[104] Drastic reductions in serum albumin should alert the physician to the possibility of concomitant pathology such as infection. Circulating elevated glucocorticoids increase clotting factors, including factor VIII, fibrinogen, and von Willebrand factor, and reduce fibrinolytic activity, resulting in a fourfold risk of thrombotic events.[105-107] Lipid abnormalities show increases in very–low density lipoprotein, low-density lipoprotein, high-density lipoprotein, and consequently total cholesterol and triglycerides. These changes probably are caused by a direct cortisol effect of increased hepatic synthesis of very low–density lipoprotein without altered clearance.[108,109]

Cushing's syndrome is characterized by insulin resistance and hyperinsulinemia, with frank diabetes mellitus occurring in 30% to 40% of patients, and glucose intolerance in a further 20% to 30%.[110,111] A recent study has suggested that as many as 2% of overweight, poorly controlled patients with diabetes may have occult Cushing's syndrome if fully investigated.[112] In the absence of clinical suspicion, the yield is probably lower.[113]

Patients with Cushing's disease show accelerated cardiovascular disease, including increased carotid artery intima-media thickness and atherosclerotic plaques on Doppler ultrasonography.[114] This increased risk is maintained even as long as 5 years after cure of the hypercortisolemia is attained.[115] It also is likely that glucocorticoids have a direct pathogenic effect on the myocardium.

Hypercortisolism suppresses the thyroidal, gonadal, and growth hormone axes. Thyrotropin-releasing hormone and thyroid-stimulating hormone release is disturbed, and particularly the nocturnal surge of thyroid-stimulating hormone is lost, resulting in reduced total thyroxine, total triiodothyronine, and free triiodothyronine levels compared with controls.[116] Others have found no differences in free thyroxine or free triiodothyronine levels but have shown a significantly increased prevalence of autoimmune thyroid disease in patients treated for Cushing's syndrome.[117,118] In both men and women, low levels of luteinizing hormone, follicle-stimulating hormone, and gonadal steroids consistent with hypogonadotropic hypogonadism are common and correlate with the degree of hypercortisolemia.[119,120] In addition, the coexistence of polycystic ovarian syndrome in Cushing's syndrome may be more common than was previously thought.[96] Hypercortisolemia causes reduced growth hormone (GH) secretion during sleep and blunted GH response to stimulation tests.[121]

The prevalence of osteoporosis as assessed by dual-energy x-ray absorptiometry is approximately 50% in adult Cushing's syndrome.[122] It appears more common in adrenal Cushing's syndrome than in Cushing's disease, and this may relate to the protective effect of increased adrenal androgens in the latter.[123]

The accentuated visceral fat distribution characteristic of Cushing's syndrome can be marked when visualized by computed tomography (CT),[75] and the liver frequently (20%) is steatotic on imaging.[124]

CLINICAL SPECTRUM

The typical patient with Cushing's disease presents at midlife complaining of the gradual development of symptoms, although males tend to present at an earlier age and with more severe clinical consequences.[125] Hypokalemia, virilization, and extremely high cortisol excretion (>10-fold normal) are distinctly uncommon and should alert the physician to an alternative cause. The clinical presentation of pituitary corticotroph macroadenomas, apart from visual field changes caused by suprasellar expansion, is not unique. By contrast, invasive pituitary adenomas present at a slightly younger age; cavernous sinus and dural involvement may result in cranial neuropathies and facial neuralgia.[126,127] Only a few case reports attest to cerebrospinal or extracranial metastasis of ACTH-producing pituitary tumors.[128]

Nelson's syndrome is characterized by the development of hyperpigmentation and high ACTH levels after bilateral adrenalectomy for Cushing's disease. Tumor growth after adrenalectomy has been attributed to the relative resistance of these tumors to physiologic glucocorticoid suppression.

An abrupt onset of severe Cushing's syndrome should prompt an evaluation for ectopic ACTH secretion. This variant of ectopic ACTH secretion classically presents as a paraneoplastic syndrome in the context of a known malignancy. The features were captured in the initial formulation of Liddle[4]: weight loss, hypokalemia, weakness, and diabetes. However, Cushing's syndrome caused by less obvious ectopic ACTH secretion often presents in the more classic way with weight gain and striae and can be difficult to differentiate clinically from Cushing's disease. It is patients with this syndrome who most often present a diagnostic dilemma. They tend to have UFC excretion in the range seen in pituitary disease and may not show hypokalemia, hyperpigmentation, or the other findings typical of severe classical ectopic ACTH secretion.

Adrenocortical carcinomas are inefficient producers of cortisol and tend to evince Cushing's syndrome when the tumor is large (>6 cm), if at all. Abdominal pain or a palpable mass suggests this cause. Feminization in a man or virilization and increased libido in a woman, indicating involvement of the zona reticularis, suggest adrenal cancer or macronodular adrenal disease, which is rarer. The typical patient with PPNAD is a child or young adult who may present with an intermittent course or a family history of associated signs: Lentigines may be the initial clue to this cause. By contrast, patients with the massive macronodular variant of ACTH-independent Cushing's syndrome tend to be older than 40 years.

DIAGNOSIS AND DIFFERENTIAL DIAGNOSIS

The diagnosis of Cushing's syndrome rests on the demonstration of both physical and biochemical features of glucocorticoid excess. Thus, the diagnosis is unequivocal in a typical patient, with many of the physical features discussed earlier in the setting of UFC levels more than fourfold above normal.[129] However, many of the signs of hypercortisolism, such as obesity, hypertension, glucose intolerance, mood changes, menstrual irregularity, and hirsutism, are common in the general population. Similarly, mild glucocorticoid excess is seen in affective disorders,[130] strenuous exercise,[59] alcoholism and alcohol withdrawal states,[131] renal failure,[132] and hypoglycemia. Diagnostic strategies for distinguishing between these pseudo-Cushing's states and true Cushing's syndrome are discussed later.

Glucocorticoid resistance is characterized by an abnormal glucocorticoid receptor number or binding, which causes compensatory increases in ACTH and excessive glucocorticoid production to maintain normal glucocorticoid-mediated effects at the target tissues. The diagnosis should be considered in the hypokalemic, hypertensive, hypercortisolemic patient without typical glucocorticoid-mediated signs of Cushing's syndrome.[133]

ESTABLISHING THE DIAGNOSIS OF CUSHING'S SYNDROME

When a careful history and physical examination reveal clinical features that could be consistent with the syndrome, exogenous

Table 16-4. Evaluation of Suspected Cushing's Syndrome

History

Increased weight
Growth retardation in children
Weakness
Easy bruising
Stretch marks
Poor wound healing
Fractures
Change in libido
Impotence/irregular or no menses
Emotional, cognitive, mood changes (fatigue, irritability, anxiety, insomnia, depression, impaired memory and concentration)

Examination

Fat distribution (centripetal obesity; rounded face; dorsocervical, supraclavicular, temporal fat pads)
Hypertension
Proximal muscle weakness and atrophy
Thin skin and ecchymoses
Purple striae
Hirsutism
Acne
Facial plethora
Edema
Impaired serial 7s/recall of three cities

Laboratory Findings

Abnormal glucose tolerance/frank diabetes mellitus, hypokalemia

First-Line Screening Tests

Elevated 24-hour urinary free cortisol (three collections)
Lack of suppression to low-dose dexamethasone (LDDST)
Elevated late-night salivary cortisol

Additional Screening Tests (if required)

Cortisol circadian rhythm
Combined dexamethasone-CRH test
Insulin tolerance test
Loperamide test

CRH, Corticotropin-releasing hormone; *LDDST,* low-dose dexamethasone suppression test.

glucocorticoid use must be excluded (Table 16-4). In addition to inquiring about the use of oral, rectal, inhaled, injected, or topical glucocorticoid administration, it is important to evaluate the use of "tonics," herbs, and skin bleaching creams, which may contain glucocorticoids. In the absence of exogenous glucocorticoids, biochemical confirmation of the diagnosis of Cushing's syndrome is needed. It is important to remember that the urgency for diagnosis and treatment of Cushing's syndrome is greatest when the symptoms are severe. In milder cases, the patient may be best served by waiting until the diagnosis is clear. Periodic reevaluation with urine screening tests and documentation of body habitus with photographs may reveal progression.

Initial Screening Tests

Hypercortisolemia, demonstrated by loss of the normal circadian rhythm of cortisol secretion, and disturbed feedback of the hypothalamic-pituitary-adrenal (HPA) axis are the cardinal biochemical features of Cushing's syndrome. Tests to confirm the diagnosis are based on these principles. To screen for Cushing's syndrome, tests of high sensitivity should be used initially to avoid missing milder cases. All of these screening tests may miss identification of mild cases of hypercortisolemia, and multiple samples or a combination of tests may be needed. A recent guideline suggests that two abnormal first-line test results should be required for the diagnosis of Cushing's syndrome.[134]

Urinary Free Cortisol

Under normal conditions, 10% of plasma cortisol is free or unbound and physiologically active. Unbound cortisol is filtered by the kidney, with most being reabsorbed in the tubules and the remainder excreted unchanged. Thus, 24-hour UFC collection produces an integrated measure of serum cortisol, smoothing out variations in cortisol during the day. UFC determinations first became clinically available in 1968[135] and have superseded the historical measurement of urinary metabolites of glucocorticoids and androgens (17-hydroxycorticosteroids [17-OHCS], 17-ketosteroids, and 17-ketogenic steroids).

The major drawback of the test is the potential for overcollection or undercollection of the 24-hour specimen, and written instructions must be given to the patient. In addition, creatinine excretion in the collection can be measured to assess completeness and should equal approximately 1 g per 24 hours in a 70 kg patient (variations depend on muscle mass). This value should not vary by more than 10% between collections in the same individual.[136] It cannot be used to correct for incomplete collection, however, because rates of cortisol and creatinine excretion are not parallel over the 24-hour period. Various groups have tried to overcome the collection issue by proposing shorter collection periods, usually at night, when the loss of circadian rhythm differs most from normal controls,[137,138] but this approach has not been widely accepted. High-performance liquid chromatography and tandem mass spectrometry are now used to measure UFC, which overcomes the previous problem of cross-reactivity of some exogenous glucocorticoids and other structurally similar steroids with conventional radioimmunoassay.[139] Occasionally, substances such as carbamazepine, digoxin, and fenofibrate can coelute with cortisol during high-performance liquid chromatography, causing falsely elevated results.[140,141]

If the previous caveats have been satisfied, the UFC measurement can be interpreted. In large series, measurement of an elevated UFC above the normal range has a high sensitivity for the diagnosis of Cushing's syndrome (≈95% to 100%).[100,142] However, it should be noted that in the latter study, 11% of 146 patients with proven Cushing's syndrome had at least one of four UFC collections within the normal range, which confirms the need for multiple collections. Values greater than fourfold normal are rare except in Cushing's syndrome. Values between this and down to the upper limit of normal are compatible with Cushing's syndrome or pseudo-Cushing's states, so that one must exclude the latter diagnosis. In summary, UFC measurements have a high sensitivity if collected correctly, and several completely normal collections make the diagnosis of Cushing's syndrome very unlikely. However, when biochemical evidence of Cushing's syndrome is not obtained in the setting of clinical features that suggest the diagnosis, repeated measurement of urine cortisol may demonstrate cyclicity or progression. The specificity is somewhat lower, thus patients with marginally elevated levels require further investigation.[55]

Late-Night Salivary Cortisol

Salivary cortisol measurement offers an excellent reflection of the plasma free cortisol concentration in health and disease because it circumvents the changes in total cortisol due to corticosteroid-binding globulin alterations.[143,144] Salivary cortisol is stable for some days at room temperature, and the simple noninvasive collection procedure means that it can be performed conveniently at home and delivered via mail. Thus, it offers a number of attractive advantages over blood collection, particularly in children. Analysis is performed using a modification of the plasma cortisol radioimmunoassay, enzyme-linked immunosorbent assay, or liquid chromatography/tandem mass spectrometry, and commercial kits are internationally available for this.[145] The diagnostic value cutoff varies between studies (0.13 μg/dL [3.6 nmol/L] to 0.55 μg/dL [15.2 nmol/L]) because of different assays and comparison groups studied.[146-153] Normal values also differ between adult and pediatric populations, and this may be affected by other comorbidities such as diabetes and hypertension.[154] However, from these studies, the sensitivity and specificity of this test appear to be relatively consistent at different centers, ranging from 92% to 100%, and from 93% to 100% respectively. It does not appear to make a difference if sampling is done at bedtime (≈23.00 hr) or at midnight, although it should be determined that the patient has a normal sleep pattern. Positive or negative results should be confirmed by repeat sampling. In summary, therefore, although late-night salivary cortisol appears to be a useful and convenient additional screening test for Cushing's syndrome, particularly in the outpatient setting, local normal ranges should be validated based on the assay used and the population studied.

Low-Dose Dexamethasone Suppression Tests

In normal individuals, administration of the potent synthetic glucocorticoid dexamethasone results in suppression of the HPA axis, whereas patients with Cushing's syndrome are resistant, at least partially, to this negative feedback. The original low-dose dexamethasone test (LDDST), as described by Liddle in 1960, measured urinary 17-OHCS before and during 48 hours of 0.5 mg dexamethasone every 6 hours, and an excretion of greater than 4 mg/day on the second day of dexamethasone treatment was considered to indicate Cushing's syndrome.[155] Dexamethasone does not cross-react with modern cortisol immunoassays, and the simpler measurement of a single plasma cortisol post dexamethasone has been validated in various series and gives the test a sensitivity of between 97% and 100% for the diagnosis of Cushing's syndrome.[156-159] The simpler overnight LDDST was proposed by Nugent and colleagues in 1965; this measured a 9:00 A.M. plasma cortisol after a single dose of 1 mg dexamethasone taken at midnight.[160] Since then, various other doses, between 0.5 and 2 mg, have been proposed for the overnight test, and various diagnostic cutoffs have been applied.[161-163] There appears to be no difference in discrimination between single doses of 1, 1.5, and 2 mg.[164] Higher doses significantly decrease the sensitivity of the test.[165] In a comprehensive review of the LDDST, both the original 2 day test and the 1 mg overnight protocol appear to have comparably high sensitivities (98% to 100%), provided a conservative postdexamethasone serum cortisol cutoff of 1.8 μg/dL (50 nmol/L) is applied. However, the specificity of the overnight test (88%) is lower compared with the 2 day test, particularly if serum cortisol is measured at both 24 and 48 hours (97% to 100%), with potential misclassification of patients with pseudo-Cushing's states and acute or chronic illnesses. Many endocrinologists use the overnight test because of its greater simplicity and lower cost, although some centers still advocate the 48-hour test because of its high sensitivity and specificity, and the information it can provide in the differential diagnosis of ACTH-dependent Cushing's syndrome (see later).[159] Written instructions should be given to the patient if the latter is to be performed on an outpatient basis. Salivary rather than serum cortisol has been evaluated as the end point for the LDDST. This offers potential benefit in terms of convenience but requires further evaluation.[149,166]

Table 16-5. Spurious Causes of Abnormal Dexamethasone Suppression Test Results

False Positive

Increased metabolism: barbiturates, phenytoin, carbamazepine, primidone, rifampicin, aminoglutethimide
Increased cortisol-binding globulin: pregnancy, oral estrogens, tamoxifen
Malabsorption
Pseudo-Cushing's states

False Negative

Reduced metabolism: high-dose benzodiazepines, indomethacin, liver disease

Factors such as variable absorption and increased or decreased dexamethasone metabolism due to other compounds (Table 16-5) can influence any oral dexamethasone test.[167] Therefore, a history of symptoms of malabsorption and a careful drug history should be taken before the test is used in a patient. Measurement of plasma dexamethasone is available in some centers and can be useful in patients of concern. One solution to overcome demonstrated malabsorption is to use one of the published intravenous dexamethasone suppression tests, recognizing that criteria for response have not been standardized.[168,169] Pregnancy and other causes of increased or decreased corticosteroid-binding globulin (such as exogenous estrogens and the nephrotic syndrome) also should be excluded because these are likely to result in false-positive and false-negative tests.[170]

Second-Line Tests

The Dexamethasone-CRH Test

In 1993, a combined dexamethasone-CRH (Dex-CRH) test was introduced for the difficult scenario of the differentiation of pseudo-Cushing's states from true Cushing's syndrome in patients with only mild hypercortisolemia and equivocal physical findings.[171] Dexamethasone 0.5 mg every 6 hours was given for eight doses, ending 2 hours before administration of ovine CRH (1 μg/kg intravenously) to 58 adults with UFC less than 360 μg/day (<1000 nmol/day). Subsequent evaluation proved that 39 had Cushing's syndrome and 19 had a pseudo-Cushing's state. The plasma cortisol value 15 minutes after CRH was less than 1.4 μg/dL (38 nmol/L) in all patients with pseudo-Cushing's states and was greater in all patients with Cushing's syndrome. A prospective follow-up study by the same group in 98 patients continued to show that the test had an impressive sensitivity and specificity of 99% and 96%, respectively.[172] However, results from a number of other smaller studies have challenged the diagnostic utility of this test over the standard LDDST.[173-175] Overall, in these reports, the specificity of the LDDST in 92 patients without Cushing's syndrome was 79%, versus 70% for the Dex-CRH. Test sensitivity in 59 patients with Cushing's syndrome was 96% for LDDST, versus 98% for the Dex-CRH group. It perhaps is not surprising that the diagnostic utility of the Dex-CRH has altered with additional studies at a greater number of centers. This might be the case for a number of reasons, including variable dexamethasone metabolism in individuals, different definitions of patients with pseudo-Cushing's, different protocols and assays, and variable diagnostic thresholds.[176] Of note, the original cortisol criteria performed poorly at these other centers, and this may have happened because many cortisol assays do not reliably measure levels <1.8 μg/dL (50 nmol/L). It does highlight that as a clinician one must be confident in the assay that is to be used for a particular test, and diagnostic criteria should be chosen that are appropriate for that assay. The Dex-CRH test remains a test that should be considered in patients with equivocal results.

Plasma Cortisol Circadian Rhythm

The normal diurnal rhythm of plasma cortisol is blunted or absent in Cushing's syndrome, with normal or increased morning values and an increase in the nighttime nadir. Although less convenient than salivary cortisol, midnight plasma cortisol levels may be useful to obtain in patients admitted for investigation. Samples are best obtained around midnight, through an indwelling line for awake patients or by direct venipuncture within 5 to 10 minutes of waking of sleeping patients. In one study, 20 normal sleeping subjects had values less than 1.8 μg/dL (50 nmol/L), whereas all 150 patients with Cushing's syndrome had midnight plasma cortisol concentrations greater than this.[158] The suggested cutoff criterion in awake patients is higher, 7.5 to 8.3 μg/dL (207 to 229 nmol/L) and less discriminatory (sensitivity 92% to 94%, and specificity 96% to 100%).[177,178] This difference probably reflects a different comparison group—patients suspected to have Cushing's but in whom it was excluded. Patients with severe medical illness, depression, and mania may have cortisol values one to three times normal.[130,164] Therefore, a sleeping midnight cortisol value less than 1.8 μg/dL (50 nmol/L) effectively excludes active Cushing's syndrome, but higher values, unless very high, are less specific for Cushing's syndrome.

Other Second-Line Tests

The insulin tolerance test has been used to distinguish Cushing's syndrome from pseudo-Cushing's states. Serum cortisol values increase in normal people after acute hypoglycemia, presumably because of central stimulation of CRH and vasopressin. The sustained hypercortisolism of Cushing's syndrome suppresses CRH and vasopressin secretion and so blunts this response. The CRH/vasopressin neurons are presumed to be overactive in pseudo-Cushing's states, particularly those that are depression associated, so a normal response to hypoglycemia (<40 mg/dL; <2.2 nmol/L) usually is maintained. Unfortunately, approximately 18% of patients with Cushing's syndrome, especially those with minimal hypercortisolism, show a normal response to adequate hypoglycemia.[164] Additionally, criteria for interpretation of results have not been established. If used, a dose of insulin of 0.3 U/kg should be used to overcome insulin resistance in these patients.[130]

The opiate agonist loperamide (16 mg orally) has been shown to inhibit CRH and thus ACTH and cortisol levels in most normal individuals, but not in patients with Cushing's syndrome. This test has not been used widely but has been evaluated in one center, revealing a sensitivity of 100% and a specificity of 95%.[179,180] However, it is unclear as to how well this test may exclude pseudo-Cushing's states because a significant proportion of patients with depression also fail to suppress the HPA axis.[181] It does not appear to be affected by drugs that affect the metabolism of dexamethasone and could potentially be useful in assessing patients on such treatment.[180]

DIFFERENTIAL DIAGNOSIS OF CUSHING'S SYNDROME

Once the diagnosis of Cushing's syndrome is made, its cause must be determined. The strategy for the differential diagnosis of Cushing's syndrome (Fig. 16-8) begins with measurement of

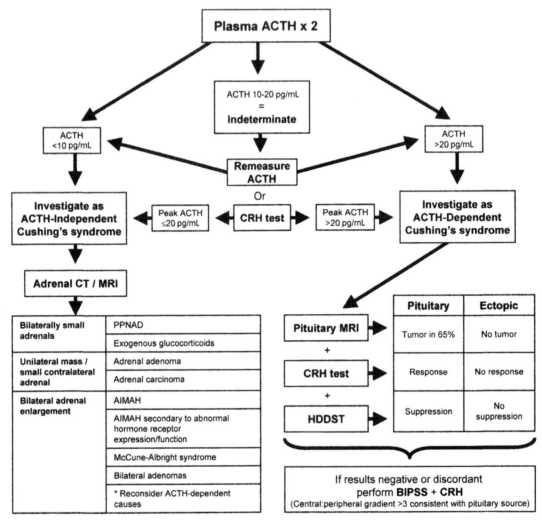

FIGURE 16-8. Suggested strategy for the differential diagnosis of Cushing's syndrome. *ACTH,* Adrenocorticotropic hormone; *AIMAH,* ACTH-independent bilateral macronodular adrenal hyperplasia; *BIPSS,* bilateral inferior petrosal sinus sampling; *CRH,* corticotropin-releasing hormone; *CT,* computed tomography; *HDDST,* high-dose dexamethasone suppression test; *MRI,* magnetic resonance imaging; *PPNAD,* primary pigmented nodular adrenal disease.

plasma ACTH to distinguish between ACTH-dependent and ACTH-independent causes. Modern two-site immunoradiometric assays are more sensitive than the older radioimmunoassays and therefore provide the best discrimination. Only assays that can reliably detect values to below 10 ng/L should be used, and appropriate collection and processing of the sample are essential, because ACTH is susceptible to degradation by peptidases; therefore the sample must be kept in an ice water bath and centrifuged, aliquoted, and frozen within a few hours to avoid a spuriously low result. Repeated measurements are usually necessary because patients with ACTH-dependent Cushing's disease have been shown to have on occasion ACTH levels less than 10 ng/L (2 pmol/L) on conventional radioimmunoassay,[182] but consistent ACTH measurements of less than 10 ng/L (2 pmol/L) at 9:00 AM with concomitant hypercortisolemia essentially confirm ACTH-independent Cushing's syndrome. When the basal ACTH level is indeterminate (10 to 20 g/L [2 to 4 pmol/L]), the response to CRH may be useful in this setting. Patients with primary adrenal disease rarely show maximal ACTH values greater than 20 ng/L (4 pmol/L), although patients with Cushing's disease usually exceed this value.

Investigating Adrenocorticotropic Hormone–Independent Cushing's Syndrome

Radiologic tests are the mainstay in differentiating between the various types of ACTH-independent Cushing's syndrome. High-resolution CT scanning of the adrenal glands has excellent diagnostic accuracy for masses greater than 1 cm and allows evaluation of the contralateral gland.[183] MRI may be useful for the differential diagnosis of adrenal masses; the T_2-weighted signal is progressively brighter in normal tissue, adenoma, carcinoma, and finally pheochromocytoma.[184] With this approach, adrenal tumors appear as a unilateral mass with an atrophic or less commonly a normal-size contralateral gland.[185] If the lesion is greater than 5 cm in diameter, it should be considered to be malignant until proven otherwise, and imaging characteristics should not be relied upon. Very rarely, bilateral adenomas may be present.[186] The adrenal glands in PPNAD appear normal or slightly lumpy from multiple small nodules but generally are not enlarged.[187] AIMAH is characterized by bilaterally huge (>5 cm) nodular or hyperplastic glands.[188] Exogenous administration of glucocorticoids results in adrenal atrophy; very small glands may provide a clue as to this entity.

The CT appearance of the adrenals in AIMAH may be similar to that of ACTH-dependent forms of Cushing's syndrome, in which adrenal enlargement is present in 70% of cases.[189] However, in our experience, the adrenal glands in Cushing's disease are smaller and usually are symmetrically enlarged with an occasional nodule, as opposed to large or huge glands with definite nodules in AIMAH. In addition, the two can usually be differentiated by the ACTH level, although some patients with the macronodular subset of Cushing's disease can develop a degree of adrenal autonomy that can cause biochemical confusion.[190] Occasionally, confusion also may arise with apparent unilateral adrenal lesions, when the biochemistry is consistent with an ACTH-dependent cause; we generally would rely on the biochemistry in this situation and would examine the contralateral gland to see whether it is hyperplastic.

Differentiating Between Adrenocorticotropic Hormone–Dependent Causes of Cushing's Syndrome

Although some patients with ectopic ACTH secretion, usually those with overt tumors, have extremely elevated values of plasma ACTH (>100 ng/L [>20 pmol/L]), complete overlap is seen between values in occult ectopic ACTH secretion and in Cushing's disease.[191] Therefore, ACTH values alone cannot differentiate reliably the ACTH-dependent forms of Cushing's syndrome.

The ACTH-dependent forms of Cushing's syndrome present the greatest diagnostic challenge. Cushing's disease accounts for by far the majority of cases of ACTH-dependent Cushing's syndrome—overall approximately 80% to 90% in most series. This percentage is gender dependent and is higher in women than in men,[192] although in prepubertal childhood, an anomalous 80% male preponderance is noted. Therefore, even before one starts further investigation, the pretest probability that the patient has Cushing's disease is very high, and any investigation must improve on this. The specificity of any test should be as close to 100% as possible for the diagnosis of Cushing's disease, to avoid inappropriate pituitary surgery in patients with ectopic ACTH production. A variety of functional tests of the HPA axis have been developed to take advantage of the differences in pathophysiology between ACTH-dependent causes of Cushing's syndrome. Some of these investigations have evolved, and others have fallen by the wayside.

Bilateral Inferior Petrosal Sinus Sampling

Bilateral inferior petrosal sinus sampling (BIPSS) is the best test for distinguishing ACTH-dependent forms of Cushing's syndrome, as long as the patient has active hypercortisolemia, which should be confirmed at the time of the procedure.[193,194] The test exploits the normal venous drainage of each half of the pituitary gland via the cavernous sinus into the corresponding petrosal sinus. Each petrosal sinus is catheterized separately via a femoral approach, and blood for measurement of ACTH is obtained simultaneously from each sinus and a peripheral vein at two timepoints before and at 3 to 5 minutes and possibly also 10 minutes after the administration of ovine or human CRH (Ferring) (1 µg/kg or 100 µg intravenously)[195] (Fig. 16-9). Where CRH is unavailable for whatever reason, recent data suggest that 10 µg desmopessin may be a suitable alternative.

ACTH concentrations are greater in the central samples in Cushing's disease and increase after CRH administration, reflecting ACTH secretion by the corticotroph adenoma. In contrast, ACTH values in the central and peripheral specimens are similar in ectopic ACTH secretion and do not increase after CRH. A ratio

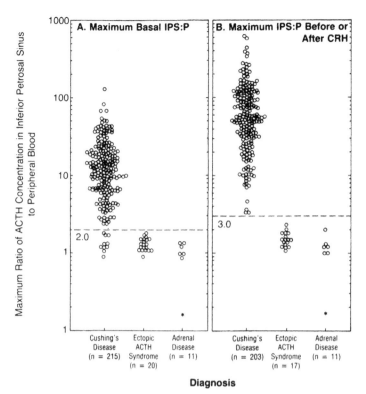

FIGURE 16-9. Maximal ratio of adrenocorticotropic hormone (ACTH) concentration in the inferior petrosal sinus to peripheral blood in patients with confirmed Cushing's disease, ectopic ACTH syndrome, or adrenal disease before corticotropin-releasing hormone (CRH) **(A)** or at any time before or after CRH administration **(B)**. A ratio of 3.0 had 100% sensitivity and specificity. (Data from Oldfield EH, Doppman JL, Nieman LK, et al: Petrosal sinus sampling with and without corticotropin-releasing hormone for the differential diagnosis of Cushing's syndrome. N Engl J Med 325:897–905, 1991.)

of central (i.e., petrosal) to peripheral ACTH values is calculated. In earlier series, pre-CRH ratios greater than 2 or post-CRH ratios greater than 3 were 100% specific for Cushing's disease,[196,197] but a small number of false positives have been reported in later series.[198,199] The sensitivity of the test is improved after CRH; however, false negatives still occur in about 6% of patients with Cushing's disease. False positives in ectopic ACTH are extremely rare.

It should be remembered that the technique is highly specialized, and allied with this are a number of important points. First, both petrosal sinuses must be cannulated adequately and catheter placement confirmed before and after sampling.[200] Second, the radiologist must confirm the venous anatomy because anomalous venous drainage can give false-negative results. Preliminary data have suggested that simultaneous measurement of prolactin can be used as an index of pituitary venous drainage, and prolactin should be measured when results indicate a noncentral source of ACTH.[201] Third, the procedure carries a small risk of complications. Transient ear discomfort or pain can occur, as can local groin hematomas. More serious transient and permanent neurologic sequelae, including brain stem infarction, have been reported, although these are rare (<1%), and most have been related to the particular type of catheter used[202,203]; if any early warning signs of such events are observed, the procedure should be halted immediately. Patients should be given heparin during sampling to prevent thrombotic events.[129] CRH itself generally is tolerated well, although patients may experience brief facial flushing and a metallic taste in the mouth. One case of CRH induced pituitary apoplexy in a patient with Cushing's disease has been reported.[204]

Another potential advantage of BIPSS involves lateralizing microadenomas within the pituitary using the inferior petrosal sinus ACTH gradient, with a basal or post-CRH intersinus ratio of at least 1.4 being the criterion used for lateralization in all large studies.[196,197,205,206] In these studies, the diagnostic accuracy of localization as assessed by operative outcome varied between 59% and 83%. This is improved if venous drainage is assessed to be symmetric.[207] Some discrepancy has been noted between studies as to whether CRH improves the predictive value of the test.[208] If a reversal of lateralization is seen pre- and post-CRH, the test cannot be relied upon.[209] Sampling of the internal jugular veins is a simpler procedure but is not as sensitive as BIPSS.[210] However, it may be a useful technique in less experienced centers, with the caveat that patients with negative results then are referred for BIPSS.[211] In our opinion, sampling from the cavernous sinus itself offers no great advantage.

High-Dose Dexamethasone Suppression Test

The original high-dose dexamethasone suppression test (HDDST) was described in the same paper as the 48-hour LDDST; 2 mg dexamethasone is used in place of 0.5 mg, with a 50% reduction in urinary 17-OHCS shown to differentiate 96% of patients with Cushing's disease rather than adrenal tumors.[155] The role of the HDDST in the differential diagnosis of ACTH-dependent Cushing's syndrome is based on the same premise, that is, that most pituitary corticotroph tumors retain some responsiveness (albeit reduced) to negative glucocorticoid feedback on ACTH secretion, whereas ectopic ACTH-secreting tumors, like adrenal tumors, typically do not. Measurement of UFC or plasma/serum cortisol has superseded that of urinary 17-OHCS, and an overnight test has been advocated, with a single dose of 8 mg dexamethasone given at 11:00 PM, and with the criterion of a 50% reduction in plasma cortisol levels on the morning after administration.[212] Despite evidence that only about 80% of patients with Cushing's disease will show suppression of plasma cortisol to less than 50% of the basal value, and large numbers of patients with ectopic Cushing's syndrome have false-positive results (≈30%),[60,213] the HDDST is still used widely. Some data suggest that that suppression to HDDST can be inferred by a greater than 30% suppression of serum cortisol to the 2 day LDDST (Fig. 16-10); therefore, in centers that use this form of the LDDST, the HDDST may not confer any extra information.[159] It should not be forgotten that patients are receiving large doses of glucocorticoids, in addition to their high endogenous cortisol production, and one should be alert for the precipitation of psychosis and/or worsening of glycemic control or other complications.

Corticotropin-Releasing Hormone Stimulation Test

The use of CRH stimulation for the differential diagnosis of ACTH-dependent Cushing's syndrome is based on two assumptions: (1) that corticotropinomas retain responsivity to CRH, whereas noncorticotroph tumors lack CRH receptors and cannot respond to the agent; and (2) that hypercortisolism has been sufficient to inhibit the normal corticotroph response. Indeed, most patients with Cushing's disease respond to CRH, either 1 μg/kg or 100 μg intravenous synthetic ovine or human sequence CRH, with increases in plasma ACTH or cortisol, and patients with ectopic ACTH secretion typically do not.[214-216] Human sequence CRH has qualitatively similar properties to ovine CRH, although it is shorter acting with a slightly smaller

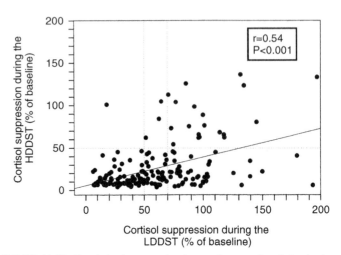

FIGURE 16-10. Correlation between the degree of suppression during the low-dose dexamethasone suppression test (LDDST) and during the high-dose dexamethasone suppression test (HDDST) in 185 patients with Cushing's disease. (Reproduced with permission from Isidori AM, Kaltsas GA, Mohammed S, et al: Discriminatory value of the low-dose dexamethasone suppression test in establishing the diagnosis and differential diagnosis of Cushing's syndrome. J Clin Endocrinol Metab 88:5299–5306, 2003. Copyright © 2003, The Endocrine Society.)

increase in plasma cortisol and ACTH in normal and obese patients and in those with Cushing's disease[217]; this may be related to the more rapid clearance of the human sequence by endogenous CRH-binding protein.[218] Availability differs worldwide, with ovine CRH predominant in North America but human CRH elsewhere.

Because different centers have used differing protocols, including different types of CRH and different sampling timepoints, little consensus has been reached on a universal criterion for interpreting the test. However, where the test has been validated in experienced centers, the diagnostic utility appears similar. For instance, in the largest published series of the use of ovine CRH in ACTH-dependent Cushing's syndrome, an increase in ACTH of at least 35% from a mean basal (5 minutes and 1 minute) to a mean of 15 and 30 minutes after ovine CRH in 100 patients with Cushing's disease and in 16 patients with ectopic ACTH syndrome (Fig. 16-11) gave the test a sensitivity of 93% for diagnosing Cushing's disease and 100% specificity. The best cortisol criterion was an increase of at least 20% at a mean of 30 and 45 minutes, revealing a sensitivity of 91% and a specificity of 88%.[219] Similarly, in the largest series involving use of the human CRH test in 101 patients with Cushing's disease and in 14 with ectopic ACTH syndrome, the best criterion used to differentiate Cushing's disease from ectopic ACTH syndrome was an increase in cortisol of at least 14% from a mean basal (15 and 0 minutes) to a mean of 15 and 30 minutes, yielding a sensitivity of 85% and a specificity of 100% (Fig. 16-12). In contrast, the best ACTH response was a maximal increase of at least 105%, indicating 70% sensitivity and 100% specificity.[192] The CRH test is a useful discriminator between causes of ACTH-dependent Cushing's syndrome; however, which cutoff to use must be evaluated at individual centers, and caution should be exercised because undoubtedly there will be patients with ectopic ACTH syndrome who respond outside these cutoffs. However, an increase in cortisol outside the normal range can differentiate Cushing's disease from normality, albeit in only approximately 50% of cases, and, as noted previously, the measurement of plasma ACTH in the test can help to discriminate ACTH-

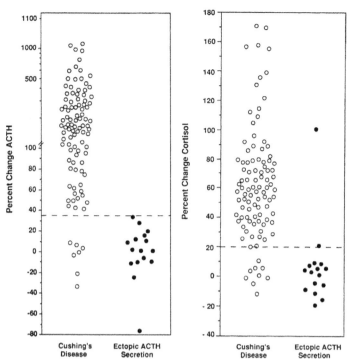

FIGURE 16-11. Response of adrenocorticotropic hormone (ACTH) and cortisol to ovine corticotropin-releasing hormone in patients with Cushing's disease and ectopic ACTH secretion. ACTH responses are expressed as the percentage of change in mean concentration 15 and 30 minutes after ovine corticotropin-releasing hormone from the mean basal value 1 and 5 minutes before the injection. The *dashed line* indicates a response of 35%, representing a diagnostic criterion with 100% specificity and 93% sensitivity. Cortisol responses are expressed as percentage of change in mean cortisol concentration 30 and 45 minutes after ovine corticotropin-releasing hormone from the mean basal value 1 and 5 minutes before the injection. The *dashed line* indicates a response of 20%, representing a diagnostic criterion with 88% specificity and 91% sensitivity. (Data from Nieman LK, Oldfield EH, Wesley R, et al: A simplified morning ovine corticotropin-releasing hormone stimulation test for the differential diagnosis of ACTH-dependent Cushing syndrome. J Clin Endocrinol Metab 77:1308–1312, 1993.)

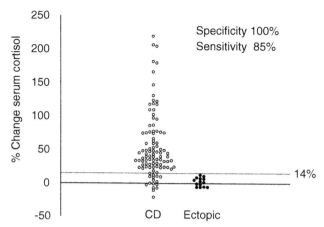

FIGURE 16-12. Percentage change in serum cortisol from a mean basal at 15 and 0 minutes to a mean value calculated from the levels at 15 and 30 minutes after the administration of human corticotropin-releasing hormone (100 mg intravenously) in 100 patients with Cushing's disease (CD) and 14 patients with ectopic adrenocorticotropic hormone syndrome. (Reproduced with permission from Newll-Price J, Morris DG, Drake WM, et al: Optimal response criteria for the human CRH test in the differential diagnosis of ACTH-dependent Cushing's syndrome. J Clin Endocrinol Metab 87:1640–1645, 2002.)

dependent from ACTH-independent causes of Cushing's syndrome when basal levels of ACTH are equivocal. We therefore believe that this test plays a useful role in the investigation of patients with Cushing's syndrome.

Other Stimulation Tests

Vasopressin and desmopressin (a synthetic long-acting vasopressin analogue without V1-mediated pressor effects) are thought to stimulate ACTH release in Cushing's disease through the corticotroph-specific V3 (or V1b) receptor. Hexarelin (a growth hormone secretagogue) also stimulates ACTH release to a sevenfold greater extent than human CRH; although the mechanism has not been entirely elucidated, this probably occurs through stimulation of vasopressin release in normal subjects,[220] and through stimulation of aberrant growth hormone secretagogue receptors in patients with corticotroph tumors.[221] These peptides all have been used in a similar manner to CRH, to try to improve the differentiation of ACTH-dependent Cushing's syndrome, but they generally have proved inferior or of no advantage.[222-225] However, desmopressin may be useful in centers where CRH is unavailable. A combined desmopressin (10 μg) and human CRH (100 μg) test initially looked extremely promising.[226] However, a later study of this combined test in 26 patients with Cushing's disease and 5 patients with ectopic ACTH syndrome showed significant overlap in responses.[227] The disappointing discrimi-

natory outcome of these stimulants is undoubtedly due to the expression of both vasopressin and growth hormone secretagogue receptors by some ectopic ACTH-secreting tumors.[129,228]

Measurement of marker peptides, such as calcitonin, gastrin, 5-hydroxyindoleacetic acid, serotonin, and catecholamines or their metabolites, may help to identify a neuroendocrine tumor.

Combined Test Strategies

Because none of the noninvasive tests have 100% diagnostic accuracy, a number of investigators have evaluated the utility of combined test strategies. The CRH and the HDDST have been paired in this way, and combined, they have a diagnostic accuracy greater than that of either test alone, yielding 98% to 100% sensitivity and 88% to 100% specificity.[229-231] Similar high accuracy has been obtained by combining the results of the LDDST and the CRH test.[159]

Imaging of the Adrenocorticotropin Hormone Source

Pituitary MRI imaging before and after gadolinium enhancement should be performed in all patients with ACTH-dependent Cushing's syndrome via T_1-weighted spin echo and/or spoiled gradient recalled acquisition (SPGR) techniques. These will identify an adenoma in up to 80% of patients with Cushing's disease,[60,232,233] and in approximately 10% of normal individuals.[234] Most adenomas (95%) exhibit a hypointense signal with no postgadolinium enhancement, and the remaining 5% show an isointense signal post gadolinium enhancement.[235] CT imaging typically shows a hypodense lesion that fails to enhance post contrast but is less sensitive than MRI in detecting small (<5 mm) adenomas and is not recommended for this reason.[60,236]

Imaging is the most helpful way to identify the source of ectopic ACTH production. Given the likely sites of tumors, CT and/or MRI of the neck, chest, and abdomen should be obtained. The most common source is a bronchial carcinoid tumor, but small (<1 cm) lesions often can prove difficult to locate. Fine-cut high-resolution CT scanning with both supine and prone images can help differentiate between tumors and vascular shadows.[55] MRI can identify chest lesions that are not evident on CT scanning and that characteristically show a high signal on T_2-weighted and short-inversion time inversion recovery (STIR) images.[237] Additionally, pheochromocytomas are bright on T_2-weighted MRI. CT-guided aspiration of masses for measurement of ACTH may provide useful functional information.[238]

Because most ectopic ACTH-secreting tumors are of neuroendocrine origin and therefore may express somatostatin receptor subtypes, radiolabeled somatostatin analogue (^{111}In-pentetreotide) scintigraphy may be useful to show functionality of identified tumors, and sporadic reports have indicated that it identifies lesions not apparent on conventional imaging.[239-241] However, in most patients, including a recent series of 35 patients with ectopic ACTH secretion, ^{111}In-pentetreotide scintigraphy was not able to detect tumors when the MRI or CT scan was negative, and significant numbers of false-positive scans resulted.[242] Thus, CT and MRI represent the best initial screening examinations, but scintigraphy may be a useful adjunctive imaging modality to help confirm abnormalities seen on CT or MRI. 18-Flurodeoxyglucose positron-emission tomography (PET) generally does not offer any advantage over conventional CT or MRI unless the tumors are metabolically active,[243] which is not usually the case.[244] However, ^{67}Ga-octreotate PET scintigraphy may show advantages over ^{111}In-pentetreotide scintigraphy.[245]

Strategy for Diagnosis and Differential Diagnosis of Cushing's Syndrome

After an international workshop in 2002, a consensus statement was published for the diagnosis and differential diagnosis of Cushing's syndrome.[129] Most of its recommendations are still valid. We would advocate that three 24-hour UFC, late-night salivary cortisols and/or the LDDST should be used as first-line screening tests. (This approach also was advocated in a recent guidelines statement issued by the Endocrine Society.[134]) False-positive results will be common, and second-line tests should be used as necessary for confirmation. Once the diagnosis of Cushing's syndrome is unequivocal, ACTH levels, the CRH test, and a dexamethasone suppression test, together with appropriate imaging, are the most useful noninvasive investigations to determine the cause. Bilateral inferior petrosal sinus sampling is recommended in cases of ACTH-dependent Cushing's syndrome in which the clinical, biochemical, or radiologic results are discordant or equivocal, although others would recommend its use in almost all cases of ACTH-dependent Cushing's syndrome.

TREATMENT

Optimal treatment for Cushing's syndrome renders the patient eucortisolemic with minimal morbidity and mortality. With the advent of synthetic glucocorticoid therapy, adrenalectomy became the treatment of choice because it conferred rapid and, in most cases, permanent resolution of Cushing's syndrome.[246] Improvements in neurosurgical techniques and appreciation of the sources of ectopic ACTH secretion have changed the therapeutic approach to Cushing's syndrome, so that surgery now is directed toward resection of abnormal tissue, whether ACTH or cortisol producing. In patients with only mild hypercortisolemia and subclinical disease, the benefits of surgical treatment have not been proved.[247] The optimal surgical approach cannot be realized if the patient is unable to safely undergo surgery, or if the tumor is occult or metastatic. Other second-line therapies that are less specific and that may have greater morbidity must be chosen in these settings. In 2007, an international meeting of endocrinologists outlined a consensus statement on the treatment of ACTH-dependent Cushing's syndrome.[248]

SURGERY

Preoperative Evaluation and Treatment

Some centers use routine preoperative medical adrenal blockade to attain a period of eucortisolemia for 4 to 6 weeks before surgery. The aim is to allow reversal of some of the metabolic and catabolic effects of the hypercortisolemia that may inhibit wound healing and cause other complications in the perioperative period. The disadvantage of this strategy is that the normal corticotrope may be disinhibited by the time of surgery, so that expected hypocortisolism after successful tumor resection does not occur, and this index of remission is not reliable. This rationale is only empirical, and a randomized trial undertaken to see whether this approach improves outcome would be welcomed.[249]

Because Cushing's syndrome is a prothrombotic state, anticoagulant prophylaxis should be considered perioperatively.[250] The lipid abnormalities, hypertension, and diabetes common in Cushing's syndrome predispose these patients to atherosclerotic cardiac disease and should be treated by conventional approaches.

Transsphenoidal Resection of Corticotropinoma

Transsphenoidal resection is regarded as the treatment of choice in Cushing's disease.[248] The procedure usually is performed via a gingival approach, as originally devised by Kanavel and Halsted and later popularized by Cushing.[251] The development of the operating microscope led to the introduction of transsphenoidal resection of pituitary microadenomas by Hardy in 1968. Additional advances have been made over the past decade with the use of rigid endoscopes and more recently flexible endoscopes. The goal of surgery is a selective adenomectomy and thus preservation of as much normal pituitary tissue as possible; the procedure should be performed by a neurosurgeon who is experienced in transsphenoidal surgery. Most large series report immediate remission rates of approximately 70% to 90%,[252-259] with lower rates noted for macroadenomas.[254,260] These reports use variable remission criteria that include normal postoperative cortisol levels, normal UFC levels, and/or a normal response to an LDDST, associated with clinical resolution of the disease. Data are insufficient regarding whether endoscopic surgery offers any benefit.[261] However, a recent report suggests that resection achieved through a technique that enucleates microadenomas via their pseudocapsule may improve remission rates to 98%.[262]

Long-term recurrence rates are as high as 20% by 10 years after surgery. Thus, in reality, transsphenoidal surgery achieves long-term cure even in the best of hands in only approximately 60% to 80% of adult patients, and therefore is somewhat disappointing; the data emphasize the need for long-term endocrinologic follow-up of these patients.[263] Favorable indicators of long-term remission are patients older than 25 years, a microadenoma detected by MRI, lack of invasion of the dura or cavernous sinus, histologic confirmation of an ACTH-secreting tumor, low postoperative cortisol levels, and long-lasting adrenal insufficiency.[248] If a tumor cannot be identified at surgery, hemihypophysectomy on the side of the gland with an ACTH gradient on petrosal sinus sampling is usually the best way to proceed, and in some series, this yields better results than those attained by selective microadenomectomy.[256,264]

The mortality associated with transsphenoidal surgery is approximately 1% to 2%.[11,258] Transient diabetes insipidus is probably the most common complication, being reported in as many as 28% of patients.[264] Other perioperative complications, including cerebrospinal fluid leak, meningitis, and profuse bleeding, occur in less than 10% of patients. Permanent complications such as persistent diabetes insipidus and injury to the optic nerve or nerves of the cavernous sinus (causing ptosis or diplopia) occur much less frequently.[11,258] However, hypopituitarism, particularly growth hormone deficiency, is common (53% to 59%), with other anterior hormone deficits occurring in approximately 35% to 45% of patients.[264,265] Such complications are more common after resection of larger tumors or with the presence of larger amounts of normal pituitary tissue (or stalk), or after repeat surgery.

Postoperative Evaluation and Management

Patients typically receive supraphysiologic doses of glucocorticoids to cover transsphenoidal surgery at initial daily doses of as high as 400 mg hydrocortisone (4 mg dexamethasone), tapering off within 1 to 3 days. Morning (9:00 AM) serum cortisol measurements then are obtained for 3 days, starting 24 hours after the last glucocorticoid administration, during which time the patient should be observed for development of signs of adrenal insufficiency. This approach allows prompt classification of likely cure, normocortisolemia, or persistent hypercortisolism. Where close perioperative supervision is possible, such glucocorticoid "cover" may be omitted, permitting a very early postoperative assessment of cure. What defines apparent cure or remission after transsphenoidal surgery is still debated. Postoperative hypocortisolemia (<1.8 μg/dL [50 nmol/L] at 9:00 AM) is probably the best indicator of the likelihood of long-term remission. However, detectable cortisol levels of <5 μg/dL (140 nmol/L) are also compatible with sustained remission.[266,267] Higher postoperative cortisol levels are more likely to be associated with failed surgery; however, cortisol levels sometimes may decline gradually over 4 to 6 weeks, reflecting gradual infarction of remnant tumor or some degree of adrenal semiautonomy. Persistent cortisol levels >5 μg/dL (140 nmol/L) 6 weeks after surgery require further investigation.

Dynamic tests have been used to predict long-term remission. The cortisol and ACTH response to CRH in the early postoperative period may provide a useful index of the risk for recurrence of Cushing's disease, the rationale being that responsiveness may indicate residual tumor.[60,268] A study of postoperative responses to CRH in 221 patients suggested that a cortisol response greater than 5 μg/dL (138 nmol/L) at 60 minutes had a positive predictive value of 42% and a negative predictive value of 94% for recurrence of disease.[269] Because patients with partial recovery of the axis would be expected to have a normal response, regardless of the risk for recurrence, the CRH test cannot be interpreted and should not be used in this setting. Some evidence suggests that persistence of the ACTH response to desmopressin postoperatively probably is linked to a higher rate of relapse.[270,271]

Patients who are hypocortisolemic should be started on glucocorticoid replacement, and 15 to 30 mg hydrocortisone (12 to 15 mg/m²) in two to three divided doses is the preferred choice. The first dose (usually half to two thirds of the total dose) should be taken before getting out of bed, and the last dose should be taken no later than 6:00 PM, because later administration of glucocorticoids may result in disordered sleep. In this situation, the lowest possible dose of hydrocortisone should be used to avoid long-term suppression of the HPA axis. All patients receiving long-term glucocorticoid replacement therapy should be instructed that they are "dependent" on taking glucocorticoids as prescribed, and that failure to take or absorb the medication will lead to adrenal crisis and possibly death. They should be prescribed a 100 mg hydrocortisone (or other high-dose

glucocorticoid) intramuscular injection pack for emergency use. They also should obtain a medical information bracelet or necklace that identifies this requirement (Medic Alert Foundation). Education should stress the effects of glucocorticoid withdrawal[272]; the need for compliance with the daily dose of glucocorticoid; the need to double the oral dose for nausea, diarrhea, and fever; and the need for parenteral administration and medical evaluation during emesis, trauma, or severe medical stress.

The patient should be told to expect desquamation of the skin and flu-like symptoms (malaise, joint aching, anorexia, and nausea) during the postoperative months, and that these are signs that indicate remission: some of these symptoms have been related to high levels of circulating interleukin-6.[273] Most patients tolerate these symptoms of glucocorticoid withdrawal much better if they are forewarned and alerted to their positive nature. Physicians should not increase the glucocorticoid dose in the absence of intercurrent illness based on these symptoms alone but should seek signs of adrenal insufficiency, such as vomiting, electrolyte abnormalities, and postural hypotension.[274] The affective and cognitive changes associated with Cushing's syndrome are particularly slow to resolve and may not normalize. Evidence of persisting physical and emotional dysfunction has been found, even after prolonged duration of cure.[275] Postoperatively, assessment for deficiencies of other pituitary hormones should be sought, and the appropriate replacement regimen initiated as necessary.

Diuresis is common after transsphenoidal surgery and may result from intraoperative or glucocorticoid-induced fluid overload or may be due to diabetes insipidus. For these reasons, assessment of paired serum and urine osmolality and the serum sodium concentration is essential. It is advisable to withhold specific therapy unless the serum osmolality is greater than 295 mOsm/kg, the serum sodium is greater than 145 mmol/L, and the urine output is greater than 200 mL/hr, with an inappropriately low urine osmolality. Desmopressin (DDAVP, Ferring) 1 μg given subcutaneously, will provide adequate vasopressin replacement for 12 hours or longer. Hyponatremia may occur in as many as 20% of patients within 10 days of surgery. This may be due to injudicious fluid replacement or inappropriate antidiuretic hormone secretion, as is frequently seen after extensive gland exploration, and fluid intake should be restricted.[276] A small minority of patients proceed to (apparently) permanent diabetes insipidus, requiring long-term treatment with a vasopressin analogue. A dose and schedule of administration should be chosen to provide unbroken sleep but allowing a period of "breakthrough" urination each day. This goal is often achieved when 10 to 20 μg desmopressin is given intranasally (or an equivalent oral dose) in the evening.

Some glucocorticoid-induced abnormalities, including hypokalemia, hypertension, and glucose intolerance, may be normalized during the postoperative period, so that preoperative treatments for these need to reassessed. Some evidence indicates that deficits in bone mass may be partially reversed after treatment of hypercortisolemia.[277,278] Bisphosphonate treatment may induce a more rapid improvement in bone mineral density[279] and should be considered (along with calcium and vitamin D supplements) in patients with osteoporosis.

Persistent hypercortisolemia after transsphenoidal exploration should prompt reevaluation of the diagnosis of Cushing's disease, especially if previous diagnostic test results were indeterminate or conflicting, or if no tumor was found on pathologic examination. Petrosal sinus sampling after transsphenoidal surgery can confirm a pituitary source of ACTH, but the rate of correct lateralization decreases, probably because of alterations in venous anatomy caused by the previous surgery; therefore, the procedure cannot be used routinely to direct a second operative search or decision for hemihypophysectomy.

Treatment options for patients with persistent Cushing's disease include repeat surgery, radiation therapy, and adrenalectomy. If immediate surgical remission is not achieved at the first exploration, early repeat transsphenoidal surgery may be worthwhile in a significant proportion of patients, at the expense of increased likelihood of hypopituitarism.[280,281] The likelihood of remission after repeat surgery is greatest when some or all of the following outcome parameters are present: The diagnosis is correct, as evidenced by previous curative surgery with pathologic confirmation of an ACTH-staining adenoma; the initial exposure or resection was incomplete; or residual tumor is seen on MRI scan without evidence of cavernous sinus invasion. Repeat sellar exploration is less likely to be helpful in patients with empty sella syndrome or very little pituitary tissue on MRI scans. Patients with cavernous sinus or dural invasion identified at the initial procedure are not candidates for repeat surgery to treat hypercortisolism and should receive radiation therapy.

Recovery of the HPA axis can be monitored by measurement of 9:00 AM serum cortisol after omission of hydrocortisone replacement. Because recovery after transsphenoidal surgery rarely occurs before 3 to 6 months and is common at 1 year, initial testing at 6 to 9 months is cost-effective.[282] If the cortisol is undetectable on 2 consecutive days, then recovery of the axis has not occurred, and glucocorticoid replacement can be restarted. If the cortisol is measurable, adequate reserve of the HPA axis can be assessed with the insulin tolerance test,[283] with a peak cortisol value of >18 μg/dL (500 nmol/L), indicating adequate reserve on modern assays.[284] Many centers use the cortisol response to 250 μg synthetic (1-24) ACTH as an alternative means of assessing HPA reserve,[285,286] but some controversy regarding its reliability in this situation has been ongoing.[287,288] If it is used instead of the insulin tolerance test, a 30 minute cortisol of 22 μg/dL (600 nmol/L) is probably more reliable than the traditional cutoff of 18 μg/dL (500 nmol).[284] Glucocorticoid replacement can be discontinued abruptly if the cortisol response is shown to be normal.

Where recovery of the HPA axis is only partial on dynamic testing, but the 9:00 AM cortisol levels are above the lower limit of the normal range (7 μg/dL [200 nmol/L]), it is reasonable to reduce the hydrocortisone unless symptoms of adrenal insufficiency occur. Patients must continue to be aware of the continuing need for additional glucocorticoids at times of stress or illness and should be given a supply of oral hydrocortisone and an intramuscular injection pack. For patients with detectable but low 9:00 AM cortisol levels, the hydrocortisone replacement dose should be adjusted down if weight loss has occurred, and a slightly lower dose may be given. Some centers assess adequate replacement of thrice daily hydrocortisone dosing by measuring serum cortisol at various points throughout the day, ensuring that levels are always sufficient (>1.8 μg/dL; 50 nmol/L) before each dose; this may mean that peak levels after each dose appear to be unphysiologic, but there is a tradeoff between mirroring a normal physiologic rhythm as far as possible and the inconvenience of multiple dosing.

Two late but unrelated conundrums may arise: the questions of recurrence and permanent lack of recovery of the axis. Patients who articulate that Cushing's syndrome has returned are often correct, even before physical and biochemical evidence is unequivocal. Assessment is warranted in a patient with these complaints or with recurrent physical signs characteristic of the hypercortisolemic phase. If this is to be done on an outpatient basis, UFC can be measured initially on dexamethasone 0.5 mg/day, if not yet weaned from glucocorticoids. Measurement of late-night salivary cortisol after omission of the afternoon dose of hydrocortisone also may be useful. However, ideally, assessment of a cortisol circadian rhythm can be done on an inpatient basis after the hydrocortisone has been stopped completely. If the UFC result is increased, evaluation of hypercortisolism should proceed. If recurrent Cushing's disease is diagnosed, the therapeutic options are the same as for persistent disease. It should be remembered when investigating recurrence that longstanding ACTH stimulation by a pituitary adenoma causing macronodular adrenal hyperplasia subsequently may involve autonomous cortisol production.[289]

If the UFC result is subnormal or low, the patient should be questioned about the actual dose of glucocorticoid that has been taken. Often, patients take additional hydrocortisone, either because they discover that this decreases the symptoms of glucocorticoid withdrawal, or because they have increased the dose "for stress," often without following strict guidelines. These patients have a suppressed axis and a very slow regression of cushingoid features because of exogenous hypercortisolism. They require education and support along with reduction in the daily dose of hydrocortisone to recommended levels. The patient who has a subnormal cortisol response to ACTH 2 years after transsphenoidal surgery (in the absence of overreplacement) may proceed to life-long ACTH deficiency.

Adrenalectomy

Resection of the affected adrenal gland(s) is the treatment of choice only for non–ACTH-dependent hypercortisolism of adrenal origin, or when a specific surgical approach to ACTH-dependent causes is not feasible. In adrenal adenomas, the cure rate is 100% when performed by experienced adrenal surgeons.[290] Surgery is the mainstay of treatment for adrenal cancer; more aggressive surgical approaches probably account for the increase in life span reported in this disease.[85,291] This approach may require multiple operations to resect primary lesions, local recurrences, and hepatic, thoracic, and, occasionally, intracranial metastases. Adjuvant medical treatment with mitotane and other chemotherapeutic agents is discussed later.

The mortality and morbidity of traditional open adrenalectomy via an anterior or posterior incision range from 1% to 20% in various series, probably reflecting differences in the severity of Cushing's syndrome and the presence of associated conditions, such as cardiovascular disease.[184,246] Apart from resection of suspected carcinoma, these approaches have been supplanted by laparoscopic resection, which has low mortality and morbidity when done by an experienced surgeon.[292] Glands as large as 7.5 cm may be removed through this approach[293] (see Chapter 15). Serum cortisol levels become undetectable after successful adrenalectomy. Early failure to achieve hypocortisolism usually is related to incomplete resection of the gland(s). Recurrence, especially in the ACTH-dependent forms of Cushing's syndrome, may be related to regrowth of adrenal cells in the surgical bed, or to growth of adrenal rest tissue.

Bilateral adrenalectomy as a second line of treatment for Cushing's disease has the advantage of providing rapid resolution of hypercortisolism and has no risk of hypopituitarism, in contrast to radiation therapy. Adrenalectomy may be chosen over radiation therapy by young patients who desire fertility, who have concerns about radiation-induced hypopituitarism and loss of reproductive function. Its disadvantages include perioperative morbidity and mortality and the life-long requirement of glucocorticoid and mineralocorticoid replacement therapy. In addition, patients with Cushing's disease have a risk for developing Nelson's syndrome, which may occur more frequently if adrenalectomy is performed at a younger age, and if a pituitary adenoma is confirmed at previous pituitary surgery.[259,294] Regular pituitary MRI and monitoring of ACTH levels are mandatory in these patients.[295] Prophylactic pituitary radiotherapy appears to reduce the risk for developing Nelson's syndrome from 50% to 25%,[296] but no consensus has been reached on this topic.

In the postoperative period after bilateral adrenalectomy, the hydrocortisone dose is maintained at approximately twice the replacement dose, and saline 0.9% is given intravenously until the patient can take oral medications. This provides sodium and sufficient mineralocorticoid activity until fludrocortisone 100 μg/day can be given by mouth. Serum cortisol measurement done to confirm adequacy of resection is assessed while the patient receives dexamethasone 0.5 mg/day and fludrocortisone. The patient then is switched back to hydrocortisone and fludrocortisone and must be advised regarding adrenal insufficiency, as previously discussed. The dose of fludrocortisone is adjusted according to the patient's blood pressure, exposure to heat, and salt intake; the usual dose is 100 μg/day but ranges from 50 to 400 μg. A normal plasma renin activity measurement provides evidence of adequate mineralocorticoid replacement and can be used to gauge therapy.

After unilateral adrenalectomy, the components of the HPA axis gradually recover after surgical cure of Cushing's syndrome. The time to recovery may be as short as 3 months and as long as 2 years.[268,282] The duration of recovery may be shorter in patients with mild hypercortisolism and in those with recurrence, and longer after resection of an adrenal adenoma.

Surgery for Ectopic Adrenocorticotropic Hormone Syndrome

If an ectopic ACTH-secreting tumor is localized and amenable to surgical excision, such as in a lobectomy for a bronchial carcinoid tumor, the chance for cure of Cushing's syndrome is high. However, if significant metastatic disease is present, surgery is unlikely to be of benefit. If the source of ACTH cannot be localized, or if metastatic disease precludes surgery, alternative treatment for hypercortisolism must be chosen. For the patient with occult disease, medical therapy allows interval tumor surveillance with the goal of eventual tumor resection. Because some tumors remain occult for as long as 20 years, this may not prove practical for all patients, and adrenalectomy is appropriate when the patient cannot tolerate the cost, medical side effects, or psychological effects of long-term medical therapy and monitoring. Long-term medical therapy also may be the treatment of choice for the patient with widely disseminated disease who is not a good surgical candidate for adrenalectomy. Bilateral adrenalectomy is the treatment of choice for any patient requiring rapid correction of hypercortisolism or when hypercortisolism cannot be controlled with medical therapy, when previously effective medical therapy must be discontinued because of significant medical side effects or intolerance, or when a severely hypercortisolemic patient is unable to take oral medications or etomidate.

RADIOTHERAPY

Pituitary

The role of radiation therapy to the pituitary gland in Cushing's disease is usually adjunctive in those who have failed transsphenoidal surgery, but it is also a good primary option for patients who cannot undergo surgery, and for those having a bilateral adrenalectomy for whom the risk for Nelson's syndrome is deemed great.

Conventional Radiotherapy

Conventional pituitary radiotherapy is delivered at a total dose of 4500 to 5000 cGy (rad) in 25 fractional doses over 35 days through a three-field (opposed lateral fields and vertex field) technique. Nowadays, this usually is based on stereotactic conformal field planning to optimize the tumor dose and to minimize radiation to other areas. This approach ensures that the daily dose to neural tissue does not exceed 180 cGy and avoids the complications of optic neuritis and cortical necrosis associated with larger total and fractional doses.[297] The latent onset of action of radiotherapy means that adjunctive medical therapy usually is instituted before or at the time of treatment. The therapeutic response is assessed at least with annual monitoring, with weaning of medical treatment if possible. When conventional radiotherapy is used as primary treatment for Cushing's disease, remission is achieved in only 40% to 60% of adult patients.[259,298-300] The response is even worse if a lower dose of radiation (2000 cGy) is used.[301] More usually, conventional radiotherapy is used in the setting of failure to cure after transsphenoidal surgery. In this regard, it performs rather better, with reported remission rates as high as 83%.[299,302] After conventional radiotherapy is given, remission usually starts by 9 months after treatment, and most patients are in remission within 2 years, although this can take much longer.[303]

Hypopituitarism is the most common side effect of pituitary radiotherapy, with growth hormone deficiency occurring in 36% to 68% of treated adults.[265,302] Gonadotropin and thyroid-stimulating hormone deficiency is seen less commonly. The risk for optic neuropathy is low and probably is less than 1% as long as low-dose fractions are used[304] (200 cGy). Similarly, the occurrence of brain necrosis is exceedingly rare.[305] The issue of secondary tumors remains contentious; although meningiomas and gliomas have been reported after pituitary radiotherapy, it is not clear whether the incidence is significantly greater than the background risk for developing such tumors in patients who already have one intracranial tumor and have undergone careful surveilllance.[304]

Stereotactic Radiosurgery

In stereotactic radiosurgery, concentrated beams of high doses of radiation are aimed precisely at the mapped discrete lesion, delivering very high doses to the tumor and relatively low doses to normal surrounding tissue. A number of techniques can be used to do this: using narrow beams from multiple gamma cobalt sources (gamma knife), using heavy charged particles (proton or helium beams), or using a single beam from a linear accelerator that is arced around the target (X-knife, SMART, Linac). The advent of high-resolution MRI for mapping has facilitated this therapy. Usually, only a single therapy dose is required, and this is biologically more effective than delivery of the same dose in fractions.[306] This technique also may be used to deliver radiation to the entire pituitary gland when a specific target is not known after surgery or MRI examination.

Probably the technique most widely used currently for Cushing's syndrome is the gamma knife. As adjunctive therapy after failed transsphenoidal surgery, it probably is no better than conventional radiotherapy.[307] Radiosurgery of the pituitary gland using proton beams has similar efficacy.[308] Linear accelerator radiotherapy for Cushing's disease is less well described, but success has been reported in small numbers of patients.[309]

As with conventional radiotherapy, the main side effect is hypopituitarism, and although the perceived risk of damage to adjacent structures such as the optic chiasm is less, additional studies and longer follow-up are needed. Some centers use it mainly for salvage of difficult recurrent tumors, for example, in the cavernous sinus or in Nelson's syndrome, whereas others have suggested it as an alternative to conventional radiotherapy in adenomas smaller than 30 mm with a minimal distance from the optic chiasm of 2 to 3 mm.[305]

Interstitial Radiotherapy

Two centers have used interstitial irradiation (yttrium-90 or gold-198 implants) as primary therapy for Cushing's disease.[310,311] Remission rates in these cohorts were high (75% to 77%), although some required a second implant. The principal side effect was hypopituitarism.

Other Tumors

No significant evidence suggests that radiotherapy improves overall survival in adrenocortical carcinoma, although sporadic reports indicate that it may be helpful adjuvant treatment to radical surgery in selected cases.[312,313] Local radiotherapy after surgical resection of an ectopic ACTH-secreting source may be beneficial, particularly in nonmetastatic thoracic carcinoid tumors.[314,315]

MEDICAL TREATMENT

Medical treatments for hypercortisolism have two broad mechanisms of action. One class of agents reduces cortisol levels through inhibition of adrenal steroidogenesis or cortisol action by antagonism at the level of the receptor. These compounds may be used in treatment for all forms of Cushing's syndrome. The second class of compounds, which generally are much less effective, modulate ACTH release and are restricted to treatment for ACTH-dependent Cushing's syndrome, principally Cushing's disease. The major current role of medical therapy is in the preoperative control of hypercortisolemia or as adjunctive treatment after failed surgical management, while other therapies such as radiotherapy are instituted.

Agents Inhibiting Steroidogenesis

The oral inhibitors of adrenal steroidogenesis are the most commonly used medical agents as treatment for Cushing's syndrome; of these, metyrapone, ketoconazole, and mitotane are the most effective. Aminoglutethimide[316] is no longer available, and trilostane[317] is now rarely used. Etomidate is the only available agent that can be given parenterally. We usually would recommend partial inhibition of cortisol production (adjusted adrenal blockade) with frequent monitoring to identify a dosing regimen that maintains eucortisolism while avoiding adrenal insufficiency or excess. However, in some patients, particularly those with variable cortisol production, it can be difficult to achieve this. In these cases, full adrenal blockade with glucocorticoid replacement to avoid symptoms of adrenal insufficiency (a block-and-replace regimen) may be advocated. In all forms of treatment,

patients and their physicians must be alert to the signs and symptoms of adrenal insufficiency.

Metyrapone

Metyrapone acts primarily to inhibit the enzyme 11β-hydroxylase,[318] and the subsequent elevation of 11-deoxycortisol can be monitored in the serum of patients treated with metyrapone. The decrease in cortisol is rapid, with trough levels at 2 hours post dose, and a test dose of 750 mg with hourly cortisol estimation for 4 hours can be used to predict response: A rapid and sustained decrease in cortisol to less than approximately 7 μg/dL (≈200 nmol/L), as is often seen with ectopic ACTH and adrenal tumors, suggests that a smaller dose of metyrapone may be appropriate, whereas a decrease 10 to 12 μg/dL (≈300 nmol/L), as often is seen in Cushing's disease, would indicate a higher dose requirement.[319] Therapy is started at 0.75 to 1.5 g/day in three to four divided doses daily. The usual requirement is approximately 2 g/day, although higher doses (as high as 6 g/day) may be needed in ectopic ACTH syndrome.[319] Metyrapone is useful in treating patients with Cushing's syndrome from adrenal tumors, ectopic ACTH syndrome, and Cushing's disease.[319,320] The principal side effects are hirsutism and acne (as predicted by the increase in adrenal androgens), dizziness, and gastrointestinal upset. The androgenic effects can be particularly problematic and may preclude its use in some younger female patients. Hypokalemia, edema, and hypertension due to increased mineralocorticoids are infrequent[319] but may require cessation of therapy. Our experience would suggest that the only major problems are associated with the increase in adrenal androgens; careful monitoring of treatment to avoid hypoadrenalism and education of the patient are required. Although not previously reported, we have seen a case of hemolysis in a patient with glucose-6-phosphate dehydrogenase deficiency.

Ketoconazole and Other Antifungals

Ketoconazole is an imidazole derivative whose primary indication is as an oral antifungal agent. However, reports of gynecomastia in some ketoconazole-treated patients led to the realization that it is an inhibitor of cytochrome P-450 enzymes, including side-chain cleavage, C17,20-lyase, 11β-hydroxylase, and 17β-hydroxylase.[321,322] It has also been reported to have a direct effect on ectopic ACTH secretion from a thymic carcinoid tumor.[323] Treatment for Cushing's syndrome usually is started at a dose of 200 mg twice daily, and its onset of action is slower than metyrapone. It has been used successfully to lower cortisol levels in patients with Cushing's syndrome of various causes, including adrenal carcinoma, ectopic ACTH syndrome, and invasive ACTH-producing pituitary carcinoma, with doses between 200 and 1200 mg/day required in as many as four divided daily doses.[324-326] The principal side effect of ketoconazole is hepatotoxicity. Reversible elevation of hepatic serum transaminases occurs in approximately 5% to 10% of patients and need not result in discontinuation of the agent if levels remain below twofold to threefold the upper normal range. The incidence of serious hepatic injury is approximately 1 in 15,000 patients,[327] and it can be fatal or may require liver transplantation.[328,329] The hepatotoxicity appears to be idiosyncratic and has been reported within 7 days of the start of treatment in a patient with Cushing's syndrome.[330] Other adverse reactions of ketoconazole include skin rashes and gastrointestinal upset, but these occur in less than 15%,[324] and one must always be wary of causing adrenal insufficiency.[331] Because of its C17-20 lyase inhibition and consequent antiandrogenic properties, ketoconazole is particularly useful in female patients in whom hirsutism, which may be worsened with metyrapone, is an issue. Conversely, gynecomastia and reduced libido in male patients may be unacceptable and may require alternative agents. One further advantage of ketoconazole is its inhibition of cholesterol synthesis, particularly low-density lipoprotein cholesterol.[332] We have found it to be particularly useful in combination with low doses of metyrapone. Fluconazole, another oral imidazole, is less well studied but has been shown to be effective, and it provides the advantage of less toxicity.[333]

Mitotane

Mitotane, or o,p'DDD, is derived from the family of insecticides that includes DDT. It inhibits adrenal steroidogenesis catalyzed by cholesterol desmolase,[334] 11- and 18-hydroxylase, and 3β-hydroxysteroid dehydrogenase.[335] It also has marked direct cytotoxic effects on the zona fasciculata and the zona reticulosa, which led to its original use in high doses (5 to 20 g/day) as treatment for inoperable adrenocortical carcinoma.[336,337] In this condition, it now is used more commonly as adjunctive treatment to surgery, and it does appear to prolong recurrence-free survival with lower doses of between 1 and 5 g/day.[338,339] At such doses, it may take a longer time to reach therapeutic levels, and where possible, monitoring of serum levels should be undertaken. It is suggested that target levels should be between 15 and 20 μg/mL.[338,340] Combined treatment of mitotane with standard chemotherapeutic agents such as cisplatin, etoposide, and doxorubicin has been used in a number of small studies in advanced adrenal carcinoma with variable benefit.[341-343]

In Cushing's disease, mitotane alone in high doses (4 to 12 g/day) can achieve remission in as many as 83% of patients, but more commonly, it is used in lower doses (0.5 to 4 g/day), sometimes in combination with radiation therapy, with clinical and biochemical remission achieved in approximately 80%.[344,345] At these doses, the onset of effect can take approximately 6 to 8 weeks, and additional adjunctive medical treatment may be needed in this interim. Similarly, the agent has a long half-life (18 to 159 days), due in part to its lipophilic properties, and it effects can last for weeks or months after discontinuation of therapy. Mitotane, alone or in combination with metyrapone or aminoglutethimide, also has proved useful as treatment for hypercortisolism associated with ectopic secretion of ACTH.[346]

The utility of mitotane is limited by its gastrointestinal and neurologic toxicity. Nausea and anorexia are common at doses as high as 4 g/day and are ubiquitous at more than 4 g/day.[347] These side effects may be avoided by beginning at a dose of 0.5 to 1.0 g/day and increasing gradually, by 0.5 to 1.0 g every 1 to 4 weeks. Doses should be taken with meals or at bedtime with food. If significant adverse effects do occur, the drug should be discontinued for 3 to 5 days and then restarted at a lower dose.[345] At higher doses and serum levels >20 μg/mL,[340] neurologic side effects are common and include drowsiness, gait disturbances, dizziness or vertigo, confusion, and problems with language. Other adverse effects at any dose include fatigue (perhaps due to decreased cortisol levels), gynecomastia, skin rash, hypouricemia, elevated liver enzymes, and abnormal platelet function.[337,348,349] The hypercholesterolemia, which is common even at low doses, can be reversed with 3-hydroxy-3-methylglutaryl coenzyme A reductase inhibitors such as simvastatin.[350] Mitotane is relatively contraindicated in women desiring fertility within 2 to 5 years. It may induce spontaneous abortion and may act as a teratogen, effects that may persist for a number of years after discontinuation because of deposition in fat.[351] Mitotane increases hormone-binding proteins (cortisol-binding globulin, sex hormone binding–globulin[352] and thyroxine-binding globulin). Therefore, total serum cortisol cannot be relied on to monitor therapy, and UFC should be used instead. The value of serum-free or salivary cortisol remains to be determined. In addition, mitotane increases the metabolic clearance of exogenously administered steroids,[353] and replacement doses of glucocorticoid must be increased by approximately one third.

Etomidate

Etomidate, an imidazole-derived anesthetic agent, was reported in 1983 to have adrenolytic effects.[354] Compared with the other imidazole derivative ketoconazole, etomidate more potently inhibits adrenocortical 11β-hydroxylase and shows similar inhibition of 17-hydroxylase, but it has less of an effect on C17-20 lyase.[355] At higher concentrations, it also appears to have an effect on cholesterol side-chain cleavage.[356] Short-term etomidate infusions can reduce severe hypercortisolemia in patients with Cushing's syndrome of various causes at doses as high as 0.3 mg/kg/hr,[357] although such high doses tend to be sedative.[358] Most case reports of long-term therapy therefore have described the use of lower nonhypnotic total doses of between 1.2 and 8.3 mg/hr to good effect.[359-362] It may be more difficult to normalize cortisol levels in patients with Cushing's disease, which probably reflects increased ACTH drive from the pituitary, as opposed to relatively fixed production from an ectopic source.[360] Clearly, etomidate is an effective adrenolytic agent that acts rapidly but is limited in its use by the fact that it has to be given parenterally. However, in this situation, it may be lifesaving. It is important to recognize that the etomidate preparations available in Europe are dissolved in an alcohol-based vehicle, although the currently available preparation in the United States uses propylene glycol, which may have potential side effects such as nephrotoxicity.[361]

Glucocorticoid Receptor Antagonists

Mifepristone (RU 486), the antiprogesterone antagonist that is marketed as an abortifacient, is also a competitive antagonist of glucocorticoid and androgen receptors. The major drawback is the lack of biochemical markers to monitor overtreatment, and its long half-life and minimal agonist activity leave the patient open to hypoadrenalism.[363]

Agents That Modulate ACTH Release

A number of agents, including the serotonin antagonists cyproheptadine[364] and ritanserin,[365] the dopamine agonists bromocriptine[366] and cabergoline,[367] and sodium valproate,[368] have been examined in Cushing's disease. The precise mechanism of action of many of these agents is incompletely understood, although most seem to reduce ACTH secretion through an effect on the hypothalamic-pituitary axis. Their efficacy in Cushing's disease seems to be variable between individual patients; therefore, we do not recommend their routine use. However, more recent data on the use of cabergoline suggest that this drug may be more effective than was previously realized.

Somatostatin Analogues

Long-acting somatostatin analogues such as octreotide and lanreotide are used widely in the therapy of various neuroendocrine tumors, and somatostatin receptors have been demonstrated on corticotroph adenomas, in addition to ectopic sources of ACTH.[369] Octreotide appears to inhibit ACTH release in Nelson's syndrome but rarely in patients with Cushing's disease, and this has been postulated to be due to somatostatin receptor down-regulation from the circulating hypercortisolemia.[370] In ectopic ACTH-secreting tumors, octreotide has produced a prolonged (>3 months) reduction in ACTH and hypercortisolemia in approximately 70% of published cases, but this high rate of response may be due to selective reporting. Preoperative assessment with pentetreotide scintigraphy may help predict which tumors might respond to treatment. Octreotide treatment produces a temporary response in GIP-dependent Cushing's syndrome but is unhelpful in other causes of ACTH-independent Cushing's syndrome.[371] So far, little experience has been reported with use of the sustained-release preparations in treating Cushing's syndrome. Much interest surrounds somatostatin analogues with a broader spectrum of activity for somatostatin receptor subtypes. Such an agent, pasireotide (SOM230; Novartis, Basel, Switzerland), has been shown in vitro to reduce human corticotroph proliferation and ACTH secretion,[372] and early results in vivo are encouraging.[373,374] Additional clinical studies are ongoing.

Thiazolidinediones

Rosiglitazone, a peroxisome-proliferator–activated receptor-γ (PPAR-γ) agonist, at suprapharmacologic doses has been shown in vitro and in animal models to suppress ACTH secretion and corticotroph tumor size.[375] However, a number of clinical trials of the thiazolidinediones rosiglitazone and pioglitazone in patients with Cushing's syndrome have generally been disappointing, with only short-term benefit seen in occasional patients even at high doses.[376-380]

Potential Novel Medical Agents

In the rare cases of Cushing's syndrome due to AIMAH and aberrant receptor expression, specific receptor antagonists have proved useful at least in the short term, and further investigation is needed.[381] Retinoic acid has been found to inhibit ACTH secretion and cell proliferation both in vitro in ACTH-producing tumor cell lines and cultured human corticotroph adenomas and in vivo in nude mice[382] and dogs.[383] The potential antisecretory and antiproliferative activities of this agent in Cushing's syndrome have not to our knowledge been investigated further in man.

Special Clinical Scenarios

CYCLIC CUSHING'S SYNDROME

Most patients with Cushing's syndrome demonstrate consistently elevated glucocorticoid values. A small subset show significant variability in glucocorticoid secretion, alternating normal and elevated values on a regular or irregular basis.[384] The few cases of spontaneous remission of Cushing's syndrome, including Cushing's first patient, may fit into this category.[2,385,386] The clinical course of patients with this type of intermittent, cyclic, or periodic Cushing's syndrome may be invariant, usually with mild signs and cushingoid symptoms, or it may parallel the biochemical abnormalities, with exacerbation of cushingoid features that parallel increased glucocorticoid production. The etiologic distribution is altered; in a recent review, Cushing's disease, ectopic ACTH secretion, and primary adrenal causes accounted for 54%, 26%, and 11%, respectively, of 65 cases, with the remainder being unclassified.[387]

Patients with periodic Cushing's syndrome often show conflicting or "inappropriate" responses to standard diagnostic tests, particularly dexamethasone suppression.[388] Discrepant urine tests have been reported in these patients, with elevated 17-OHCS and normal UFC excretion.[389] If studied during a quiescent period, patients with nonpituitary disease may be misclassified as having Cushing's disease, and those with "normal" responses to the LDDST may be incorrectly diagnosed as not having Cushing's syndrome.[390] Dynamic testing should be performed only during a sustained period of hypercortisolism, as documented by failure to suppress on an LDDST, concurrent increased evening salivary or plasma cortisol, and/or elevated UFC excretion.

IATROGENIC AND FACTITIOUS CUSHING'S SYNDROME

Appropriate therapeutic but supraphysiologic doses of glucocorticoids given for a medical condition cause most cases of iatrogenic Cushing's syndrome, which usually is an expected, unavoidable adverse effect of therapy. Exogenous hypercortisolism may result also when a prescribed dose of glucocorticoid is increased inappropriately by the patient. Although most common with oral agents, Cushing's syndrome may result from glucocorticoids administered to the nasal or rectal mucosa, the tracheobronchial tree, or the skin.[391-393] The use of all prescription drugs, over-the-counter medications, and herbal remedies,[394] including nasal drops, inhalants, and topical agents, should be assessed in all cushingoid patients. Agents not given for their glucocorticoid activity, such as fludrocortisone acetate and megestrol,[395] also may produce cushingoid features on occasion. Agents sold for cosmetic skin whitening may contain potent glucocorticoids.

Factitious Cushing's syndrome, which may be a form of Münchausen's syndrome, is rare. The typical suppression of plasma ACTH and dehydroepiandrosterone sulfate may lead to a mistaken diagnosis of primary adrenal disease.[396] Plasma and urine cortisol values vary, depending on the route, schedule, and type of glucocorticoid ingested. For example, intravenous injection of hydrocortisone may suppress ACTH values and increase UFC levels without increasing single random plasma cortisol values.[397] If basal urine or plasma cortisol values are low, it may be useful to screen the urine for synthetic glucocorticoids.[396]

Treatment for exogenous Cushing's syndrome consists of discontinuing glucocorticoid ingestion. If this is possible, a weaning schedule should be followed until a replacement dose of hydrocortisone is reached, at which point the patient may be weaned very gradually, as discussed earlier for postoperative treatment. If the degree of suppression of the axis cannot be estimated from the medication and dose received, the response to synthetic ACTH can be used as a rough gauge of adrenal suppression.

For the patient in whom glucocorticoids cannot be discontinued, a change in dose or schedule may ameliorate symptoms of Cushing's syndrome. Patients who require supraphysiologic glucocorticoid therapy should undergo measurement of bone density and should be counseled to maintain adequate calcium and vitamin D intake, to exercise, and to receive bisphosphonate therapy when appropriate.

CHRONIC RENAL FAILURE

Cushing's syndrome has been described in the setting of chronic renal failure only rarely.[398-400] Plasma levels of cortisol are normal in chronic renal failure when assessed with radioimmunoassays using an organic extraction procedure,[401,402] but they may be increased if other assay techniques are used.[403] ACTH levels are increased.[401] Glomerular filtration rates of less than 30 mL/min result in decreased cortisol excretion, and the UFC may be normal despite excessive cortisol production.[404] ACTH and cortisol responses to ovine CRH may be suppressed in patients with renal failure, except for those undergoing continuous ambulatory peritoneal dialysis.[402] The metabolism of dexamethasone is normal in chronic renal failure, but oral absorption can be altered in some patients, which may necessitate measurement of plasma dexamethasone levels.[405,406] The reduced degree of suppression of cortisol by dexamethasone suggests a prolonged half-life of cortisol. Normal suppression of the overnight 1 mg LDDST is uncommon, and the 2 day LDDST does better in this regard.[132,406,407] The cortisol response to insulin-induced hypoglycemia is normal or absent.[405,408]

PEDIATRIC CUSHING'S SYNDROME

The most common presentation of Cushing's syndrome in children is growth retardation, often with a decrease in height percentile over time as the weight percentile increases.[409-411] However, hypercortisolemic patients with virilizing adrenal tumors may show growth acceleration; thus, the absence of growth failure does not exclude the diagnosis of Cushing's syndrome.[412] Other virilizing signs such as acne and hirsutism are seen in approximately 50% of patients regardless of etiology.[411] Hypertension and striae are seen in approximately 50% of cases.[413] Muscle weakness may be less common in the pediatric patient.[70] This may reflect the effect of exercise rather than age because older patients who follow an exercise program tend to maintain strength. In addition to the spectrum of psychiatric and cognitive changes seen in adults, which can affect school performance, children may show "compulsive diligence" and actually do well academically.[409] Depression is less common in children than in adults. Headache and fatigue are common.[411] Cushing's disease accounts for between 75% and 80% of Cushing's syndrome in children and adolescents, but before the age of 10 years, ACTH-independent causes of Cushing's syndrome are more common. Cushing's disease has a male predominance in prepubertal children. Two primary adrenal causes of Cushing's syndrome, McCune-Albright syndrome and PPNAD, are typically diseases of childhood or young adulthood. Signs of virilization or feminization in the very young (<4 years) suggest adrenal carcinoma. Ectopic secretion of ACTH occurs rarely in the pediatric population and usually is due to bronchial or thymic carcinoids.[414]

As mentioned previously, late-night salivary cortisol measurement has particular logistical benefits in children. Study of its utility in the pediatric population has been limited, and diagnostic criteria are not clear, although a cutoff of 0.27 μg/dL (7.5 nmol/L) has been suggested if the sample is taken around midnight.[166,415] Serum cortisol measurement in inpatients has high sensitivity.[416] In children, UFC should be corrected for body surface area (×1.72 m²).[417] The standard 2 day LDDST adult protocol can be used in children weighing 40 kg or more, otherwise the dexamethasone dose is adjusted to 30 μg/kg/day.[410] As in adults, there is good correlation between cortisol suppression on the LDDST and on the HDDST for the differential diagnosis; thus, the latter is not necessary.[418] Although it can be argued that the ectopic ACTH syndrome is so rare in children that the CRH test or BIPSS is not necessary, they do add reassurance in those with a negative pituitary MRI, which is the case in more than 50% of cases. In addition, BIPSS has arguably better

accuracy in lateralization of the pituitary tumor.[414] MRI is at least as useful as CT in the evaluation of adrenal causes.[419]

Adrenalectomy, either unilateral or bilateral depending on the cause, is first-line therapy in ACTH-independent Cushing's syndrome. Transsphenoidal surgery is the treatment of choice in children with Cushing's disease, with similar rates of remission as in adults in expert hands.[420] Conventional radiotherapy used in the setting of failure to cure after transsphenoidal surgery performs even better than in adults with reported remission rates as high as 100%, with cure occurring within 12 months.[421] Following pituitary surgery, plus or minus radiotherapy, the incidence of growth hormone deficiency is high, but prompt diagnosis and treatment with human growth hormone ensure acceptable growth acceleration and catch-up growth, although an abnormal body composition often persists.[422] Similarly, normalization of reduced bone mineral density can be achieved.[423]

CUSHING'S SYNDROME IN PREGNANCY

The pregnant woman with possible Cushing's syndrome presents a diagnostic challenge to the physician because of the physical and biochemical changes that are common to both conditions, including weight gain, fatigue, striae, hypertension, and glucose intolerance. The investigative screening process has to be based on the recognition of physiologic changes in pregnancy.[424] Total serum cortisol levels increase in pregnancy, beginning in the first trimester and peaking at 6 months, with a decrease only after delivery, probably reflecting increased induction of hepatic corticosteroid-binding globulin production by estrogen. UFC excretion is normal in the first trimester and then rises up to threefold by term. Thus, only UFC values greater than threefold normal are diagnostic in the last two trimesters. Suppression to dexamethasone is blunted, but not because of reduced bioavailability of dexamethasone. The cortisol diurnal rhythm is maintained in pregnancy but with a higher nadir, and appropriate diagnostic cutoffs in pregnancy have yet to be established. Adrenal adenomas are frequently the cause of Cushing's syndrome in pregnancy (40% to 50%), but it is interesting to note that ACTH levels may not be suppressed in these patients, possibly because of placental CRH stimulation of the pituitary corticotrophs or placental ACTH secretion. The HDDST may be useful in distinguishing these patients from those with Cushing's disease. The CRH test also has been used to identify patients with Cushing's disease, and no evidence of harm has been found in animal studies and in the small number of pregnant patients studied with this drug. MRI without gadolinium enhancement is considered safe in the third trimester, and its use in combination with the noninvasive tests discussed earlier should resolve most diagnostic issues. IPSS with appropriate additional radiation protection for the fetus should be reserved only for cases in which diagnostic uncertainty remains.

Although Cushing's syndrome is rare in pregnancy, maternal hypercortisolism is associated with poor outcomes, both maternal and fetal. Definitive surgical treatment for adrenal or pituitary disease is recommended to achieve eucortisolemia, although adverse fetal outcomes may persist: The second trimester is probably the safest time for operative intervention. Medical treatment carries potential risk for the fetus and should be considered only as second-line therapy when the benefit outweighs the risk, and then generally only as an interim measure. Metyrapone is probably the adrenolytic agent of choice, although its association with preeclampsia has been reported. Ketoconazole has been utilized successfully in a small number of patients but is teratogenic in animals and therefore should be used cautiously.[425]

Prognosis

The life expectancy of patients with nonmalignant causes of Cushing's syndrome, at one time a uniformly fatal illness, has improved dramatically with effective surgical and medical treatments and the availability of antibiotics, antihypertensive agents, and glucocorticoids. In a 1952 review, Plotz[67] reported a 5-year mortality rate of 50% in actively hypercortisolemic patients, with 46% caused by bacterial infection and 40% due to cardiovascular complications (cardiac failure, cardiovascular accidents, or renal insufficiency). In 1961, the mortality rate was similar, but the causes had changed: Two thirds were due to postoperative adrenal crisis before cortisone was available or from metastatic adrenal cancer. Cardiovascular events related to hypertension (stroke, heart failure, renal failure, myocardial infarction) led to death in approximately 20%; infectious causes decreased to approximately 15%.[71] Ten years later, in 1971, 30% of patients with benign causes of Cushing's syndrome died within 5 years of diagnosis, most from cardiovascular disease or infection, despite decreased postoperative mortality.[426] In 1979, a lower incidence of death (6%) was noted within 2 to 10 years of radiation therapy, mitotane, or combination treatment for Cushing's disease.[344] This improvement may reflect earlier detection of Cushing's syndrome and better treatment for hypercortisolism and associated medical complications, such as hypertension, or lower perioperative mortality. Three studies on long-term survival in Cushing's disease treated in the era of transsphenoidal surgery have been completed; two were epidemiologic studies from northern Spain[66] and Denmark,[61] and the third was a series from a single neurosurgical center where all patients had undergone transsphenoidal surgery.[255] Investigators report varying standardized mortality ratios of 3.8, 1.7, and 0.98, respectively. The discrepancy in findings between the three series is not completely clear, but it is difficult to make absolute comparisons, not least because the study by Swearingen and colleagues undoubtedly is affected by selection bias. However, the latter two studies do appear to show that after curative transsphenoidal surgery, long-term mortality is not significantly different from that in the general population. This is perhaps surprising because increased cardiovascular risk markers and evidence of atherosclerotic disease persist when measured 5 years after remission of Cushing's disease.[115] The outcome of pediatric Cushing's disease is excellent if treated at centers with appropriate experience.[413]

Cushing's syndrome results in significant impairment in quality of life. Unfortunately, in the long term, this is improved only partially with treatment.[275,427]

The prognosis of the potentially malignant causes of Cushing's syndrome is variable. Adrenal cancer, as reviewed earlier, has an extremely poor prognosis. Tumors that produce ACTH ectopically tend to have a poor prognosis, particularly when compared with tumors from the same tissue that do not produce ACTH. Small cell lung cancer, islet cell tumors, and thymic carcinoids[428] illustrate this phenomenon. As many as 82% of patients with small cell lung cancer and Cushing's syndrome die within 2 weeks from the start of chemotherapy.[63] Among the causes of ectopic ACTH syndrome, pheochromocytoma and bronchial carcinoid appear to offer the best prognosis after tumor resection, but this is not universal.

REFERENCES

1. Cushing HW: The pituitary body and its disorders, Philadelphia, 1912, JB Lippincott.
2. Cushing HW: The basophil adenomas of the pituitary body and their clinical manifestations (pituitary basophilism), Bulletin of the Johns Hopkins Hospital 1:137–195, 1932.
3. Walters W, Wilder RM, Kepler EJ: The suprarenal cortical syndrome with presentation of ten cases, Ann Surg 100:670–688, 1934.
4. Liddle GW, Nicholson WE, Island DP, et al: Clinical and laboratory studies of ectopic humoral syndromes, Recent Prog Horm Res 25:283–314, 1969.
5. Howlett TA, Rees LH, Besser GM: Cushing's syndrome, Clin Endocrinol Metab 14:911–945, 1985.
6. Bertagna X: New causes of Cushing's syndrome, N Engl J Med 327:1024–1025, 1992.
7. Reznik Y, Allali-Zerah V, Chayvialle JA, et al: Food-dependent Cushing's syndrome mediated by aberrant adrenal sensitivity to gastric inhibitory polypeptide, N Engl J Med 327:981–986, 1992.
8. Lacroix A, Bolte E, Tremblay J, et al: Gastric inhibitory polypeptide-dependent cortisol hypersecretion—a new cause of Cushing's syndrome, N Engl J Med 327:974–980, 1992.
9. Malchoff CD, Orth DN, Abboud C, et al: Ectopic ACTH syndrome caused by a bronchial carcinoid tumor responsive to dexamethasone, metyrapone, and corticotropin-releasing factor, Am J Med 84:760–764, 1988.
10. Biller BM, Alexander JM, Zervas NT, et al: Clonal origins of adrenocorticotropin-secreting pituitary tissue in Cushing's disease, J Clin Endocrinol Metab 75:1303–1309, 1992.
11. Mampalam TJ, Tyrrell JB, Wilson CB: Transsphenoidal microsurgery for Cushing disease. A report of 216 cases, Ann Intern Med 109:487–493, 1988.
12. Young WF Jr, Scheithauer BW, Gharib H, et al: Cushing's syndrome due to primary multinodular corticotrope hyperplasia, Mayo Clin Proc 63:256–262, 1988.
13. Asa SL, Ezzat S: The cytogenesis and pathogenesis of pituitary adenomas, Endocr Rev 19:798–827, 1998.
14. Dahia PL, Grossman AB: The molecular pathogenesis of corticotroph tumors, Endocr Rev 20:136–155, 1999.
15. Rabbitt EH, Ayuk J, Boelaert K, et al: Abnormal expression of 11 beta-hydroxysteroid dehydrogenase type 2 in human pituitary adenomas: a prereceptor determinant of pituitary cell proliferation, Oncogene 22:1663–1667, 2003.
16. Korbonits M, Chahal HS, Kaltsas G, et al: Expression of phosphorylated p27(Kip1) protein and Jun activation domain-binding protein 1 in human pituitary tumors, J Clin Endocrinol Metab 87:2635–2643, 2002.
17. Trautmann K, Thakker RV, Ellison DW, et al: Chromosomal aberrations in sporadic pituitary tumors, Int J Cancer 91:809–814, 2001.
18. Metzger AK, Mohapatra G, Minn YA, et al: Multiple genetic aberrations including evidence of chromosome 11q13 rearrangement detected in pituitary adenomas by comparative genomic hybridization, J Neurosurg 90:306–314, 1999.
19. Fan X, Paetau A, Aalto Y, et al: Gain of chromosome 3 and loss of 13q are frequent alterations in pituitary adenomas, Cancer Genet Cytogenet 128:97–103, 2001.
20. Evans CO, Young AN, Brown MR, et al: Novel patterns of gene expression in pituitary adenomas identified by complementary deoxyribonucleic acid microarrays and quantitative reverse transcription-polymerase chain reaction, J Clin Endocrinol Metab 86:3097–3107, 2001.
21. Imura H: Ectopic hormone syndromes, Clin Endocrinol Metab 9:235–260, 1980.
22. de Bustros A, Baylin SB: Hormone production by tumours: biological and clinical aspects, Clin Endocrinol Metab 14:221–256, 1985.
23. Pearse AG: Common cytochemical and ultrastructural characteristics of cells producing polypeptide hormones (the APUD series) and their relevance to thyroid and ultimobranchial C cells and calcitonin, Proc R Soc Lond B Biol Sci 170:71–80, 1968.
24. Pullan PT, Clement-Jones V, Corder R, et al: ACTH LPH and related peptides in the ectopic ACTH syndrome, Clin Endocrinol (Oxf) 13:437–445, 1980.
25. Rees LH, Bloomfield GA, Gilkes JJ, et al: ACTH as a tumor marker, Ann N Y Acad Sci 297:603–620, 1977.
26. Stewart MF, Crosby SR, Gibson S, et al: Small cell lung cancer cell lines secrete predominantly ACTH precursor peptides not ACTH, Br J Cancer 60:20–24, 1989.
27. White A, Clark AJ, Stewart MF: The synthesis of ACTH and related peptides by tumours, Bailliere's Clin Endocrinol Metab 4:1–27, 1990.
28. DeBold CR, Menefee JK, Nicholson WE, et al: Proopiomelanocortin gene is expressed in many normal human tissues and in tumors not associated with ectopic adrenocorticotropin syndrome, Mol Endocrinol 2:862–870, 1988.
29. de Keyzer Y, Bertagna X, Luton JP, et al: Variable modes of proopiomelanocortin gene transcription in human tumors, Mol Endocrinol 3:215–223, 1989.
30. Clark AJ, Lavender PM, Besser GM, et al: Pro-opiomelanocortin mRNA size heterogeneity in ACTH-dependent Cushing's syndrome, J Mol Endocrinol 2:3–9, 1989.
31. Clark AJ, Stewart MF, Lavender PM, et al: Defective glucocorticoid regulation of proopiomelanocortin gene expression and peptide secretion in a small cell lung cancer cell line, J Clin Endocrinol Metab 70:485–490, 1990.
32. Roth KA, Newell DC, Dorin RI, et al: Aberrant production and regulation of proopiomelanocortin-derived peptides in ectopic Cushing's syndrome, Horm Metab Res 20:225–229, 1988.
33. Melmed S, Yamashita S, Kovacs K, et al: Cushing's syndrome due to ectopic proopiomelanocortin gene expression by islet cell carcinoma of the pancreas, Cancer 59:772–778, 1987.

34. Limper AH, Carpenter PC, Scheithauer B, et al: The Cushing syndrome induced by bronchial carcinoid tumors, Ann Intern Med 117:209–214, 1992.
35. Asa SL, Kovacs K, Vale W, et al: Immunohistologic localization of corticotrophin-releasing hormone in human tumors, Am J Clin Pathol 87:327–333, 1987.
36. Jessop DS, Cunnah D, Millar JG, et al: A phaeochromocytoma presenting with Cushing's syndrome associated with increased concentrations of circulating corticotrophin-releasing factor, J Endocrinol 113:133–138, 1987.
37. Zangeneh F, Young WF Jr, Lloyd RV, et al: Cushing's syndrome due to ectopic production of corticotropin-releasing hormone in an infant with ganglioneuroblastoma, Endocr Pract 9:394–399, 2003.
38. Wajchenberg BL, Mendonca BB, Liberman B, et al: Ectopic adrenocorticotropic hormone syndrome, Endocr Rev 15:752–787, 1994.
39. Sidhu S, Gicquel C, Bambach CP, et al: Clinical and molecular aspects of adrenocortical tumourigenesis, ANZ J Surg 73:727–738, 2003.
40. Beuschlein F, Reincke M, Karl M, et al: Clonal composition of human adrenocortical neoplasms, Cancer Res 54:4927–4932, 1994.
41. Weiss LM, Medeiros LJ, Vickery AL Jr: Pathologic features of prognostic significance in adrenocortical carcinoma, Am J Surg Pathol 13:202–206, 1989.
42. Travis WD, Tsokos M, Doppman JL, et al: Primary pigmented nodular adrenocortical disease. A light and electron microscopic study of eight cases, Am J Surg Pathol 13:921–930, 1989.
43. Stratakis CA, Boikos SA: Genetics of adrenal tumors associated with Cushing's syndrome: a new classification for bilateral adrenocortical hyperplasias, Nat Clin Pract Endocrinol Metab 3:748–757, 2007.
44. Kirk JM, Brain CE, Carson DJ, et al: Cushing's syndrome caused by nodular adrenal hyperplasia in children with McCune-Albright syndrome, J Pediatr 134:789–792, 1999.
45. Weinstein LS, Shenker A, Gejman PV, et al: Activating mutations of the stimulatory G protein in the McCune-Albright syndrome, N Engl J Med 325:1688–1695, 1991.
46. Boston BA, Mandel S, LaFranchi S, et al: Activating mutation in the stimulatory guanine nucleotide-binding protein in an infant with Cushing's syndrome and nodular adrenal hyperplasia, J Clin Endocrinol Metab 79:890–893, 1994.
47. Swords FM, Baig A, Malchoff DM, et al: Impaired desensitization of a mutant adrenocorticotropin receptor associated with apparent constitutive activity, Mol Endocrinol 16:2746–2753, 2002.
48. Findlay JC, Sheeler LR, Engeland WC, et al: Familial adrenocorticotropin-independent Cushing's syndrome with bilateral macronodular adrenal hyperplasia, J Clin Endocrinol Metab 76:189–191, 1993.
49. Christopoulos S, Bourdeau I, Lacroix A: Aberrant expression of hormone receptors in adrenal Cushing's syndrome, Pituitary 7:225–235, 2004.
50. Maschler I, Rosenmann E, Ehrenfeld EN: Ectopic functioning adrenocortico-myelolipoma in longstanding Nelson's syndrome, Clin Endocrinol (Oxf) 10:493–497, 1979.
51. Lalau JD, Vieau D, Tenenbaum F, et al: A case of pseudo-Nelson's syndrome: cure of ACTH hypersecretion by removal of a bronchial carcinoid tumor responsible for Cushing's syndrome, J Endocrinol Invest 13:531–537, 1990.
52. Adeyemi SD, Grange AO, Giwa-Osagie OF, et al: Adrenal rest tumour of the ovary associated with isosexual precocious pseudopuberty and cushingoid features, Eur J Pediatr 145:236–238, 1986.
53. Contreras P, Altieri E, Liberman C, et al: Adrenal rest tumor of the liver causing Cushing's syndrome: treatment with ketoconazole preceding an apparent surgical cure, J Clin Endocrinol Metab 60:21–28, 1985.
54. Marieb NJ, Spangler S, Kashgarian M, et al: Cushing's syndrome secondary to ectopic cortisol production by an ovarian carcinoma, J Clin Endocrinol Metab 57:737–740, 1983.
55. Newell-Price J, Trainer P, Besser M, et al: The diagnosis and differential diagnosis of Cushing's syndrome and pseudo-Cushing's states, Endocr Rev 19:647–672, 1998.
56. Chrousos GP, Schuermeyer TH, Doppman J, et al: NIH conference. Clinical applications of corticotropin-releasing factor, Ann Intern Med 102:344–358, 1985.
57. Gold PW, Gwirtsman H, Avgerinos PC, et al: Abnormal hypothalamic-pituitary-adrenal function in anorexia nervosa. Pathophysiologic mechanisms in underweight and weight-corrected patients, N Engl J Med 314:1335–1342, 1986.
58. Gold PW, Loriaux DL, Roy A, et al: Responses to corticotropin-releasing hormone in the hypercortisolism of depression and Cushing's disease. Pathophysiologic and diagnostic implications, N Engl J Med 314:1329–1335, 1986.
59. Luger A, Deuster PA, Kyle SB, et al: Acute hypothalamic-pituitary-adrenal responses to the stress of treadmill exercise. Physiologic adaptations to physical training, N Engl J Med 316:1309–1315, 1987.
60. Invitti C, Giraldi FP, de Martin M, et al: Diagnosis and management of Cushing's syndrome: results of an Italian multicentre study. Study Group of the Italian Society of Endocrinology on the Pathophysiology of the Hypothalamic-Pituitary-Adrenal Axis, J Clin Endocrinol Metab 84:440–448, 1999.
61. Lindholm J, Juul S, Jorgensen JO, et al: Incidence and late prognosis of Cushing's syndrome: a population-based study, J Clin Endocrinol Metab 86:117–123, 2001.
62. Abeloff MD, Trump DL, Baylin SB: Ectopic adrenocorticotrophic (ACTH) syndrome and small cell carcinoma of the lung-assessment of clinical implications in patients on combination chemotherapy, Cancer 48:1082–1087, 1981.
63. Dimopoulos MA, Fernandez JF, Samaan NA, et al: Paraneoplastic Cushing's syndrome as an adverse prognostic factor in patients who die early with small cell lung cancer, Cancer 69:66–71, 1992.
64. Janssen-Heijnen ML, Coebergh JW: The changing epidemiology of lung cancer in Europe, Lung Cancer 41:245–258, 2003.
65. Ambrosi B, Faglia G: Epidemiology of pituitary tumours. In Faglia G, Beck-Peccoz P, Ambrosi B, Travaglini P, Spada A, editors: Pituitary adenomas: New trends in basic and clinical research, Amsterdam, 1991, Excerpta Medica.
66. Etxabe J, Vazquez JA: Morbidity and mortality in Cushing's disease: an epidemiological approach, Clin Endocrinol (Oxf) 40:479–484, 1994.
67. Plotz CM, Knowlton AI, Ragan C: The natural history of Cushing's syndrome, Am J Med 13:597–614, 1952.
68. Leinung MC, Young WF Jr, Whitaker MD, et al: Diagnosis of corticotropin-producing bronchial carcinoid tumors causing Cushing's syndrome, Mayo Clin Proc 65:1314–1321, 1990.
69. Ross EJ, Linch DC: Cushing's syndrome—killing disease: discriminatory value of signs and symptoms aiding early diagnosis, Lancet 2:646–649, 1982.
70. Urbanic RC, George JM: Cushing's disease—18 years' experience, Medicine (Baltimore) 60:14–24, 1981.
71. Soffer LJ, Iannaccone A, Gabrilove JL: Cushing's syndrome *1: A study of fifty patients, The American Journal of Medicine 30:129–146, 1961.
72. Sprague RG, Randall RV, Salassa RM: Cushing's syndrome: review of 100 cases, Arch Intern Med 98:389–398, 1956.
73. Nugent CA, Warner HR, Dunn JT, et al: PROBABILITY THEORY IN THE DIAGNOSIS OF CUSHING'S SYNDROME, J Clin Endocrinol Metab 24:621–627, 1964.
74. Pecori GF, Pivonello R, Ambrogio AG, et al: The dexamethasone-suppressed corticotropin-releasing hormone stimulation test and the desmopressin test to distinguish Cushing's syndrome from pseudo-Cushing's states, Clin Endocrinol (Oxf) 66:251–257, 2007.
75. Rockall AG, Sohaib SA, Evans D, et al: Computed tomography assessment of fat distribution in male and female patients with Cushing's syndrome, Eur J Endocrinol 149:561–567, 2003.
76. Roy-Camille R, Mazel C, Husson JL, et al: Symptomatic spinal epidural lipomatosis induced by a long-term steroid treatment. Review of the literature and report of two additional cases, Spine 16:1365–1371, 1991.
77. Noel P, Pepersack T, Vanbinst A, et al: Spinal epidural lipomatosis in Cushing's syndrome secondary to an adrenal tumor, Neurology 42:1250–1251, 1992.
78. Healy ME, Hesselink JR, Ostrup RC, et al: Demonstration by magnetic resonance of symptomatic spinal epidural lipomatosis, Neurosurgery 21:414–415, 1987.
79. Pleasure DE, Walsh GO, Engel WK: Atrophy of skeletal muscle in patients with Cushing's syndrome, Arch Neurol 22:118–125, 1970.
80. Muller R, Kugelberg E: Myopathy in Cushing's syndrome, J Neurol Neurosurg Psychiatry 22:314–319, 1959.
81. Afifi AK, Bergman RA, Harvey JC: Steroid myopathy. Clinical, histologic and cytologic observations, Johns Hopkins Med J 123:158–173, 1968.
82. Vertebral compression fractures with accelerated bone turnover in a patient with Cushing's disease, Am J Med 68:932–940, 1980.
83. Kingsley GH, Hickling P: Polyarthropathy associated with Cushing's disease, Br Med J (Clin Res Ed) 292:1363, 1986.
84. Phillips KA, Nance EP Jr, Rodriguez RM, et al: Avascular necrosis of bone: a manifestation of Cushing's disease, South Med J 79:825–829, 1986.
85. Bertagna C, Orth DN: Clinical and laboratory findings and results of therapy in 58 patients with adrenocortical tumors admitted to a single medical center (1951 to 1978), Am J Med 71:855–875, 1981.
86. Starkman MN, Schteingart DE: Neuropsychiatric manifestations of patients with Cushing's syndrome. Relationship to cortisol and adrenocorticotropic hormone levels, Arch Intern Med 141:215–219, 1981.
87. Starkman MN, Schteingart DE, Schork MA: Correlation of bedside cognitive and neuropsychological tests in patients with Cushing's syndrome, Psychosomatics 27:508–511, 1986.
88. Haskett RF: Diagnostic categorization of psychiatric disturbance in Cushing's syndrome, Am J Psychiatry 142:911–916, 1985.
89. Hudson JI, Hudson MS, Griffing GT, et al: Phenomenology and family history of affective disorder in Cushing's disease, Am J Psychiatry 144:951–953, 1987.
90. Rubinow DR, Post RM, Savard R, et al: Cortisol hypersecretion and cognitive impairment in depression, Arch Gen Psychiatry 41:279–283, 1984.
91. Kathol RG: Etiologic implications of corticosteroid changes in affective disorder, Psychiatr Med 3:135–162, 1985.
92. Fallo F, Sonino N, Barzon L, et al: Effect of surgical treatment on hypertension in Cushing's syndrome, Am J Hypertens 9:77–80, 1996.
93. Bakker RC, Gallas PR, Romijn JA, et al: Cushing's syndrome complicated by multiple opportunistic infections, J Endocrinol Invest 21:329–333, 1998.
94. Graham BS, Tucker WS Jr: Opportunistic infections in endogenous Cushing's syndrome, Ann Intern Med 101:334–338, 1984.
95. Sarlis NJ, Chanock SJ, Nieman LK: Cortisolemic indices predict severe infections in Cushing syndrome due to ectopic production of adrenocorticotropin, J Clin Endocrinol Metab 85:42–47, 2000.
96. Kaltsas GA, Korbonits M, Isidori AM, et al: How common are polycystic ovaries and the polycystic ovarian syndrome in women with Cushing's syndrome? Clin Endocrinol (Oxf) 53:493–500, 2000.
97. Halbreich U, Zumoff B, Kream J, et al: The mean 1300–1600 h plasma cortisol concentration as a diagnostic test for hypercortisolism, J Clin Endocrinol Metab 54:1262–1264, 1982.
98. Liu JH, Kazer RR, Rasmussen DD: Characterization of the twenty-four hour secretion patterns of adrenocorticotropin and cortisol in normal women and patients with Cushing's disease, J Clin Endocrinol Metab 64:1027–1035, 1987.
99. Refetoff S, Van Cauter E, Fang VS, et al: The effect of dexamethasone on the 24-hour profiles of adrenocorticotropin and cortisol in Cushing's syndrome, J Clin Endocrinol Metab 60:527–535, 1985.
100. Mengden T, Hubmann P, Muller J, et al: Urinary free cortisol versus 17-hydroxycorticosteroids: a comparative study of their diagnostic value in Cushing's syndrome, Clin Investig 70:545–548, 1992.
101. Evans PJ, Peters JR, Dyas J, et al: Salivary cortisol levels in true and apparent hypercortisolism, Clin Endocrinol (Oxf) 20:709–715, 1984.
102. Christy NP, Laragh JH: Pathogenesis of hypokalemic alkalosis in Cushing's syndrome, Nord Hyg Tidskr 265:1083–1088, 1961.
103. Stewart PM, Krozowski ZS: 11 beta-Hydroxysteroid dehydrogenase, Vitam Horm 57:249–324, 1999.
104. Putignano P, Kaltsas GA, Korbonits M, et al: Alterations in serum protein levels in patients with Cushing's

syndrome before and after successful treatment, J Clin Endocrinol Metab 85:3309–3312, 2000.
105. Ambrosi B, Sartorio A, Pizzocaro A, et al: Evaluation of haemostatic and fibrinolytic markers in patients with Cushing's syndrome and in patients with adrenal incidentaloma, Exp Clin Endocrinol Diabetes 108:294–298, 2000.
106. Casonato A, Pontara E, Boscaro M, et al: Abnormalities of von Willebrand factor are also part of the prothrombotic state of Cushing's syndrome, Blood Coagul Fibrinolysis 10:145–151, 1999.
107. Patrassi GM, Dal Bo ZR, Boscaro M, et al: Further studies on the hypercoagulable state of patients with Cushing's syndrome, Thromb Haemost 54:518–520, 1985.
108. Taskinen MR, Nikkila EA, Pelkonen R, et al: Plasma lipoproteins, lipolytic enzymes, and very low density lipoprotein triglyceride turnover in Cushing's syndrome, J Clin Endocrinol Metab 57:619–626, 1983.
109. Friedman TC, Mastorakos G, Newman TD, et al: Carbohydrate and lipid metabolism in endogenous hypercortisolism: shared features with metabolic syndrome X and NIDDM, Endocr J 43:645–655, 1996.
110. Biering H, Knappe G, Gerl H, et al: [Prevalence of diabetes in acromegaly and Cushing syndrome], Acta Med Austriaca 27:27–31, 2000.
111. Krassowski J, Godziejewska M, Kurta J, et al: [Glucose tolerance in adrenocortical hyperfunction. Analysis of 100 cases], Pol Arch Med Wewn 92:70–75, 1994.
112. Catargi B, Rigalleau V, Poussin A, et al: Occult Cushing's syndrome in type-2 diabetes, J Clin Endocrinol Metab 88:5808–5813, 2003.
113. Newsome S, Chen K, Hoang J, et al: Cushing's syndrome in a clinic population with diabetes, Intern Med J 38:178–182, 2008.
114. Faggiano A, Pivonello R, Spiezia S, et al: Cardiovascular risk factors and common carotid artery caliber and stiffness in patients with Cushing's disease during active disease and 1 year after disease remission, J Clin Endocrinol Metab 88:2527–2533, 2003.
115. Colao A, Pivonello R, Spiezia S, et al: Persistence of increased cardiovascular risk in patients with Cushing's disease after five years of successful cure, J Clin Endocrinol Metab 84:2664–2672, 1999.
116. Bartalena L, Martino E, Petrini L, et al: The nocturnal serum thyrotropin surge is abolished in patients with adrenocorticotropin (ACTH)-dependent or ACTH-independent Cushing's syndrome, J Clin Endocrinol Metab 72:1195–1199, 1991.
117. Colao A, Pivonello R, Faggiano A, et al: Increased prevalence of thyroid autoimmunity in patients successfully treated for Cushing's disease, Clin Endocrinol (Oxf) 53:13–19, 2000.
118. Niepomniszcze H, Pitoia F, Katz SB, et al: Primary thyroid disorders in endogenous Cushing's syndrome, Eur J Endocrinol 147:305–311, 2002.
119. Luton JP, Thieblot P, Valcke JC, et al: Reversible gonadotropin deficiency in male Cushing's disease, J Clin Endocrinol Metab 45:488–495, 1977.
120. Lado-Abeal J, Rodriguez-Arnao J, Newell-Price JD, et al: Menstrual abnormalities in women with Cushing's disease are correlated with hypercortisolemia rather than raised circulating androgen levels, J Clin Endocrinol Metab 83:3083–3088, 1998.
121. Giustina A, Bossoni S, Bussi AR, et al: Effect of galanin on the growth hormone (GH) response to GH-releasing hormone in patients with Cushing's disease, Endocr Res 19:47–56, 1993.
122. Kaltsas G, Manetti L, Grossman AB: Osteoporosis in Cushing's syndrome, Front Horm Res 30:60–72, 2002.
123. Ohmori N, Nomura K, Ohmori K, et al: Osteoporosis is more prevalent in adrenal than in pituitary Cushing's syndrome, Endocr J 50:1–7, 2003.
124. Rockall AG, Sohaib SA, Evans D, et al: Hepatic steatosis in Cushing's syndrome: a radiological assessment using computed tomography, Eur J Endocrinol 149:543–548, 2003.
125. Giraldi FP, Moro M, Cavagnini F: Gender-related differences in the presentation and course of Cushing's disease, J Clin Endocrinol Metab 88:1554–1558, 2003.
126. King AB: The diagnosis of carcinoma of the pituitary gland, Bull Johns Hopkins Hosp 89:339–353, 1951.
127. Martins AN, Hayes GJ, Kempe LG: INVASIVE PITUITARY ADENOMAS, J Neurosurg 22:268–276, 1965.
128. Della CS, Corsello SM, Satta MA, et al: Intracranial and spinal dissemination of an ACTH secreting pituitary neoplasia. Case report and review of the literature, Ann Endocrinol (Paris) 58:503–509, 1997.
129. Arnaldi G, Angeli A, Atkinson AB, et al: Diagnosis and complications of Cushing's syndrome: a consensus statement, J Clin Endocrinol Metab 88:5593–5602, 2003.
130. Besser GM, Edwards CRW: Cushing's Syndrome, Clin Endocrinol Metab 1:451–490, 1972.
131. Lamberts SW, Klijn JG, de Jong FH, et al: Hormone secretion in alcohol-induced pseudo-Cushing's syndrome. Differential diagnosis with Cushing disease, JAMA 242:1640–1643, 1979.
132. Wallace EZ, Rosman P, Toshav N, et al: Pituitary-adrenocortical function in chronic renal failure: studies of episodic secretion of cortisol and dexamethasone suppressibility, J Clin Endocrinol Metab 50:46–51, 1980.
133. Werner S, Thoren M, Gustafsson JA, et al: Glucocorticoid receptor abnormalities in fibroblasts from patients with idiopathic resistance to dexamethasone diagnosed when evaluated for adrenocortical disorders, J Clin Endocrinol Metab 75:1005–1009, 1992.
134. Nieman LK, Biller BM, Findling JW, et al: The diagnosis of Cushing's syndrome: an Endocrine Society Clinical Practice Guideline, J Clin Endocrinol Metab 93:1526–1540, 2008.
135. Murphy BE: Clinical evaluation of urinary cortisol determinations by competitive protein-binding radioassay, J Clin Endocrinol Metab 28:343–348, 1968.
136. Orth DN: Cushing's syndrome, N Engl J Med 332:791–803, 1995.
137. Contreras LN, Hane S, Tyrrell JB: Urinary cortisol in the assessment of pituitary-adrenal function: utility of 24-hour and spot determinations, J Clin Endocrinol Metab 62:965–969, 1986.
138. Laudat MH, Billaud L, Thomopoulos P, et al: Evening urinary free corticoids: a screening test in Cushing's syndrome and incidentally discovered adrenal tumours, Acta Endocrinol (Copenh) 119:459–464, 1988.
139. Lin CL, Wu TJ, Machacek DA, et al: Urinary free cortisol and cortisone determined by high performance liquid chromatography in the diagnosis of Cushing's syndrome, J Clin Endocrinol Metab 82:151–155, 1997.
140. Turpeinen U, Markkanen H, Valimaki M, et al: Determination of urinary free cortisol by HPLC, Clin Chem 43:1386–1391, 1997.
141. Meikle AW, Findling J, Kushnir MM, et al: Pseudo-Cushing Syndrome Caused by Fenofibrate Interference with Urinary Cortisol Assayed by High-Performance Liquid Chromatography, J Clin Endocrinol Metab 88:3521–3524, 2003.
142. Nieman LK, Cutler GB Jr: The sensitivity of the urine free cortisol measurement as a screening test for Cushing's syndrome, Program of the 72nd Annual Meeting of The Endocrine Society, Atlanta GA (Abstract P-822) 1990.
143. Laudat MH, Cerdas S, Fournier C, et al: Salivary cortisol measurement: a practical approach to assess pituitary-adrenal function, J Clin Endocrinol Metab 66:343–348, 1988.
144. Putignano P, Dubini A, Toja P, et al: Salivary cortisol measurement in normal-weight, obese and anorexic women: comparison with plasma cortisol, Eur J Endocrinol 145:165–171, 2001.
145. Raff H, Homar PJ, Skoner DP: New enzyme immunoassay for salivary cortisol, Clin Chem 49:203–204, 2003.
146. Papanicolaou DA, Mullen N, Kyrou I, et al: Nighttime salivary cortisol: a useful test for the diagnosis of Cushing's syndrome, J Clin Endocrinol Metab 87:4515–4521, 2002.
147. Putignano P, Toja P, Dubini A, et al: Midnight salivary cortisol versus urinary free and midnight serum cortisol as screening tests for Cushing's syndrome, J Clin Endocrinol Metab 88:4153–4157, 2003.
148. Raff H, Raff JL, Findling JW: Late-night salivary cortisol as a screening test for Cushing's syndrome, J Clin Endocrinol Metab 83:2681–2686, 1998.
149. Castro M, Elias PC, Quidute AR, et al: Out-patient screening for Cushing's syndrome: the sensitivity of the combination of circadian rhythm and overnight dexamethasone suppression salivary cortisol tests, J Clin Endocrinol Metab 84:878–882, 1999.
150. Viardot A, Huber P, Puder JJ, et al: Reproducibility of nighttime salivary cortisol and its use in the diagnosis of hypercortisolism compared with urinary free cortisol and overnight dexamethasone suppression test, J Clin Endocrinol Metab 90:5730–5736, 2005.
151. Trilck M, Flitsch J, Ludecke DK, et al: Salivary cortisol measurement–a reliable method for the diagnosis of Cushing's syndrome, Exp Clin Endocrinol Diabetes 113:225–230, 2005.
152. Yaneva M, Mosnier-Pudar H, Dugue MA, et al: Midnight salivary cortisol for the initial diagnosis of Cushing's syndrome of various causes, J Clin Endocrinol Metab 89:3345–3351, 2004.
153. Baid SK, Sinaii N, Wade M, et al: Radioimmunoassay and tandem mass spectrometry measurement of bedtime salivary cortisol levels: a comparison of assays to establish hypercortisolism, J Clin Endocrinol Metab 92:3102–3107, 2007.
154. Liu H, Bravata DM, Cabaccan J, et al: Elevated late-night salivary cortisol levels in elderly male type 2 diabetic veterans, Clin Endocrinol (Oxf) 63:642–649, 2005.
155. Liddle GW: Tests of pituitary-adrenal suppressibility in the diagnosis of Cushing's syndrome, J Clin Endocrinol Metab 20:1539–1560, 1960.
156. Kennedy L, Atkinson AB, Johnston H, et al: Serum cortisol concentrations during low dose dexamethasone suppression test to screen for Cushing's syndrome, Br Med J (Clin Res Ed) 289:1188–1191, 1984.
157. Hankin ME, Theile HM, Steinbeck AW: An evaluation of laboratory tests for the detection and differential diagnosis of Cushing's syndrome, Clin Endocrinol (Oxf) 6:185–196, 1977.
158. Newell-Price J, Trainer P, Perry L, et al: A single sleeping midnight cortisol has 100% sensitivity for the diagnosis of Cushing's syndrome, Clin Endocrinol (Oxf) 43:545–550, 1995.
159. Isidori AM, Kaltsas GA, Mohammed S, et al: Discriminatory value of the low-dose dexamethasone suppression test in establishing the diagnosis and differential diagnosis of Cushing's syndrome, J Clin Endocrinol Metab 88:5299–5306, 2003.
160. Nugent CA, Nichols T, Tyler FH: Diagnosis of Cushing's syndrome—single dose dexamethasone suppression test, Arch Intern Med 172–176, 1965.
161. Shimizu N, Yoshida H: Studies on the "low dose" suppressible Cushing's disease, Endocrinol Jpn 23:479–484, 1976.
162. McHardy-Young S, Harris PW, Lessof MH, et al: Single dose dexamethasone suppression test for Cushing's Syndrome, Br Med J 2:740–744, 1967.
163. Seidensticker JF, Folk RL, Wieland RG, et al: Screening test for Cushing's syndrome with plasma 11-hydroxycorticosteroids, JAMA 202:87–90, 1967.
164. Crapo L: Cushing's syndrome: a review of diagnostic tests, Metabolism 28:955–977, 1979.
165. Odagiri E, Demura R, Demura H, et al: The changes in plasma cortisol and urinary free cortisol by an overnight dexamethasone suppression test in patients with Cushing's disease, Endocrinol Jpn 35:795–802, 1988.
166. Martinelli CE Jr, Sader SL, Oliveira EB, et al: Salivary cortisol for screening of Cushing's syndrome in children, Clin Endocrinol (Oxf) 51:67–71, 1999.
167. Putignano P, Kaltsas GA, Satta MA, et al: The effects of anti-convulsant drugs on adrenal function, Horm Metab Res 30:389–397, 1998.
168. Abou Samra AB, Dechaud H, Estour B, et al: Beta-lipotropin and cortisol responses to an intravenous infusion dexamethasone suppression test in Cushing's syndrome and obesity, J Clin Endocrinol Metab 61:116–119, 1985.
169. Atkinson AB, McAteer EJ, Hadden DR, et al: A weight-related intravenous dexamethasone suppression test distinguishes obese controls from patients with Cushing's syndrome, Acta Endocrinol (Copenh) 120:753–759, 1989.
170. Klose M, Lange M, Rasmussen AK, et al: Factors influencing the adrenocorticotropin test: role of contemporary cortisol assays, body composition, and oral contraceptive agents, J Clin Endocrinol Metab 92:1326–1333, 2007.
171. Yanovski JA, Cutler GB Jr, Chrousos GP, et al: Corticotropin-releasing hormone stimulation following low-dose dexamethasone administration. A new test to distinguish Cushing's syndrome from pseudo-Cushing's states, JAMA 269:2232–2238, 1993.
172. Yanovski JA, Cutler GB Jr, Chrousos GP, et al: Prospective evaluation of the dexamethasone-suppressed corticotrophin-releasing hormone test in the differential

diagnosis of Cushing's syndrome and pseudo-Cushing's states, Program of the 77th Annual Meeting of the Endocrine Society, Washington DC p 99 (abstract):1995.

173. Martin NM, Dhillo WS, Banerjee A, et al: Comparison of the dexamethasone-suppressed corticotropin-releasing hormone test and low-dose dexamethasone suppression test in the diagnosis of Cushing's syndrome, J Clin Endocrinol Metab 91:2582–2586, 2006.

174. Gatta B, Cortet C, Martinie M, et al: Reevaluation of the dex-CRH test for the differential diagnosis between Cushing's disease and pseudo-Cushing's syndrome. Program of the 88th Annual Meeting of The Endocrine Society, Boston, MA, 2006, P2–734 2006.

175. Erickson D, Natt N, Nippoldt T, et al: Dexamethasone-suppressed corticotropin-releasing hormone stimulation test for diagnosis of mild hypercortisolism, J Clin Endocrinol Metab 92:2972–2976, 2007.

176. Nieman L: Editorial: The dexamethasone-suppressed corticotropin-releasing hormone test for the diagnosis of Cushing's syndrome: what have we learned in 14 years? J Clin Endocrinol Metab 92:2876–2878, 2007.

177. Papanicolaou DA, Yanovski JA, Cutler GB Jr, et al: A single midnight serum cortisol measurement distinguishes Cushing's syndrome from pseudo-Cushing states, J Clin Endocrinol Metab 83:1163–1167, 1998.

178. Reimondo G, Allasino B, Bovio S, et al: Evaluation of the effectiveness of midnight serum cortisol in the diagnostic procedures for Cushing's syndrome, Eur J Endocrinol 153:803–809, 2005.

179. Ambrosi B, Bochicchio D, Ferrario R, et al: Effects of the opiate agonist loperamide on pituitary-adrenal function in patients with suspected hypercortisolism, J Endocrinol Invest 12:31–35, 1989.

180. Ambrosi B, Bochicchio D, Colombo P, et al: Loperamide to diagnose Cushing's syndrome, JAMA 270:2301–2302, 1993.

181. Bernini GP, Argenio GF, Cerri F, et al: Comparison between the suppressive effects of dexamethasone and loperamide on cortisol and ACTH secretion in some pathological conditions, J Endocrinol Invest 17:799–804, 1994.

182. Lytras N, Grossman A, Perry L, et al: Corticotrophin releasing factor: responses in normal subjects and patients with disorders of the hypothalamus and pituitary, Clin Endocrinol (Oxf) 20:71–84, 1984.

183. Fig LM, Gross MD, Shapiro B, et al: Adrenal localization in the adrenocorticotropic hormone-independent Cushing syndrome, Ann Intern Med 109:547–553, 1988.

184. Perry RR, Nieman LK, Cutler GB Jr, et al: Primary adrenal causes of Cushing's syndrome. Diagnosis and surgical management, Ann Surg 210:59–68, 1989.

185. Doppman JL, Miller DL, Dwyer AJ, et al: Macronodular adrenal hyperplasia in Cushing disease, Radiology 166:347–352, 1988.

186. Mimou N, Sakato S, Nakabayashi H, et al: Cushing's syndrome associated with bilateral adrenal adenomas, Acta Endocrinol (Copenh) 108:245–254, 1985.

187. Doppman JL, Travis WD, Nieman L, et al: Cushing syndrome due to primary pigmented nodular adrenocortical disease: findings at CT and MR imaging, Radiology 172:415–420, 1989.

188. Doppman JL, Nieman LK, Travis WD, et al: CT and MR imaging of massive macronodular adrenocortical disease: a rare cause of autonomous primary adrenal hypercortisolism, J Comput Assist Tomogr 15:773–779, 1991.

189. Sohaib SA, Hanson JA, Newell-Price JD, et al: CT appearance of the adrenal glands in adrenocorticotrophic hormone-dependent Cushing's syndrome, AJR Am J Roentgenol 172:997–1002, 1999.

190. Aron DC, Findling JW, Fitzgerald PA, et al: Pituitary ACTH dependency of nodular adrenal hyperplasia in Cushing's syndrome. Report of two cases and review of the literature, Am J Med 71:302–306, 1981.

191. Howlett TA, Drury PL, Perry L, et al: Diagnosis and management of ACTH-dependent Cushing's syndrome: comparison of the features in ectopic and pituitary ACTH production, Clin Endocrinol (Oxf) 24:699–713, 1986.

192. Newell-Price J, Morris DG, Drake WM, et al: Optimal response criteria for the human CRH test in the differential diagnosis of ACTH-dependent Cushing's syndrome, J Clin Endocrinol Metab 87:1640–1645, 2002.

193. Yamamoto Y, Davis DH, Nippoldt TB, et al: False-positive inferior petrosal sinus sampling in the diagnosis of Cushing's disease. Report of two cases, J Neurosurg 83:1087–1091, 1995.

194. Yanovski JA, Cutler GB Jr, Doppman JL, et al: The limited ability of inferior petrosal sinus sampling with corticotropin-releasing hormone to distinguish Cushing's disease from pseudo-Cushing states or normal physiology, J Clin Endocrinol Metab 77:503–509, 1993.

195. Miller DL, Doppman JL: Petrosal sinus sampling: technique and rationale, Radiology 178:37–47, 1991.

196. Oldfield EH, Doppman JL, Nieman LK, et al: Petrosal sinus sampling with and without corticotropin-releasing hormone for the differential diagnosis of Cushing's syndrome, N Engl J Med 325:897–905, 1991.

197. Kaltsas GA, Giannulis MG, Newell-Price JD, et al: A critical analysis of the value of simultaneous inferior petrosal sinus sampling in Cushing's disease and the occult ectopic adrenocorticotropin syndrome, J Clin Endocrinol Metab 84:487–492, 1999.

198. Colao A, Faggiano A, Pivonello R, et al: Inferior petrosal sinus sampling in the differential diagnosis of Cushing's syndrome: results of an Italian multicenter study, Eur J Endocrinol 144:499–507, 2001.

199. Swearingen B, Katznelson L, Miller K, et al: Diagnostic errors after inferior petrosal sinus sampling, J Clin Endocrinol Metab 89:3752–3763, 2004.

200. McCance DR, McIlrath E, McNeill A, et al: Bilateral inferior petrosal sinus sampling as a routine procedure in ACTH-dependent Cushing's syndrome, Clin Endocrinol (Oxf) 30:157–166, 1989.

201. Findling JW, Kehoe ME, Raff H: Identification of patients with Cushing's disease with negative pituitary adrenocorticotropin gradients during inferior petrosal sinus sampling: prolactin as an index of pituitary venous effluent, J Clin Endocrinol Metab 89:6005–6009, 2004.

202. Miller DL: Neurologic complications of petrosal sinus sampling, Radiology 183:878, 1992.

203. Lefournier V, Gatta B, Martinie M, et al: One transient neurological complication (sixth nerve palsy) in 166 consecutive inferior petrosal sinus samplings for the etiological diagnosis of Cushing's syndrome, J Clin Endocrinol Metab 84:3401–3402, 1999.

204. Rotman-Pikielny P, Patronas N, Papanicolaou DA: Pituitary apoplexy induced by corticotrophin-releasing hormone in a patient with Cushing's disease, Clin Endocrinol (Oxf) 58:545–549, 2003.

205. Tabarin A, Greselle JF, San Galli F, et al: Usefulness of the corticotropin-releasing hormone test during bilateral inferior petrosal sinus sampling for the diagnosis of Cushing's disease, J Clin Endocrinol Metab 73:53–59, 1991.

206. Landolt AM, Schubiger O, Maurer R, et al: The value of inferior petrosal sinus sampling in diagnosis and treatment of Cushing's disease, Clin Endocrinol (Oxf) 40:485–492, 1994.

207. Lefournier V, Martinie M, Vasdev A, et al: Accuracy of bilateral inferior petrosal or cavernous sinuses sampling in predicting the lateralization of Cushing's disease pituitary microadenoma: influence of catheter position and anatomy of venous drainage, J Clin Endocrinol Metab 88:196–203, 2003.

208. Morris DG, Grossman AB: Dynamic tests in the diagnosis and differential diagnosis of Cushing's syndrome, J Endocrinol Invest 26:64–73, 2003.

209. Miller DL, Doppman JL, Nieman LK, et al: Petrosal sinus sampling: discordant lateralization of ACTH-secreting pituitary microadenomas before and after stimulation with corticotropin-releasing hormone, Radiology 176:429–431, 1990.

210. Erickson D, Huston J, III, Young WF Jr, et al: Internal jugular vein sampling in adrenocorticotropic hormone-dependent Cushing's syndrome: a comparison with inferior petrosal sinus sampling, Clin Endocrinol (Oxf) 60:413–419, 2004.

211. Ilias I, Chang R, Pacak K, et al: Jugular venous sampling: an alternative to petrosal sinus sampling for the diagnostic evaluation of adrenocorticotropic hormone-dependent Cushing's syndrome, J Clin Endocrinol Metab 89:3795–3800, 2004.

212. Tyrrell JB, Findling JW, Aron DC, et al: An overnight high-dose dexamethasone suppression test for rapid differential diagnosis of Cushing's syndrome, Ann Intern Med 104:180–186, 1986.

213. Aron DC, Raff H, Findling JW: Effectiveness versus efficacy: the limited value in clinical practice of high dose dexamethasone suppression testing in the differential diagnosis of adrenocorticotropin-dependent Cushing's syndrome, J Clin Endocrinol Metab 82:1780–1785, 1997.

214. Kaye TB, Crapo L: The Cushing syndrome: an update on diagnostic tests, Ann Intern Med 112:434–444, 1990.

215. Giraldi FP, Invitti C, Cavagnini F: The corticotropin-releasing hormone test in the diagnosis of ACTH-dependent Cushing's syndrome: a reappraisal, Clin Endocrinol (Oxf) 54:601–607, 2001.

216. Ilias I, Torpy DJ, Pacak K, et al: Cushing's syndrome due to ectopic corticotropin secretion: twenty years' experience at the National Institutes of Health, J Clin Endocrinol Metab 90:4955–4962, 2005.

217. Trainer PJ, Faria M, Newell-Price J, et al: A comparison of the effects of human and ovine corticotropin-releasing hormone on the pituitary-adrenal axis, J Clin Endocrinol Metab 80:412–417, 1995.

218. Trainer PJ, Woods RJ, Korbonits M, et al: The pathophysiology of circulating corticotropin-releasing hormone-binding protein levels in the human, J Clin Endocrinol Metab 83:1611–1614, 1998.

219. Nieman LK, Oldfield EH, Wesley R, et al: A simplified morning ovine corticotropin-releasing hormone stimulation test for the differential diagnosis of adrenocorticotropin-dependent Cushing's syndrome, J Clin Endocrinol Metab 77:1308–1312, 1993.

220. Korbonits M, Kaltsas G, Perry LA, et al: The growth hormone secretagogue hexarelin stimulates the hypothalamo-pituitary-adrenal axis via arginine vasopressin, J Clin Endocrinol Metab 84:2489–2495, 1999.

221. Korbonits M, Bustin SA, Kojima M, et al: The expression of the growth hormone secretagogue receptor ligand ghrelin in normal and abnormal human pituitary and other neuroendocrine tumors, J Clin Endocrinol Metab 86:881–887, 2001.

222. Tabarin A, San Galli F, Dezou S, et al: The corticotropin-releasing factor test in the differential diagnosis of Cushing's syndrome: a comparison with the lysine-vasopressin test, Acta Endocrinol (Copenh) 123:331–338, 1990.

223. Malerbi DA, Mendonca BB, Liberman B, et al: The desmopressin stimulation test in the differential diagnosis of Cushing's syndrome, Clin Endocrinol (Oxf) 38:463–472, 1993.

224. Ghigo E, Arvat E, Ramunni J, et al: Adrenocorticotropin- and cortisol-releasing effect of hexarelin, a synthetic growth hormone-releasing peptide, in normal subjects and patients with Cushing's syndrome, J Clin Endocrinol Metab 82:2439–2444, 1997.

225. Castinetti F, Morange I, Dufour H, et al: Desmopressin test during petrosal sinus sampling: a valuable tool to discriminate pituitary or ectopic ACTH-dependent Cushing's syndrome, Eur J Endocrinol 157:271–277, 2007.

226. Newell-Price J, Perry L, Medbak S, et al: A combined test using desmopressin and corticotropin-releasing hormone in the differential diagnosis of Cushing's syndrome, J Clin Endocrinol Metab 82:176–181, 1997.

227. Tsagarakis S, Tsigos C, Vasiliou V, et al: The desmopressin and combined CRH-desmopressin tests in the differential diagnosis of ACTH-dependent Cushing's syndrome: constraints imposed by the expression of V2 vasopressin receptors in tumors with ectopic ACTH secretion, J Clin Endocrinol Metab 87:1646–1653, 2002.

228. Korbonits M, Jacobs RA, Aylwin SJB, et al: Expression of the Growth Hormone Secretagogue Receptor in Pituitary Adenomas and Other Neuroendocrine Tumors, J Clin Endocrinol Metab 83:3624–3630, 1998.

229. Nieman LK, Chrousos GP, Oldfield EH, et al: The ovine corticotropin-releasing hormone stimulation test and the dexamethasone suppression test in the differential diagnosis of Cushing's syndrome, Ann Intern Med 105:862–867, 1986.

230. Hermus AR, Pieters GF, Pesman GJ, et al: The corticotropin-releasing-hormone test versus the high-dose dexamethasone test in the differential diagnosis of Cushing's syndrome, Lancet 2:540–544, 1986.

231. Grossman AB, Howlett TA, Perry L, et al: CRF in the differential diagnosis of Cushing's syndrome: a comparison with the dexamethasone suppression test, Clin Endocrinol (Oxf) 29:167–178, 1988.

232. Doppman JL, Frank JA, Dwyer AJ, et al: Gadolinium DTPA enhanced MR imaging of ACTH-secreting microadenomas of the pituitary gland, J Comput Assist Tomogr 12:728–735, 1988.
233. Patronas N, Bulakbasi N, Stratakis CA, et al: Spoiled gradient recalled acquisition in the steady state technique is superior to conventional postcontrast spin echo technique for magnetic resonance imaging detection of adrenocorticotropin-secreting pituitary tumors, J Clin Endocrinol Metab 88:1565–1569, 2003.
234. Hall WA, Luciano MG, Doppman JL, et al: Pituitary magnetic resonance imaging in normal human volunteers: occult adenomas in the general population, Ann Intern Med 120:817–820, 1994.
235. Findling JW, Doppman JL: Biochemical and radiologic diagnosis of Cushing's syndrome, Endocrinol Metab Clin North Am 23:511–537, 1994.
236. Escourolle H, Abecassis JP, Bertagna X, et al: Comparison of computerized tomography and magnetic resonance imaging for the examination of the pituitary gland in patients with Cushing's disease, Clin Endocrinol (Oxf) 39:307–313, 1993.
237. Doppman JL, Pass HI, Nieman LK, et al: Detection of ACTH-producing bronchial carcinoid tumors: MR imaging vs CT, AJR Am J Roentgenol 156:39–43, 1991.
238. Doppman JL, Nieman L, Miller DL, et al: Ectopic adrenocorticotropic hormone syndrome: localization studies in 28 patients, Radiology 172:115–124, 1989.
239. de Herder WW, Lamberts SW: Octapeptide somatostatin-analogue therapy of Cushing's syndrome, Postgrad Med J 75:65–66, 1999.
240. Tabarin A, Valli N, Chanson P, et al: Usefulness of somatostatin receptor scintigraphy in patients with occult ectopic adrenocorticotropin syndrome, J Clin Endocrinol Metab 84:1193–1202, 1999.
241. Tsagarakis S, Christoforaki M, Giannopoulou H, et al: A reappraisal of the utility of somatostatin receptor scintigraphy in patients with ectopic adrenocorticotropin Cushing's syndrome, J Clin Endocrinol Metab 88:4754–4758, 2003.
242. Torpy DJ, Chen CC, Mullen N, et al: Lack of utility of (111)In-pentetreotide scintigraphy in localizing ectopic ACTH producing tumors: follow-up of 18 patients, J Clin Endocrinol Metab 84:1186–1192, 1999.
243. Kumar J, Spring M, Carroll PV, et al: 18Fluorodeoxyglucose positron emission tomography in the localization of ectopic ACTH-secreting neuroendocrine tumours, Clin Endocrinol (Oxf) 64:371–374, 2006.
244. Pacak K, Ilias I, Chen CC, et al: The role of [(18)F]fluorodeoxyglucose positron emission tomography and [(111)In]-diethylenetriaminepentaacetate-D-Phe-pentetreotide scintigraphy in the localization of ectopic adrenocorticotropin-secreting tumors causing Cushing's syndrome, J Clin Endocrinol Metab 89:2214–2221, 2004.
245. Sarkar R, Thompson NW, McLeod MK: The role of adrenalectomy in Cushing's syndrome, Surgery 108:1079–1084, 1990.
246. Terzolo M, Reimondo G, Bovio S, et al: Subclinical Cushing's syndrome, Pituitary 7:217–223, 2004.
247. Biller BM, Grossman AB, Stewart PM, et al: Treatment of Adrenocorticotropin-Dependent Cushing's Syndrome: A Consensus Statement, J Clin Endocrinol Metab 93:2454–2462, 2008.
248. Lamberts SW, van der Lely AJ, de Herder WW: Transsphenoidal selective adenomectomy is the treatment of choice in patients with Cushing's disease. Considerations concerning preoperative medical treatment and the long-term follow-up, J Clin Endocrinol Metab 80:3111–3113, 1995.
249. Boscaro M, Sonino N, Scarda A, et al: Anticoagulant prophylaxis markedly reduces thromboembolic complications in Cushing's syndrome, J Clin Endocrinol Metab 87:3662–3666, 2002.
250. Welbourn RB: The evolution of transsphenoidal pituitary microsurgery, Surgery 100:1185–1190, 1986.
251. Fahlbusch R, Buchfelder M, Muller OA: Transsphenoidal surgery for Cushing's disease, J R Soc Med 79:262–269, 1986.
252. Knappe UJ, Ludecke DK: Persistent and recurrent hypercortisolism after transsphenoidal surgery for Cushing's disease, Acta Neurochir Suppl 65:31–34, 1996.
253. Stevenaert A, Perrin G, Martin D, et al: [Cushing's disease and corticotrophic adenoma: results of pituitary microsurgery], Neurochirurgie 48:234–265, 2002.
254. Swearingen B, Biller BM, Barker FG, et al: Long-term mortality after transsphenoidal surgery for Cushing disease, Ann Intern Med 130:821–824, 1999.
255. Hammer GD, Tyrrell JB, Lamborn KR, et al: Transsphenoidal microsurgery for Cushing's disease: initial outcome and long-term results, J Clin Endocrinol Metab 89:6348–6357, 2004.
256. Hofmann BM, Fahlbusch R: Treatment of Cushing's disease: a retrospective clinical study of the latest 100 cases, Front Horm Res 34:158–184, 2006.
257. Bochicchio D, Losa M, Buchfelder M: Factors influencing the immediate and late outcome of Cushing's disease treated by transsphenoidal surgery: a retrospective study by the European Cushing's Disease Survey Group, J Clin Endocrinol Metab 80:3114–3120, 1995.
258. Sonino N, Zielezny M, Fava GA, et al: Risk factors and long-term outcome in pituitary-dependent Cushing's disease, J Clin Endocrinol Metab 81:2647–2652, 1996.
259. Blevins LS Jr, Christy JH, Khajavi M, et al: Outcomes of therapy for Cushing's disease due to adrenocorticotropin-secreting pituitary macroadenomas, J Clin Endocrinol Metab 83:63–67, 1998.
260. Netea-Maier RT, van Lindert EJ, den Heijer M, et al: Transsphenoidal pituitary surgery via the endoscopic technique: results in 35 consecutive patients with Cushing's disease, Eur J Endocrinol 154:675–684, 2006.
261. Oldfield EH, Vortmeyer AO: Development of a histological pseudocapsule and its use as a surgical capsule in the excision of pituitary tumors, J Neurosurg 104:7–19, 2006.
262. Atkinson AB, Kennedy A, Wiggam MI, et al: Long-term remission rates after pituitary surgery for Cushing's disease: the need for long-term surveillance, Clin Endocrinol (Oxf) 63:549–559, 2005.
263. Rees DA, Hanna FW, Davies JS, et al: Long-term follow-up results of transsphenoidal surgery for Cushing's disease in a single centre using strict criteria for remission, Clin Endocrinol (Oxf) 56:541–551, 2002.
264. Hughes NR, Lissett CA, Shalet SM: Growth hormone status following treatment for Cushing's syndrome, Clin Endocrinol (Oxf) 51:61–66, 1999.
265. Pereira AM, van Aken MO, van Dulken H, et al: Long-term predictive value of postsurgical cortisol concentrations for cure and risk of recurrence in Cushing's disease, J Clin Endocrinol Metab 88:5858–5864, 2003.
266. Esposito F, Dusick JR, Cohan P, et al: Clinical review: Early morning cortisol levels as a predictor of remission after transsphenoidal surgery for Cushing's disease, J Clin Endocrinol Metab 91:7–13, 2006.
267. Avgerinos PC, Chrousos GP, Nieman LK, et al: The corticotropin-releasing hormone test in the postoperative evaluation of patients with Cushing's syndrome, J Clin Endocrinol Metab 65:906–913, 1987.
268. Nieman LK, Gumowski J, DeVroom H, et al: Prediction of long-term remission of Cushing's disease after successful transsphenoidal resection of ACTH-secreting tumor. Presented at the 80th Annual Meeting of the Endocrine Society P345: New Orleans, LA, 1998.
269. Colombo P, Dall'Asta C, Barbetta L, et al: Usefulness of the desmopressin test in the postoperative evaluation of patients with Cushing's disease, Eur J Endocrinol 143:227–234, 2000.
270. Losa M, Mortini P, Dylgjeri S, et al: Desmopressin stimulation test before and after pituitary surgery in patients with Cushing's disease, Clin Endocrinol (Oxf) 55:61–68, 2001.
271. Byyny RL: Withdrawal from glucocorticoid therapy, N Engl J Med 295:30–32, 1976.
272. Papanicolaou DA, Tsigos C, Oldfield EH, et al: Acute glucocorticoid deficiency is associated with plasma elevations of interleukin-6: does the latter participate in the symptomatology of the steroid withdrawal syndrome and adrenal insufficiency? J Clin Endocrinol Metab 81:2303–2306, 1996.
273. Leshin M: Acute adrenal insufficiency: recognition, management, and prevention, Urol Clin North Am 9:229–235, 1982.
274. Lindsay JR, Nansel T, Baid S, et al: Long-term impaired quality of life in Cushing's syndrome despite initial improvement after surgical remission, J Clin Endocrinol Metab 91:447–453, 2006.
275. Olson BR, Rubino D, Gumowski J, et al: Isolated hyponatremia after transsphenoidal pituitary surgery, J Clin Endocrinol Metab 80:85–91, 1995.
276. Manning PJ, Evans MC, Reid IR: Normal bone mineral density following cure of Cushing's syndrome, Clin Endocrinol (Oxf) 36:229–234, 1992.
277. Di Somma C, Pivonello R, Loche S, et al: Effect of 2 years of cortisol normalization on the impaired bone mass and turnover in adolescent and adult patients with Cushing's disease: a prospective study, Clin Endocrinol (Oxf) 58:302–308, 2003.
278. Di Somma C, Colao A, Pivonello R, et al: Effectiveness of chronic treatment with alendronate in the osteoporosis of Cushing's disease, Clin Endocrinol (Oxf) 48:655–662, 1998.
279. Ram Z, Nieman LK, Cutler GB Jr, et al: Early repeat surgery for persistent Cushing's disease, J Neurosurg 80:37–45, 1994.
280. Locatelli M, Vance ML, Laws ER: Clinical review: the strategy of immediate reoperation for transsphenoidal surgery for Cushing's disease, J Clin Endocrinol Metab 90:5478–5482, 2005.
281. Doherty GM, Nieman LK, Cutler GB Jr, et al: Time to recovery of the hypothalamic-pituitary-adrenal axis after curative resection of adrenal tumors in patients with Cushing's syndrome, Surgery 108:1085–1090, 1990.
282. Plumpton FS, Besser GM: The adrenocortical response to surgery and insulin-induced hypoglycemia in corticosteroid-treated and normal subjects, Br J Surg 55:857, 1968.
283. Bangar V, Clayton RN: How reliable is the short synacthen test for the investigation of the hypothalamic-pituitary-adrenal axis? Eur J Endocrinol 139:580–583, 1998.
284. Kehlet H, Lindholm J, Bjerre P: Value of the 30 min ACTH-test in assessing hypothalamic-pituitary-adrenocortical function after pituitary surgery in Cushing's disease, Clin Endocrinol (Oxf) 20:349–353, 1984.
285. Stewart PM, Corrie J, Seckl JR, et al: A rational approach for assessing the hypothalamo-pituitary-adrenal axis, Lancet 1:1208–1210, 1988.
286. Orme SM, Peacey SR, Barth JH, et al: Comparison of tests of stress-released cortisol secretion in pituitary disease, Clin Endocrinol (Oxf) 45:135–140, 1996.
287. Ammari F, Issa BG, Millward E, Scanion MF: A comparison between short ACTH and insulin stress tests for assessing hypothalamo-pituitary-adrenal function, Clin Endocrinol (Oxf) 44:473–476, 1996.
288. Timmers HJ, van Ginneken EM, Wesseling P, et al: A patient with recurrent hypercortisolism after removal of an ACTH-secreting pituitary adenoma due to an adrenal macronodule, J Endocrinol Invest 29:934–939, 2006.
289. Valimaki M, Pelkonen R, Porkka L, et al: Long-term results of adrenal surgery in patients with Cushing's syndrome due to adrenocortical adenoma, Clin Endocrinol (Oxf) 20:229–236, 1984.
290. Bellantone R, Ferrante A, Boscherini M, et al: Role of reoperation in recurrence of adrenal cortical carcinoma: results from 188 cases collected in the Italian National Registry for Adrenal Cortical Carcinoma, Surgery 122:1212–1218, 1997.
291. McCallum RW, Connell JM: Laparoscopic adrenalectomy, Clin Endocrinol (Oxf) 55:435–436, 2001.
292. Wells SA, Merke DP, Cutler GB Jr, et al: Therapeutic controversy: The role of laparoscopic surgery in adrenal disease, J Clin Endocrinol Metab 83:3041–3049, 1998.
293. Kemink L, Pieters G, Hermus A, et al: Patient's age is a simple predictive factor for the development of Nelson's syndrome after total adrenalectomy for Cushing's disease, J Clin Endocrinol Metab 79:887–889, 1994.
294. Assie G, Bahurel H, Coste J, et al: Corticotroph tumor progression after adrenalectomy in Cushing's Disease: A reappraisal of Nelson's Syndrome, J Clin Endocrinol Metab 92:172–179, 2007.
295. Jenkins PJ, Trainer PJ, Plowman PN, et al: The long-term outcome after adrenalectomy and prophylactic pituitary radiotherapy in adrenocorticotropin-dependent Cushing's syndrome, J Clin Endocrinol Metab 80:165–171, 1995.
296. Sheline GE, Wara WM, Smith V: Therapeutic irradiation and brain injury, Int J Radiat Oncol Biol Phys 6:1215–1228, 1980.
297. Orth DN, Liddle GW: Results of treatment in 108 patients with Cushing's syndrome, N Engl J Med 285:243–247, 1971.

298. Howlett TA, Plowman PN, Wass JA, et al: Megavoltage pituitary irradiation in the management of Cushing's disease and Nelson's syndrome: long-term follow-up, Clin Endocrinol (Oxf) 31:309–323, 1989.
299. Murayama M, Yasuda K, Minamori Y, et al: Long term follow-up of Cushing's disease treated with reserpine and pituitary irradiation, J Clin Endocrinol Metab 75:935–942, 1992.
300. Littley MD, Shalet SM, Beardwell CG, et al: Long-term follow-up of low-dose external pituitary irradiation for Cushing's disease, Clin Endocrinol (Oxf) 33:445–455, 1990.
301. Estrada J, Boronat M, Mielgo M, et al: The long-term outcome of pituitary irradiation after unsuccessful transsphenoidal surgery in Cushing's disease, N Engl J Med 336:172–177, 1997.
302. Mahmoud-Ahmed AS, Suh JH: Radiation therapy for Cushing's disease: a review, Pituitary 5:175–180, 2002.
303. Plowman PN: Pituitary adenoma radiotherapy—when, who and how? Clin Endocrinol (Oxf) 51:265–271, 1999.
304. Becker G, Kocher M, Kortmann RD, et al: Radiation therapy in the multimodal treatment approach of pituitary adenoma, Strahlenther Onkol 178:173–186, 2002.
305. Marks LB: Conventional fractionated radiation therapy vs. radiosurgery for selected benign intracranial lesions (arteriovenous malformations, pituitary adenomas, and acoustic neuromas), J Neurooncol 17:223–230, 1993.
306. Jagannathan J, Sheehan JP, Pouratian N, et al: Gamma Knife surgery for Cushing's disease, J Neurosurg 106:980–987, 2007.
307. Petit JH, Biller BM, Yock TI, et al: Proton stereotactic radiotherapy for persistent adrenocorticotropin-producing adenomas, J Clin Endocrinol Metab 93:393–399, 2008.
308. Swords FM, Allan CA, Plowman PN, et al: Stereotactic Radiosurgery XVI: A Treatment for Previously Irradiated Pituitary Adenomas, J Clin Endocrinol Metab 88:5334–5340, 2003.
309. Sandler LM, Richards NT, Carr DH, et al: Long term follow-up of patients with Cushing's disease treated by interstitial irradiation, J Clin Endocrinol Metab 65:441–447, 1987.
310. Molinatti GM, Limone P, Porta M: Treatment of Cushing's disease by interstitial pituitary irradiation: short- and long-term follow-up, Panminerva Med 37:1–7, 1995.
311. Magee BJ, Gattamaneni HR, Pearson D: Adrenal cortical carcinoma: survival after radiotherapy, Clin Radiol 38:587–588, 1987.
312. de Castro F, Isa W, Aguera L, et al: [Primary adrenal carcinoma], Actas Urol Esp 17:30–34, 1993.
313. He J, Zhou J, Lu Z: Radiotherapy of ectopic ACTH syndrome due to thoracic carcinoids, Chin Med J (Engl) 108:338–341, 1995.
314. Andres R, Mayordomo JI, Cajal S, et al: Paraneoplastic Cushing's syndrome associated to locally advanced thymic carcinoid tumor, Tumori 88:65–67, 2002.
315. Misbin RI, Canary J, Willard D: Aminoglutethimide in the treatment of Cushing's syndrome, J Clin Pharmacol 16:645–651, 1976.
316. Semple CG, Beastall GH, Gray CE, et al: Trilostane in the management of Cushing's syndrome, Acta Endocrinol (Copenh) 102:107–110, 1983.
317. Carballeira A, Fishman LM, Jacobi JD: Dual sites of inhibition by metyrapone of human adrenal steroidogenesis: correlation of in vivo and in vitro studies, J Clin Endocrinol Metab 42:687–695, 1976.
318. Verhelst JA, Trainer PJ, Howlett TA, et al: Short and long-term responses to metyrapone in the medical management of 91 patients with Cushing's syndrome, Clin Endocrinol (Oxf) 35:169–178, 1991.
319. Jeffcoate WJ, Rees LH, Tomlin S, et al: Metyrapone in long-term management of Cushing's disease, Br Med J 2:215–217, 1977.
320. Feldman D: Ketoconazole and other imidazole derivatives as inhibitors of steroidogenesis, Endocr Rev 7:409–420, 1986.
321. Engelhardt D, Weber MM, Miksch T, et al: The influence of ketoconazole on human adrenal steroidogenesis: incubation studies with tissue slices, Clin Endocrinol (Oxf) 35:163–168, 1991.
322. Steen RE, Kapelrud H, Haug E, et al: In vivo and in vitro inhibition by ketoconazole of ACTH secretion from a human thymic carcinoid tumour, Acta Endocrinol (Copenh) 125:331–334, 1991.
323. Sonino N, Boscaro M, Paoletta A, et al: Ketoconazole treatment in Cushing's syndrome: experience in 34 patients, Clin Endocrinol (Oxf) 35:347–352, 1991.
324. Tabarin A, Navarranne A, Guerin J, et al: Use of ketoconazole in the treatment of Cushing's disease and ectopic ACTH syndrome, Clin Endocrinol (Oxf) 34:63–69, 1991.
325. Ahmed M, Kanaan I, Alarifi A, et al: ACTH-producing pituitary cancer: experience at the King Faisal Specialist Hospital & Research Centre, Pituitary 3:105–112, 2000.
326. Lewis JH, Zimmerman HJ, Benson GD, et al: Hepatic injury associated with ketoconazole therapy. Analysis of 33 cases, Gastroenterology 86:503–513, 1984.
327. Duarte PA, Chow CC, Simmons F, et al: Fatal hepatitis associated with ketoconazole therapy, Arch Intern Med 144:1069–1070, 1984.
328. Knight TE, Shikuma CY, Knight J: Ketoconazole-induced fulminant hepatitis necessitating liver transplantation, J Am Acad Dermatol 25:398–400, 1991.
329. McCance DR, Ritchie CM, Sheridan B, et al: Acute hypoadrenalism and hepatotoxicity after treatment with ketoconazole, Lancet 1:573, 1987.
330. Tucker WS Jr, Snell BB, Island DP, et al: Reversible adrenal insufficiency induced by ketoconazole, JAMA 253:2413–2414, 1985.
331. Miettinen TA: Cholesterol metabolism during ketoconazole treatment in man, J Lipid Res 29:43–51, 1988.
332. Riedl M, Maier C, Zettinig G, et al: Long term control of hypercortisolism with fluconazole: case report and in vitro studies, Eur J Endocrinol 154:519–524, 2006.
333. Hart MM, Swackhamer ES, Straw JA: Studies on the site of action of o,p′-DDD in the dog adrenal cortex. II, Steroids 17:575–586, 1971.
334. Ojima M, Saitoh M, Itoh N, et al: [The effects of o,p′-DDD on adrenal steroidogenesis and hepatic steroid metabolism], Nippon Naibunpi Gakkai Zasshi 61:168–178, 1985.
335. Bergenstal DM, Hertz R, Lipsett MB, et al: Chemotherapy of adrenocortical cancer with O,p′DDD, Ann Intern Med 53:672–682, 1960.
336. Gutierrez ML, Crooke ST: Mitotane (o,p′-DDD), Cancer Treat Rev 7:49–55, 1980.
337. Kasperlik-Zaluska AA: Clinical results of the use of mitotane for adrenocortical carcinoma, Braz J Med Biol Res 33:1191–1196, 2000.
338. Terzolo M, Angeli A, Fassnacht M, et al: Adjuvant mitotane treatment for adrenocortical carcinoma, N Engl J Med 356:2372–2380, 2007.
339. van Slooten H, Moolenaar AJ, van Seters AP, et al: The treatment of adrenocortical carcinoma with o,p′-DDD: prognostic implications of serum level monitoring, Eur J Cancer Clin Oncol 20:47–53, 1984.
340. Bukowski RM, Wolfe M, Levine HS, et al: Phase II trial of mitotane and cisplatin in patients with adrenal carcinoma: a Southwest Oncology Group study, J Clin Oncol 11:161–165, 1993.
341. Berruti A, Terzolo M, Pia A, et al: Mitotane associated with etoposide, doxorubicin, and cisplatin in the treatment of advanced adrenocortical carcinoma. Italian Group for the Study of Adrenal Cancer, Cancer 83:2194–2200, 1998.
342. Williamson SK, Lew D, Miller GJ, et al: Phase II evaluation of cisplatin and etoposide followed by mitotane at disease progression in patients with locally advanced or metastatic adrenocortical carcinoma: a Southwest Oncology Group Study, Cancer 88:1159–1165, 2000.
343. Luton JP, Mahoudeau JA, Bouchard P, et al: Treatment of Cushing's disease by O,p′DDD. Survey of 62 cases, N Engl J Med 300:459–464, 1979.
344. Schteingart DE, Tsao HS, Taylor CI, et al: Sustained remission of Cushing's disease with mitotane and pituitary irradiation, Ann Intern Med 92:613–619, 1980.
345. Carey RM, Orth DN, Hartmann WH: Malignant melanoma with ectopic production of adrenocorticotropic hormone. Palliative treatment with inhibitors of adrenal steroid biosynthesis, J Clin Endocrinol Metab 36:482–487, 1973.
346. Hutter AM Jr, Kayhoe DE: Adrenal cortical carcinoma. Results of treatment with o,p′DDD in 138 patients, Am J Med 41:581–592, 1966.
347. Luton JP, Cerdas S, Billaud L, et al: Clinical features of adrenocortical carcinoma, prognostic factors, and the effect of mitotane therapy, N Engl J Med 322:1195–1201, 1990.
348. Haak HR, Caekebeke-Peerlinck KM, van Seters AP, et al: Prolonged bleeding time due to mitotane therapy, Eur J Cancer 27:638–641, 1991.
349. Maher VM, Trainer PJ, Scoppola A, et al: Possible mechanism and treatment of o,p′DDD-induced hypercholesterolaemia, Q J Med 84:671–679, 1992.
350. Leiba S, Weinstein R, Shindel B, et al: The protracted effect of o,p′-DDD in Cushing's disease and its impact on adrenal morphogenesis of young human embryo, Ann Endocrinol (Paris) 50:49–53, 1989.
351. van Seters AP, Moolenaar AJ: Mitotane increases the blood levels of hormone-binding proteins, Acta Endocrinol (Copenh) 124:526–533, 1991.
352. Hague RV, May W, Cullen DR: Hepatic microsomal enzyme induction and adrenal crisis due to o,p′DDD therapy for metastatic adrenocortical carcinoma, Clin Endocrinol (Oxf) 31:51–57, 1989.
353. Ledingham IM, Watt I: Influence of sedation on mortality in critically ill multiple trauma patients, Lancet 1:1270, 1983.
354. Weber MM, Lang J, Abedinpour F, et al: Different inhibitory effect of etomidate and ketoconazole on the human adrenal steroid biosynthesis, Clin Investig 71:933–938, 1993.
355. Lamberts SW, Bons EG, Bruining HA, et al: Differential effects of the imidazole derivatives etomidate, ketoconazole and miconazole and of metyrapone on the secretion of cortisol and its precursors by human adrenocortical cells, J Pharmacol Exp Ther 240:259–264, 1987.
356. Schulte HM, Benker G, Reinwein D, et al: Infusion of low dose etomidate: correction of hypercortisolemia in patients with Cushing's syndrome and dose-response relationship in normal subjects, J Clin Endocrinol Metab 70:1426–1430, 1990.
357. Allolio B, Schulte HM, Kaulen D, et al: Nonhypnotic low-dose etomidate for rapid correction of hypercortisolaemia in Cushing's syndrome, Klin Wochenschr 66:361–364, 1988.
358. Herrmann BL, Mitchell A, Saller B, et al: [Transsphenoidal hypophysectomy of a patient with an ACTH-producing pituitary adenoma and an "empty sella" after pretreatment with etomidate], Dtsch Med Wochenschr 126:232–234, 2001.
359. Drake WM, Perry LA, Hinds CJ, et al: Emergency and prolonged use of intravenous etomidate to control hypercortisolemia in a patient with Cushing's syndrome and peritonitis, J Clin Endocrinol Metab 83:3542–3544, 1998.
360. Krakoff J, Koch CA, Calis KA, et al: Use of a parenteral propylene glycol-containing etomidate preparation for the long-term management of ectopic Cushing's syndrome, J Clin Endocrinol Metab 86:4104–4108, 2001.
361. Greening JE, Brain CE, Perry LA, et al: Efficient short-term control of hypercortisolaemia by low-dose etomidate in severe paediatric Cushing's disease, Horm Res 64:140–143, 2005.
362. Sartor O, Cutler GB Jr: Mifepristone: treatment of Cushing's syndrome, Clin Obstet Gynecol 39:506–510, 1996.
363. Waveren Hogervorst CO, Koppeschaar HP, Zelissen PM, et al: Cortisol secretory patterns in Cushing's disease and response to cyproheptadine treatment, J Clin Endocrinol Metab 81:652–655, 1996.
364. Sonino N, Fava GA, Fallo F, et al: Effect of the serotonin antagonists ritanserin and ketanserin in Cushing's disease, Pituitary 3:55–59, 2000.
365. Mercado-Asis LB, Yasuda K, Murayama M, et al: Beneficial effects of high daily dose bromocriptine treatment in Cushing's disease, Endocrinol Jpn 39:385–395, 1992.
366. Pivonello R, Ferone D, de Herder WW, et al: Dopamine receptor expression and function in corticotroph pituitary tumors, J Clin Endocrinol Metab 89:2452–2462, 2004.
367. Colao A, Pivonello R, Tripodi FS, et al: Failure of long-term therapy with sodium valproate in Cushing's disease, J Endocrinol Invest 20:387–392, 1997.
368. Greenman Y, Melmed S: Heterogeneous expression of two somatostatin receptor subtypes in pituitary tumors, J Clin Endocrinol Metab 78:398–403, 1994.
369. Lamberts SW, de Herder WW, Krenning EP, et al: A role of (labeled) somatostatin analogs in the differential diagnosis and treatment of Cushing's syndrome, J Clin Endocrinol Metab 78:17–19, 1994.

370. de Herder WW, Lamberts SW: Is there a role for somatostatin and its analogs in Cushing's syndrome? Metabolism 45:83–85, 1996.

371. Batista DL, Zhang X, Gejman R, et al: The effects of SOM230 on cell proliferation and adrenocorticotropin secretion in human corticotroph pituitary adenomas, J Clin Endocrinol Metab 91:4482–4488, 2006.

372. Boscaro M, Atkinson AB, Bertherat J, et al: SOM230 Cushing's disease study group. Early data on the efficacy and safety of the novel multi-ligand somatostatin analog SOM230 in patients with Cushing's disease. 87th Annual Meeting of The Endocrine Society, San Diego, CA, June 4–7, 2005, P2-672 2005.

373. Boscaro M, Glusman JE, Ludlam W, et al: Treatment of pituitary dependent Cushing's disease with the multi-receptor ligand somatostatin analog pasireotide (SOM230): A multicenter, phase II trial, J Clin Endocrinol Metab 94:115–122, 2009.

374. Heaney AP, Fernando M, Yong WH, et al: Functional PPAR-gamma receptor is a novel therapeutic target for ACTH-secreting pituitary adenomas, Nat Med 8:1281–1287, 2002.

375. Suri D, Weiss RE: Effect of pioglitazone on adrenocorticotropic hormone and cortisol secretion in Cushing's disease, J Clin Endocrinol Metab 90:1340–1346, 2005.

376. Ambrosi B, Dall'Asta C, Cannavo S, et al: Effects of chronic administration of PPAR-gamma ligand rosiglitazone in Cushing's disease, Eur J Endocrinol 151:173–178, 2004.

377. Pecori GF, Scaroni C, Arvat E, et al: Effect of protracted treatment with rosiglitazone, a PPARgamma agonist, in patients with Cushing's disease, Clin Endocrinol (Oxf) 64:219–224, 2006.

378. Morcos M, Fohr B, Tafel J, et al: Long-term treatment of central Cushing's syndrome with rosiglitazone, Exp Clin Endocrinol Diabetes 115:292–297, 2007.

379. Munir A, Song F, Ince P, et al: Ineffectiveness of rosiglitazone therapy in Nelson's syndrome, J Clin Endocrinol Metab 92:1758–1763, 2007.

380. Sonino N, Boscaro M, Fallo F: Pharmacologic management of Cushing syndrome: new targets for therapy, Treat Endocrinol 4:87–94, 2005.

381. Paez-Pereda M, Kovalovsky D, Hopfner U, et al: Retinoic acid prevents experimental Cushing syndrome, J Clin Invest 108:1123–1131, 2001.

382. Castillo V, Giacomini D, Paez-Pereda M, et al: Retinoic acid as a novel medical therapy for Cushing's disease in dogs, Endocrinology 147:4438–4444, 2006.

383. Shapiro MS, Shenkman L: Variable hormonogenesis in Cushing's syndrome, Q J Med 79:351–363, 1991.

384. Kammer H, Barter M: Spontaneous remission of Cushing's disease. A case report and review of the literature, Am J Med 67:519–523, 1979.

385. Hayslett JP, Cohn GL: Spontaneous remission of Cushing's disease. Report of a case, N Engl J Med 276:968–970, 1967.

386. Meinardi JR, Wolffenbuttel BH, Dullaart RP: Cyclic Cushing's syndrome: a clinical challenge, Eur J Endocrinol 157:245–254, 2007.

387. Brown RD, Van Loon GR, Orth DN, et al: Cushing's disease with periodic hormonogenesis: one explanation for paradoxical response to dexamethasone, J Clin Endocrinol Metab 36:445–451, 1973.

388. Vagnucci AH, Evans E: Cushing's disease with intermittent hypercortisolism, Am J Med 80:83–88, 1986.

389. Kreze A, Veleminsky J, Spirova E: A follow-up of the "low dose suppressible" hypercortisolism, Endocrinol Exp 17:119–123, 1983.

390. Tsuruoka S, Sugimoto K, Fujimura A: Drug-induced Cushing syndrome in a patient with ulcerative colitis after betamethasone enema: evaluation of plasma drug concentration, Ther Drug Monit 20:387–389, 1998.

391. Findlay CA, Macdonald JF, Wallace AM, et al: Childhood Cushing's syndrome induced by betamethasone nose drops, and repeat prescriptions, BMJ 317:739–740, 1998.

392. Quddusi S, Browne P, Toivola B, et al: Cushing syndrome due to surreptitious glucocorticoid administration, Arch Intern Med 158:294–296, 1998.

393. McConkey B: Adrenal corticosteroids in Chinese herbal remedies, QJM 96:81–82, 2003.

394. Mann M, Koller E, Murgo A, et al: Glucocorticoidlike activity of megestrol. A summary of Food and Drug Administration experience and a review of the literature, Arch Intern Med 157:1651–1656, 1997.

395. Cizza G, Nieman LK, Doppman JL, et al: Factitious Cushing syndrome, J Clin Endocrinol Metab 81:3573–3577, 1996.

396. O'Hare JP, Vale JA, Wood S, et al: Factitious Cushing's syndrome, Acta Endocrinol (Copenh) 111:165–167, 1986.

397. Sharp NA, Devlin JT, Rimmer JM: Renal failure obfuscates the diagnosis of Cushing's disease, JAMA 256:2564–2565, 1986.

398. Otokida K, Fujiwara T, Oriso S, et al: Cortisol and its metabolites in the plasma and urine in Cushing's syndrome with chronic renal failure (CRF), compared to Cushing's syndrome without CRF, Nippon Jinzo Gakkai Shi 31:651–656, 1989.

399. Jain S, Sakhuja V, Bhansali A, et al: Corticotropin-dependent Cushing's syndrome in a patient with chronic renal failure–a rare association, Ren Fail 15:563–566, 1993.

400. Luger A, Lang I, Kovarik J, et al: Abnormalities in the hypothalamic-pituitary-adrenocortical axis in patients with chronic renal failure, Am J Kidney Dis 9:51–54, 1987.

401. Siamopoulos KC, Dardamanis M, Kyriaki D, et al: Pituitary adrenal responsiveness to corticotropin-releasing hormone in chronic uremic patients, Perit Dial Int 10:153–156, 1990.

402. Nolan GE, Smith JB, Chavre VJ, et al: Spurious overestimation of plasma cortisol in patients with chronic renal failure, J Clin Endocrinol Metab 52:1242–1245, 1981.

403. Sederberg-Olsen P, Binder C, Kehlet H: Urinary excretion of free cortisol in impaired renal function, Acta Endocrinol (Copenh) 78:86–90, 1975.

404. Ramirez G, Gomez-Sanchez C, Meikle WA, et al: Evaluation of the hypothalamic hypophyseal adrenal axis in patients receiving long-term hemodialysis, Arch Intern Med 142:1448–1452, 1982.

405. Workman RJ, Vaughn WK, Stone WJ: Dexamethasone suppression testing in chronic renal failure: pharmacokinetics of dexamethasone and demonstration of a normal hypothalamic-pituitary-adrenal axis, J Clin Endocrinol Metab 63:741–746, 1986.

406. Rosman PM, Farag A, Peckham R, et al: Pituitary-adrenocortical function in chronic renal failure: blunted suppression and early escape of plasma cortisol levels after intravenous dexamethasone, J Clin Endocrinol Metab 54:528–533, 1982.

407. Rodger RS, Dewar JH, Turner SJ, et al: Anterior pituitary dysfunction in patients with chronic renal failure treated by hemodialysis or continuous ambulatory peritoneal dialysis, Nephron 43:169–172, 1986.

408. Streeten DH, Faas FH, Elders MJ, et al: Hypercortisolism in childhood: shortcomings of conventional diagnostic criteria, Pediatrics 56:797–803, 1975.

409. Magiakou MA, Mastorakos G, Oldfield EH, et al: Cushing's syndrome in children and adolescents. Presentation, diagnosis, and therapy, N Engl J Med 331:629–636, 1994.

410. Weber A, Trainer PJ, Grossman AB, et al: Investigation, management and therapeutic outcome in 12 cases of childhood and adolescent Cushing's syndrome, Clin Endocrinol (Oxf) 43:19–28, 1995.

411. Lee PD, Winter RJ, Green OC: Virilizing adrenocortical tumors in childhood: eight cases and a review of the literature, Pediatrics 76:437–444, 1985.

412. Savage MO, Lienhardt A, Lebrethon MC, et al: Cushing's disease in childhood: presentation, investigation, treatment and long-term outcome, Horm Res 55(Suppl 1):24–30, 2001.

413. Storr HL, Chan LF, Grossman AB, et al: Paediatric Cushing's syndrome: epidemiology, investigation and therapeutic advances, Trends Endocrinol Metab 18:167–174, 2007.

414. Gafni RI, Papanicolaou DA, Nieman LK: Nighttime salivary cortisol measurement as a simple, noninvasive, outpatient screening test for Cushing's syndrome in children and adolescents, J Pediatr 137:30–35, 2000.

415. Batista DL, Riar J, Keil M, et al: Diagnostic tests for children who are referred for the investigation of Cushing syndrome, Pediatrics 120:e575–e586, 2007.

416. Carpenter PC: Diagnostic evaluation of Cushing's syndrome, Endocrinol Metab Clin North Am 17:445–472, 1988.

417. Dias R, Storr HL, Perry LA, et al: The discriminatory value of the low-dose dexamethasone suppression test in the investigation of paediatric Cushing's syndrome, Horm Res 65:159–162, 2006.

418. Hanson JA, Weber A, Reznek RH, et al: Magnetic resonance imaging of adrenocortical adenomas in childhood: correlation with computed tomography and ultrasound, Pediatr Radiol 26:794–799, 1996.

419. Storr HL, Afshar F, Matson M, et al: Factors influencing cure by transsphenoidal selective adenomectomy in paediatric Cushing's disease, Eur J Endocrinol 152:825–833, 2005.

420. Storr HL, Plowman PN, Carroll PV, et al: Clinical and endocrine responses to pituitary radiotherapy in pediatric Cushing's disease: an effective second-line treatment, J Clin Endocrinol Metab 88:34–37, 2003.

421. Davies JH, Storr HL, Davies K, et al: Final adult height and body mass index after cure of paediatric Cushing's disease, Clin Endocrinol (Oxf) 62:466–472, 2005.

422. Scommegna S, Greening JP, Storr HL, et al: Bone mineral density at diagnosis and following successful treatment of pediatric Cushing's disease, J Endocrinol Invest 28:231–235, 2005.

423. Lindsay JR, Nieman LK: The hypothalamic-pituitary-adrenal axis in pregnancy: challenges in disease detection and treatment, Endocr Rev 26:775–799, 2005.

424. Lindsay JR, Jonklaas J, Oldfield EH, et al: Cushing's syndrome during pregnancy: personal experience and review of the literature, J Clin Endocrinol Metab 90:3077–3083, 2005.

425. Welbourn RB, Montgomery DA, Kennedy TL: The natural history of treated Cushing's syndrome, Br J Surg 58:1–16, 1971.

426. Heald AH, Ghosh S, Bray S, et al: Long-term negative impact on quality of life in patients with successfully treated Cushing's disease, Clin Endocrinol (Oxf) 61:458–465, 2004.

427. Wick MR, Rosai J: Neuroendocrine neoplasms of the thymus, Pathol Res Pract 183:188–199, 1988.

428. Jex RK, van Heerden JA, Carpenter PC, et al: Ectopic ACTH syndrome, Diagnostic and therapeutic aspects, Am J Surg 149:276–282, 1985.

429. Torpy DJ, Mullen N, Ilias I, et al: Association of hypertension and hypokalemia with Cushing's syndrome caused by ectopic ACTH secretion: a series of 58 cases, Ann N Y Acad Sci 970:134–144, 2002.

430. Morris DG, Grossman AB: Cushing's syndrome—The diagnosis and differential diagnosis. In Gaillard RC, editor: The ACTH Axis: Pathogenesis, Diagnosis and Treatment, Hingham, 2003, Kluwer, p. 270.

Index

Page numbers followed by 'f' indicate figures and 't' indicate tables

Printed and bound by CPI Group (UK) Ltd, Croydon, CR0 4YY

03/10/2024

01040364-0013